Cancer of the Head and Neck

Editor: Katelyn Harding

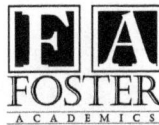

FOSTER
ACADEMICS

www.fosteracademics.com

www.fosteracademics.com

FA
FOSTER
ACADEMICS

Cataloging-in-Publication Data

Cancer of the head and neck / edited by Katelyn Harding.
    p. cm.
Includes bibliographical references and index.
ISBN 978-1-63242-742-7
1. Head--Cancer. 2. Neck--Cancer. 3. Oncology. I. Harding, Katelyn.
RC280.H4 C35 2019
616.994 91--dc23

© Foster Academics, 2019

Foster Academics,
118-35 Queens Blvd., Suite 400,
Forest Hills, NY 11375, USA

ISBN 978-1-63242-742-7 (Hardback)

Contents

Permissions

List of Contributors

Index

Preface

Head and neck cancer refers to a group of cancers that originate in the mouth, throat, sinuses, nose, larynx or salivary glands. Some of its common symptoms are a persistent sore throat, change in the voice, trouble swallowing and a lump or sore, which does not heal. Nearly 75% of all cases of head and neck cancer can be attributed to alcohol and tobacco consumption. Other risk factors include the consumption of betel quid, radiation exposure, Epstein-Barr virus, etc. Advancements in the diagnosis and local management of head and neck cancer and targeted therapy have resulted in the improvement in the quality of life and survival. Treatment generally follows a combination of radiation therapy, surgery, chemotherapy and targeted therapy. This book is a valuable compilation of topics, ranging from the basic to the most complex principles and practices in the management of cancer of the head and neck. It presents the complex subject of head and neck cancer in the most comprehensible language. The readers would gain knowledge that would broaden their perspective about this disease.

After months of intensive research and writing, this book is the end result of all who devoted their time and efforts in the initiation and progress of this book. It will surely be a source of reference in enhancing the required knowledge of the new developments in the area. During the course of developing this book, certain measures such as accuracy, authenticity and research focused analytical studies were given preference in order to produce a comprehensive book in the area of study.

This book would not have been possible without the efforts of the authors and the publisher. I extend my sincere thanks to them. Secondly, I express my gratitude to my family and well-wishers. And most importantly, I thank my students for constantly expressing their willingness and curiosity in enhancing their knowledge in the field, which encourages me to take up further research projects for the advancement of the area.

Editor

Myoepithelial carcinoma with RB1 mutation: remarkable chemosensitivity to carcinoma of unknown origin therapy

Timothy M. Hoggard[1], Evita Henderson-Jackson[2,6], Marilyn M. Bui[2,6], Jamie Caracciolo[3], Jamie K. Teer[4], Sean Yoder[5], Odion Binitie[6,8], Ricardo J. Gonzalez[6], Andrew S. Brohl[6] and Damon R. Reed[6,7,8*]

Abstract

Background: Myoepithelial carcinoma of soft tissue is a rare, malignant neoplasm that is morphologically and immunophenotypically similar to its counterpart in salivary gland. It demonstrates myoepithelial differentiation, possessing both epithelial and myogenic characteristics. Thought to be chemotherapy insensitive, the optimal treatment regimen of this tumor has yet to be established and only a select few cases in the literature discuss treatment efficacy in detail.

Case presentation: Here we present a case of a young adult with metastatic myoepithelial carcinoma with an initial excellent response to systemic therapy utilizing carboplatin and paclitaxel with continued complete response after 3 years. The patient also underwent complete surgical excision and received adjuvant radiation to the primary site of disease. Exome sequencing revealed an inactivating mutation in *RB1* which we believe to be the first such mutation to be reported in this cancer type.

Conclusions: Given increasing evidence suggesting RB1 loss is associated with responsiveness to conventional chemotherapies, particularly platinum-based regimens, we hypothesize that this genetic feature predisposed chemosensitivity in our patient's tumor.

Keywords: Myoepthelioid carcinoma, RB1, Chemotherapy, Paclitaxel, Carboplatin

Background

Myoepithelial tumors are rare salivary gland tumors classically found in the parotid gland. Most are benign myoepitheliomas. The malignant counterpart, myoepithelial carcinoma, is even more rare and represents less than 2% of salivary gland carcinomas [1]. Most cases of myoepithelial carcinoma are de novo in origin but may occasionally arise in association with a preexisting myoepithelioma or benign mixed tumor (pleomorphic adenoma) [2]. These malignant tumors also occur in non-salivary sites, such the nasopharynx, lung, breast, and skin [3–6]. About 50 cases of soft tissue locations of this tumor, both benign and malignant, have been described most often located in deep subcutaneous, intramuscular, or subfascial tissue of the limbs and limb girdles [1, 6–10]. Compared to their salivary equivalent these tumors demonstrate increasing tendency for metastasis as well as aggressive histologic features, particularly within the pediatric population [1, 11]. These tumors exhibit a heterogenous histomorphology and variable immunophenotypic findings, in turn, proving difficult to diagnosis [1]. Several recurrent molecular underpinnings unique to soft tissue myoepithelial carcinoma have been described, including *EWSR1* gene rearrangements in up to 45% of cases [12]. Additionally, homozygous deletion of *SMARCB1* has been reported in 3/5 cases that lack the *EWSR1* gene rearrangement [13]. Comprehensive molecular analysis of this rare tumor type, however, has not been performed.

* Correspondence: damon.reed@moffitt.org
[6]Sarcoma Department, 12901 Bruce B Downs Blvd., Tampa, FL 33612, USA
[7]Chemical Biology and Molecular Medicine Program, 12901 Bruce B Downs Blvd., Tampa, FL 33612, USA
Full list of author information is available at the end of the article

Materials and methods

A chart review was conducted under IRB approval (MCC15003, University of South Florida IRB). To further evaluate our patient for a potential molecular explanation for dramatic chemotherapy response, we performed whole exome sequencing on the initial left popliteal mass resection, prior to any radiation or chemotherapy. Paired-end sequencing was performed on Illumina NextSeq 500 (76 × 2) instrument, generating 214,044,758 total read pairs, resulting in 107× mean coverage across the capture region after duplication removal and mapping. 99.6% of targeted bases achieved at least 10× depth of coverage. Burrows-Wheeler Aligner was used to align sequence reads to the human reference [14]. The Genome Analysis Toolkit was used for insertion/deletion realignment, quality score recalibration, and identification of single nucleotide and insertion/deletion variants [15]. To enrich for somatic mutations, we restricted our analysis to variants that are rare or absent in population databases (MAF <0.01 in 1000 Genomes Project, the NHLBI Exome Sequencing Project, and ExAC database). To further limit our findings to those most likely to be oncogenic, we utilized curated databases including COSMIC and the Cancer Gene Census to manually review variants for functional consequence and known status as an oncogene/tumor suppressor gene.

Case presentation

A 34-year-old male presented to our institution for evaluation of a left popliteal mass that was present and growing over 1 year with increasing pain. There was no neurologic or vascular compromise distal to the lesion. The patient developed inguinal pain 1 month prior to presentation. Otherwise the review of systems was negative.

Left knee MRI demonstrated a large, lobulated nonspecific T2-weighted hyperintense soft tissue mass in the popliteal fossa with local mass effect and surrounding soft tissue edema suspicious for soft tissue sarcoma (Fig. 1a). Contrast-enhanced computed tomography of the chest, abdomen, and pelvis performed for tumor staging demonstrated evidence of necrotic left external iliac lymphadenopathy (Fig. 1b), along with a right lung mass and a pulmonary nodule (Fig. 1c) most consistent with distant metastatic disease.

Tumor cells obtained from CT-guided core biopsy of the popliteal mass and then subsequently of the inguinal lymph nodes showed a proliferation of rounded epithelioid to spindle shaped cells with hyperchromatic nuclei arranged in trabecular-like architecture within hyalinized stroma. Ultimately, complete surgical resection of the primary, popliteal site was performed. Immunohistochemical evaluation revealed reactivity for vimentin, CAM5.2 as well as focal reactivity for CKAE1/3, EMA

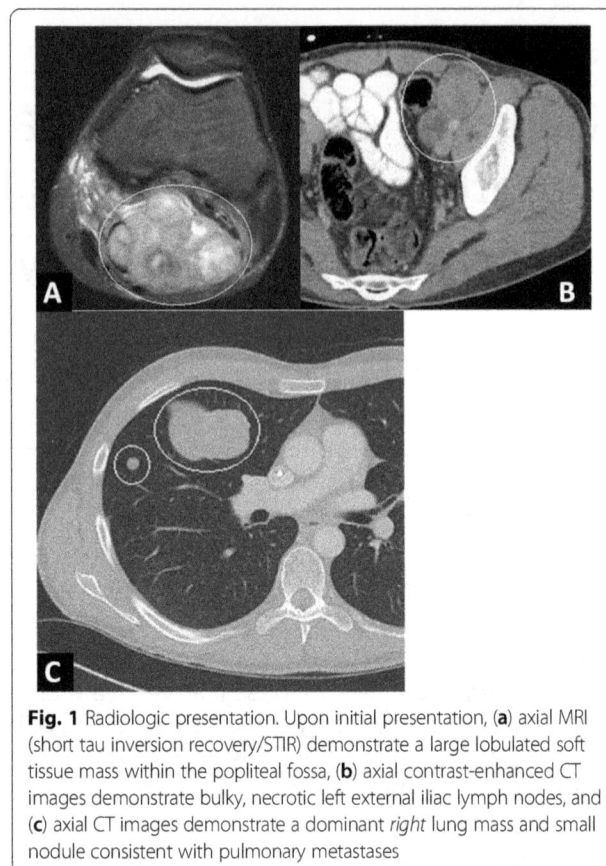

Fig. 1 Radiologic presentation. Upon initial presentation, (**a**) axial MRI (short tau inversion recovery/STIR) demonstrate a large lobulated soft tissue mass within the popliteal fossa, (**b**) axial contrast-enhanced CT images demonstrate bulky, necrotic left external iliac lymph nodes, and (**c**) axial CT images demonstrate a dominant *right* lung mass and small nodule consistent with pulmonary metastases

and synaptophysin. The tumor was negative for S-100, desmin, chromogranin and CD45. Further immunohistochemical analysis following external consultation revealed pankeratin and focal EMA positivity while staining for GFAP, calponin, p63, CD99, FLI-1, CD34, MUC-4, ERG and TLE-1 was negative. Given the limited sample, the lesion was tentatively termed "atypical spindle and round cell neoplasm, possibly myoepithelial in type" (Fig. 2a-f). The patient underwent radical resection of the popliteal mass with a positive margin allowing sufficient tissue to confirm the diagnosis. Grossly, the tumor measured 9.0 × 7.8 × 5.0 cm and cut sections showed an encapsulated, pale white, rubbery, lobulated mass. Histopathologic examination revealed a lobulated, multinodular, infiltrative malignant neoplasm composed of cellular nodules of epithelioid tumor cells with hyperchromatic nuclei showing frequent mitoses arranged in a trabecular fashion. Small proportions of the nodules were hypocellular with tumor cells exhibiting less nuclear atypia and more prominent myxoid stroma. Tumor necrosis was present. The specimen was again sent for consultation and the staining profile mirrored that of the biopsy specimens, aside from focal desmin positivity. Molecular analysis was notably negative for rearrangement of *EWSR1* (22q12) locus and rearrangement of SS18

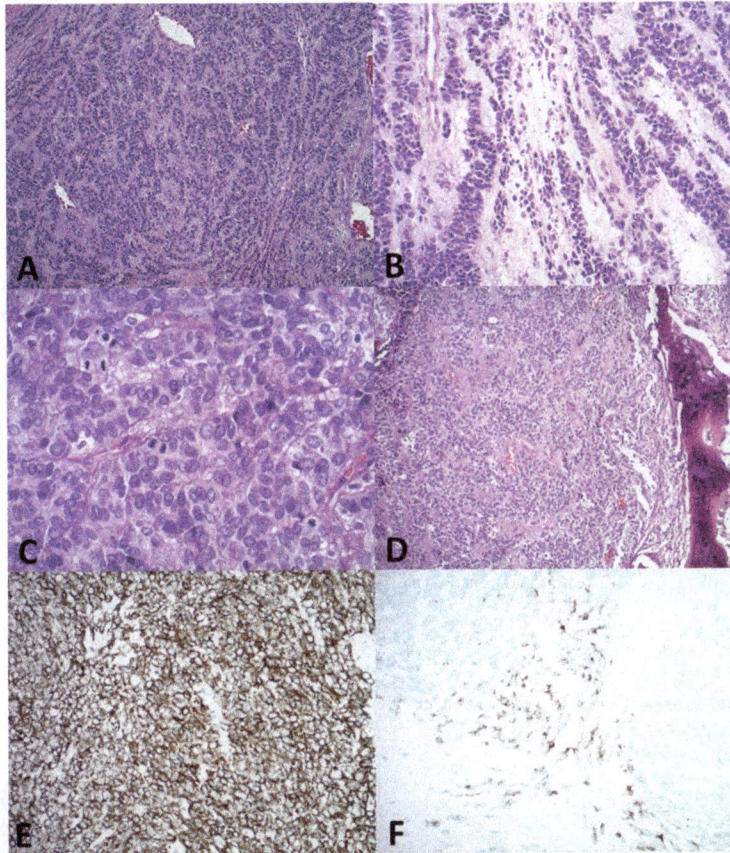

Fig. 2 Histologic analysis of tumor specimen at (**a**) 10× and (**b**) 20× magnification demonstrates rounded epithelioid to spindle shaped cells arranged in a trabecular-like fashion. (**c**) High power field demonstrates mitotic activity. (**d**) Bone formation is also noted. (**e**) Immunohistochemical analysis at 20× magnification reveals CKAE1/3 and CAM5.2 reactivity in addition to (**f**) focal EMA reactivity

(SYT; 18q11.2) locus. Additional molecular testing (FISH analysis) performed revealed no rearrangement of NR4A3. In view of the histomorphologic features and reactivity for epithelial markers, a final diagnosis of high-grade myoepithelial carcinoma was rendered both locally and by outside consultation, although the immunophenotype was not definitive in that regard.

Because of the systemic disease burden and limited reported activity of traditional sarcoma chemotherapeutic regimens, the case was discussed amongst medical and pediatric oncologists within and outside our institution without a clear consensus. We elected to treat with 3 cycles of carboplatin and paclitaxel initially with an almost immediate clinical response. Surveillance CT imaging of the chest, abdomen and pelvis demonstrated decreased size of iliac lymph nodes and pulmonary metastases consistent with tumor response to neoadjuvant therapy while MRI demonstrated surgical changes without clear, active disease (Fig. 3a-d).

The patient underwent a completion lymphadenectomy of the left superficial femoral and deep pelvic nodes without evidence of residual tumor in 25 examined lymph nodes. The patient received an additional 2 cycles of carboplatin and paclitaxel. Due to incomplete radiographic response the patient underwent a wedge resection, which also confirmed pathologic complete remission without malignancy identified. Hemorrhage and areas containing epithelioid macrophages with foamy and/or hemosiderin laden cytoplasm along focal adjacent hyaline fibrosis were seen. This was interpreted to be compatible with chemotherapy effect. The patient received adjuvant radiation therapy with 2 Gy fractions ×33 doses to the popliteal fossa. The patient remains in radiographic remission 36 months from completion of chemotherapy. Molecular studies were undertaken to elucidate the mechanism responsible for the durable response to systemic therapy.

Results

From whole exome sequencing, we identified 509 high-confidence coding variants in our tumor specimen, including 45 truncating (missense, frameshift, or splice site) and 464 nonsynonymous. Of these, we identified 2 truncating mutations in well-described tumor suppressor genes, *RB1* and *MED12*. We additionally note several

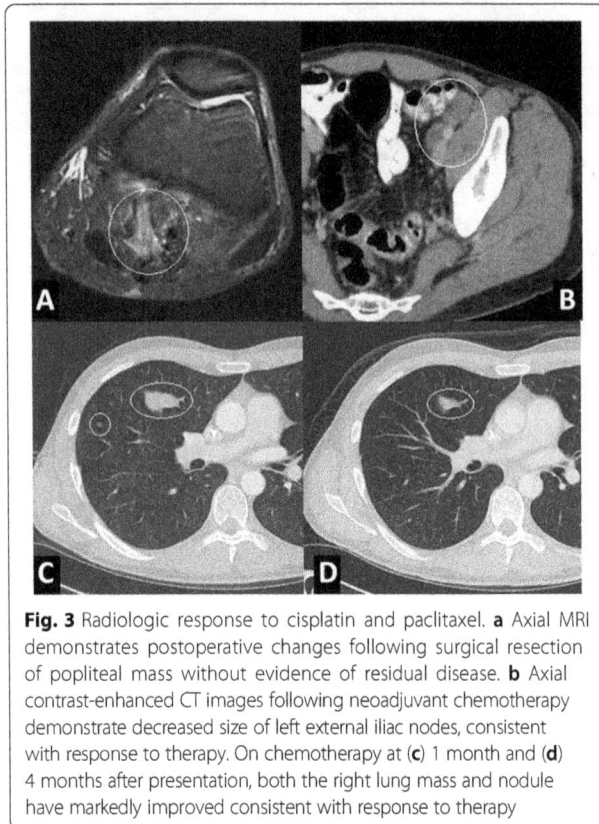

Fig. 3 Radiologic response to cisplatin and paclitaxel. **a** Axial MRI demonstrates postoperative changes following surgical resection of popliteal mass without evidence of residual disease. **b** Axial contrast-enhanced CT images following neoadjuvant chemotherapy demonstrate decreased size of left external iliac nodes, consistent with response to therapy. On chemotherapy at (**c**) 1 month and (**d**) 4 months after presentation, both the right lung mass and nodule have markedly improved consistent with response to therapy

mutations of less clear oncogenic consequence, including a truncating mutation in *ITGA2*, a possible tumor suppressor, and a nonsynonymous mutation in *PDGFRA* that has been reported in several cancer cases, but is also an uncommon population polymorphism [16–18]. Further description of these notable mutations is provided in Table 1.

Discussion

We report an exceptional and sustained response to chemotherapy in a young adult with myoepithelial carcinoma arising from the popliteal fossa with lymph node and pulmonary metastasis. While it is difficult to identify literature with a response rate for this rare malignancy or with a denominator of non-responders, there are at least case reports where chemotherapy regimens with broad activity have been attempted. Two such reports have shown either complete or partial response to

carboplatin/paclitaxel [5, 6]. Partial response in two adult patients is briefly mentioned in a myoepithelial tumor review from 2008, whereas a second report details a patient with a metastatic vulvar mass. Diagnosis in this case was made based upon immunohistochemical staining profile, which similarly was notable for CAM5.2 and focal CKAE1/3 reactivity. The patient was treated initially with excision of the mass and bilateral inguinal lymph node dissection followed by pelvic radiation, but a broad chemotherapy regimen utilizing carboplatin and paclitaxel was initiated after the development of pulmonary metastasis. A complete pathologic response was noted and the patient remained in complete remission over 3 years. An additional study showed complete response to both ifosfamide and melphalan in a patient with metastatic soft tissue disease [19]. In this report, the patient initially presented with a tumor in their toe, which subsequently recurred in the ipsilateral lower extremity following radical disarticulation. Hyperthermic isolated limb perfusion using tumor necrosis factor and melphalan was initiated with a complete response. Pelvic metastases were later noted, successfully treated with ifosfamide and radiation. Chemotherapeutic response in the pediatric population is similarly difficult to identify. In a series of 29 pediatric patients with soft tissue myoepithelial carcinoma, approximately half received chemotherapy [1]. Of these, only one patient demonstrated a clinical response, seen after multiple cycles of doxorubicin and ifosfamide due to metastasis following initial tumor excision. An additional series of 7 non-metastatic, pediatric patients reported favorable outcomes following a regimen utilizing cisplatin with six patients remaining without evidence of disease at a mean follow-up of 2.5 years [20]. Three of the seven tumors had *EWSR1* rearrangement which was previously identified in series where it was associated with superficial location and more likely to be benign [12, 21]. Our sequencing methodology would be unlikely to have detected an *EWRS1* structural variation but clinical testing as mentioned above was negative.

Local surgical tumor excision with wide margins is recommended for myoepithelial carcinoma of soft tissues, although the optimal approach to treatment has yet to be established [6]. The efficacy of radiation or chemotherapy, either as an adjuvant therapy or in metastatic disease, also has not been consistently demonstrated [1, 6, 11]. As is common with rare malignancies, there is a lack of consensus guidelines and multiple options for care. In this case chemotherapy was incorporated because of the patients young age and metastatic presentation, but there are likely many scenarios whereby chemotherapy may be of benefit for patients with a similar malignancy whereby chemotherapy may not be considered. In fact, myoepithelial carcinoma is currently incorporated into a cooperative group clinical

Table 1 Notable mutations in Myoepithelial Carcinoma tumor sample

Gene	Mutation	dbSNP
RB1	NM_000321:exon1:c.38_66del:p.A13fs	-
MED12	NM_005120:exon13:c.C1861T:p.R621X	-
ITGA2	NM_002203:exon17:c.G2155 T:p.E719X	-
PDGFRA	NM_006206:exon5:c.C661T:p.L221F	rs139913632

trial for soft tissue sarcomas as a chemotherapy resistant tumor eligible only for the "non-chemotherapy cohort" (NCT02180867).

Histologically, myoepithelial tumors often display a variety of cellular morphologies, making identification and diagnosis more difficult. The tumors may be composed exclusively of a single cell type, but are more frequently present as a combination of epithelioid, spindle cell, plasmacytoid or clear cell types [9]. Immunohistochemical staining serves as a key step in differentiating from similar appearing tumors. Myoepithelial carcinomas are generally positive for S-100, cytokeratin, epithelial membrane antigen (EMA) and α-smooth muscle actin [9]. The differential diagnosis include carcinoma, melanoma, epithelioid sarcoma, extraskeletal myxoid chondrosarcoma and chordoma. *EWSR1* gene rearrangement is identified in only 50% of the soft tissue myoepithlelial carcinoma [22].

Using whole exome sequencing, we examined our patient's tumor for possible oncogenic variants that may help elucidate a mechanism for chemotherapy sensitivity. Given that matched germline DNA was not available for comparison, we expect many of variants uncovered to be rare or private germline mutations or passenger somatic mutations and therefore of little oncogenic consequence. We were able to identify, however, truncating mutations in *RB1* and *MED12* that are very likely to be somatic oncogenic drivers in this patient given the well-established role of these two genes as tumor suppressors across multiple tumor types. To our knowledge, this is the first description of inactivating mutation in either of these two genes reported in this cancer type.

The retinoblastoma protein (*RB1*) is one of the most frequently affected tumor suppressors across multiple cancer histologies and plays a critical role in regulation of cell cycle and apoptosis [23]. *RB1* pathway deregulation has been reported in various benign and malignant salivary tumors, including malignant myoepithelioma [24]. Interestingly, preclinical and clinical evidence in multiple cancer types suggest that RB1 expressional loss is associated with increased responsiveness to conventional chemotherapies [23]. Additionally, a recent genomic study in small cell lung cancer showed that presence of *RB1* inactivating mutation was highly predictive of good response to platinum-based chemotherapy [25]. Childhood retinoblastoma, almost invariably caused by either germline or somatic mutational inactivation of *RB1*, is also highly responsive to platinum-based chemotherapy [26]. Given this mounting evidence, we hypothesize that *RB1* mutation in our patient's tumor predisposed to chemosensitivity. In contrast, loss of the RNA polymerase II mediator complex member *MED12* has been shown to induce drug resistance, particularly to tyrosine kinase inhibitor therapy, via activation of transforming growth factor B receptor signaling [27].

In summary, we report a case of myoepithelial carcinoma with a *RB1* inactivating mutation that experienced a dramatic response to platinum-based chemotherapy. We believe that our case adds to growing evidence across multiple cancer types that RB1 loss is predictive of chemosensitivity, perhaps in particular to platinum-based regimens. Given the rarity of this tumor type, the optimal systemic therapy approach is not well defined. Further study should be undertaken to evaluate whether RB1 loss is a recurring feature in this histology and whether platinum-based chemotherapy is more broadly effective in this tumor type outside of this case.

Conclusion

While formal recommendations are difficult to make based on a case report, our review of the literature would suggest that continued consideration for systemic carcinoma therapy, more specifically with paclitaxel and carboplatin, should be considered in myoepithelial carcinoma patients presenting with stage 4 disease and extremity primary locations.

Abbreviations
COSMIC: Catalogue of Somatic Mutations in Cancer; CT: Computed Tomography; ExAC: Exome Aggregation Consortium; IRB: Institutional Review Board; MAF: Minor allele frequency; MRI: Magnetic Resonance Imaging; NCT: National Clinical Trial; NHLBI: National Heart, Lung, and Blood Institute

Acknowledgements
Our study received assistance from the Tissue Core, Molecular Genomics Core, and Cancer Informatics Core Facilities at the H. Lee Moffitt Cancer Center & Research Institute, an NCI designated Comprehensive Cancer Center, supported under NIH grant P30-CA76292.

Funding
The study was funded by the Gonzmart Family Foundation. The funding body played no role in the design, conduct, interpretation, or writing of this research and manuscript.

Authors' contributions
Substantial Contributions to conception and design, acquisition of data, analysis and interpretation of data: TMH, EH, MMB, JC, SY, OB, RJG, JKT, ASB and DRR. Been involved in drafting manuscript or revising it critically: TMH, EH, MMB, JC, JKT, ASB and DRR. Given final approval for version to be published: TMH, EH, MMB, JC, SY, OB, RJG, JKT, ASB and DRR. Agree to be accountable: TMH, EH, MMB, JC, SY, OB, RJG, JKT, ASB and DRR. All authors read and approved the final manuscript.

Competing interests
The authors declare that they have no competing interests.

Author details
[1]University of South Florida Morsani College of Medicine, 12901 Bruce B Downs Blvd., Tampa, FL 33612, USA. [2]Department of Anatomic Pathology, 12901 Bruce B Downs Blvd., Tampa, FL 33612, USA. [3]Department of Diagnostic Imaging, 12901 Bruce B Downs Blvd., Tampa, FL 33612, USA. [4]Department of Biostatistics and Bioinformatics, 12901 Bruce B Downs Blvd., Tampa, FL 33612, USA. [5]Molecular Genomics Core Facility, 12901 Bruce B Downs Blvd., Tampa, FL 33612, USA. [6]Sarcoma Department, 12901 Bruce B Downs Blvd., Tampa, FL 33612, USA. [7]Chemical Biology and Molecular Medicine Program, 12901 Bruce B Downs Blvd., Tampa, FL 33612, USA. [8]Adolescent and Young Adult Program; H. Lee Moffitt Cancer Center and Research Institute, 12901 Bruce B Downs Blvd., Tampa, FL 33612, USA.

References

1. Gleason BC, Fletcher CD. Myoepithelial carcinoma of soft tissue in children: an aggressive neoplasm analyzed in a series of 29 cases. Am J Surg Pathol. 2007;31:1813–24.

2. McCluggage WG, Primrose WJ, Toner PG. Myoepithelial carcinoma (malignant myoepithelioma) of the parotid gland arising in a pleomorphic adenoma. J Clin Pathol. 1998;51:552–6.

3. Miura K, Harada H, Aiba S, Tsutsui Y. Myoepithelial carcinoma of the lung arising from bronchial submucosa. Am J Surg Pathol. 2000;24:1300–4.

4. Dhawan A, Shenoy A, Sriprakash D. Myoepithelial carcinoma of the nasopharynx: case report of a rare entity. Natl J Maxillofac Surg. 2011;2:207–9.

5. Noronha V, Cooper DL, Higgins SA, Murren JR, Kluger HM. Metastatic myoepithelial carcinoma of the vulva treated with carboplatin and paclitaxel. Lancet Oncol. 2006;7:270–1.

6. Gleason BC, Hornick JL. Myoepithelial tumours of skin and soft tissue: an update. Diagnostic Histopathology. 2008;14:552–62.

7. Michal M, Miettinen M. Myoepitheliomas of the skin and soft tissues. Report of 12 cases. Virchows Arch. 1999;434:393–400.

8. Kilpatrick SE, Hitchcock MG, Kraus MD, Calonje E, Fletcher CD. Mixed tumors and myoepitheliomas of soft tissue: a clinicopathologic study of 19 cases with a unifying concept. Am J Surg Pathol. 1997;21:13–22.

9. Jo VY, Fletcher CD. Myoepithelial neoplasms of soft tissue: an updated review of the clinicopathologic, immunophenotypic, and genetic features. Head Neck Pathol. 2015;9:32–8.

10. Hornick JL, Fletcher CD. Myoepithelial tumors of soft tissue: a clinicopathologic and immunohistochemical study of 101 cases with evaluation of prognostic parameters. Am J Surg Pathol. 2003;27:1183–96.

11. Lee JR, Georgi DE, Wang BY. Malignant myoepithelial tumor of soft tissue: a report of two cases of the lower extremity and a review of the literature. Ann Diagn Pathol. 2007;11:190–8.

12. Antonescu CR, Zhang L, Chang NE, Pawel BR, Travis W, Katabi N, Edelman M, Rosenberg AE, Nielsen GP, Dal Cin P, Fletcher CD. EWSR1-POU5F1 fusion in soft tissue myoepithelial tumors. A molecular analysis of sixty-six cases, including soft tissue, bone, and visceral lesions, showing common involvement of the EWSR1 gene. Genes Chromosomes Cancer. 2010;49:1114–24.

13. Le Loarer F, Zhang L, Fletcher CD, Ribeiro A, Singer S, Italiano A, Neuville A, Houlier A, Chibon F, Coindre JM, Antonescu CR. Consistent SMARCB1 homozygous deletions in epithelioid sarcoma and in a subset of myoepithelial carcinomas can be reliably detected by FISH in archival material. Genes Chromosomes Cancer. 2014;53:475–86.

14. Li H, Durbin R. Fast and accurate short read alignment with burrows-wheeler transform. Bioinformatics. 2009;25:1754–60. doi:10.1093/bioinformatics/btp1324. Epub 2009 May 1718

15. DePristo MA, Banks E, Poplin R, Garimella KV, Maguire JR, Hartl C, Philippakis AA, del Angel G, Rivas MA, Hanna M, et al. A framework for variation discovery and genotyping using next-generation DNA sequencing data. Nat Genet. 2011;43:491–8. doi:10.1038/ng.1806. Epub 2011 Apr 1010

16. Jeck WR, Parker J, Carson CC, Shields JM, Sambade MJ, Peters EC, Burd CE, Thomas NE, Chiang DY, Liu W, et al. Targeted next generation sequencing identifies clinically actionable mutations in patients with melanoma. Pigment Cell Melanoma Res. 2014;27:653–63.

17. Cassier PA, Fumagalli E, Rutkowski P, Schoffski P, Van Glabbeke M, Debiec-Rychter M, Emile JF, Duffaud F, Martin-Broto J, Landi B, et al. Outcome of patients with platelet-derived growth factor receptor alpha-mutated gastrointestinal stromal tumors in the tyrosine kinase inhibitor era. Clin Cancer Res. 2012;18:4458–64.

18. Ding W, Fan XL, Xu X, Huang JZ, Xu SH, Geng Q, Li R, Chen D, Yan GR. Epigenetic silencing of ITGA2 by MiR-373 promotes cell migration in breast cancer. PLoS One. 2015;10:e0135128.

19. Rastrelli M, Passuello N, Cecchin D, Basso U, Tosi AL, Rossi CR. Metastatic malignant soft tissue myoepithelioma: a case report showing complete response after locoregional and systemic therapy. J Surg Case Rep. 2013;16(12). doi:10.1093/jscr/rjt109.

20. Bisogno G, Tagarelli A, Schiavetti A, Scarzello G, Ferrari A, Cecchetto G, Alaggio R. Myoepithelial carcinoma treatment in children: a report from the TREP project. Pediatr Blood Cancer. 2014;61:643–6.

21. Rekhi B, Sable M, Jambhekar NA. Histopathological, immunohistochemical and molecular spectrum of myoepithelial tumours of soft tissues. Virchows Arch. 2012;461:687–97.

22. Fletcher CDM, World Health Organization. International Agency for Research on Cancer.: WHO classification of tumours of soft tissue and bone. Lyon: IARC Press; 2013.

23. Indovina P, Pentimalli F, Casini N, Vocca I, Giordano A. RB1 dual role in proliferation and apoptosis: cell fate control and implications for cancer therapy. Oncotarget. 2015;6:17873–90.

24. Etges A, Nunes FD, Ribeiro KC, Araujo VC. Immunohistochemical expression of retinoblastoma pathway proteins in normal salivary glands and in salivary gland tumours. Oral Oncol. 2004;40:326–31.

25. Dowlati A, Lipka MB, McColl K, Dabir S, Behtaj M, Kresak A, Miron A, Yang M, Sharma N, Fu P, Wildey G. Clinical correlation of extensive-stage small-cell lung cancer genomics. Ann Oncol. 2016;27:642–7.

26. Rodriguez ML, Juarez CP, Luna JD. Intravitreal triamcinolone acetonide injection in blind painful eyes. Intraocular steroids as a treatment for blind painful red eyes. Eur J Ophthalmol. 2003;13:292–7.

27. Huang S, Holzel M, Knijnenburg T, Schlicker A, Roepman P, McDermott U, Garnett M, Grernrum W, Sun C, Prahallad A, et al. MED12 controls the response to multiple cancer drugs through regulation of TGF-beta receptor signaling. Cell. 2012;151:937–50.

2

Moesin expression by tumor cells is an unfavorable prognostic biomarker for oral cancer

Francisco Bárbara Abreu Barros[1], Agnes Assao[1], Natália Galvão Garcia[1], Suely Nonogaki[2], André Lopes Carvalho[3], Fernando Augusto Soares[4], Luiz Paulo Kowalski[5] and Denise Tostes Oliveira[1*]

Abstract

Background: Moesin is a member of the ERM (ezrin, radixin and moesin) proteins that participate in cell migration and tumor invasion through transductional signals sent to actin filaments by glycoproteins, such as podoplanin.

Methods: This study aimed to evaluate the participation of moesin and podoplanin in the invasive tumor front of oral squamous cell carcinomas, and their influence on patients' prognosis. Podoplanin and moesin immunoexpressions were evaluated by a semi-quantitative score method, based on the capture of 10 microscopic fields, at 400X magnification, in the invasive tumor front of oral squamous cell carcinomas. The association of moesin and podoplanin expression with clinicopathological variables was analyzed by the chi-square, or Fisher's exact test. The 5 and 10 years survival rates were calculated by the Kaplan-Meier method and the survival curves were compared by using the log-rank test.

Results: The immunohistochemical expression of moesin in the invasive front of oral squamous cell carcinomas was predominantly strong, homogenously distributed on the membrane and in the cytoplasm of tumor cells. The expression of moesin was not associated with clinical, demographic and microscopic features of the patients. Otherwise, podoplanin expression by malignant epithelial cells was predominantly strong and significantly associated with radiotherapy ($p = 0.004$), muscular invasion ($p = 0.006$) and lymph node involvement ($p = 0.013$). Strong moesin expression was considered an unfavorable prognostic factor for patients with oral squamous cell carcinomas, clinical stage II and III ($p = 0.024$).

Conclusions: These results suggested that strong moesin expression by malignant cells may help to determine patients with oral squamous cell carcinoma and poor prognosis.

Keywords: Oral cancer, Squamous cell carcinoma, Podoplanin, Moesin, Biomarkers

Background

Moesin is a member of the ERM (ezrin, radixin and moesin) family of proteins that plays a role in cellular morphology, cell adhesion, controlling adherent junctions and cell motility, the key events of the carcinogenesis processes [1–3]. Specifically, the metastatic process involves moesin and other ERM proteins, leading to changes in cell morphology, cell to cell adhesion and in actin filament reorganization [4].

Recently, the overexpression of moesin in tumors has been correlated with metastasis and poor prognosis for the patient [5–8], including those with oral squamous cell carcinomas [9, 10]. Moesin probably participates in necessary conformational changes for an appropriate cell configuration, flexible enough to allow extravasation [11]. These processes occur through the phosphorylation of the C-terminal domain of moesin, which binds to actin filaments [12]. In the other domain, N-terminal, transmembrane molecules, such as podoplanin, are able to activate it, consequently inducing Rho phosphorylation. These

* Correspondence: denisetostes@usp.br
[1]Department of Stomatology, Area of Pathology, Bauru School of Dentistry, University of São Paulo, Alameda Octávio Pinheiro Brisolla, 9-75, Bauru, São Paulo 17012-901, Brazil
Full list of author information is available at the end of the article

downstream signals result in loss of adhesion, motility and higher rates of cell proliferation [13].

Podoplanin is a transmembrane glycoprotein and its overexpression has been associated with enhanced cancer cell motility, tumor invasion and poor patient prognosis in head and neck tumors [14–21]. The role of podoplanin in the tumor invasion process was first hypothesized by Martin-Villar et al. (2005), who reported the activation of ERM proteins by podoplanin through Rho-A phosphorylation. This connection is responsible for the maintanance of the ERM proteins in an open and active state conformation, strengthening the anchorage of podoplanin to cytoskeleton filaments.

To gain further understanding of the participation of moesin in tumor invasion process and its association with podoplanin in this pathway, for the first time, we analyzed the immunohistochemical association of moesin and podoplanin in oral squamous cell carcinomas with clinicopathological features and patients' prognosis.

Methods

This study was based on the analysis of eighty-four surgical specimens of patients who underwent surgical treatment for primary oral squamous cell carcinoma (OSCC) at the Head and Neck Surgery and Otorhinolaryngology Department of the A.C. Camargo Cancer Hospital, São Paulo, Brazil, from 1963 to 2012. Tumors were selected according to the following inclusion criteria: (1) oral squamous cell carcinoma located in the tongue, floor of the mouth, inferior gingiva and retromolar area, confirmed by biopsy; (2) patients not submitted to other previous treatment; (3) complete clinical data and follow up; (4) tumor tissue available for microscopic analysis. Clinical data were obtained from the medical records of the A.C. Camargo Cancer Hospital and included age, ethnic group, gender, tobacco and alcohol consumption, TNM stage (UICC: union for international cancer control, 2004), treatment (surgery, post-operative adjuvant radiotherapy), localization of the tumor and clinical follow-up (local recurrence, regional recurrence and death). Histopathological analysis included the following variables: vascular embolization, perineural infiltration, muscular infiltration, bone infiltration and lymph node involvement (pN+). Additionally, the histopathological grade of malignancy of oral squamous cell carcinomas was determined in hematoxylin & eosin stained sections [22].

Podoplanin and moesin immunoexpression in oral squamous cell carcinomas

The immunohistochemistry technique followed the protocol of the Department of Pathology of the A.C. Camargo Cancer Hospital used previously by Faustino et al. (2008). The tumors sections were incubated with

following primary monoclonal anti-podoplanin antibody: D2-40 clone, Dako North America Inc., M3619, Glostrup, Denmark, dilution 1:200 and with anti-moesin antibody 38/87 clone, Neomarkers, USA, dilution 1:400. Palatine tonsil was used as positive control for anti-podoplanin antibody and placenta for anti-moesin antibody. The lymphatic vessels were used as internal control.

Immunohistochemistry evaluation

Approximately, 10 microscopic fields of each tumor specimen were captured with a digital camera (AxiocamMRc, Zeiss) attached to a microscope (Axioskop 2 Plus, Zeiss), at 400X magnification to evaluate the immunoexpression of podoplanin and moesin. Images of each tumor field were sequentially captured in the invasive tumor front and recorded in a computer program system (Axiovision 4.9, Zeiss, Jena, Germany).

Two experienced pathologists evaluated podoplanin and moesin expressions by malignant cells, based on a semi-quantitative score system, previously established by Faustino et al. (2008). The final score was determined by the sum of the immunostaining intensity and the percentage of positive immunostaining cells. Subsequently, the oral squamous cell carcinomas were classified into 3 groups: 0 = absent immunostaining; 1 = weak immunostaining; 2 = strong immunostaining [23].

Statistical analyses

The statistical analyses were performed using SPSS Statistical software version 21.0 (SPSS Inc., Chicago, IL, USA). The association of podoplanin and moesin immunoexpression by neoplastic cells with the clincopathological variables was verified by the Chi-square (x^2), or Fischer's exact tests. For these analyses, the absent and weak immunoexpressions were grouped together, obtaining a final group of absent/weak tumor immunoexpression and strong tumor immunoexpression. The overall survival probability in 5 and 10 years was estimated using the Kaplan-Meier method, and survival curves were compared by log-rank test. The follow-up period considered for overall survival consisted of the time between the date of surgery and death or the date of the last information about the patient. Cox regression analysis of the survival data was performed to test any statistical significance of regression coefficients. For all statistical analyses applied, p values of less than 0.05 were considered statistically significant.

Results

For the present study, the sample consisted of 84 patients with oral squamous cell carcinomas, predominantly male (85.7%), white (95.2%), with ages varying from 33 to 95 years (mean of 58 years). According to risk factors for OSCC, alcohol (67.9%) and tobacco (84.5%) consumption were reported by the majority of the patients. The most common location for OSCC was the tongue (54.8%), followed by floor of the mouth (28.6%). Moreover, most patients were clinically classified as T2 (59.5%) or T3 (40.5%), and N+ (48.8%), at the time of physical examination.

Only three patients (3.6%) were not submitted to elective neck dissection, 78.6% were submitted to ipsilateral neck dissection and 17.8% were dissected bilaterally. Thirty-eight patients (45.2%) who were submitted to neck dissection were positive for lymph node metastasis (pN+), shown by histopathological analysis.

Local recurrence occurred in 25% of the patients, while regional recurrence was present in 16.7% and local and regional recurrences, simultaneously, occurred in 6% of the patients.

Most tumors, 86.9% were classified as well/moderately differentiated; and 13.1% were classified as poorly differentiated, according to the histopathological grade of tumor malignancy [22].

Immunohistochemical expression of moesin in oral squamous cell carcinomas

Immunohistochemical expression of moesin in the invasive front of oral squamous cell carcinomas was weak in 40 tumors, while in 44 tumors the expression was strong. A predominantly cytoplasmic moesin expression

was observed in most of the tumors. The keratin pearls and some areas with more differentiated neoplastic cells showed weak/negative moesin immunoexpression (Fig. 1).

Clinical, demographic and microscopic features analyzed were not statistically associated with moesin expression (Tables 1 and 2).

Immunohistochemical expression of podoplanin in oral squamous cell carcinomas

The expression of podoplanin in oral squamous cell carcinomas was weak in 49 tumors and strong in 35 tumors. Membranous and cytoplasmic podoplanin expression was observed in oral squamous cell carcinomas with a predominance of the membranous expression (Fig. 1).

The strong podoplanin expression was associated with post-operative radiotherapy ($p = 0.004$) in those patients diagnosed with squamous cell carcinomas. Podoplanin expression was not associated with the demographic and clinical features analyzed (Table 1).

Concerning microscopic features analyzed, podoplanin expression in patients with muscle infiltration was weak compared with those without infiltration ($p = 0.006$). Moreover, the podoplanin expression was significantly associated with lymph node metastasis (pN+). In other words, most patients with lymph node metastasis presented weak expression of podoplanin ($p = 0.013$), as illustrated in Table 2.

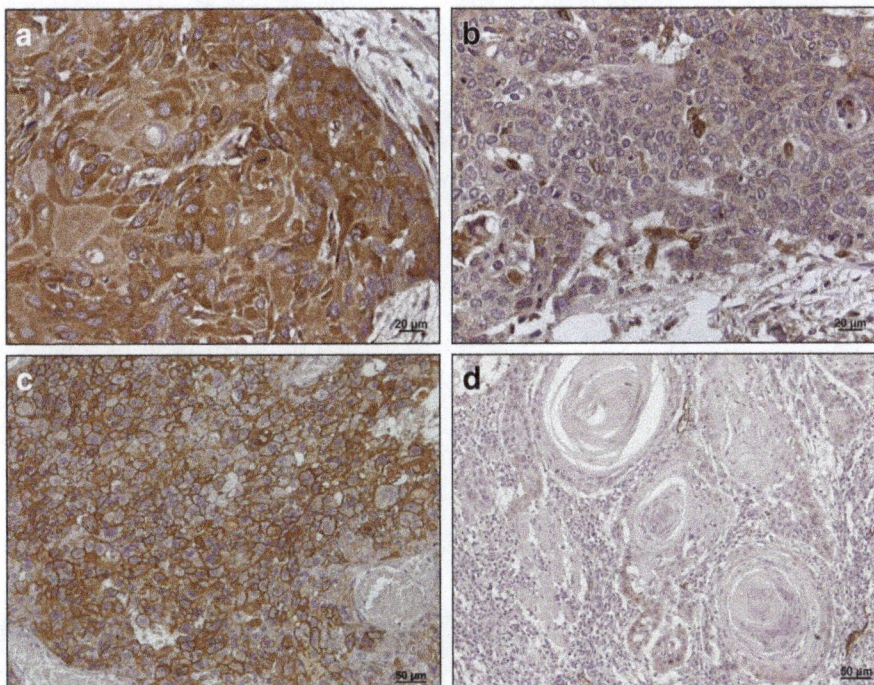

Fig. 1 Immunohistochemical expression of moesin in oral squamous cell carcinomas. Strong (a) and weak cytoplasmic (b) moesin expression (a, IHQ 400X; (b, IHQ 200X). Membranous strong (c) and weak/absent podoplanin expression (d) (c, IHQ 200X; d, IHQ 200X)

Table 1 Expression of podoplanin and moesin at invasive tumor front of 84 oral squamous cell carcinoma, according to clinical data and follow-up. A.C. Camargo Cancer Hospital, São Paulo, Brazil, 1963 to 2012

Variable	Moesin				p	Podoplanin				p
	Weak		Strong			Weak		Strong		
	N	%	N	%		N	%	N	%	
Gender										
Male	35	87.5	37	84.1	0.656	45	91.8	27	77.1	0.058
Female	5	12.5	7	15.9		4	8.2	8	22.9	
Age										
≤ 58 years	22	55	20	45.5	0.382	24	49	18	51.4	0.825
> 58 years	18	45	24	54.5		25	51	17	48.6	
White	39	97,5	41	93.2	0.618	46	93.9	34	97.1	0.637
Non-white	1	2,5	3	6.8		3	6.1	1	2.9	
Tobacco[a]										
Yes	31	93.9	40	95.2	0.999	43	95.6	28	93.3	0.999
No	2	6.1	2	4.8		2	4.4	2	6.7	
Alcohol[a]										
Yes	26	76.5	31	73.8	0.790	32	71.1	25	80.6	0.346
No	8	23.5	11	26.2		13	28.9	6	19.4	
T Stage										
T2	25	62.5	25	56.8	0.596	27	55.1	23	65.7	0.329
T3	15	37.5	19	43.2		22	44.9	12	34.3	
N Stage										
N0	22	55	21	47.7	0.505	24	49	19	54.3	0.631
N+	18	45	23	52.3		25	51	16	45.7	
Lymph Node Involvement										
No	2	5	1	2.3	0.679	1	2	2	5.7	0.669
Ipsilateral	30	75	36	81.8		39	79.6	27	77.1	
Contralateral	8	20	7	15.9		9	18.4	6	17.1	
Radiotherapy										
Yes	20	50	17	38.6	0.295	21	42.9	26	74.3	**0.004**
No	20	50	27	61.4		28	57.1	9	25.7	
Recurrence										
Yes	22	55	21	47.7	0.505	26	53.1	15	42.9	0.356
No	18	45	23	52.3		23	46.9	20	57.1	
Second Tumor										
Yes	10	25	4	9.1	0.061	6	12.2	8	22.9	0.198
No	30	75	40	90.0		43	87.8	27	77.1	
TOTAL	40	100	44	100		36	100	55	100	

N: Number of tumors; p: value obtained by chi-squares test or Fischer's exact test
[a]Excluded patients with lost records
p<0.05 was considered statistically significant

Overall analysis of podoplanin and moesin expression in oral squamous cell carcinomas was not statistically associated (p = 0.460).

Table 2 Immunohistochemical distribution of moesin and podoplanin at invasive front tumor of 84 oral squamous cell carcinoma, according to microscopical variables. A.C. Camargo Cancer Hospital, São Paulo, Brazil, 1963 to 2012

Variable	Moesin				p	Podoplanin				p
	Weak		Strong			Weak		Strong		
	N	%	N	%		N	%	N	%	
Vascular Embolization										
Yes	25	64.5	28	63.6	0.914	35	71.4	18	51.4	0.061
No	15	37.5	16	36.4		14	28.6	17	48.6	
Perineural Infiltration										
Yes	28	70	29	65.9	0.688	34	69.4	23	65.7	0.722
No	12	30	15	43.1		15	30.6	12	34.3	
Muscular Infiltration										
Yes	31	77.5	38	86.4	0.289	45	91.8	24	68.6	**0.006**
No	9	22.5	6	13.6		4	8.2	11	31.4	
Bone Infiltration										
Yes	2	5	3	6.8	0.999	1	2	4	11.4	0.155
No	38	95	41	93.2		48	98	31	88.6	
Lymph node Involvement[a]										
pN0	21	55.3	22	51.2	0.712	20	41.7	23	69.7	**0.013**
pN+	17	44.7	21	48.8		28	58.3	10	30.3	
TOTAL	40	100	44	100		49	100	35	100	

N: Number of tumors; p: value obtained by chi-squares test or Fischer's exact test. pN0: patients without node metastasis; pN+: patients with node metastasis
[a]Excluded patients who were not submitted to elective neck dissection
p<0.05 was considered statistically significant

Overall survival analysis

Overall survival rates varied from 0.01 to 288 months, mean of 57.2 months. Only moesin expression showed statistically significant differences (p = 0.024). The overall survival rate, in 5 years and 10 years, for patients with oral squamous cell carcinomas and strong moesin expression was reduced from 38.5%, to 23.8%, respectively. For oral squamous cell carcinomas in patients with weak moesin expression the survival rate varied from 22.7% in 5 years to 6.8% in 10 years. These differences in oral cancer patients' survival rates for moesin expression were statistically significant (Table 3 and Fig. 2).

Based on Cox regression analysis, patients with oral squamous cell carcinomas and strong moesin expression by neoplastic epithelial cells had 1.737-fold higher chance of relative risk of death (p = 0.022), as illustrated in Table 4.

Discussion

To date, the intracellular location of moesin during oral carcinogenesis has been poorly understood. Moesin translocation from plasma membrane to the cytoplasm of neoplastic cells has been demonstrated in a previous study [24] and it may reduce the ability to form cell-cell

Table 3 Overall survival rates in 5 and 10 years of 84 patients with oral squamous cell carcinoma according to demographic features, risk factors, lymph node metastasis (pN), moesin and podoplanin, expression. A.C. Camargo Cancer Center, São Paulo, Brazil, 1963 to 2012

Variable	Overall Survival		p
	5 years (%)	10 years (%)	
Gender			
Male	33.8	15.4	0.145
Female	8.3	8.3	
Age			
≤ 58 years	38.1	19.3	0.075
> 58 years	22	9.8	
Tobacco			
Yes	28.6	11.2	0.282
No	25	25	
Alcohol			
Yes	25	9.6	0.512
No	31.6	12.6	
Radioterapy			
Yes	32.4	11.8	0.802
No	28.4	16.5	
Muscle Infiltration			
Yes	30.9	11.5	0.313
No	26.7	26.7	
Pn			
pN0	39.5	21.2	0.081
pN+	21.7	8.1	
Moesin			
Weak	38.5	23.8	*0.024*
Strong	22.7	6.8	
Podoplanin			
Weak	27.1	5.0	0.133
Strong	34.3	25.7	

*pN+: Histopathological lymph node metastasis; pN0: Absence of lymph node metastasis, histopathologically
p = value obtained by log-rank test
p<0.05 was considered statistically significant

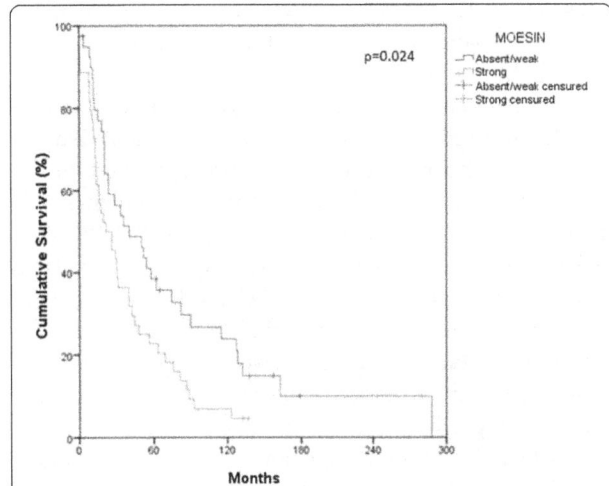

Fig. 2 Prognostic value for moesin expression in oral squamous cell carcinomas. Cumulative overall survival rates by Kaplan-Meier method. ($p = 0.024$)

contacts, as well as, influence the cytoskeleton remodeling and tumor invasion process, when overexpressed in the cytoplasm [24]. Furthermore, podoplanin linkage with the N-terminal moesin domain activates the ERM proteins, consequently inducing Rho-A phosphorylation and in the maintenance of the ERM proteins in an active form (open conformation), in the cytoplasm [25].

The moesin immunoprofile in the invasive front of oral squamous cell carcinomas, clinical stages II and III, was predominantly cytoplasmic and strong. Keratin pearls and some areas with more differentiated neoplastic cells

showed negative moesin expression. Confirming these results, other authors described the membranous and cytoplasmic moesin expression in oral squamous cell carcinomas, [5, 9, 10]. Belbin et al. (2005) showed that membranous and cytoplasmic moesin expression increased when normal epithelium was compared with dysplastic epithelium and/or with tumor samples [10]. The authors affirmed that moesin expression was significantly associated with head and neck squamous cell carcinomas progression. In addition, as found in the present study, the loss of moesin expression in more differentiated cells was found in keratin pearls [5, 26].

The expression of moesin was not associated with the clinical, demographic and microscopic features analyzed ($p > 0.05$), reinforcing previous findings [5, 7, 9, 26]. Kobayashi et al. (2004) found a significant association of moesin with the size of the tumor, but the sample analyzed varied from T1 to T4 tumors. Differently, the present study was composed of T2 and T3 tumors and no association could be found with moesin expression, as it was restricted to a limited size of tumors. According to our previous experiences with analyses of protein expression by oral neoplastic cells, the OSCCs clinically

Table 4 Moesin expression analysis by Cox proportional hazard model. A.C. Camargo Cancer Hospital, São Paulo, Brazil, 1963 to 2012

Variable	Overall Survival		
		p	HR (95%CI)
Moesin	Weak (0)	0.022	1.737 (1.083- 2.788)
	Strong (1)		

HR: Hazard according to gender, age, lymph node metastasis, radiotherapy, muscle infiltration, tobacco, alcohol, moesin and podoplanin expression by neoplastic cells. CI: Confidence Interval classified as T2 and T3 are better for verifying their influence on patients' prognosis, than T1 (initial tumors) or T4 (advanced tumors).

Regarding podoplanin expression by tumor cells, as previously observed by de Vicente et al. (2015) and Tsuneki et al. (2013), the present results showed higher podoplanin expression in the earlier stages of tumors and in highly differentiated malignant cells. These studies [27–29] verified that podoplanin expression was inversely correlated with the degree of neoplastic epithelial cell differentiation. In agreement with the cited studies, the results found in the present study confirmed a weak/absent podoplanin expression in the majority of tumors with muscular infiltration and lymph node involvement (pN+).

Initial studies about podoplanin related strong podoplanin expression to the worst prognosis and more advanced stages of oral squamous cell carcinomas [14–16, 30, 31]. Instead, the present results showed the opposite side of those findings, and the authors suggest further studies should be conducted about podoplanin expression in less differentiated tumors to validate these findings.

Considering demographic and clinical features, the strong expression of podoplanin was observed mainly in those patients submitted to post-operative radiotherapy ($p = 0.004$) [14, 18, 19, 28, 30]; however, further studies are necessary for better evaluation of radiotherapy and podoplanin expression.

Concerning clinical stages T and N, our results failed to find an association between podoplanin expression and the clinical stages of the tumor, probably because we included only T2 and T3 tumors, while in other studies, the tumor stages varied from I to IV [14, 16, 19, 20, 30].

No statistically significant association ($p = 0.460$) was found between podoplanin and moesin immunoexpression by malignant cells in the invasive front of oral squamous cell carcinomas. As this was the first study about the joint expression of podoplanin and moesin in oral cancer, further investigations based on in vitro assays are necessary for better evaluation of the participation of these molecules together in the tumor invasion process.

The overall survival and the prognostic value of moesin and podoplanin expression in oral squamous cell carcinomas were analyzed in this study. Moesin expression was considered a significant prognostic factor for oral squamous cell carcinomas. The overall survival rate in 5 years was 22.7% for those patients with the strong moesin expression, while for patients with weaker moesin expression, the overall survival rates in 5 years was 38.5%. In ten years, overall survival rates for strong moesin expression were 6.8% and 23.8% for weak expression. Moreover, the patient with strong moesin expression presented a 1737 times higher risk of dying, compared with those with the weak expression. These results are consistent with those found by Kobayashi et al. (2004) and Schlecht et al. (2012) in oral squamous cell carcinomas and in breast cancer [6, 32].

Interestingly and corroborating the above results, a recent study conducted by Li et al. (2015) observed the knockdown of moesin in oral squamous cell carcinomas cell lines and a significantly reduction in migration and invasion [33]. Furthermore, moesin silencing showed an increase in cell-cell adhesion. By cell spreading assay, moesin inhibition reduced filopodia formation, indicating the role of moesin in cytoskeletal modifications. This study was in agreement with the present results, which indicated that the weak expression of moesin could be related to higher survival rates in oral squamous cell carcinoma patients.

Podoplanin expression, in turn, was not considered as a significant prognostic factor for oral squamous cell carcinomas, as related by de Vicente et al. (2015) and Dos Santos Almeida et al. (2013). Although previous results considered [14–16, 30, 31] that strong podoplanin expression was related to poor prognosis, we could not predict the prognostic significance of podoplanin in those tumors, probably because strong podoplanin expression was related to initial tumors in earlier stages of the neoplastic cell differentiation process [27–29]. Therefore, considering the latest controversial studies concerning podoplanin expression, we suggest that further studies with a larger sample should be conducted to confirm the potential prognostic value of this protein in oral squamous cell carcinomas.

Conclusions

The weak immunohistochemical expression of moesin by neoplastic epithelial cells could be used as a favorable prognostic marker for oral squamous cell carcinomas. Additionally, the weaker expression of podoplanin was associated with lymph node involvement and muscular infiltration in oral squamous cell carcinomas, indicating that podoplanin expression occurs in more differentiated cells and at earlier stages of the tumors. Moreover, malignant cells of oral squamous cell carcinomas expressed both podoplanin and moesin, but these proteins probably act individually in tumor invasion process.

Abbreviations
ERM: Ezrin, radixin, moesin; OSCC: Oral squamous cell carcinoma; SPSS: Statistical Package for the Social Sciences; TNM: Tumor size, lymph nodes and metastasis; UICC: Union for international cancer control

Acknowledgements
We would like to thank the São Paulo Research Foundation (FAPESP grant#2012/13411-6) and the National Council for Scientific and Technological Development (CNPq) for supporting the present study and the involved researchers.

Funding

This study was supported by São Paulo Research Foundation (FAPESP grant#2012/13411-6) and by the National Council for Scientific and Technological Development (CNPq). The funding body had no influence on the design of the study, the collection, analysis, and interpretation of data and the manuscript.

Authors' contributions

FBAB, AA, FAS, LPK contributed to the conception and design of this project, acquisition, interpretation of data and critical revision of the manuscript. NGG contributed obtaining tumor images and revision of the manuscript. SN conducted the immunohistochemical technique. ALC contributed to the study design, statistical critical analysis and data interpretation. DTO contributed to the conception and design of this project, critical interpretation of data and critical revision of the manuscript. All authors read and approved the final manuscript.

Competing interests

The authors declare that they have no competing interests.

Author details

[1]Department of Stomatology, Area of Pathology, Bauru School of Dentistry, University of São Paulo, Alameda Octávio Pinheiro Brisolla, 9-75, Bauru, São Paulo 17012-901, Brazil. [2]Adolfo Lutz Institute, Pathology Division, São Paulo, Brazil. [3]Fundação Pio XII Institution – Cancer Hospital of Barretos, Barretos, São Paulo, Brazil. [4]Rede D'Or Hospitals Network - Pathology Division São Paulo, Brazil. [5]Department of Head and Neck Surgery and Otorhinolaringology, A.C.Camargo Cancer Center Hospital, São Paulo, Brazil.

References

1. Deng W, Cho S, Li R. FERM domain of moesin desorbs the basic-rich cytoplasmic domain of l-selectin from the anionic membrane surface. J Mol Biol. 2013;425(18):3549–62. https://doi.org/10.1016/j.jmb.2013.06.008.
2. Jiang L, Phang JM, Yu J, Harrop SJ, Sokolova AV, Duff AP, et al. CLIC proteins, ezrin, radixin, moesin and the coupling of membranes to the actin cytoskeleton: a smoking gun? Biochim Biophys Acta. 2014;1838(2):643–57. https://doi.org/10.1016/j.bbamem.2013.05.025.
3. Li YY, Zhou CX, Gao Y. Podoplanin promotes the invasion of oral squamous cell carcinoma in coordination with MT1-MMP and rho GTPases. Am J Cancer Res. 2015;5(2):514–29.
4. Yilmaz M, Christofori G. EMT, the cytoskeleton, and cancer cell invasion. Cancer Metastasis Rev. 2009;28(1-2):15–33. https://doi.org/10.1007/s10555-008-9169-0.
5. Madan R, Brandwein-Gensler M, Schlecht NF, Elias K, Gorbovitsky E, Belbin TJ, et al. Differential tissue and subcellular expressionof ERM proteins in normal and malignant tissues: cytoplasmic ezrin expression has prognostic signficance for head and neck squamous cell carcinoma. Head Neck. 2006;28(11):1018–27. https://doi.org/10.1002/hed.20435.
6. Charafe-Jauffret E, Monville F, Bertucci F, Esterni B, Ginestier C, Finetti P, et al. Moesin expression is a marker of basal breast carcinomas. Int J Cancer. 2007;121(8):1779–85. https://doi.org/10.1002/ijc.22923.
7. Schlecht NF, Brandwein-Gensler M, Smith RV, Kawachi N, Broughel D, Lin J, et al. Cytoplasmic ezrin and moesin correlate with poor survival in head and neck squamous cell carcinoma. Head Neck Pathol. 2012; 6(2):232–43. https://doi.org/10.1007/s12105-011-0328-1.
8. Wang X, Liu M, Zhao CY. Expression of ezrin and moesin related to invasion, metastasis and prognosis of laryngeal squamous cell carcinoma. Genet Mol Res. 2014;13(3):8002–13. https://doi.org/10.4238/2014.September.29.13.
9. Kobayashi H, Sagara J, Kurita H, Morifuji M, Ohishi M, Kurashina K, et al. Clinical significance of cellular distribution of moesin in patients with oral squamous cell carcinoma. Clin Cancer Res. 2004;10(2):572–80.
10. Belbin TJ, Singh B, Smith RV, Socci ND, Wreesmann VB, Sanchez-Carbayo M, et al. Molecular profiling of tumor progression in head and neck cancer. Arch Otolaryngol Head Neck Surg. 2005;131(1):10–8. https://doi.org/10.1001/archotol.131.1.10.
11. Jung WY, Kang Y, Lee H, Mok YJ, Kim HK, Kim A, et al. Expression of moesin and CD44 is associated with poor prognosis in gastric adenocarcinoma. Histopathology. 2013;63(4):474–81. https://doi.org/10.1111/his.12202.
12. Matsui T, Maeda M, Doi Y, Yonemura S, Amano M, Kaibuchi K, et al. Rho-kinase phosphorylates COOH-terminal threonines of ezrin/radixin/moesin (ERM) proteins and regulates their head-to-tail association. J Cell Biol. 1998; 140(3):647–57.
13. Martin-Villar E, Scholl FG, Gamallo C, Yurrita MM, Munoz-Guerra M, Cruces J, et al. Characterization of human PA2.26 antigen (T1alpha-2, podoplanin), a small membrane mucin induced in oral squamous cell carcinomas. Int J Cancer. 2005;113(6):899–910. https://doi.org/10.1002/ijc.20656.
14. Yuan P, Temam S, El-Naggar A, Zhou X, Liu DD, Lee JJ, et al. Overexpression of podoplanin in oral cancer and its association with poor clinical outcome. Cancer. 2006;107(3):563–9. https://doi.org/10.1002/cncr.22061.
15. Vormittag L, Thurnher D, Geleff S, Pammer J, Heiduschka G, Brunner M, et al. Co-expression of Bmi-1 and podoplanin predicts overall survival in patients with squamous cell carcinoma of the head and neck treated with radio(chemo)therapy. Int J Radiat Oncol Biol Phys. 2009;73(3):913–8. https://doi.org/10.1016/j.ijrobp.2008.10.040.
16. Kreppel M, Scheer M, Drebber U, Ritter L, Zoller JE. Impact of podoplanin expression in oral squamous cell carcinoma: clinical and histopathologic correlations. Virchows Arch. 2010;456(5):473–82. https://doi.org/10.1007/s00428-010-0915-7.
17. Funayama A, Cheng J, Maruyama S, Yamazaki M, Kobayashi T, Syafriadi M, et al. Enhanced expression of podoplanin in oral carcinomas in situ and squamous cell carcinomas. Pathobiology. 2011;78(3):171–80. https://doi.org/10.1159/000324926.
18. Huber GF, Fritzsche FR, Zullig L, Storz M, Graf N, Haerle SK, et al. Podoplanin expression correlates with sentinel lymph node metastasis in early squamous cell carcinomas of the oral cavity and oropharynx. Int J Cancer. 2011;129(6):1404–9. https://doi.org/10.1002/ijc.25795.
19. Kreppel M, Drebber U, Wedemeyer I, Eich HT, Backhaus T, Zoller JE, et al. Podoplanin expression predicts prognosis in patients with oral squamous cell carcinoma treated with neoadjuvant radiochemotherapy. Oral Oncol. 2011;47(9):873–8. https://doi.org/10.1016/j.oraloncology.2011.06.508.
20. Bartuli FN, Luciani F, Caddeo F, Compagni S, Piva P, Ottria L, et al. Podoplanin in the development and progression of oral cavity cancer: a preliminary study. Oral Implantol. 2012;5(2-3):33–41.
21. dos Santos AA, Oliveira DT, Pereira MC, Faustino SE, Nonogaki S, Carvalho AL, et al. Podoplanin and VEGF-C immunoexpression in oral squamous cell carcinomas: prognostic significance. Anticancer Res. 2013;33(9):3969–76.
22. Bryne M, Koppang HS, Lilleng R, Stene T, Bang G, Dabelsteen E. New malignancy grading is a better prognostic indicator than Broders' grading in oral squamous cell carcinomas. J Oral Pathol Med. 1989;18(8):432–7.
23. Faustino SE, Oliveira DT, Nonogaki S, Landman G, Carvalho AL, Kowalski LP. Expression of vascular endothelial growth factor-C does not predict occult lymph-node metastasis in early oral squamous cell carcinoma. Int J Oral Maxillofac Surg. 2008;37(4):372–8. https://doi.org/10.1016/j.ijom.2007.11.021.
24. Clucas J, Valderrama F. ERM proteins in cancer progression. J Cell Sci. 2014; 127(Pt 2):267–75. https://doi.org/10.1242/jcs.133108.
25. Martin-Villar E, Fernandez-Munoz B, Parsons M, Yurrita MM, Megias D, Perez-Gomez E, et al. Podoplanin associates with CD44 to promote directional cell migration. Mol Biol Cell. 2010;21(24):4387–99. https://doi.org/10.1091/mbc.E10-06-0489.
26. Kobayashi H, Sagara J, Masumoto J, Kurita H, Kurashina K, Taniguchi S. Shifts in cellular localization of moesin in normal oral epithelium, oral epithelial dysplasia, verrucous carcinoma and oral squamous cell carcinoma. J Oral Pathol Med. 2003;32(6):344–9.
27. de Vicente JC, Santamarta TR, Rodrigo JP, Garcia-Pedrero JM, Allonca E, Blanco-Lorenzo V. Expression of podoplanin in the invasion front of oral squamous cell carcinoma is not prognostic for survival. Virchows Arch. 2015; 466(5):549–58. https://doi.org/10.1007/s00428-015-1746-3.
28. Ohta M, Abe A, Ohno F, Hasegawa Y, Tanaka H, Maseki S, et al. Positive and negative regulation of podoplanin expression by TGF-beta and histone deacetylase inhibitors in oral and pharyngeal squamous cell carcinoma cell lines. Oral Oncol. 2013;49(1):20–6. https://doi.org/10.1016/j.oraloncology.2012.06.017.
29. Tsuneki M, Yamazaki M, Maruyama S, Cheng J, Saku T. Podoplanin-mediated cell adhesion through extracellular matrix in oral squamous cell carcinoma. Lab Invest. 2013;93(8):921–32. https://doi.org/10.1038/labinvest.2013.86.

3

Neutrophil-lymphocyte ratio complements volumetric staging as prognostic factor in patients treated with definitive radiotherapy for oropharyngeal cancer

Cédric Panje[1], Oliver Riesterer[1], Christoph Glanzmann[1] and Gabriela Studer[1,2]*

Abstract

Background: Volumetric tumor staging has been shown as superior prognostic tool compared to the conventional TNM system in patients undergoing definitive intensity-modulated radiotherapy (IMRT) for head and neck cancer. Recently, clinical immunoscores such as the neutrophil-lymphocyte ratio (NLR) have been investigated as prognostic markers in several tumor entities. The aim of this study was to assess the combined prognostic value of NLR and tumor volume in patients treated with IMRT for oropharyngeal cancer (OC).

Methods: Data on all consecutive patients treated for locally advanced or inoperable OC with IMRT from 2002–2011 was prospectively collected. Tumor volume was assessed based on the total gross tumor volume (tGTV) calculated by the treatment planning system volume algorithm. The NLR was collected by a retrospective analysis of differential blood count before initiation of therapy.

Results: Overall, 187 eligible patients were treated with a median IMRT dose of 69.6 Gy. Three-year recurrence-free survival (RFS) for low, intermediate, high and very high tumor volume groups was 88%, 74%, 62% and 25%, respectively (p = 0.007). Patients with elevated NLR (>4.68) showed a significantly decreased 3-year RFS of 44% vs. 81% (p < 0.001) and 3-year OS of 56% vs. 84% (p < 0.001). The NLR remained a significant prognostic factor for RFS and OS when tested among tumor volume groups. Univariate and multivariate regression analysis confirmed both tumor volume and NLR as independent prognostic factors. The NLR offered further statistically significant prognostic differentiation of the small/intermediate/large tumor volume groups.

Conclusion: The NLR remains an independent prognostic factor for patients with OC undergoing radiotherapy independent of the tumor volume.

Keywords: Radiotherapy, IMRT, Head and neck cancer, Oropharyngeal cancer, Volumetric staging, Neutrophil-lymphocyte ratio, NLR

Background

Definitive intensity-modulated radiotherapy (IMRT) with or without concomitant chemotherapy has been established as standard treatment for locally advanced and inoperable oropharyngeal cancer [1]. Several investigators have previously shown that for non-surgical definitive IMRT collectives of head neck cancer patients volumetric staging may provide a prognostic benefit over the conventional Union for International Cancer Control (UICC) staging system (7th edition) and its T and N categories with regard to all disease control outcome parameters [2–6]. It is known for decades that tumor volume and, in consequence, the number of clonogenic cells is one of the most important predictors for tumor control in radiotherapy [7, 8]. As anatomically (i.e. surgically) defined system, the T and N categories of the standard TNM system are predominantly based on the extent of invasion into adjacent structures, number and site of

* Correspondence: gabriela.studer@luks.ch
[1]Department of Radiation Oncology, University Hospital Zurich, Rämistrasse 100, CH-8091 Zürich, Switzerland
[2]Cantonal Hospital Lucerne, Spitalstrasse, CH-6000 Lucerne, Switzerland

Neutrophil-lymphocyte ratio complements volumetric staging as prognostic factor in patients treated...

15

involved nodes. Included size parameters are one-dimensional diameter measurement, which may not correlate well with tumor volume [9]. Consequently, it has been shown that there is a significant variability in tumor volume and, in consequence, in outcome within a single T category in head and neck cancer [10, 11].

More recently, immunological scores such as the neutrophil-lymphocyte ratio (NLR) have been introduced as prognostic markers for several tumor entities including various sites of head neck cancer [12–17].

Increased blood neutrophils and tumor associated neutrophils have been linked to inferior outcome in cancer [18], particularly the immunosuppressive subset of myeloid-derived suppressor cells [19, 20]. In contrary, several studies have shown that tumor-infiltrating lymphocytes may represent increased anti-tumor immunity with improved local control and long-term prognosis [21–23]. Blood lymphocytes have consequently been identified as significant prognostic marker in head and neck cancer alone as well as part of clinical immuno-scores such as the neutrophil-lymphocyte ratio [13].

However, it is not clear yet whether an elevated NLR represents a surrogate parameter for increased tumor burden in advanced disease [24] or rather tumor-associated immunological processes which are mainly volume-independent.

The aim of our study was therefore to explore the correlation between the NLR and the tumor volume in patients with oropharyngeal cancer undergoing definitive IMRT. The hypothesis was that the NLR may offer additional prognostic information to the previously tested volumetric staging system.

Methods

Data on all consecutive patients with locally advanced or inoperable oropharyngeal cancer (OC) treated with IMRT at our institution from 2002 to 2011 was prospectively collected. Approval of the Local Ethics Committee (Cantonal Ethics Committee Zurich, Nr. 709) is available.

Patients were treated with normofractionated or slightly hypofractionated (2.11 Gy per fraction) definitive IMRT over 6–7 weeks and, if there was no medical contraindication, with weekly cycles of concomitant cisplatin chemotherapy (40 mg/m2/week) or immunotherapy with cetuximab as previously prescribed [3, 25]. Recurrence-free survival and overall survival rates were evaluated. The following clinical parameters were assessed: age at diagnosis, gender, performance status (Eastern Cooperative Oncology Group, ECOG), histology, TN tumor and nodal stage, UICC stage, smoking history, and total tumor volume. Tumor volume was based on the total (nodal and primary) gross tumor volume (tGTV) using information from clinical examination, endoscopy, planning

CT as well as magnetic resonance imaging (MRI) and, if available, positron emission tomography (PET) [3]. Tumor volume definition was reviewed by two board-certified authors (GS and CG). Volumetric three-dimensional tGTV measurements in cubic centimeters (cm^3) were automatically calculated by the treatment planning system volume algorithm (Eclipse® V8.5, Varian Medical Systems, Palo Alto, CA).

Retrospectively collected NLR was obtained from the most recent available differential blood count after diagnosis and before initiation of radiochemotherapy, or, if applicable, before induction chemotherapy by dividing the number of neutrophils by the number of lymphocytes. Neutrophils and lymphocytes were counted in 10^9/ml. Patients with acute infections, traumatic injuries, or invasive biopsies within two weeks before the blood count were excluded from further analysis.

Statistics

Statistical analysis was performed using R software (version 3.2) [26] and the packages "survival" and "prodlim". For comparisons between different groups, the Chi-square and Mann Whitney U test were used. Spearman correlation test was used to analyze correlation between individual factors. Survival analysis was performed using the Kaplan-Meier method and the log-rank test to assess statistical significance. Univariate and multivariate analysis for prognostic factors were investigated using the Cox proportional hazard regression model and the significance level was set to 0.05.

Results

Patient and treatment characteristics

Overall, 194 patients treated with IMRT for oropharyngeal cancer at our institution between 2002 and 2011 were identified. Seven patients were excluded due to primary metastatic disease, missing pretreatment differential blood count or inflammatory or traumatic disease within 2 weeks before the pre-IMRT blood count in order to avoid interference with the NLR. Table 1 shows demographic and tumor related characteristics for the remaining 187 eligible patients.

Median IMRT prescription dose to macroscopic tumor was 69.6 Gy (range 66–72 Gy in 30–35 fractions).

Tumor volume and NLR

Median tGTV was 40 cm^3 (range 3–216 cm^3). Based on a previously reported prognostic tumor volumetric staging [2], 14% of the patients ($n = 26$) belong to the low-volume group (<15 cm^3), 60% ($n = 112$) to the intermediate-volume group (15–70 cm^3) and 26% ($n = 49$) to the high-volume group (>70 cm^3). A previously reported forth prognostic subgroup of tumors

Table 1 Patient and treatment characteristics

Parameter	
Age	median 61.6 years (range 36.9–91.4)
Gender	72% male ($n = 134$) 28% female ($n = 53$)
Histology	100% squamous cell carcinoma
Oropharyngeal subsite	52% tonsil ($n = 97$) 40% base of tongue ($n = 75$) 5% vallecula ($n = 9$) 2% soft palate ($n = 4$) 1% posterior wall ($n = 2$)
T stage (UICC 7th edition)	12% T1 ($n = 22$) 31% T2 ($n = 59$) 19% T3 ($n = 36$) 33% T4 ($n = 61$) 5% not available/recurrent disease ($n = 9$)
N stage (UICC 7th edition)	16% N0 ($n = 30$) 12% N1 ($n = 22$) 4% N2a ($n = 7$) 32% N2b ($n = 60$) 29% N2c ($n = 55$) 4% N3 ($n = 7$) 3% not available/recurrent disease ($n = 6$)
UICC Stage (7th edition)	8% Stage II ($n = 15$) 19% Stage III ($n = 35$) 67% Stage IVA ($n = 122$) 4% Stage IVB ($n = 7$) 2% Recurrent disease ($n = 3$)
ECOG performance score	80% ECOG 0 ($n = 149$) 15% ECOG 1 ($n = 28$) 5% ECOG 2 ($n = 9$)
Tumor volume (combined nodal and primary volume); n = events (any recurrence)	median 40 cm³ (range 3–216 cm³); overall 52 events subgroup 1–15 cm³: 14% ($n = 26$); 3 events subgroup 15–70 cm³: 60% ($n = 112$); 28 events subgroup 70–130 cm³: 23% ($n = 43$); 17 events subgroup >130 cm³: 3% ($n = 6$); 4 events
Smoking status	active = 62% ($n = 116$) stopped =25% ($n = 46$) never smoked = 13% ($n = 25$)
NLR	median 3.33 (range 0.91–33.71)
IMRT dose prescription	median 69.6 Gy (66–72 Gy) single dose 2–2.11 Gy
Concomitant systemic therapy	42% cisplatin weekly ($n = 78$) 47% reduced number of cisplatin cycles ($n = 87$) 7% cetuximab ($n = 14$) 4% no systemic therapy ($n = 7$)
Induction chemotherapy	8% of patients ($n = 15$)
Follow-up	median 61.2 months (range 1.7–169)

>130 cm³ volume [3] was not separately analyzed due to limited sample size ($n = 6$).

Median NLR was 3.33 (range 0.91–33.71, lower and upper quartile 2.34 and 4.68, respectively). In the high-tumor volume group (> 70 cm³), median NLR was significantly higher than in the low-volume groups with 3.7 versus 3.12 ($p = 0.035$) and NRL correlated significantly with the tumor volume in the whole study population ($p = 0.006$, rho = 0.2, Fig. 1).

Outcome related to tumor volume and NLR: Recurrence-free survival and overall survival

Recurrence-free survival (RFS) for the entire cohort was 72% at three years and remained unchained at five years. Overall survival (OS) was 77% at three years and 70% at five years, respectively.

Three-year RFS rates were 88%, 74%, 62% and 25% for the low-volume (<15 cm³), intermediate-volume (15–70 cm³), high-volume (>70–130 cm³) and very high-volume group (>130 cm³), respectively ($p = 0.007$, see Fig. 2a-b). Corresponding 5-year RFS rates for the prognostic volume groups were 88%, 74%, 62%, and 25%, respectively.

There was also a significant correlation of tumor volume with OS($p < 0.001$), with 3-year OS rates for the prognostic volume groups of 87%, 79%, 74% and 17%, respectively, and 5-year OS of 87%, 71%, 69% and 17%, respectively.

Using the upper quartile of 4.68 as cut-off value for further analysis, the subgroup with elevated NLR showed a significantly reduced RFS and OS with a difference for RFS at 3-years of 44% vs. 81% ($p < 0.001$) and at 3-years for OS of 56% vs. 84% ($p < 0.001$), respectively (Fig. 2c-d).

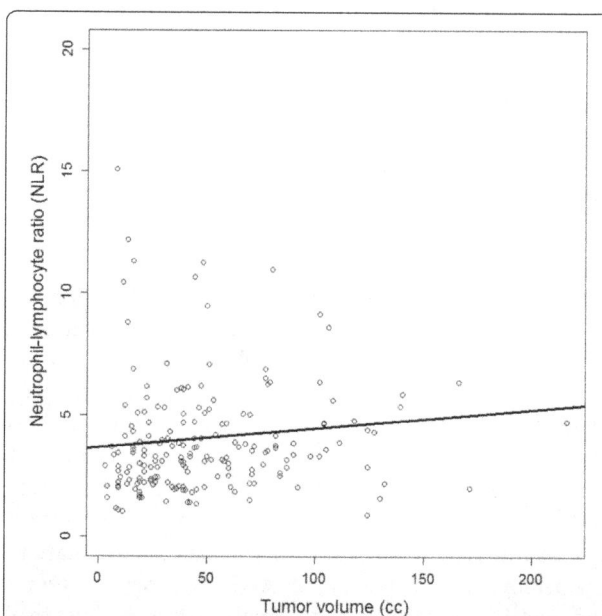

Fig. 1 Correlation analysis demonstrates a statistically significant correlation between neutrophil-lymphocyte ratio and total tumor volume ($p = 0.0059$, rho = 0.20)

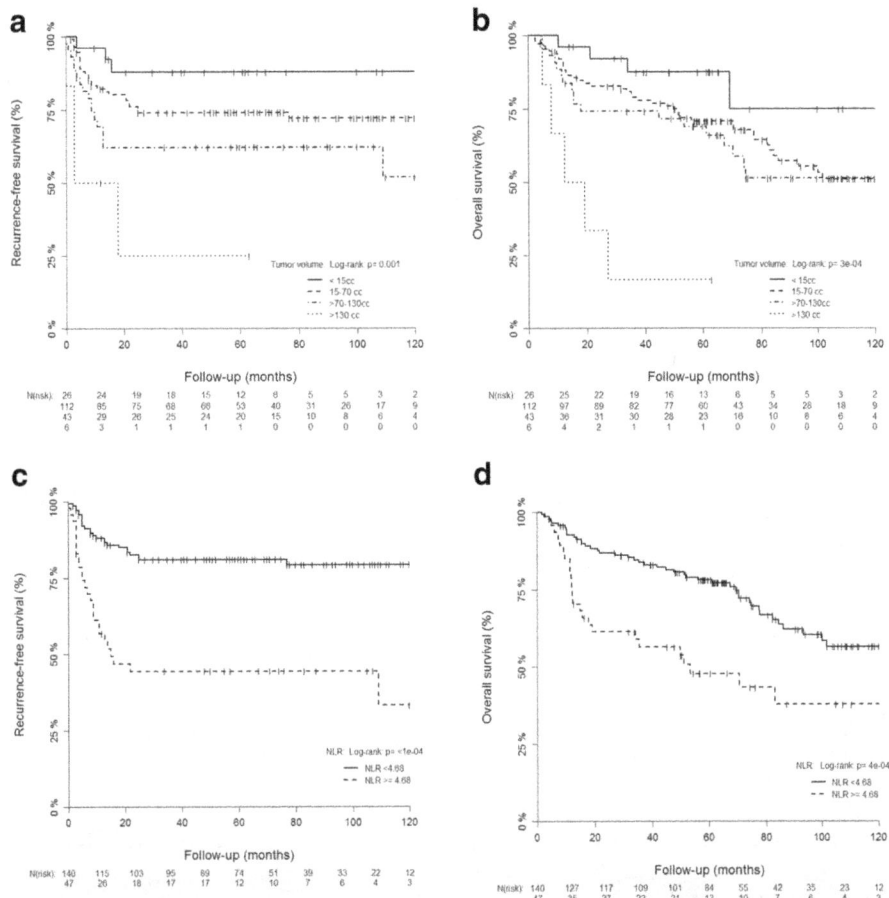

Fig. 2 Recurrence-free survival and overall survival is significantly affected by tumor volume group (**a-b**) and elevated NLR (> = 4.68) **c-d**

The NLR remained a significant prognostic factor when used for each volume group separately: Patients with elevated NLR (> = 4.68) showed a significantly reduced recurrence-free survival in all tumor volume groups (15 cm^3, 15-70 cm^3, >70 cm^3) as well as a significantly inferior overall survival in the high-tumor volume group and a trend towards significance for the intermediate volume group (Fig. 3). Three-year OS and RFS for all tumor volume groups with and without elevated NLR is summarized in Table 2.

Univariate and multivariate regression analysis

Univariate analysis showed significantly increased hazard ratios for OS and RFS for elevated NLR and tumor volume, and a significantly reduced hazard ratio for normal ECOG, and the absence of smoking history. The application of full-dose cisplatin chemotherapy ($\geq$ 200 mg per square meter body surface total dose) was significantly associated only with OS, and showed a trend towards significance for RFS (p = 0.052, Table 3).

For multivariate Cox regression analysis, all significant factors from univariate analysis were included. Tumor volume, elevated NLR and ECOG status remained significant on multivariate testing, whereas chemotherapy and smoking status did not (Table 4).

Discussion

Volumetric tumor staging has been previously established by our group and others as superior prognostic factor compared to the TNM and UICC staging systems for patients with locally advanced head and neck cancer undergoing IMRT [3–5]. As previously reported, we have identified distinct cut-off values for volumetric staging in a prospective patient cohort which correlate well with recurrence-free survival and overall survival [3]. However, there is still a considerable difference in oncological outcome within the pre-defined volume groups, which supports the use of additional prognostic factors such as HPV status [27], advanced imaging [28] or clinical immunoscores [15, 29] to determine the individual risk group of a patient.

Our aim was to analyze the prognostic impact of the NLR in addition to the previously established volumetric risk groups in a cohort of patients undergoing definitive

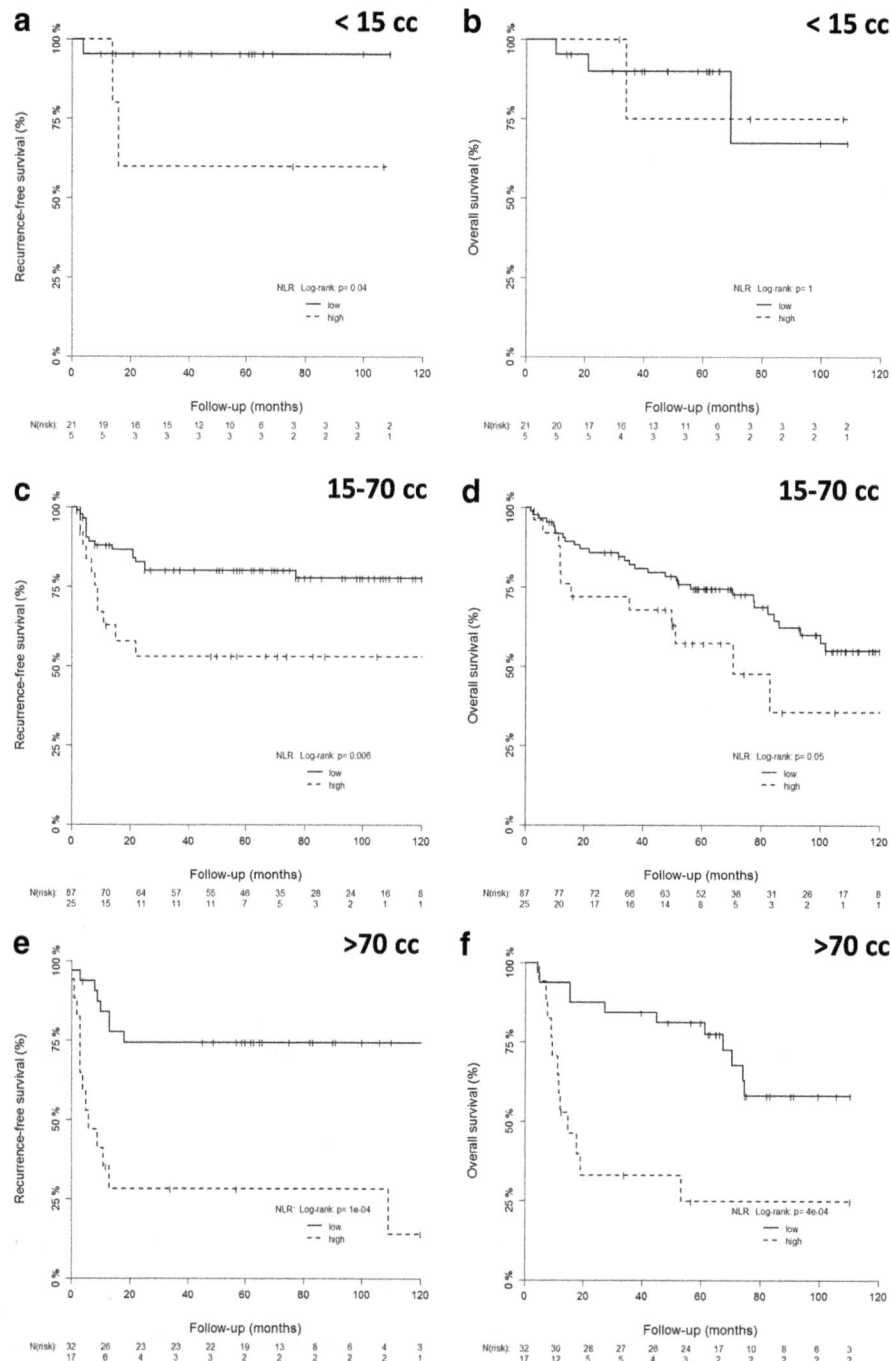

Fig. 3 Stratification for NLR in different tumor volume groups. Patients with elevated NLR (> = 4.68) showed a significantly reduced recurrence-free survival in all tumor volume groups as well as inferior overall survival in the intermediate and high-tumor volume group (**a-b**: <15 cm^3, **c-d**: 15-70 cm^3, **e-f**: >70 cm^3). NLR resulted in an additional statistically significant prognostic differentiation of the volumetric cohorts with respect to RFS and OS rates (except of the 'small tumor volume' cohort with only 4 events, Fig. 3b)

radio(chemo)therapy for oropharyngeal cancer. Our hypothesis was that the use of the NLR may further refine the prognostic volumetric groups which could be confirmed based on a significant association with RFS in all volume groups and with OS in the high tumor volume group. While several authors have investigated the role of the NLR alone in head neck cancer [12, 13, 15], this study is, to our knowledge, the first analysis which combines the prognostic factors of tumor volume and the NLR.

Our data of a large non-surgical cohort of OC treated with IMRT confirms the findings of other

Table 2 Prognostic value of the NLR in different tumor volume risk groups. Cut-off for the NLR was 4.68

	3-year recurrence-free survival				3-year overall survival			
	High NLR	Low NLR	Hazard ratio	P value	High NLR	Low NLR	Hazard ratio	P value
Small tumor volume (< 15 cm^3)	60%	95%	8.16	**0.041**	75%	90%	0.95	0.964
Intermediate tumor volume (15–70 cm^3)	53%	80%	2.77	**0.006**	68%	82%	1.95	0.052
High tumor volume (>70 cm^3)	28%	74%	5.04	**< 0.001**	33%	84%	4.16	**< 0.001**

groups [12, 13, 15] that one of the most commonly investigated immunoscores, the NLR, was significantly associated with recurrence-free survival and overall survival (see Table 5). Although the NLR showed a weak, but statistically significant correlation with tumor volume, the NLR remained a significant independent prognostic marker in all tumor volume subgroups.

Sun et al. [15] previously demonstrated the prognostic significance of NLR in different UICC-stage-based subgroups in nasopharyngeal cancer with no significant impact in stage I and II disease. Similarly, our data for OC shows a significant correlation with RFS, but not with OS in small tumor volumes (<15 cm^3), which, however, may also be due to the small sample size (n = 26) and the limited number of events (n = 4).

Our study was limited by the following facts:

- While the tumor volume was assessed prospectively since 2004, the NLR was collected retrospectively from electronic patient records and blood samples were not taken systematically for this purpose at a specific time point.
- A general limitation of the NLR is that is affected by any inflammatory condition such as infections or invasive procedures as well as by myelosuppressive conditions such as (induction) chemotherapy which led to the exclusion of several patients in our analysis. Future clinical immunoscores may therefore include more cancer-specific hematological markers and identify specific leucocyte subgroups. For instance, it

was found that head and neck cancer patients showed an increased number of immature granulocytes in the peripheral blood [30] as well as unique immunophenotypes of immunosuppressive neutrophils (CD11c bright/CD62L dim/CD11b bright/CD16 bright), which were found in cancer patients but not in healthy donors [31].

- The major limitation of our study is the fact that included patients were not systematically screened for HPV infection, which has been recently established as strong prognostic factor in OC [27, 32, 33], but which had not yet been established as standard at our institution in the investigated period (2002–2011). A subset analysis of OC patients with available p16 status has recently shown that p16-positive patients presented with significantly lower NLR, but the NLR remained a significant prognostic factor both in the p16-positive and p16-negative group [13]. Additionally, other studies confirmed blood neutrophils and lymphocytes as strong prognostic factors in p16-positive OC with significantly lowered blood neutrophils compared to the p16-negative group [34, 35]. These findings are complemented by current immunological research in head and neck cancer which suggests an increased anti-tumor immunity, particularly increased numbers of tumor-infiltrating lymphocytes in p16 positive tumors [36]. Future studies on larger OC cohorts including p16 status will have to clarify the role and correlation of p16 status and NLR as prognostic factors.

Table 3 Univariate Analysis for recurrence-free survival (RFS) and overall survival (OS)

	RFS			OS		
	HR	Conf. int.	p-value	HR	Conf. int.	p-value
Age	1.001	0.9729–1.03	0.942	1.018	0.9932–1.043	0.157
Sex	0.7161	0.3755–1.366	0.308	0.755	0.4312–1.321	0.323
Normal ECOG	0.3812	0.213–0.6823	**0.002**	0.333	0.2009–0.5518	**< 0.001**
UICC stage	1.14	0.6254–2.079	0.668	1.163	0.6781–1.996	0.582
No smoking history	0.2293	0.05573–0.9431	**0.026**	0.314	0.1142–0.8635	**0.018**
Chemotherapy (full dose)	0.5653	0.3158–1.012	0.052	0.555	0.335–0.9195	**0.021**
Tumor volume	1.015	1.008–1.021	**< 0.001**	1.011	1.005–1.017	**< 0.001**
NLR	4.059	2.315–7.117	**< 0.001**	2.311	1.438–3.714	**< 0.001**

Table 4 Multivariate analysis for recurrence-free survival (RFS) and overall survival (OS)

	RFS			OS		
	HR	Conf. int.	p-value	HR	Conf. int.	p-value
Normal ECOG	0.5212	0.28515 0.9526	0.521	0.4027	0.2384 0.6804	**< 0.001**
No smoking history	0.4191	0.09899 1.7739	0.237	0.4887	0.1733 1.3786	0.176
Chemotherapy (full dose)	0.9337	0.50318 1.7328	0.828	0.8130	0.4757 1.3892	0.449
Tumor volume	1.0111	1.00454 1.0177	**0.036**	1.0077	1.0016 1.0138	**0.013**
NLR	3.0218	1.67305 5.4579	**< 0.001**	1.7333	1.0462 2.8718	**0.033**

Recent advances in cancer research have identified inflammatory response as crucial factor for tumor development and progression, and, on the other hand, the presence of tumor-infiltrating lymphocytes as positive prognostic markers in several tumor entities [37]. The NLR is a clinical immunoscore which can be easily deducted from a differential blood count, which is frequently available in patients receiving chemoradiotherapy. It has been established as prognostic marker in several tumor entities [24] including several cohorts of different head and neck cancer subgroups treated with surgery or radiotherapy [12, 15, 17, 38].

We decided to use a single, representative cut-off value for the NLR instead of a subdivision into several prognostic groups, as our major aim was to demonstrate *in principle* the prognostic impact of the NLR in each prognostic tumor volume group. The cut-off value for the NLR in this study of 4.68 is in the same range as in previous publications on NLR in OC (see Table 5). Additionally, a further subdivision with several NLR cut-offs would have resulted in too small subgroups in our single institution cohort which may not allow to draw a significant conclusion.

Table 5 Summary of studies investigating the prognostic role of the neutrophil-lymphocyte ratio (NLR) in oropharyngeal cancer (OC)

Study	Cohort and treatment	NLR cut-off	Results	p16 status
Rachidi et al. [13]	n = 543 HNSCC (170 OC), any treatment (2000–2012)	4.39 (upper tertile)	- Increased mortality for high NLR (HR = 2.39) - NLR prognostic factor both in p16-pos. And neg. Pts. - NLR significantly lower in p16-pos. Patients	yes (89/543)
Charles et al. [29]	n = 145 (76 OC), radio(chemo)therapy (2005–2012)	5.0 (based on review [39])	- High NLR associated in OC with inferior OS (HR = 4.6) and RFS (HR = 3.01) - No subgroup analysis for p16 pos. Pts.	yes (95/145)
Kano et al. [40]	n = 285 HNSCC (116 OC), radiochemotherapy (2003–2012)	1.92 (based on ROC analysis)	- High NLR associated with inferior OS and DFS, but not significant on multivariate analysis	no
Valero et al. [35]	n = 824 (203 OC), any treatment (2010–2012)	1.35 and 3.86 (three groups based on RPA)	- High NLR associated with inferior DSS - Lower neutrophil number in p16 pos. Pts.	yes (125/824)
Selzer et al. [14]	n = 170 (74 OC), primary radio(chemo)therapy or radioimmunotherapy (2002–2012)	5.0	- High NLR associated with inferior median OS (17 vs. 27 months)	no
Moon et al. [41]	n = 153 (51 OC), HNSCC prospective study (2010–2012)	not described	- High NLR associated with inferior PFS (HR = 2.20) and OS (HR = 3.22)	no
Huang et al. [34]	n = 510, OC, radio(chemo)therapy (2000–2010)	not applied (neutrophils and lymphocytes were analyzed separately)	- High neutrophils and low lymphocytes are associated with inferior prognosis - Reduced neutrophil count and similar lymphocyte count in p16-pos. Pts.	yes (all)
Young et al. [42]	n = 249, OC, radio(chemo)therapy (2004–2010)	5.0	- High NLR associated with inferior locoregional control (HR = 2.072)	no

HNSCC squamous cell carcinoma of the head and neck, *pts.* patients, *ROC* receiver-operating characteristic, *RPA* recursive partitioning analysis, *OS* Overall survival, *PFS* progression-free survival, *DFS* disease-free survival, *DSS* disease-specific survival

Conclusion

In summary, our results demonstrate that the NLR is an independent prognostic factor for patients with OC undergoing radio(chemo)therapy regarding RFS in all tumor volume subgroups and regarding OS in high-volume groups. The NLR and tumor volume represent two easily available clinical parameters that impose no additional diagnostic burden to the patients. Future prospective studies are needed to validate our findings. In addition, blood assays are needed that identify more specific subtypes of circulating leukocytes in order to improve the accuracy of oncological immunoscores.

Abbreviations

CT: Computed tomography; DFS: Disease-free survival; DSS: Disease-specific survival; ECOG: Eastern Cooperative Oncology Group; HNSCC: Squamous cell carcinoma of the head and neck; HPV: Human papilloma virus; IMRT: Intensity-modulated radiotherapy; NLR: Neutrophil-lymphocyte ratio; OC: Oropharyngeal cancer; OS: Overall survival; PET: Positron emission tomography; RFS: Recurrence-free survival; ROC: Receiver operating characteristic; tGTV: Total gross tumor volume; UICC: Union for International Cancer Control

Funding

This work was not supported by any external funding.

Authors' contributions

GS and CP conceived of the study and wrote the manuscript with OR. GS and CG performed the volumetric analysis. GS and CG collected the clinical data within a prospective database. CP did the statistical analysis. All authors read and approved the final manuscript.

Competing interests

The authors declare that they have no competing interests.

References

1. Marur S, Forastiere AA. Head and neck squamous cell carcinoma: update on epidemiology, diagnosis, and treatment. Mayo Clin Proc. 2016;91(3):386–96.
2. Studer G, Lutolf UM, El-Bassiouni M, Rousson V, Glanzmann C. Volumetric staging (VS) is superior to TNM and AJCC staging in predicting outcome of head and neck cancer treated with IMRT. Acta Oncol. 2007;46(3):386–94.
3. Studer G, Glanzmann C. Volumetric staging in oropharyngeal cancer patients treated with definitive IMRT. Oral Oncol. 2013;49(3):269–76.
4. Strongin A, Yovino S, Taylor R, Wolf J, Cullen K, Zimrin A, Strome S, Regine W, Suntharalingam M. Primary tumor volume is an important predictor of clinical outcomes among patients with locally advanced squamous cell cancer of the head and neck treated with definitive chemoradiation. Int J Radiat Oncol Biol Phys. 2012;82(5):1823–30.
5. Knegjens JL, Hauptmann M, Pameijer FA, Balm AJ, Hoebers FJ, de Bois JA, Kaanders JH, van Herpen CM, Verhoef CG, Wijers OB, et al. Tumor volume as prognostic factor in chemoradiation for advanced head and neck cancer. Head Neck. 2011;33(3):375–82.
6. Studer G, Seifert B, Glanzmann C. Prediction of distant metastasis in head neck cancer patients: implications for induction chemotherapy and pre-treatment staging? Strahlenther Onkol. 2008;184(11):580–5.
7. Johnson CR, Thames HD, Huang DT, Schmidt-Ullrich RK. The tumor volume and clonogen number relationship: tumor control predictions based upon tumor volume estimates derived from computed tomography. Int J Radiat Oncol Biol Phys. 1995;33(2):281–7.
8. Brenner DJ. Dose, volume, and tumor-control predictions in radiotherapy. Int J Radiat Oncol Biol Phys. 1993;26(1):171–9.
9. Sorensen AG, Patel S, Harmath C, Bridges S, Synnott J, Sievers A, Yoon YH, Lee EJ, Yang MC, Lewis RF, et al. Comparison of diameter and perimeter methods for tumor volume calculation. J Clin Oncol. 2001;19(2):551–7.
10. Studer G, Glanzmann C. Volumetric stratification of cT4 stage head and neck cancer. Strahlenther Onkol. 2013;189(10):867–73.
11. Pameijer FA, Balm AJ, Hilgers FJ, Muller SH. Variability of tumor volumes in T3-staged head and neck tumors. Head Neck. 1997;19(1):6–13.
12. Haddad CR, Guo L, Clarke S, Guminski A, Back M, Eade T. Neutrophil-to-lymphocyte ratio in head and neck cancer. J Med Imaging Radiat Oncol. 2015;59(4):514–9.
13. Rachidi S, Wallace K, Wrangle JM, Day TA, Alberg AJ, Li Z. Neutrophil-to-lymphocyte ratio and overall survival in all sites of head and neck squamous cell carcinoma. Head Neck. 2016;38(Suppl 1):E1068–74.
14. Selzer E, Grah A, Heiduschka G, Kornek G, Thurnher D. Primary radiotherapy or postoperative radiotherapy in patients with head and neck cancer: comparative analysis of inflammation-based prognostic scoring systems. Strahlenther Onkol. 2015;191(6):486–94.
15. Sun W, Zhang L, Luo M, Hu G, Mei Q, Liu D, Long G, Hu G. Pretreatment hematologic markers as prognostic factors in patients with nasopharyngeal carcinoma: neutrophil-lymphocyte ratio and platelet-lymphocyte ratio. Head Neck. 2016;38(Suppl 1):E1332–40.
16. Tu XP, Qiu QH, Chen LS, Luo XN, Lu ZM, Zhang SY, Chen SH. Preoperative neutrophil-to-lymphocyte ratio is an independent prognostic marker in patients with laryngeal squamous cell carcinoma. BMC Cancer. 2015;15:743.
17. Wong BY, Stafford ND, Green VL, Greenman J. Prognostic value of the neutrophil-to-lymphocyte ratio in patients with laryngeal squamous cell carcinoma. Head Neck. 2016;38(Suppl 1):E1903–8.
18. Moses K, Brandau S. Human neutrophils: their role in cancer and relation to myeloid-derived suppressor cells. Semin Immunol. 2016;28(2):187–96.
19. Montero AJ, Diaz-Montero CM, Kyriakopoulos CE, Bronte V, Mandruzzato S. Myeloid-derived suppressor cells in cancer patients: a clinical perspective. J Immunother. 2012;35(2):107–15.
20. Freiser ME, Serafini P, Weed DT. The immune system and head and neck squamous cell carcinoma: from carcinogenesis to new therapeutic opportunities. Immunol Res. 2013;57(1–3):52–69.
21. Uppaluri R, Dunn GP, Lewis JS Jr. Focus on TILs: prognostic significance of tumor infiltrating lymphocytes in head and neck cancers. Cancer Immun. 2008;8:16.
22. Ward MJ, Thirdborough SM, Mellows T, Riley C, Harris S, Suchak K, Webb A, Hampton C, Patel NN, Randall CJ, et al. Tumour-infiltrating lymphocytes predict for outcome in HPV-positive oropharyngeal cancer. Br J Cancer. 2014;110(2):489–500.
23. Balermpas P, Michel Y, Wagenblast J, Seitz O, Weiss C, Rodel F, Rodel C, Fokas E. Tumour-infiltrating lymphocytes predict response to definitive chemoradiotherapy in head and neck cancer. Br J Cancer. 2014;110(2):501–9.
24. Templeton AJ, McNamara MG, Seruga B, Vera-Badillo FE, Aneja P, Ocana A, Leibowitz-Amit R, Sonpavde G, Knox JJ, Tran B, et al. Prognostic role of neutrophil-to-lymphocyte ratio in solid tumors: a systematic review and meta-analysis. J Natl Cancer Inst. 2014;106(6):dju124.
25. Studer G, Rordorf T, Glanzmann C. Impact of tumor volume and systemic therapy on outcome in patients undergoing IMRT for large volume head neck cancer. Radiat Oncol. 2011;6:120.
26. R: A Language and Environment for Statistical Computing [http://www.R-project.org]. Accessed 28 Nov 2016.
27. Ang KK, Harris J, Wheeler R, Weber R, Rosenthal DI, Nguyen-Tan PF, Westra WH, Chung CH, Jordan RC, Lu C, et al. Human papillomavirus and survival of patients with oropharyngeal cancer. N Engl J Med. 2010;363(1):24–35.
28. Nesteruk M, Lang S, Veit-Haibach P, Studer G, Stieb S, Glatz S, Hemmatazad H, Ikenberg K, Huber G, Pruschy M, et al. Tumor stage, tumor site and HPV dependent correlation of perfusion CT parameters and [18F]-FDG uptake in head and neck squamous cell carcinoma. Radiother Oncol. 2015;117(1):125–31.
29. Charles KA, Harris BD, Haddad CR, Clarke SJ, Guminski A, Stevens M, Dodds T, Gill AJ, Back M, Veivers D, et al. Systemic inflammation is an independent predictive marker of clinical outcomes in mucosal squamous cell carcinoma of the head and neck in oropharyngeal and non-oropharyngeal patients. BMC Cancer. 2016;16(1):124.
30. Trellakis S, Farjah H, Bruderek K, Dumitru CA, Hoffmann TK, Lang S, Brandau S. Peripheral blood neutrophil granulocytes from patients with head and neck squamous cell carcinoma functionally differ from their counterparts in healthy donors. Int J Immunopathol Pharmacol. 2011;24(3):683–93.
31. Hao S, Andersen M, Yu H. Detection of immune suppressive neutrophils in peripheral blood samples of cancer patients. Am J Blood Res. 2013;3(3):239–45.

32. Ragin CC, Taioli E. Survival of squamous cell carcinoma of the head and neck in relation to human papillomavirus infection: review and meta-analysis. Int J Cancer. 2007;121(8):1813–20.

33. Rosenthal DI, Harari PM, Giralt J, Bell D, Raben D, Liu J, Schulten J, Ang KK, Bonner JA. Association of Human Papillomavirus and p16 status with outcomes in the IMCL-9815 phase III registration trial for patients with Locoregionally advanced oropharyngeal squamous cell carcinoma of the head and neck treated with radiotherapy with or without Cetuximab. J Clin Oncol. 2016;34(12):1300–8.

34. Huang SH, Waldron JN, Milosevic M, Shen X, Ringash J, Su J, Tong L, Perez-Ordonez B, Weinreb I, Bayley AJ, et al. Prognostic value of pretreatment circulating neutrophils, monocytes, and lymphocytes in oropharyngeal cancer stratified by human papillomavirus status. Cancer. 2015;121(4):545–55.

35. Valero C, Pardo L, Lopez M, Garcia J, Camacho M, Quer M, Leon X. Pretreatment count of peripheral neutrophils, monocytes, and lymphocytes as independent prognostic factor in patients with head and neck cancer. Head Neck. 2016;39(2):219–26.

36. Saber CN, Gronhoj Larsen C, Dalianis T, von Buchwald C. Immune cells and prognosis in HPV-associated oropharyngeal squamous cell carcinomas: review of the literature. Oral Oncol. 2016;58:8–13.

37. Grivennikov SI, Greten FR, Karin M. Immunity, inflammation, and cancer. Cell. 2010;140(6):883–99.

38. Salim DK, Mutlu H, Eryilmaz MK, Salim O, Musri FY, Tural D, Gunduz S, Coskun HS. Neutrophil to lymphocyte ratio is an independent prognostic factor in patients with recurrent or metastatic head and neck squamous cell cancer. Mol Clin Oncol. 2015;3(4):839–42.

39. Guthrie GJ, Charles KA, Roxburgh CS, Horgan PG, McMillan DC, Clarke SJ. The systemic inflammation-based neutrophil-lymphocyte ratio: experience in patients with cancer. Crit Rev Oncol Hematol. 2013;88(1):218–30.

40. Kano S, Homma A, Hatakeyama H, Mizumachi T, Sakashita T, Kakizaki T, Fukuda S. Pretreatment lymphocyte-to-monocyte ratio as an independent prognostic factor for head and neck cancer. Head Neck. 2017;39(2):247–53.

41. Moon H, Roh JL, Lee SW, Kim SB, Choi SH, Nam SY, Kim SY. Prognostic value of nutritional and hematologic markers in head and neck squamous cell carcinoma treated by chemoradiotherapy. Radiother Oncol. 2016;118(2):330–4.

42. Young CA, Murray LJ, Karakaya E, Thygesen HH, Sen M, Prestwich RJ. The prognostic role of the neutrophil-to-lymphocyte ratio in oropharyngeal carcinoma treated with Chemoradiotherapy. Clin Med Insights Oncol. 2014;8:81–6.

4

Prevalence and types of high-risk human papillomaviruses in head and neck cancers from Bangladesh

Mushfiq H. Shaikh[1,2,3], Aminul I. Khan[4], Anwar Sadat[5], Ahmed H. Chowdhury[6], Shahed A. Jinnah[7], Vinod Gopalan[8], Alfred K. Lam[8], Daniel T. W. Clarke[2,3], Nigel A. J. McMillan[2,3] and Newell W. Johnson[1,3,9,10*]

Abstract

Background: There is a dramatic rise in the incidence of Human papillomavirus (HPV) – associated head and neck squamous cell carcinoma (HNSCC) in the world, with considerable variation by geography, gender and ethnicity. Little is known about the situation in Bangladesh, where tobacco- and areca nut-related head and neck cancers (HNCs) are the most common cancers in men. We aimed to determine the prevalence of HPV in HNSCC in Bangladesh and to explore the possible value of cell cycle markers in clinical diagnostic settings.

Methods: One hundred and ninety six archival HNSCC tissue samples were analysed for the presence of HPV DNA. The DNA quality was assured, and then amplified using a nested PCR approach. The typing of HPV was performed by automated DNA sequencing. Cellular markers p53, Cyclin D1 and pRb were tested on all samples by immunohistochemistry (IHC), as well as p16 as a putative surrogate for the detection of HPV.

Results: HPV DNA was detected in 36/174 (~21%) samples: 36% of cancers from the oropharynx; 31% of oral cancers, and 22% from the larynx. HPV-16 was most common, being present in 33 samples, followed by HPV-33 (2 samples) and HPV-31 (1 sample). Twenty-eight out of 174 samples were positive for p16, predominantly in HPV-positive tissues ($p < 0.001$). No statistically significant association was observed between the cellular markers and HPV DNA positive cases. However, p16 positivity had excellent predictive value for the presence of HPV by PCR.

Conclusion: There is a significant burden of HPV-associated HNSCC in Bangladesh, particularly in the oropharynx but also in oral and laryngeal cancers. Whilst a combination of PCR-based DNA detection and p16 IHC is useful, the latter has excellent specificity, acceptable sensitivity and good predictive value for carriage of HPV in this population and should be used for prognostic evaluation and treatment planning of all HNSCC patients in South Asia, as in the Western world.

Keywords: Head and neck squamous cell carcinoma (HNSCC), Human papillomavirus (HPV), Nested polymerase chain reaction (PCR), Immunohistochemistry (IHC), South Asia, Bangladesh

Background

Head and neck cancer (HNC) is a major health problem worldwide, with an annual incidence of approximately 600,000 cases and close to 300,000 deaths, mostly in less developed countries (GLOBOCAN 2012) [1]. Whilst most – 80-90% in some countries - are squamous cell carcinomas

and variants thereof, neoplasms in this region are diverse at clinical and biological levels, which make them difficult to manage. Although tobacco, areca nut and alcohol are the major risk factors for HNSCC, infection with high-risk types of Human papillomavirus (HPV) has been shown to be strongly associated with a significant proportion of cases [2]. This association varies by anatomical site/subsite, with a predilection for mucosa associated with the lymphoid aggregations of Waldeyer's ring, and are thus seen in the oro-pharynx, especially base of tongue and palatine tonsils, compared to the oral cavity, larynx and hypo-pharynx [3].

* Correspondence: n.johnson@griffith.edu.au
[1]School of Dentistry and Oral Health, Griffith University, Gold Coast, QLD 4222, Australia
[3]Understanding Chronic Conditions Program, Menzies Health Institute Queensland, Gold Coast, QLD 4222, Australia
Full list of author information is available at the end of the article

Recently, the International Agency for Research on Cancer (IARC) has acknowledged HPV as an aetiological factor for oropharyngeal squamous cell carcinoma (OPSCC) [4, 5]. HPV-associated HNSCC represents a distinct entity with increase in incidence over the last three decades, mostly in developed countries and commonly affecting young adult males who tend to be non-smokers, non- or light- drinkers and many have relatively high socioeconomic status [6]. It is suggested that this is related to changing sexual behaviour, with an increase in oral-genital contact [7], sexual debut at early age and a high number of lifetime sex partners [8]. Because HPV-related HNC patients have significantly better treatment response and 3-year overall survival rates (82.4% vs 57.1%) irrespective of age, gender or tumour stage [9, 10], knowledge of HPV status is mandatory in most tumour boards for the planning of treatment.

Approximately one-third of the total HNC cases in the world have been shown to be associated with high-risk HPV infection, but wide geographic variation exists [9, 11].

The prevalence of HPV in HNC, especially, OPSCC is much higher in North America (~70%) and Europe (~50%) compared to rest of the world [12]. An increasing trend is noticed in Australia, where HPV-positive OPSCC rose from 20% to 63% of cases over the last two decades [13]. South Asia (including the Indian subcontinent) has the highest incidence rates and disease burden of HNSCC in the world with approximately 200,000 new cases each year and more than 100,000 deaths (GLOBOCAN 2012) [1, 11]. However, relevant studies in South Asian populations are few and inconsistent. HNSCC is *the leading* cancer in males and 3rd most common in females in India [14]. Bangladesh shares similar cultural & social norms as India. Likewise, HNSCC is also the most common cancer in males in Bangladesh, surpassing lung cancer [15]. As extensive use of tobacco (in smoking and smokeless forms) and chewing of areca nut dominate the risks for head and neck cancer across South Asia, less attention has been given to the role of HPV. There are no comprehensive data from Bangladesh. Because of the high burden of this disease in South and South East Asia it is essential to have accurate data on the role of HPV across the region.

The primary objective of our study was to investigate the prevalence of high risk HPV in HNSCC in a Bangladeshi cohort of patients assembling tumours from different sites of the head and neck region. We also determined the concordance between commonly used HPV detection methods, namely polymerase chain reaction (detects the presence of HPV DNA in tumour tissue) and p16 immunohistochemistry (IHC), a commonly used surrogate marker for HPV-associated cancers. Increased p16 expression is a direct consequence of E7 (HPV oncoprotein) -induced retinoblastoma (pRb) protein inactivation (no/low expression)

[16], and Cyclin D1 protein expression is dependent on intact pRb expression [17]. Thus, analyzing the expression of both pRb and Cyclin D1 could provide useful prognostic information about the biological activity of HPV in HNSCC. Further, HPV-positive HNSCC is associated with low level of p53 expression due to the suppressing action of another viral oncoprotein, HPV E6 [18]. Based on these considerations, here we address the correlation of the potential prognostic markers p16, p53, pRb and Cyclin D1 with HPV status. Our data provide insights into the relative burden and aetiology of HNCs in Bangladesh, likely generalizable to South Asia as a whole.

Methods
Study population and data collection
A total of 196 de-identified HNSCC cases were included. Patients were from Dhaka Medical College Hospital (DMCH), A.I. Khan Laboratory and Millennium Dental Clinic in the city. All were over 20 years of age, clinically and pathologically diagnosed with head and neck cancer between December 2014 and May 2016. The cancers were classified into different subsites of the head and neck following the ICD-10 classification. The borders of tongue (C02.1), gingiva (C03), floor of the mouth (C04), hard palate (C05.0), buccal mucosa (C06.0), vestibular fold (C06.1) and retromolar area (C06.2) were grouped under 'oral cavity' (C02-C06), while the base of the tongue (C01), soft palate (C05.1), tonsils (C09.9), vallecula (C10.0) and pharyngeal walls (C10.2 & C10.3) were congregated under 'oropharynx' (C01, C09 & C10). Further, pyriform fossa (C12) and cricoid region (C13) were classified under 'hypopharynx' (C12, C13) and the supraglottic (C32.1), vocal cord (C32.0), epiglottic (C32.1) and aryepiglottic fold (C32.1) were grouped under 'larynx' (C32). Cancers of the salivary glands and nasopharynx were excluded. Diagnostic biopsy specimens were preserved as formalin fixed paraffin embedded (FFPE) blocks in the Department of Pathology, DMCH and in A. I. Khan Pathology Laboratory, Dhanmondi, and Dhaka. Clinico-pathological data of tumour sites, tumour differentiation, and demography of patients were retrieved from the pathological records.

The study was approved by the Griffith University Human Research Ethics Committee in Australia (GU Ref No: DOH/13/14/HREC) and DMCH Human Ethics Committee (Memo No. DMC/ECC/2016/32) in Bangladesh.

HPV DNA detection & type determination
DNA isolation and testing of sample integrity
The FFPE blocks were sectioned whilst maintaining utmost precautions to avoid inter-block contamination of DNA. This was achieved by pre-chilling and moistening each block in a separate ice container before sectioning, thorough cleaning of the microtome, single use of brush

and forceps, changing gloves in between each block, changing the water bath for each block and using a new blade for each block. Genomic DNA was extracted from a 10 um thick section, using GeneRead FFPE kit (Qiagen, Germany). A section from a blank paraffin block was cut and processed along with the sections from the cases to check for any contamination. DNA concentrations were determined with a NanoDrop 2000 spectrophotometer (Thermo Scientific, Waltham, MA). DNA integrity was assessed for 150 bp fragments of the Beta-actin housekeeping gene by PCR using the GoTaq Green PCR kit (Promega, Madison, WI). Nuclease free water was used as negative control, while genomic DNA from the HPV16 positive head and neck cancer cell line, UDSCC-2 (kindly provided by Dr. Silke Schwarz and Prof. Thomas Hoffman, University of Ulm, Germany) and HPV-negative head and neck cancer cell line, SCC25 were used as a positive control and a negative tissue control, respectively, in the first PCR run. From the 2nd PCR run onwards, samples that had shown positivity and negativity in the first PCR run were used as positive and negative controls, respectively.

Detection of HPV DNA by PCR

Nested PCR, consisting of two sets of degenerative/consensus primer pairs, MY09/11 and GP5+/GP6+ (Sigma-Aldrich, St. Louis, MO, USA) were used [19–21]. A gradient PCR was performed to optimise the annealing temperature for each primer set. The HPV $L1$ gene was amplified using primers MY09/11 in the first round, followed by GP5+/GP6+ in the second round. The PCR reaction mix contained forward and reversed primers (0.5 µM of each), 1 × PCR buffer (containing 1.5 mM MgCl$_2$) (Phusion High-Fidelity 5 × PCR Buffer, New England Biolabs, MA, USA), 200 µM of dNTPs (10 mM dNTP Mix, New England Biolabs, MA, USA), 1.0 unit of Phusion DNA polymerase (Taq polymerase 1unit/50 µl, New England Biolabs, MA, USA) and nuclease-free water, up to a final volume of 20 µl. Positive and negative reaction controls were included in each PCR run. DNA amplification was carried out in an automated thermal cycler (Takara Bio Inc., Japan). Reactions were brought to 98 °C for 30 s (initial denaturation), followed by forty cycles consisting of a denaturing step for 10 s at 98 °C, an annealing step for 30 s at 55.5 °C (MY09/11 in first round) or 55 °C (GP5+/GP6+ second round), and an extension step for 20 s at 72 °C. A final extension step at 72 °C was carried out for 5 min. A total of 2 µl of the first-round PCR product was used in the second round of amplifications.

The PCR products of the samples from both rounds were electrophoresed in 2% agarose gel prepared with 1× TAE (Tris-acetate-EDTA) buffer (DNA Agar, Marine Bio Products Inc., Quincy, MA, USA), stained with 0.5 g/mol of ethidium bromide (Merck, KGaA, Darmstadt, Germany) and visualized under ultraviolet light using the Chemi-Doc machine (BioRad, USA). The size of the amplified product was determined by comparing with a reference molecular weight DNA marker, (Quick Load, 100 bp DNA Ladder, New England Biolab, MA, USA). Any sample that showed a positive band in the gel for both first (band size 450 bp) and second (band size 150 bp) round of PCR was taken as an HPV-positive sample and purified for sequencing.

Sequencing for HPV type

A PCR DNA purification kit (Qiagen, Germany) was used to purify the PCR product of the HPV-DNA positive samples detected in gel electrophoresis. These were submitted to the Australian Genome Research Facility (AGRF) for automated sequencing. Sequences were compared with available HPV genome sequences in Genebank using the NCBI (National Center for Biotechnology Information) Blast programme.

Histological diagnosis

Adjacent haematoxylin and eosin (H&E) stained sections were used to confirm diagnoses and to grade. Grades 1, 2 and 3 were referred to as well, moderately and poorly differentiated, respectively [22].

Immunohistochemical analysis

Immunohistochemistry (IHC) for p16, p53, pRb and Cyclin D1 was performed in the laboratories of Menzies Health Institute Queensland (MHIQ) and/or Gold Coast University Hospital, using DAKO histology kits (EnVision FLEX Mini Kit, High pH) (DAKO, Agilent, Santa Clara, CA), some manually, others in an Intellipath (Biocare Medical, Concord, CA) autostainer. Briefly, from each FFPE block, a 4um thick section was cut and affixed to Menzel-Gläser super-frost plus slides (Thermo Fisher Scientific, Waltham, MA) and air-dried at 37 °C for 48 h. Slides were preheated at 60 °C, followed by dewaxing and re-hydration using xylene, ethanol and water. Antigen retrieval was performed with the DAKO EnVision Kit (DAKO, Agilent, Santa Clara, CA) followed by wash with Tris-Buffer Saline (TBS) mixed with 0.1% Tween 20. Staining with primary antibodies was carried out according to the protocol recommended by DAKO, using an Intellipath autostainer, where staining steps and incubation times were programmed according to the DAKO EnVision FLEX Mini Kit protocol. A similar procedure was followed for manual staining. The primary antibodies mouse anti-p16^{INK4a} (#2D9A12; DAKO, Agilent, Santa Clara, CA), mouse anti-human p53 (#DO-7; DAKO, Agilent, Santa Clara, CA), rabbit anti-human Cyclin D1 (#EP12, DAKO, Agilent, Santa Clara, CA), and rabbit anti-human pRB (#9308; Cell Signaling,

Danvers, MA) were optimized for antibody concentration and incubation time according to their respective company protocols. Positive and negative IHC controls were used in every run. A tonsillar SCC with high p16 expression was taken as positive control for p16 IHC; for p53 a positive colon cancer; for Cyclin D1 and pRb, a known positive tonsillar carcinoma.

IHC slides were scored independently by three head and neck pathologists (AL, MS & VG). Discordant cases were few and agreed by discussion. Cases with moderate to strong staining of all neoplastic areas were recorded as positive, while sections with weak and focal staining were regarded as negative. To be regarded as p16 positive, sections had to show both nuclear and cytoplasmic staining in 50% or more of neoplastic cells [23, 24]. For p53, Cyclin D1 and pRb proteins, in which reaction product is present in nuclei only, slides were scored dichotomously, negative being <10% of cells staining, positive being >10% [25–27]. Typical staining patterns of each cellular marker are presented in Fig. 1 (a–d).

Statistical analysis

This was carried out using SPSS version 22 (IBM Corporation, Armonk, NY). To compare the characteristics of HPV-positive and -negative patients, χ^2 or Fischer's exact tests were used. However, to determine the mean age differences between HPV-positive and -negative groups, an independent t-test were used. Spearman's rank coefficient was used to analyse possible correlations among and between p16, p53, pRb and cyclin D1 expression levels. All analyses were two-sided and p-values below 0.05 were regarded as significant. In addition, the predictive values of p16 and PCR-determined HPV status were examined by standard 2X2 table analyses, and the sensitivity and specificity calculated [28, 29].

Results

Patient demography and histology

A total of 174 of the 196 blocks were analysed: 22 did not contain PCR-amplifiable DNA as determined by β-actin. The mean age of all patients was 56.6 years (Table 1): 138 (~80%) were men and 36 (~20%) women. Primary tumour sites, as given in pathology records, were: oral cavity 55 (31.6%), oropharynx 35 (20.1%), larynx 64 (36.8%) and hypopharynx 20 (11.5%). The majority, 98 (56.3%), were moderately differentiated; followed by well- 66 (37.9%) and poorly differentiated 10 (5.7%) (Table 1).

Presence of HPV DNA and HPV type

Overall, 36/174 (~21%) of blocks were positive for HPV DNA. The HPV prevalence was significantly higher for tumours in the oropharynx, 13/35 (37.1%), followed by oral cavity, 11/55 (20.0%) and larynx, 8/64 (12.5%) and hypopharynx (20.0%). Sequencing showed that HPV-16 was most common, 33/36 (~92%) of the HPV-positive tumours, followed by HPV-31 (2 cases) (~6%) and HPV-33 (1 case) (~3%).

HPV-positive patients were younger (mean ~54 years) than HPV-negative cases (mean ~ 57 years) and HPV prevalence was inversely correlated with age, ($p = 0.014$). A higher proportion of cases in men were HPV-positive (30/138, 21.7% cf. 6/36, 16.6% for women) but this was not statistically significant (Table 1). Among the HPV-positive cases, a significantly higher proportion fell into the moderately differentiated group ($p = 0.011$) (Table 1) (Fig. 2).

Correlation between presence of HPV DNA and p16 expression

Only 28 of 174 samples (16.1%) exhibited p16 overexpression, mostly in HPV positive cases ($p < 0.0001$) (Table 2). Of the 36 cases positive for HPV DNA, 26 (72%) showed

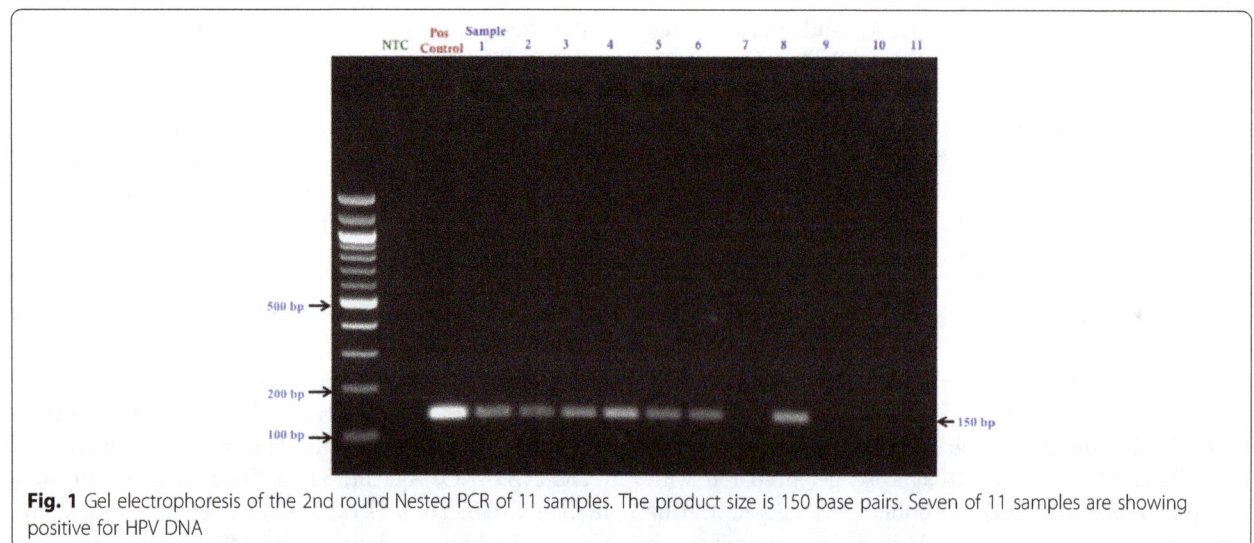

Fig. 1 Gel electrophoresis of the 2nd round Nested PCR of 11 samples. The product size is 150 base pairs. Seven of 11 samples are showing positive for HPV DNA

Table 1 Demographic and clinical characteristics of patients

Characteristics	All patients ($n = 174$) (%)	HPV DNA + ve ($n = 36$) (%)	HPV DNA-ve ($n = 138$)(%)	X^2 (Chi-square)	p-value
Mean Age	56.6	54.2	57.2		0.143
Age groups (years)					
20–59	94 (54.1)	26 (72.2)	68 (49.3)	6.053*	0.014
60 and above	80 (45.9)	10 (27.8)	70 (50.7)		
Gender					
Male	138 (79.3)	30 (83.3)	108 (78.3)	0.448	0.503
Female	36 (20.7)	6 (16.7)	30 (21.7)		
Primary Tumour sites					
Oral Cavity (C02-C06)	55 (31.6)	11 (30.6)	44 (31.9)	8.412*	0.038
Oropharynx (C01, C09 & C10)	35 (20.1)	13 (36.1)	22 (15.9)		
Larynx (C32)	64 (36.8)	8 (22.2)	56 (40.6)		
Hypopharynx (C13)	20 (11.5)	4 (11.1)	16 (11.6)		
Histopathological Grading					
Well differentiated	48 (27.6)	4 (11.1)	44 (31.9)	8.947*	0.011
Moderately differentiated	92 (52.9)	20 (55.6)	72 (52.2)		
Poorly differentiated	34 (19.5)	12 (33.3)	22 (15.9)		
Immunohistochemistry (IHC) Analysis					
p16 expression					
Positive	28 (16.1)	26 (72.2)	2 (1.4)	105.914*	0.0001
Negative	146 (83.9)	10 (27.8)	136 (98.6)		
p53 expression					
Positive	86 (49.4)	23 (63.9)	63 (45.7)	3.799	0.051
Negative	88 (51.6)	13 (36.1)	75 (54.3)		
Cyclin D1 expression					
Positive	62 (35.6)	13 (36.1)	49 (35.5)	0.05	0.946
Negative	112 (64.4)	23 (63.9)	89 (64.5)		
pRb expression					
Positive	66 (37.9)	15 (41.7)	51 (37.0)	0.269	0.604
Negative	108 (62.1)	21 (58.3)	87 (63.0)		

*indicates statistical significance

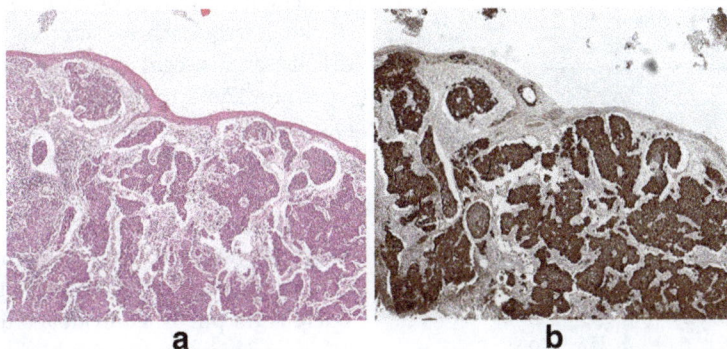

Fig. 2 a Poorly differentiated HPV-associated SCC of tonsil (H&E), in this area beneath an intact surface, (**b**) Intense staining of nuclei and cytoplasm for p16 in the same tumour (20X magnification of original image)

Table 2 Concordance between HPV positive nested PCR and p16 IHC results

P16 by IHC	HPV DNA detection by PCR		
	HPV positive	HPV negative	Total
Positive	26 (14.9%)	2 (1.2%)	28 (16.1%)
Negative	10 (5.7%)	136 (78.2%)	146 (83.9%)
Total	36	138	174

p16 overexpression (true positive), whereas 138 (94%) of the 146 cases were negative for both HPV DNA and p16 (true negative). From the oropharynx, 13 cases showed HPV-positivity, 11 of which were also positive for p16. Similarly, from the oral cavity, 11 cases were HPV-positive but only 6 cases showed p16 positivity. From the larynx, 8 cases were HPV positive, 6 of which were also p16 positive. From the hypopharynx, 4 cases were HPV positive, 3 of which were also p16 positive. Taking PCR data as the standard, p16 as a surrogate marker for presence of HPV showed excellent specificity of almost 99%, an acceptable sensitivity of 72%, with both Positive and Negative Predictive Values of 93% (Table 3).

Expression of cell cycle proteins: (Fig. 3)
Strong expression of p53 was seen in overall half of cases, 86/174 (~49%), a higher proportion in the HPV-positive cases 23/36 (63.9%) compared to HPV negative cases 63/138 (45.7%). The positive cases for Cyclin D1 and pRb were 62/174 (35.6%) and 66/174 (37.9%) respectively, predominantly in HPV-negative cases: 49/62 (79%) and 51/66 (77.3%), respectively. However, none of these differences were statistically significant (Table 1).

Correlations between over-expressions of cell cycle proteins and presence of high-risk HPV infection are presented in Table 4. There was a substantial and highly significant agreement between HPV and p16 status ($p < 0.01$) and slight agreement between HPV status and p53 expression (r value 0.132). There was no agreement between HPV status and pRb expression, and

Table 3 Sensitivity and specificity between HPV DNA detection by PCR ("positive result defined as disease for statistical testing") and p16 by IHC

Point estimate		Confidence limits (95% CI)
Types	Value	Lower, upper
Sensitivity	72.22%	54.81% to 85.80%
Specificity	98.55%	94.86% to 99.82%
Positive Likelihood Ratio	49.83	12.40 to 200.21
Negative Likelihood Ratio	0.28	0.17 to 0.48
"Disease" prevalence	20.69% [a]	14.93% to 27.47%
Positive Predictive Value	92.86% [a]	76.50% to 99.12%
Negative Predictive Value	93.15% [a]	87.76% to 96.67%

[a]Does not reflect real prevalence of the "disease"

disagreement between HPV status and Cyclin D1 expression (r value − 0.005). However, there was no significant correlation between the HPV status and expressions of p53, pRb and Cyclin D1 markers (Table 4).

Among the cell cycle proteins, a significant but weak agreement (r value 0.224) was observed between p16 and p53 expression ($p < 0.01$). However, no significant interrelationship has been identified among p16, Cyclin D1 and pRb expression. There were significant correlations between p53 & Cyclin D1 ($p < 0.05$), and between p53 & pRb ($p < 0.01$) but at weak to moderate levels (r values 0.170 and 0.216, respectively) (Table 4). A significant association is also seen between Cyclin D1 and pRb proteins but at a weak level.

Discussion
Epidemiological, clinical & molecular studies indicate that high-risk HPV plays a pivotal role in the aetiopathogenesis of some HNSCCs. It is well documented that HPV-associated HNSCC are mostly seen in the oropharyngeal region due to the presence of lymphoid tissue, which makes it vulnerable to HPV infection [3]. An increasing trend of HPV-associated HNSCC, especially oropharyngeal cancer, is seen in developed countries, where tobacco and alcohol related HNSCC cases are decreasing [30]. Similar trends are not yet clear in South Asia, South East Asia or East Asia, because there are so far few data from these regions. Such studies as have been published have small sample sizes and have examined mostly cancers of the oral cavity, possibly because this is the dominant site for HNSCC, most of which are tobacco, areca nut and alcohol related [11].

Bangladesh, being the 3rd most populous country in South Asia and 8th in the world (~160 million), has the highest HNSCC incidence in the region, 21/100,000 per annum (approximately 25,000 p.a. new cases), mostly affecting males [31].The mortality rate is very high, approximately 16,500 deaths annually (15/100,000 p.a.), about half of which are from cancers of the oropharynx (~ 8500 p.a.) [31]. A survey by WHO in 2004 estimated that ~130,000 head and neck cancer patients existed in Bangladesh [32]. Although tobacco (smokeless or smoked), frequently together with areca nut, is the major risk factor, a recent study gives a reduction of tobacco use from 42.4% to 36.3% between years 2009 and 2012, [33] among those aged 15 and above; in the 40–54 year age group, this fell from 64% to 54%. Bangladesh is a rapidly "progressing" country, embracing much of the good and bad characteristics of western culture. This is associated with reductions in the use of smokeless tobacco and areca products, and increasing smoking rates. There is no published evidence to assess changes in sexual behaviours, and it has become necessary to investigate the true prevalence of HPV-associated HNSCC in the country and the wider region.

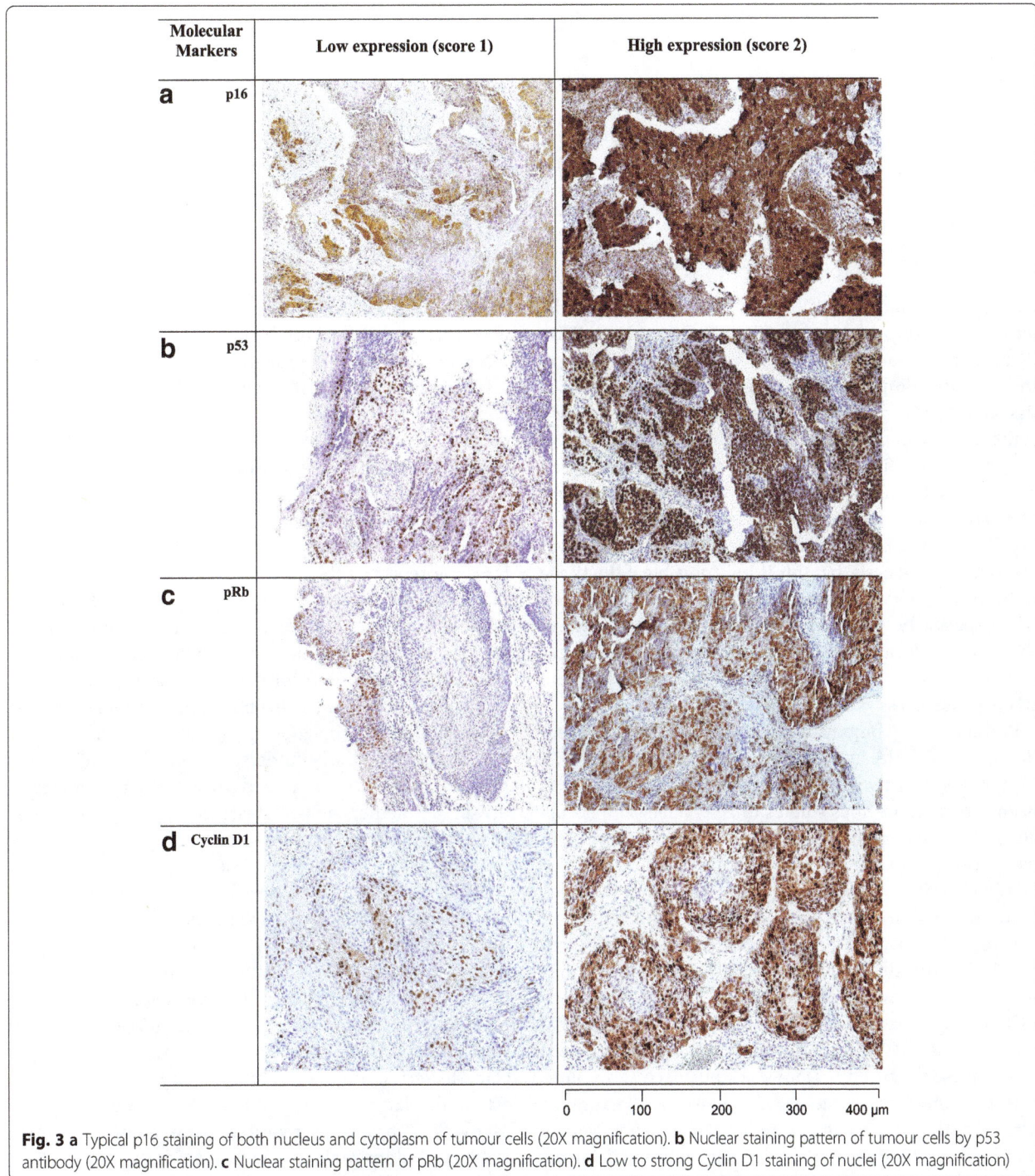

Fig. 3 a Typical p16 staining of both nucleus and cytoplasm of tumour cells (20X magnification). **b** Nuclear staining pattern of tumour cells by p53 antibody (20X magnification). **c** Nuclear staining pattern of pRb (20X magnification). **d** Low to strong Cyclin D1 staining of nuclei (20X magnification)

The reported prevalence of HPV-associated HNSCC varies widely across the world [34]. Possible reasons for this include geographical location, differences in sexual behaviours and other lifestyle factors, inclusion of mixed ethnicities and, importantly, differences in laboratory detection methods. Sensitivities of the latter are critical, so that lesions with low copy numbers of HPV may fail to be correctly ascribed. It is necessary to use a highly sensitive but controlled detection system, a well-characterised study population and site-specific tissue samples for accurate estimation of HPV prevalence in HNSCC. Although PCR-based assays, in situ hybridization (ISH) and p16 IHC are widely available, there is no consensus on the optimum technique for routine screening. Recent studies have largely used PCR, which is sensitive and cost effective [34, 35]. However, these can be too sensitive and may

Table 4 Agreement between HPV status and cell-cycle proteins in HNSCC tumours

	HPV	p16	p53	Cyclin D1	pRb
HPV	1.00				
p16	0.766**	1.00			
p53	0.132	0.224**	1.00		
Cyclin D1	- 0.005	0.01	0.177*	1.00	
pRb	- 0.001	0.077	0.222**	0.160*	1.00

**$p < 0.01$, **correlation is significant at 0.01 level (2-tailed)
*$p < 0.05$, *correlation is significant at 0.05 level (2-tailed)

amplify contaminant HPV from the laboratory environment if appropriate measures are not taken. With PCR, most laboratories use the L1 gene of HPV as the amplification target, as it is more stable in fixed tissues and its product is equivalent to whole HPV genome. It is important to realise that whatever gene is chosen for amplification, be it L1 or the E6/E7 oncogenes, positive results merely indicate the presence of the virus: they show association, not causation. Thus targeting E6/E7 mRNA is, conceptually, ideal as these are the driver genes for oncogenesis, but this is only possible if the tissue is fresh as such RNA degrades quickly over time. ISH offers specificity, particular in the sense of being able to show nuclear location, and thus presumptive viral integration, but this is time consuming, often has background staining and is less sensitive [36].

We applied a combination of nested PCR- for detection of HPV DNA and IHC for expression of p16 [37]. Combination of two sets of primers in nested PCR has been shown in previous studies to be efficient and accurate with oro-pharyngeal tissue [38–40]. The p16 protein has recently emerged as an important biomarker for HPV in HNSCC. In healthy cells, pRb (a cell cycle check point protein) normally supresses the transcription of p16 protein. However, in HPV-related cancers, pRb protein is functionally inactivated by HPV E7 protein, leading to overexpression of p16 [41, 42]. While consensus PCR is highly sensitive, without p16 IHC, the clinical relevance of HPV infection might be falsely interpreted as the presence of HPV DNA does not necessarily indicate that the virus is biologically active in the tumour [36]. On the other hand, simplicity, cost effectiveness and high sensitivity make p16 IHC attractive as a surrogate marker, even in the absence of a direct mechanistic association between HPV integration and p16 overexpression. Moreover, SCC of the oral cavity and of the larynx typically bear low numbers of transcriptionally active HPVs, suggesting that the expression of p16 at these sites may be elevated via a non-viral mechanism, leading to a false positive interpretation [43]. In spite of this, the specificity of p16, and its acceptable sensitivity, makes it a valuable tool. If there were no cost limitations, both methods would be used.

A recent study from Australia showed greater discordance than we report here between the detection of HPV DNA in HNSCC tissue samples [50/248 (20%)] and p16 IHC [61/248 (28%)] [44]. A study from the USA was discordant in the opposite direction, with 54/79 (61%) of cases HPV DNA positive by PCR but only 19/79 (24%) p16 positive [45]. The reasons for these discordances could be either the high sensitivity of nested PCR or the low sensitivity of p16 IHC (especially in the oral cavity and larynx) due to somatic alterations in chromosome 9 [46]. Moreover, subjective evaluation/lack of standardised p16 scoring criteria make comparison of different studies dangerous. Although a high cut-off point for p16 staining (> 50% tumour cells moderately or strongly stained) has been used for cervical cancer, a low cut-off point, used for cases with limited p16 staining, has the potential for over-diagnosing the involvement of HPV [47]. It is not clearly understood whether HPV DNA positive cancers with limited p16 positivity are HPV-driven or whether the p16 is silenced by mutations or by DNA methylation of promoter regions, as has been reported in cervical cancers [48].

The overall worldwide prevalence of HPV in HNSCC averages approximately 30% with wide variation depending on geographical location and tumour sites [34]. Few studies from South Asia have been published; the majority of them from India, and these suggest an overall prevalence of approximately 37% [11]. We found 21% of total HNSCC cases positive for HPV DNA in this Bangladeshi series, highest in the oropharynx (~ 37%), lowest in the larynx (~ 12.5 %). High prevalence in oral cavity SCC has been reported from South East Asia (~48%), Eastern Asia (~43%) and South Asia (~38%) [11]; whereas our study shows slightly lower HPV frequencies in OCSCC (~20%). In oropharyngeal cancer, our study shows the prevalence of HPV to be higher compared to a recent Indian study, where the proportion was approximately 23% [49].Our findings for laryngeal cancer (~ 12.5%) are lower than the overall HPV-positive laryngeal cancer prevalence so far reported in the Asia-Pacific region (23.6%) [11] .

To our knowledge, there is only one published study from Bangladesh describing the prevalence of HPV in

HNSCC, using conventional PCR methods. This had a small sample size ($n = 34$), included samples only from the oral cavity and found just 3% of HPV positive cases [50]. Possible reasons for this discordance could be a less sensitive detection method or samples having poor DNA quality: it was also published several years ago, and the prevalence may well be rising nowadays in Bangladesh, as elsewhere in the world.

HPV16 is the most commonly detected HPV type, being present in 90% of cases of HPV-positive HNSCCs worldwide [51]. Our data are similar: 33 out of 36 (~92%) were HPV16 and all were single HPV infections. Similar findings are reported from North America, Europe and the Asia-Pacific [11, 34]. This is likely to be related to social norms, as a relatively high proportion of men in western countries tend to have multiple sexual – including the practice of oral sex – partners [52]. Our data show the prevalence of HPV to be inversely correlated with age, a significantly higher prevalence being seen in those less than 60 yrs. old (mean age 54.2), compared with older patients ($p = 0.025$). This accords with the mean age reported from Australia (55.2 years), North America (58 years) and Europe (< 60 years), although the mean age of our Bangladeshi HPV-positive HNSCC patients was slightly higher than reported from other South Asian countries (52.8 years), especially India [6, 11].

In our study, HPV-positive cases tended to have high expression of p16, an association which was statistically significant: however, our HPV-positive cases had low to moderate expression of Cyclin D1, pRb and p53 proteins, none of which were statistically significant. The negative correlation between HPV status and Cyclin D & pRb perhaps indicates that malignancy may not need both aberrant Cyclin D1 and pRb pathways. Our findings in this respect match previously reported studies from China, India and Australia [44, 53, 54].

Several recent studies have demonstrated the prognostic value of cell cycle markers in HPV-positive HNSCC patients. A recent cohort study suggests that high p16 expression is correlated with better survival: p16 positive and HPV-positive cases had a 2 year disease free survival of 86.2%, (95% CI 79–91.1) compared to p16 negative and HPV–negative cases of only 44.2%, (CI 30.2–58.1) [55]. Some studies have suggested that high expressions of p53, Cyclin D1 or pRb also relate to poor prognosis. For example a study from Sweden suggests that patients with HPV + ve DNA and low/absent p53 had a 5-year survival of 88.2% compared to 33.3% for HPV + ve cases with high p53 expression. Patients with HPV-negative and low/absent p53 had a better survival than HPV-negative but high p53 cases (52.6% vs 9.1%) [56].

A comprehensive study of 226 patients from Australia suggests a strong association between HPV positivity and downregulation or absent expression of Cyclin D1.In an HPV-positive tumour group, Cyclin D1-positive cancers had 8 fold-increased risk of poor prognosis compared to Cyclin D1-negative cancers with 3.3 years overall survival. However, the effect of Cyclin D1 was small in HPV-negative HNSCC [57]. A strong inverse relationship between pRb and p16 expressions has also been reported: cases with low pRb and high p16 expression had better survival [58].

There are several limitations to the present study. We have a modest cohort size, with small numbers in some anatomical subsites. Use of FFPE archival samples resulted in poor quality of DNA in some samples, which had to be excluded. Nevertheless, most amplified the L1 target satisfactorily. Expression of E6/E7 mRNA could not be explored in FFPE tissues, as fresh or frozen tissues were not available. We also have limited information on tobacco, areca nut and alcohol habits, and on the sexual lives of our cases. Most importantly no treatment and patient outcome information was available to us.

This is the first comprehensive study from Bangladesh and one of the first studies from South Asia to use a combination of detection methods for HPV and their interrelationship with cell cycle markers of putative prognostic value. Nevertheless our cases were derived from a single pathology laboratory, which may limit generalizability. However, this is the largest public laboratory in the nation and receives a wide range of patients and tissue samples from all corners of Bangladesh.

Conclusion

Our data show that HPV is associated with, and probably responsible for ~21% of HNSCC in Bangladesh. Because it is now well known that such cases respond comparatively well to treatment, routine assessment of HPV status in HNSCC should be mandated. We strongly recommend the use of ICD-10 for proper site-specific classification of cases. We urge the Bangladesh Government to mandate Tumour Boards and perform longitudinal studies on HNC to confirm the importance of HPV in treatment planning. We recommend the use of both p16 IHC and PCR-based detection of virus, though p16 alone is a useful surrogate marker. Routine use of IHC for the status of p53, pRb and cyclin D1, does not seem to be indicated.

Abbreviations
FFPE: Formalin fixed paraffin embedded; HNC : Head and neck cancer; HNSCC: Head and neck squamous cell carcinoma; HPV: Human papillomavirus; IARC: International Agency for Research on Cancer; ICD –10: International Classification of Disease Version 10; IHC: Immunohistochemistry; OCSCC: Oral cavity squamous cell carcinoma; OPSCC: Oropharyngeal squamous cell carcinoma; PCR: Polymerase chain reaction

Acknowledgements
Special thanks to Mr. Chris Philippa (Gold Coast University Hospital, Australia) for kind assistance with the p16 immunohistochemistry. Thanks to Dr. Helen Rogers, Mrs. Wendy Kelly and Sura Fallaha for assistance with histology.

Funding
MHS was funded by a Griffith University International Scholarship. The project had no specific funding.

Authors' contributions
The study was initiated by NWJ and MHS. AIK, AS, SAJ and AHC provided the tissue samples and case data. MHS designed the experimental protocols and performed all laboratory procedures. Histopathological interpretation and histochemical scoring were performed by AL and VG. NAJM, NWJ and DTWC advised on laboratory methods and data interpretation. MHS performed statistical analyses and wrote the first draft of the manuscript, which was revised and agreed by all authors.

Competing interests
The authors declare that they have no competing interests.

Author details
[1]School of Dentistry and Oral Health, Griffith University, Gold Coast, QLD 4222, Australia. [2]School of Medical Science, Griffith University, Gold Coast, QLD 4222, Australia. [3]Understanding Chronic Conditions Program, Menzies Health Institute Queensland, Gold Coast, QLD 4222, Australia. [4]Department of Pathology, National Medical College and Hospital, Dhaka 1100, Bangladesh. [5]Department of Oral and Maxillo-facial Surgery, Dhaka Dental College & Hospital, Dhaka 1216, Bangladesh. [6]Department of Neuro-medicine, Dhaka Medical College and Hospital, Dhaka 1000, Bangladesh. [7]Department of Pathology, Dhaka Medical College and Hospital, Dhaka 1000, Bangladesh. [8]School of Medicine, Griffith University, Gold Coast, QLD 4222, Australia. [9]Dental Institute, King's College London, London, UK. [10]Menzies Health Institute Queensland and School of Dentistry and Oral Health, Griffith University, Building G40, Room 9.16, Gold Coast Campus, Gold Coast, QLD 4222, Australia.

References
1. Ferlay J, Soerjomataram I, Dikshit R, Eser S, Mathers C, Rebelo M, Parkin DM, Forman D, Bray F. Cancer incidence and mortality worldwide: sources, methods and major patterns in GLOBOCAN 2012. Int J Cancer. 2015;136(5):E359–86.
2. Gillison ML, Shah KV. Human papillomavirus-associated head and neck squamous cell carcinoma: mounting evidence for an etiologic role for human papillomavirus in a subset of head and neck cancers. Curr Opin Oncol. 2001;13(3):183–8.
3. Rautava J, Syrjanen S. Biology of human papillomavirus infections in head and neck carcinogenesis. Head neck pathol. 2012;6(Suppl 1):S3–15.
4. Dalianis T. Human papillomavirus (HPV) and oropharyngeal squamous cell carcinoma. Presse Med. 2014;43(12 Pt 2):e429–34.
5. IARC Working group on the Evaluation of Carcinogenic risks to humans. Biological agents. Volume 100 B. A review of human carcinogens. IARC Monogr Eval Carcinog Risks Hum. 2012;100(Pt B):1–441.
6. Gillison ML, Chaturvedi AK, Anderson WF, Fakhry C. Epidemiology of human Papillomavirus-positive head and neck Squamous cell carcinoma. J Clin Oncol. 2015;33(29):3235–42.
7. D'Souza G, Agrawal Y, Halpern J, Bodison S, Gillison ML. Oral sexual behaviors associated with prevalent oral human papillomavirus infection. J Infect Dis. 2009;199(9):1263–9.
8. Schwartz SM, Daling JR, Doody DR, Wipf GC, Carter JJ, Madeleine MM, Mao EJ, Fitzgibbons ED, Huang S, Beckmann AM, et al. Oral cancer risk in relation to sexual history and evidence of human papillomavirus infection. J Natl Cancer Inst. 1998;90(21):1626–36.
9. Ang KK, Harris J, Wheeler R, Weber R, Rosenthal DI, Nguyen-Tan PF, Westra WH, Chung CH, Jordan RC, Lu C, et al. Human papillomavirus and survival of patients with oropharyngeal cancer. N Engl J Med. 2010;363(1):24 35.
10. Bonilla-Velez J, Mroz EA, Hammon RJ, Rocco JW. Impact of human papillomavirus on oropharyngeal cancer biology and response to therapy: implications for treatment. Otolaryngol Clin N Am. 2013;46(4):521–43.
11. Shaikh MH, McMillan NA, Johnson NW. HPV-associated head and neck cancers in the Asia Pacific: a critical literature review & meta-analysis. Cancer Epidemiol. 2015;39(6):923–38.
12. Stein AP, Saha S, Kraninger JL, Swick AD, Yu M, Lambert PF, Kimple RJ. Prevalence of human Papillomavirus in Oropharyngeal cancer: a systematic review. Cancer J. 2015;21(3):138–46.
13. Hong A, Lee CS, Jones D, Veillard AS, Zhang M, Zhang X, Smee R, Corry J, Porceddu S, Milross C, et al. Rising prevalence of human papillomavirus-related oropharyngeal cancer in Australia over the last 2 decades. Head & neck. 2016;38(5):743–50.
14. Badwe RA, Dikshit R, Laversanne M, Bray F. Cancer incidence trends in India. Jpn J Clin Oncol. 2014;44(5):401–7.
15. Hussain SM. Comprehensive update on cancer scenario of Bangladesh. South Asian J Cancer. 2013;2(4):279–84.
16. Boyer SN, Wazer DE, Band V. E7 protein of human papilloma virus-16 induces degradation of retinoblastoma protein through the ubiquitin-proteasome pathway. Cancer Res. 1996;56(20):4620–4.
17. Bates S, Parry D, Bonetta L, Vousden K, Dickson C, Peters G. Absence of cyclin D/cdk complexes in cells lacking functional retinoblastoma protein. Oncogene. 1994;9(6):1633–40.
18. Scheffner M, Werness BA, Huibregtse JM, Levine AJ, Howley PM. The E6 oncoprotein encoded by human papillomavirus types 16 and 18 promotes the degradation of p53. Cell. 1990;63(6):1129–36.
19. de Roda Husman AM, Walboomers JM, van den Brule AJ, Meijer CJ, Snijders PJ. The use of general primers GP5 and GP6 elongated at their 3' ends with adjacent highly conserved sequences improves human papillomavirus detection by PCR. J Gen Virol. 1995;76(Pt 4):1057–62.
20. Depuydt CE, Boulet GA, Horvath CA, Benoy IH, Vereecken AJ, Bogers JJ. Comparison of MY09/11 consensus PCR and type-specific PCRs in the detection of oncogenic HPV types. J Cell Mol Med. 2007;11(4):881–91.
21. Gravitt PE, Peyton CL, Alessi TQ, Wheeler CM, Coutlee F, Hildesheim A, Schiffman MH, Scott DR, Apple RJ. Improved amplification of genital human papillomaviruses. J Clin Microbiol. 2000;38(1):357–61.
22. WHO: IARC WHO classification of Tumours, vol. 9, 3rd edn. WHO Publications center, NY, USA.: WHO; 2005.
23. Lewis JS Jr. p16 Immunohistochemistry as a standalone test for risk stratification in oropharyngeal squamous cell carcinoma. Head Neck Pathol. 2012;6(Suppl 1):S75–82.
24. Liu SZ, Zandberg DP, Schumaker LM, Papadimitriou JC, Cullen KJ. Correlation of p16 expression and HPV type with survival in oropharyngeal squamous cell cancer. Oral Oncol. 2015;51(9):862–9.
25. Shiraki M, Odajima T, Ikeda T, Sasaki A, Satoh M, Yamaguchi A, Noguchi M, Nagai I, Hiratsuka H. Combined expression of p53, cyclin D1 and epidermal growth factor receptor improves estimation of prognosis in curatively resected oral cancer. Mod Pathol. 2005;18(11):1482–9.
26. Rodriguez-Pinilla M, Rodriguez-Peralto JL, Hitt R, Sanchez JJ, Ballestin C, Diez A, Sanchez-Verde L, Alameda F, Sanchez-Cespedes M. Cyclin a as a predictive factor for chemotherapy response in advanced head and neck cancer. Clin Cancer Res. 2004;10(24):8486–92.
27. Shin DM, Lee JS, Lippman SM, Lee JJ, Tu ZN, Choi G, Heyne K, Shin HJ, Ro JY, Goepfert H, et al. p53 expressions: predicting recurrence and second primary tumors in head and neck squamous cell carcinoma. J Natl Cancer Inst. 1996; 88(8):519–29.
28. Gardner IA, Greiner M. Receiver-operating characteristic curves and likelihood ratios: improvements over traditional methods for the evaluation and application of veterinary clinical pathology tests. Vet Clin Pathol. 2006;35(1):8–17.
29. Altman DGMD, Bryant TN, Gardner MJ. Statistics with confidence, vol. 2nd: BMJ Books. New Jersey: Wiley; 2000.
30. Chaturvedi AK, Anderson WF, Lortet-Tieulent J, Curado MP, Ferlay J, Franceschi S, Rosenberg PS, Bray F, Gillison ML. Worldwide trends in incidence rates for oral cavity and oropharyngeal cancers. J Clin Oncol. 2013;31(36):4550–9.
31. Ferlay JSI, Ervik M, Dikshit R, Eser S, Mathers C, Rebelo M, Parkin DM, Forman D, Bray F. Cancer incidence and mortality worldwide : IARC CancerBase no. 11. In: GLOBOCAN 2012. vol. 1.0. IARC, Lyon, France: International Agency for Research on Cancer (IARC); 2013.

32. Hussain SA, Sullivan R. Cancer control in Bangladesh. Jpn J Clin Oncol. 2013; 43(12):1159–69.

33. Nargis N, Thompson ME, Fong GT, Driezen P, Hussain AK, Ruthbah UH, Quah AC, Abdullah AS. Prevalence and patterns of tobacco use in Bangladesh from 2009 to 2012: evidence from international tobacco control (ITC) study. PLoS One. 2015;10(11):e0141135.

34. Ndiaye C, Mena M, Alemany L, Arbyn M, Castellsague X, Laporte L, Bosch FX, de Sanjose S, Trottier H. HPV DNA, E6/E7 mRNlA, and p16INK4a detection in head and neck cancers: a systematic review and meta-analysis. Lancet Oncol. 2014;15(12):1319–31.

35. Venuti A, Paolini F. HPV detection methods in head and neck cancer. Head Neck Pathol. 2012;6(Suppl 1):S63–74.

36. Smeets SJ, Hesselink AT, Speel EJ, Haesevoets A, Snijders PJ, Pawlita M, Meijer CJ, Braakhuis BJ, Leemans CR, Brakenhoff RH. A novel algorithm for reliable detection of human papillomavirus in paraffin embedded head and neck cancer specimen. Int J Cancer. 2007;121(11):2465–72.

37. Braakhuis BJ, Brakenhoff RH, Meijer CJ, Snijders PJ, Leemans CR. Human papilloma virus in head and neck cancer: the need for a standardised assay to assess the full clinical importance. Eur J Cancer. 2009;45(17):2935–9.

38. Winder DM, Ball SL, Vaughan K, Hanna N, Woo YL, Franzer JT, Sterling JC, Stanley MA, Sudhoff H, Goon PK. Sensitive HPV detection in oropharyngeal cancers. BMC Cancer. 2009;9:440.

39. Fuessel Haws AL, He Q, Rady PL, Zhang L, Grady J, Hughes TK, Stisser K, Konig R, Tyring SK. Nested PCR with the PGMY09/11 and GP5(+)/6(+) primer sets improves detection of HPV DNA in cervical samples. J Virol Methods. 2004;122(1):87–93.

40. Syrjanen S. The role of human papillomavirus infection in head and neck cancers. Ann Oncol. 2010;21(Suppl 7):vii243–5.

41. Klussmann JP, Gultekin E, Weissenborn SJ, Wieland U, Dries V, Dienes HP, Eckel HE, Pfister HJ, Fuchs PG. Expression of p16 protein identifies a distinct entity of tonsillar carcinomas associated with human papillomavirus. Am J Pathol. 2003;162(3):747–53.

42. Adelstein DJ, Ridge JA, Gillison ML, Chaturvedi AK, D'Souza G, Gravitt PE, Westra W, Psyrri A, Kast WM, Koutsky LA, et al. Head and neck squamous cell cancer and the human papillomavirus: summary of a National Cancer Institute state of the science meeting, November 9-10, 2008, Washington DC. Head Neck. 2009;31(11):1393–422.

43. Bishop JA, Ma XJ, Wang H, Luo Y, Illei PB, Begum S, Taube JM, Koch WM, Westra WH. Detection of transcriptionally active high-risk HPV in patients with head and neck squamous cell carcinoma as visualized by a novel E6/E7 mRNA in situ hybridization method. Am J Surg Pathol. 2012;36(12):1874–82.

44. Antonsson A, Neale RE, Boros S, Lampe G, Coman WB, Pryor DI, Porceddu SV, Whiteman DC. Human papillomavirus status and p16(INK4A) expression in patients with mucosal squamous cell carcinoma of the head and neck in Queensland, Australia. Cancer Epidemiol. 2015;39(2):174–81.

45. Weinberger PM, Yu Z, Haffty BG, Kowalski D, Harigopal M, Brandsma J, Sasaki C, Joe J, Camp RL, Rimm DL, et al. Molecular classification identifies a subset of human papillomavirus–associated oropharyngeal cancers with favorable prognosis. J Clin Oncol. 2006;24(5):736–47.

46. Combes JD, Franceschi S. Role of human papillomavirus in non-oropharyngeal head and neck cancers. Oral Oncol. 2014;50(5):370–9.

47. Sano T, Oyama T, Kashiwabara K, Fukuda T, Nakajima T. Expression status of p16 protein is associated with human papillomavirus oncogenic potential in cervical and genital lesions. Am J Pathol. 1998;153(6):1741–8.

48. Nuovo GJ, Plaia TW, Belinsky SA, Baylin SB, Herman JG. In situ detection of the hypermethylation-induced inactivation of the p16 gene as an early event in oncogenesis. Proc Natl Acad Sci U S A. 1999;96(22):12754–9.

49. Bahl A, Kumar P, Dar L, Mohanti BK, Sharma A, Thakar A, Karthikeyan V, Sikka K, Singh C, Poo K, et al. Prevalence and trends of human papillomavirus in oropharyngeal cancer in a predominantly north Indian population. Head Neck. 2014;36(4):505–10.

50. Akhter M, Ali L, Hassan Z, Khan I. Association of human papilloma virus infection and oral squamous cell carcinoma in Bangladesh. J Health Popul Nutr. 2013;31(1):65–9.

51. Kreimer AR, Bhatia RK, Messeguer AL, Gonzalez P, Herrero R, Giuliano AR. Oral human papillomavirus in healthy individuals: a systematic review of the literature. Sex Transm Dis. 2010;37(6):386–91.

52. D'Souza G, Gross ND, Pai SI, Haddad R, Anderson KS, Rajan S, Gerber J, Gillison ML, Posner MR. Oral human papillomavirus (HPV) infection in HPV-positive patients with oropharyngeal cancer and their partners. J Clin Oncol. 2014;32(23):2408–15.

53. Ma XL, Ueno K, Pan ZM, Hi SZ, Ohyama M, Eizuru Y. Human papillomavirus DNA sequences and p53 over-expression in laryngeal squamous cell carcinomas in Northeast China. J Med Virol. 1998;54(3):186–91.

54. Mitra S, Banerjee S, Misra C, Singh RK, Roy A, Sengupta A, Panda CK, Roychoudhury S. Interplay between human papilloma virus infection and p53 gene alterations in head and neck squamous cell carcinoma of an Indian patient population. J Clin Pathol. 2007;60(9):1040–7.

55. Lewis JS Jr, Thorstad WL, Chernock RD, Haughey BH, Yip JH, Zhang Q, El-Mofty SK. p16 positive oropharyngeal squamous cell carcinoma:an entity with a favorable prognosis regardless of tumor HPV status. Am J Surg Pathol. 2010;34(8):1088–96.

56. Sivars L, Nasman A, Tertipis N, Vlastos A, Ramqvist T, Dalianis T, Munck-Wikland E, Nordemar S. Human papillomavirus and p53 expression in cancer of unknown primary in the head and neck region in relation to clinical outcome. Cancer Med. 2014;3(2):376–84.

57. Hong AM, Dobbins TA, Lee CS, Jones D, Fei J, Clark JR, Armstrong BK, Harnett GB, Milross CG, Tran N, et al. Use of cyclin D1 in conjunction with human papillomavirus status to predict outcome in oropharyngeal cancer. Int J Cancer. 2011;128(7):1532–45.

58. Holzinger D, Flechtenmacher C, Henfling N, Kaden I, Grabe N, Lahrmann B, Schmitt M, Hess J, Pawlita M, Bosch FX. Identification of oropharyngeal squamous cell carcinomas with active HPV16 involvement by immunohistochemical analysis of the retinoblastoma protein pathway. Int J Cancer. 2013;133(6):1389–99.

5

Diagnostic accuracy of ^{18}F–FDG PET/CT and MR imaging in patients with adenoid cystic carcinoma

Verena Ruhlmann[1]* , Thorsten D. Poeppel[1], Johannes Veit[2], James Nagarajah[3], Lale Umutlu[4], Thomas K. Hoffmann[2], Andreas Bockisch[1], Ken Herrmann[1] and Wolfgang Sauerwein[5]

Abstract

Background: The aim of this study was to evaluate the value of 18F–FDG PET/CT (PET/CT) and MRI for local and/or whole-body restaging of adenoid cystic carcinoma of the head and neck (ACC).

Methods: Thirty-six patients with ACC underwent conventional MRI of the head and neck and a whole-body PET/CT and were analysed with regards to detection of a local tumor recurrence, lymph node or distant metastases. A consensus interpretation of all available imaging data was used as reference standard. Sensitivity, specificity, diagnostic accuracy, positive and negative predictive values were calculated for MRI and PET/CT.

Results: The sensitivity of PET/CT and MRI was 96% (89%), specificity 89% (89%), PPV 96% (96%), NPV 89% (73%) and accuracy 94% (89%) for detection of local tumors. Additionally, PET/CT revealed lymph node metastases in one patient and distant metastases in 9/36 patients. In three patients secondary primaries were found.

Conclusions: Whole-body PET/CT in addition to MRI of the head and neck improves detection of local tumour and metastastic spread in ACC.

Keywords: PET/CT, MRI, Adenoid cystic carcinoma

Background

Adenoid cystic carcinoma (ACC) is a rare type of cancer mainly located within secretory glands, most commonly the minor but also the major salivary glands of the head and neck [1]. Each year, about 1200 people are diagnosed with ACC in the United States. ACC is a (generally) well-differentiated and slowly growing tumour with a relatively indolent but relentless course. The tumour is characterised by a marked tendency for perineural invasion with the risk of incomplete resection and (late) local and distant recurrences [2–4].

Due to the tendency of this tumour to spread along nerve tracts, the complete radical resection of the primary tumour as the main therapeutic approach is very challenging and results in frequent local recurrences. Adjuvant

radiotherapy is commonly applied after surgery and leads to improved local control. Furthermore, in some cases, surgery is not feasible to tumour location, therefore primary radiation (e.g. using high linear energy transfer (LET) beams (fast neutrons or carbon ions) [5–7] is the only treatment option. Chemotherapy has only limited effects in trials so far [8–10]. Sub-cellular and genetic characteristics of the ACC can be used for targeted systemic therapy efforts and have in part already been considered in clinical trials [11]. Hence, so far no breakthrough has been achieved in systemic therapy for this entity.

In contrast to 10- to 20-year survival rates (about 40% at 15 years), 5-year survival rates in patients with ACC are high with around 89% [12, 13], reflecting a prolonged course of metastatic disease and late local recurrences. Another specific feature of ACC is the relatively rare occurrence of regional lymph nodes metastases although micro metastases might be detected in a relevant number of patients if neck dissection is performed [14]. Even after

---
* Correspondence: verena.ruhlmann@uk-essen.de; verena@ruhlmann.de
[1]Department of Nuclear Medicine, University Duisburg-Essen, Medical Faculty, University Hospital Essen, Hufelandstrasse 55, 45147 Essen, Germany
Full list of author information is available at the end of the article

successful local therapy distant metastases often occur metachronously in lung and sometimes in the liver and limit long-term prognosis. According to the existing literature, distant metastases in ACC are rare at initial diagnosis and depend on disease duration and primary site, although some authors state that current diagnostic means might not be sensitive enough to detect them [15, 16].

Due to the diffuse growth pattern the detection of local recurrence, especially differentiation between scar formation, radiation effects and vital tumour is limited and routine imaging techniques (computed tomography (CT), magnetic resonance imaging (MRI) and ultrasound (US)) suffer from low specificity [17–19]. Thus, in case of suspected recurrence it is anticipated that metabolic information provided by ^{18}F–fluorodeoxyglucose (FDG) positron emission tomography (PET) could improve the distinction between benign and malignant lesions [17, 20, 21]. Published reports on FDG uptake in ACC are rare [22–25], and many of these are only case series with a small number of patients. The existing literature hints that most squamous cell carcinomas are intensely FDG avid, whereas adenoid cystic carcinoma and mucoepidermoid carcinoma show variable uptake depending on the grade of differentiation [26]. In a recently published study by Kim et al. [27] the pretreatment SUVmax of FDG-PET was as a predictor of distant metastasis in ACC of the head and neck.

In this study we evaluate the diagnostic accuracy of FDG PET/CT and MRI for restaging ACC patients in a relatively large population with particular focus on local and whole-body staging.

Materials and methods
Patient population
Imaging data of 36 consecutive patients (19 females, 17 males, mean age 57 ± 12 years) suffering from ACC of the head and neck (histologically confirmed initial localisations: salivary glands (parotid and submandibular gland; $n = 18$), small salivary glands: oropharynx ($n = 7$), trachea ($n = 2$), paranasal sinus ($n = 4$), eye socket ($n = 2$) and upper jaw ($n = 3$)) were retrospectively analysed. The diagnostic imaging procedures were performed within the context of routine clinical procedures within a short time interval in the case of restaging of ACC when suspecting recurrences ($n = 16$) or approximately two months after local tumour resection prior to adjuvant radiation therapy ($n = 20$). Therefore, ethics approval was waived.

MRI studies
All patients underwent a conventional MRI of the head and neck. MRI was performed in a whole-body 1.5 Tesla MR scanner using the following sequence protocol:

1. A T1-weighted Spin Echo (T1 SE) in coronal slice orientation (time of repetition (TR) 425 ms, echo time TE) 15 ms, slice thickness 5 mm, matrix size 512, field of view (FOV) 280).
2. An axial T1-weighted SE (TR 455 ms, TE 11 ms, slice thickness 5 mm, matrix size 512, FOV 230).
3. An axial T2-weighted SE (TR 3900 ms, TE 87 ms, slice thickness 5 mm, matrix size 512, FOV 260).
4. An axial post contrast T1-weighted SE with fat saturation (TR 474 ms, TE 11 ms, slice thickness 5 mm, matrix size 512, FOV 230) after i.v. administration of 0.1 mmol/kg body weight of gadobutrol (Gadovist, Bayer Healthcare, Leverkusen, Germany).
5. A coronal post-contrast T1-weighted SE TR (TR 710 ms, TE 15 ms, slice thickness 5 mm, matrix size 512, FOV 280).

PET/CT studies
Dedicated head and neck and whole-body FDG PET/CT scans were performed using a Biograph mCT™ (Siemens AG, Healthcare Sector, Erlangen, Germany). The head and neck scan was performed 60 ± 5 min after tracer injection (weight-dependent FDG dose, mean activity 290 ± 45 MBq) and 40 s after intravenous contrast agent injection (60 ml Ultravist®; Bayer Healthcare Deutschland, Leverkusen, Germany) from the skull base to the aortic arch (slice thickness 3 mm). To minimize artefacts, the patient's arms were placed beside the body. Afterwards, the patients were encouraged to place the arms over their head for the following whole-body examination. The scan ranged from the upper thorax to the thighs and was performed 70 s after injection of an additional dose of 70 ml contrast agent (slice thickness 5 mm). In both protocols, the manufacturer-supplied dose reduction techniques CareDose 4D™and CareKV™ were used (presets 210 mAs, 120 kV; Siemens AG). Blood glucose was below 150 mg/dl at the time of tracer injection. PET data were acquired for 4 min per bed position in the head and neck area and for 2 min per bed position in the rest of the body. For reconstruction, attenuation weighted ordered-subsets expectation maximization (AW-OSEM) iterative algorithm with 4 iterations and 8 subsets, Gaussian filter with 4.0 mm full width at half maximum (FWHM) and scatter correction were used.

Immediately after the PET scan a thoracic full-dose CT scan was performed in the forced inspiratory position with the following parameters: 120 kV, automatic mA/s adjustment (Care Dose 4D™, preset: 70 mAs), 5-mm slice thickness; reconstruction in lung window.

Image analysis
Board certified physicians in nuclear medicine and radiology visually interpreted the PET/CT and MRI data,

being blinded to the results of the other imaging examinations. The presence of residual/recurrent tumours, number of regional lymph node metastases and distant metastases were counted separately in both CT and MRI.

On MR images, a lesion in a suspected site of tumour with a hypo- to isotense signal in the T1-weighted image, a slightly to markedly hyperintense signal in the T2-weighted image and an enhancement in the contrast-enhanced T1-weighted image was considered as malignant. On CT and MR images, increased short-axis diameter (>10 mm), central necrosis, irregular shape and the lack of a fatty hilus sign and increased contrast agent uptake were considered as signs of malignancy in lymph nodes.

On the hybrid images (PET/CT), central necrosis, focal soft tissue increase and focal FDG-uptake were considered as indicators of malignancy in local cancer recurrence. In a PET-specific semi-quantitative approach, the maximum standardized uptake values (SUVmax) of all tumour lesions/suspected sites of metastasis or focally increased tracer uptake visually defined above the mediastinal blood pool were determined by drawing spherical volumes of interest (VOI) that closely encircled a lesion.

Reference standard

A consensus interpretation of all available imaging data (prior examinations and follow-up examinations (median 12, range 3–105 months): MRI of the head and neck, thoracic CT, whole-body-PET/CT, ultrasound) adopted by all readers was used as reference standard.

Statistical analysis

Sensitivity, specificity, positive predictive value (PPV), negative predictive value (NPV) and diagnostic accuracy were calculated for MRI, PET, CT and PET/CT using Microsoft Excel (15.29.1).

Results

Recurrent or residual tumour

A recurrent or residual tumour was present in 27 of the 36 patients according to the reference standard. MRI detected 24 of 27 tumour lesions. In the remaining three cases with tumour recurrence the MRI findings were indistinct (an illustrative example is given in Fig. 1). MRI was negative in 8 of 9 the patients without signs of tumour and indistinct in one patient (Fig. 2). Thus, the sensitivity was 89%, specificity 89%, PPV 96%, NPV 73% and accuracy 89%.

PET/CT detected 26 of 27 tumour lesions with increased FDG uptake (Fig. 3). One patient did not show any pathologically increased tracer uptake in the tumour lesion (in the former parotid gland area with penetration of the base of the skull, the mastoid and neurocranium) that was only detected on MRI (Fig. 4). Mean SUVmax across all lesions was 6.8 ± 3.4 (median 5.7, range 2.0–15.0). PET/CT was negative in 8 of 9 patients without a tumour. PET/CT was false-positive in one patient (Fig. 5). Thus, the corresponding sensitivity was 96%, specificity 89% and accuracy 94%. PPV and NPV calculated to 96% and 89%, respectively.

Lymph node metastases

In one patient, regional cervical lymph node metastases were dectected in accordance with the reference standard. On the PET component this patient with the primary tumour in the right parotid gland presented increased FDG uptake (SUVmax 6.0), whereas the the lymph node was according to CT and MRI size criteria not suspicious.

Distant metastases

PET/CT detected distant metastases in 9 out of 36 patients with manifestations in the lung ($n = 8$), bone ($n = 5$), adrenal gland ($n = 1$), kidney ($n = 1$), and liver ($n = 1$), as well as distant lymph node metastases ($n = 1$) in the mediastinum (primary localisation in the submandibular

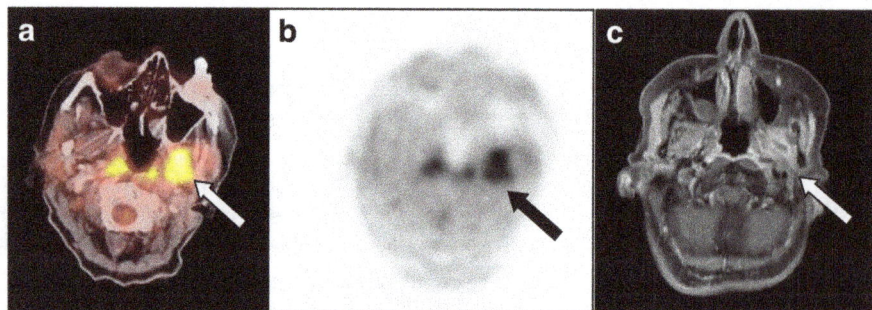

Fig. 1 ACC recurrence: PET/CT imaging was true-positive, indistinctive finding on MRI. Patient after resection of an adenoid cystic carcinoma in the left parotid gland and after combined neutron/proton therapy. Recurrence is seen on the fused PET/CT (**a**) and PET image (**b**) with a focally increased FDG-uptake (arrow), but not on the contrast-enhanced T1-weighted MR image (**c**). In MRI, the finding was evaluated as radiation necrosis

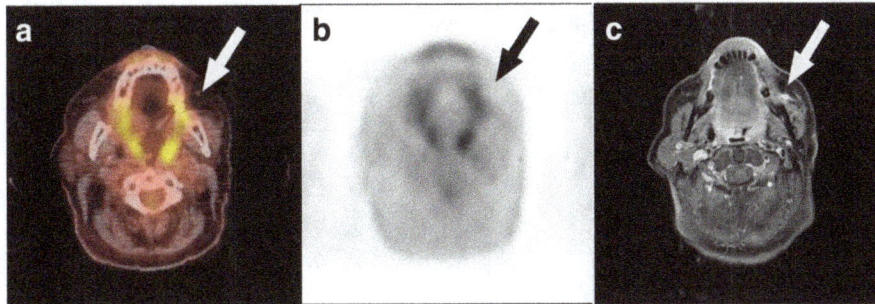

Fig. 2 No tumour recurrence: PET/CT imaging was true-negative, indistinctive finding on MRI. Patient after multiple resections of recurrent tumours of a left buccal adenoid cystic carcinoma. A hyperintense lesion is seen on the contrast-enhanced T1-weighted MR image (**c**) (arrow), but there was no pathological finding on the fused PET/CT (**a**) and PET image (**b**). The follow-up confirmed no recurrence

gland). Corresponding mean SUVmax was 3.9 ± 2.3 (median 3.8, range 1.2–9.9). Four patients presented lung metastases that were not known at time of first diagnosis but discriminated by PET/CT after local tumour resection prior to adjuvant radiation therapy.

In all patients with distant metastases, the lesions could be defined as malignant on combined PET/CT. In case of lung metastases the CT was indistinctive in 2 patients (differential diagnosis: granuloma), but the PET component helped the lesion characterization as malignant. In two cases with disseminated lung metastases, the smallest malignant lesions could only be detected on CT.

All patients with distant metastases had no synchronical regional lymph node metastases, and 4/9 patients had no local recurrence.

In addition to the main diagnosis a secondary primary carcinoma was found in three patients. In these cases with histopathologically confirmed cervical carcinoma, prostate carcinoma and breast cancer preferential treatment was conducted.

Discussion

This study demonstrates the high sensitivity of whole-body FDG PET/CT in detecting both recurrent/residual tumours and regional metastatic spread in patients with ACC. FDG PET/CT also outperformed head neck MRI for local staging and restaging. Moreover, the whole body imaging approach enables the detection of distant metastases even at an early stage and in the follow up.

Local tumours were present in 75% of the patients in our study population. Of these, 63% had residual tumours, and 37% had tumour recurrence. The detection rate of a residual or recurrent tumour on PET/CT was highly accurate with only one false-negative and one false-positive finding. PET/CT was only false-negative in one patient with tumour recurrence in the head and neck area. PET/CT was false-positive in only one case in the head and neck area, possibly due to a physiological hyperfunctional pharyngeal reaction and perfusion after contralateral resection of the primary tumour. MRI had four indistinct findings in the former local tumour region. The diagnostic performance of PET/CT was

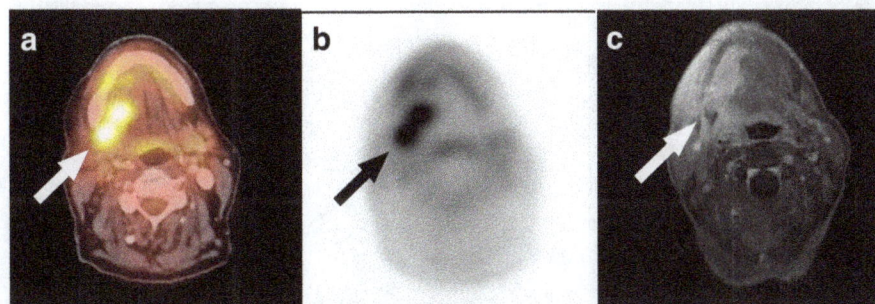

Fig. 3 ACC tumour remaining: PET/CT and MR imaging was true-positive. Patient after resection of an adenoid cystic carcinoma, now with a tumour remnant on the right root of the tongue prior to neutron therapy. The tumour mass is seen on the fused PET/CT (**a**) and PET image (**b**) with a focally increased FDG-uptake (SUVmax 14.1) and contrast-enhanced T1-weighted MR image (**c**) (arrow)

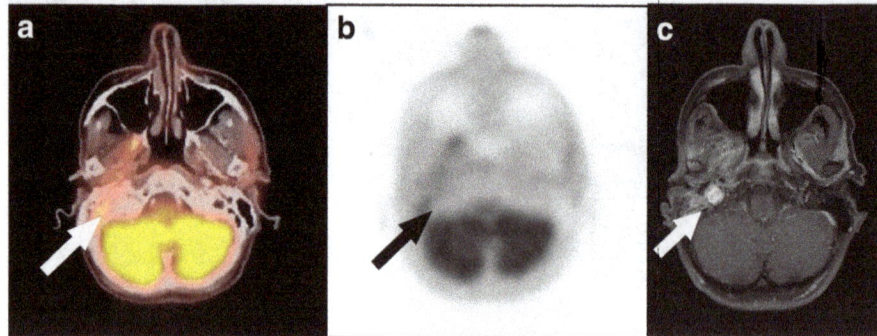

Fig. 4 ACC recurrence: PET/CT imaging was false-negative and MRI true-positive. Patient after multiple resections of the primary and recurrent tumours of an ACC in the right parotid gland area. A false-negative finding is seen on the on the fused PET/CT (**a**) and PET image (**b**), but there was a true-positive finding on the contrast-enhanced T1-weighted MR image (**c**) with a hyperintense tumour recurrence (arrow)

comparable to MRI in local restaging with a higher sensitivity (96% v. 89%) and diagnostic accuracy (94% vs. 89%) due to less indistinct findings.

Locoregional lymph node metastases were present in only one patient in our study population with a true-positive finding on PET and false-negative finding on CT or MRI due to size criteria. This low incidence of locoregional lymph node metastases is in line with previous reports that described that an ACC rarely metastasises to regional lymph nodes [28, 29]. The ability of PET to detect metastases in lymph nodes that are inconspicuous in morphologic imaging has been shown in a variety of cancers [17, 30, 31].

Combined whole-body PET/CT detected all distant metastases in our study. There were only two cases with disseminated metastases of the lung in which not all of the CT-detectable lesions were also FDG positive due to the limited spatial resolution. In two patients the lung metastases showed a pathologically increased FDG uptake, whereas the CT was indistinctive (differential diagnosis: granuloma). Distant metastases were present in 25% of the patients in our study population. Surprisingly,

in the patient group with the primary examination after local tumour resection prior to radiation therapy, 11% of the patients already showed distant metastases in the lung. In three patients secondary carcinomas were found with PET/CT allowing early therapeutic interventions. Previous reports have described overall rate of distant metastases in 25 to 50% of patients with ACC [29], but the occurrence mainly depends on the follow-up period. In fact, in 35 to 50% of patients with ACC, distant metastases were usually found within a follow-up period of more than 15 to 20 years [32]. These studies, which were published several years ago, used conventional diagnostics such as X-ray with comparably low specificity and sensitivity for staging the lung of ACC patients. Therefore, slow-growing metastases might have been misinterpreted as newly occurred metastases at a late time point, although other diagnostic imaging methods like CT might have shown a metastatic disease at an earlier time point in their clinical course or even at time of initial diagnosis.

According to Spiro et al. [29], large primary tumour size and locoregional treatment failure are the most

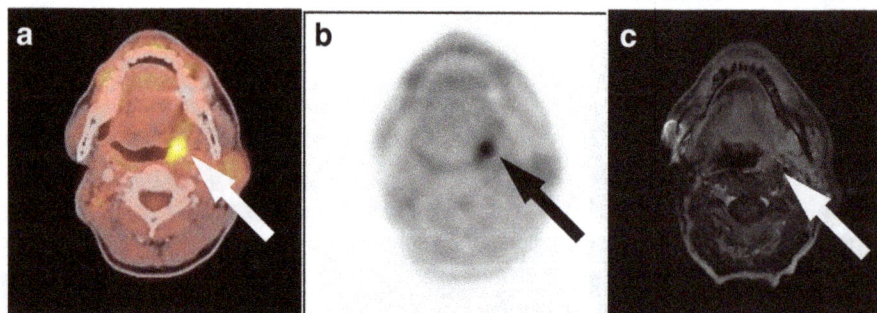

Fig. 5 No tumour recurrence: PET/CT imaging was false-positive and MRI true-negative. Patient after resection of an ACC in the right parotid gland and mandibula. A contralateral false-positive finding is seen on the PET (**b**) and fused PET/CT image (**a**) with a focally increased FDG-uptake (SUVmax 5.4; arrow), but there was no pathological finding on the contrast-enhanced T1-weighted MR image (**c**)

important predisposing factors for outcome. However, distant metastases may develop despite successful locoregional tumour therapy. As in our study, the lungs are the most commonly reported sites to harbour distant metastases. These patients may remain asymptomatic for a long time during their clinical course. However, the onset of symptoms or the development of other visceral metastases usually results in a short survival period. Thus, whole body imaging seems advisable in restaging and follow-up of ACC patients to better understand the course of disease and find optimal therapy strategies, as was recently highlighted in a report from Tewari et al. [33].

In our study, almost all lesions were FDG-avid, and the majority showed a moderately to high FDG uptake. Previously published literature predominantly case reports or case series on FDG uptake in this advancing but relentlessly growing tumour with a propensity for perineural invasion comprise only very few patients [22–25]. In larger studies ACC often represent only a minority within a group of mixed head and neck cancers [25]. The existing literature of experience with PET imaging show that adenoid cystic carcinoma and mucoepidermoid carcinoma showed variable FDG-uptake depending on the grade of differentiation [26] in comparison to most squamous cell carcinomas that showed high uptake. Due to the complex development of the disease in patients with ACC an appropiate diagnostic imaging is required. The evaluation of changes in tissues and structures in the tumour environment, especially after extended tumour resection in the head and neck area, surgical procedures with transplants or external beam radiotherapy, is a big challenge since US, conventional CT and MRI provide mainly just morphological information and exactly here PET imaging can improve the diagnostic work-up as a tool that depict metabolism information.

A limitation of this study is the nevertheless limited number of patients due to the rarity of this malignant disease. This study cohort comprised 36 patients which is more than any other study. The small sample size did not permit an analysis of the FDG uptake depending on the histopathological ACC subtypes (cribriform, solid and tubular). Another limitation is the reference standard lacking histopathological confirmation. However, the consensus interpretation (adopted by all readers) based on profound imaging data including prior and follow-up examinations (median 12, range 3–105 months).

Interestingly, FDG PET/CT depicted all lesions visualized by the standard imaging tools head and neck is MRI and if applicable thoracic CT. This underlines the potential of whole-body FDG-PET/CT improving the diagnostic accuracy of restaging ACC. Whereas MRI is commonly needed preoperatively for the assessment of

tumour delineation and relevant tumour invasion of surrounding structures it is not a routine whole-body imaging technique. The advantages of FDG-PET/CT are the examination of the whole body at one time and at a high sensitivity. Furthermore, our study demonstrates that due to certain weaknesses the conventional CT and MR imaging of the head and neck could benefit from the additional metabolism information provided by the PET component. Thus, in the time of installation of integrated whole-body PET/MR systems, it would be of interest to determine whether a single whole-body PET/MRI could replace a whole-body PET/CT by combining the advantages of both modalities.

Conclusions
Our study demonstrates the potential of FDG-PET/CT as important diagnostic tool in the restaging of ACC patients. FDG PET/CT has a higher sensitivity and diagnostic accuracy than MRI for the loco-regional tumour staging and provides valuable additional information as a whole-body technique.

Acknowledgements
Not applicable.

Funding
No specific funding was received for this study.

Authors' contributions
VR, WS, KH, TH, LU, TP, JV, JN, AB made substantial contributions to conception and design of the study. VR, WS, JN, TP made substantial contributions to acquisition of patient and imaging data. VR, LU, TP made substantial contributions to (statistically) analysis and interpretation of PET/CT and MRI data. VR, WS, KH, TH, LU, JN, TP, JV, AB have been involved in drafting the manuscript and revising it critically for important intellectual content. All authors read and approved the final manuscript.

Competing interests
Prof. Ken Herrmann is a member of the editorial board (Consulting Editor) of this journal. The authors declare that they have no competing interests.

Author details
[1]Department of Nuclear Medicine, University Duisburg-Essen, Medical Faculty, University Hospital Essen, Hufelandstrasse 55, 45147 Essen, Germany. [2]Department of Oto-Rhino-Laryngology, Head and Neck Surgery, University Hospital Ulm, Frauensteige 12, 89070 Ulm, Germany. [3]Department of Nuclear Medicine, Radboud University Nijmegen Medical Centre, Geert Grooteplein 8, 6525, GA, Nijmegen, the Netherlands. [4]Department of Diagnostic and Interventional Radiology and Neuroradiology, University Duisburg-Essen, University Hospital Essen, Hufelandstrasse 55, 45147 Essen, Germany. [5]Department of Radiation Oncology, University Duisburg-Essen, University Hospital Essen, Hufelandstrasse 55, 45147 Essen, Germany.

References

1. Barnes L, Eveson JW, Reichart P, Sidransky D. World Health Organization Classification of Tumours. Pathology and Genetics of Head and Neck Tumours. Lyon: IARC Press; 2005.
2. Garden AS, Weber RS, Morrison WH, Ang KK, Peters LJ. The influence of positive margins and nerve invasion in adenoid cystic carcinoma of the head and neck treated with surgery and radiation. Int J Rad Oncol. 1995;32:619–26.
3. Chummun S, McLean NR, Kelly CG, Dawes PJDK, Fellows S, Meikle D, et al. Adenoid cystic carcinoma of the head and neck. Br J Plast Surg. 2001;54:476–80.
4. Dubergé T, Bénézery K, Resbeut M, Azria D, Minsat M, Ellis S, et al. Carcinomes adénoïdes kystiques ORL : étude rétrospective multicentrique de 169 cas. Cancer/Radiothérapie. 2012;16:247–56.
5. Schulz-Ertner D, Nikoghosyan A, Didinger B, Münter M, Jäkel O, Karger CP, et al. Therapy strategies for locally advanced adenoid cystic carcinomas using modern radiation therapy techniques. Cancer. 2005;104:338–44.
6. Huber PE, Debus J, Latz D, Zierhut D, Bischof M, Wannenmacher M, et al. Radiotherapy for advanced adenoid cystic carcinoma: neutrons, photons or mixed beam? Radiother Oncol. 2001;59:161–7.
7. Prott FJ, Micke O, Haverkamp U, Willich N, Schüller P, Pötter R. Results of fast neutron therapy of adenoid cystic carcinoma of the salivary glands. Anticancer Res. 2000;20:3743–9.
8. Laurie SA, Ho AL, Fury MG, Sherman E, Pfister DG. Systemic therapy in the management of metastatic or locally recurrent adenoid cystic carcinoma of the salivary glands: a systematic review. Lancet Oncol. 2011;12:815–24.
9. Papaspyrou G, Hoch S, Rinaldo A, Rodrigo JP, Takes RP, van Herpen C, et al. Chemotherapy and targeted therapy in adenoid cystic carcinoma of the head and neck: a review. Head Neck. 2010;33:905–11.
10. Samant S, van den Brekel MW, Kies MS, Wan J, Robbins KT, Rosenthal DI, et al. Concurrent chemoradiation for adenoid cystic carcinoma of the head and neck. Head Neck. 2011;34:1263–8.
11. Büchsenschütz K, Veit JA, Schuler PJ, Thierauf J, Laban S, Fahimi F, et al. Molecular approaches to systemic therapy of adenoid cystic carcinoma of the head and neck area. Laryngorhinootologie. 2014;93:657–64.
12. Westra WH. The surgical pathology of salivary gland neoplasms. Otolaryngol Clin N Am. 1999;32:919–43.
13. Fordice J, Kershaw C, El-Naggar A, Goepfert H. Adenoid cystic carcinoma of the head and neck. Arch Otolaryngol Head Neck Surg. 1999;125:149.
14. Coca-Pelaz A, Rodrigo JP, Bradley PJ, Vander Poorten V, Triantafyllou A, Hunt JL, et al. Adenoid cystic carcinoma of the head and neck – an update. Oral Oncol. 2015;51:652–61.
15. Huang M, Ma D, Sun K, Yu G, Guo C, Gao F. Factors influencing survival rate in adenoid cystic carcinoma of the salivary glands. Int J Oral Maxillofac Surg. 1997;26:435–9.
16. Ciccolallo L, Licitra L, Cantú G, Gatta G. Survival from salivary glands adenoid cystic carcinoma in European populations. Oral Oncol. 2009;45:669–74.
17. Adams S, Baum RP, Stuckensen T, Bitter K, Hör G. Prospective comparison of 18 F-FDG PET with conventional imaging modalities (CT, MRI, US) in lymph node staging of head and neck cancer. Eur J Nucl Med Mol Imaging. 1998; 25:1255–60.
18. Wu S, Liu G, Chen R, Guan Y. Role of ultrasound in the assessment of benignity and malignancy of parotid masses. Dentomaxillofac Radiol. 2012; 41:131–5.
19. Kato H, Kanematsu M, Sakurai K, Mizuta K, Aoki M, Hirose Y, et al. Adenoid cystic carcinoma of the maxillary sinus: CT and MR imaging findings. Jpn J Radiol. 2013;31:744–9.
20. Freudenberg LS, Antoch G, Schütt P, Beyer T, Jentzen W, Müller SP, et al. FDG-PET/CT in re-staging of patients with lymphoma. Eur J Nucl Med Mol Imaging. 2004;31:325–9.
21. Riegger C, Herrmann J, Nagarajah J, Hecktor J, Kuemmel S, Otterbach F, et al. Whole-body FDG PET/CT is more accurate than conventional imaging for staging primary breast cancer patients. Eur J Nucl Med Mol Imaging. 2012; 39:852–63.
22. Naswa N, Sharma P, Gupta SK, Karunanithi S, Reddy RM, Patnecha M, et al. Dual tracer functional imaging of Gastroenteropancreatic neuroendocrine tumors using 68Ga-DOTA-NOC PET-CT and 18F-FDG PET-CT. Clin Nucl Med. 2014;39:e27–34.
23. Bhagat N, Zuckier LS, Hameed M, Cathcart C, Baredes S, Ghesani NV. Detection of recurrent adenoid cystic carcinoma with PET-CT. Clin Nucl Med. 2007;32:574–7.
24. Treglia G, Bertagna F, Ceriani L, Giovanella LA. Rare case of adenoid cystic carcinoma of the breast detected by 18F-FDG PET/CT. Revista Española de Medicina Nuclear e Imagen Molecular. 2015;34:205–6.
25. Otsuka H, Graham MM, Kogame M, Nishitani H. The impact of FDG-PET in the management of patients with salivary gland malignancy. Ann Nucl Med. 2005;19:691–4.
26. Park CM, Goo JM, Lee HJ, Kim MA, Lee CH, Kang M-J. Tumors in the tracheobronchial tree: CT and FDG PET Features1. Radiographics. 2009; 29:55–71.
27. Kim D, Kim W, Lee J, Ki Y, Lee B, Cho K, et al. Pretreatment maximum standardized uptake value of 18F-fluorodeoxyglucose positron emission tomography as a predictor of distant metastasis in adenoid cystic carcinoma of the head and neck. Head Neck. 2015;38:755–61.
28. Bradley PJ. Adenoid cystic carcinoma of the head and neck: a review. Curr Opin Otolaryngol Head Neck Surg. 2004;12:127–32.
29. Spiro H, Distant R. Metastasis in adenoid cystic carcinoma of salivary origin. Am J Surg. 1997;174:495–8.
30. Zanation AM, Sutton DK, Couch ME, Weissler MC, Shockley WW, Shores CG. Use, accuracy, and implications for patient management of [18F]-2-Fluorodeoxyglucose-positron emission/computerized tomography for head and neck tumors. Laryngoscope. 2005;115:1186–90.
31. Murakami R, Uozumi H, Hirai T, Nishimura R, Shiraishi S, Ota K, et al. Impact of FDG-PET/CT imaging on nodal staging for head-and-neck squamous cell carcinoma. Int J Radiation Oncol Biol Phys. 2007;68:377–82.
32. Bradley PJ. Distant metastases from salivary glands cancer. ORL J Otorhinolaryngol Relat Spec. 2001;63:233–42.
33. Tewari A, Padma S, Sundaram P. Detection of atypical metastases in recurrent adenoid cystic carcinoma of parotid gland. J Can Res Ther. 2013;9:148.

6

Droplet digital PCR for detection and quantification of circulating tumor DNA in plasma of head and neck cancer patients

Joost H. van Ginkel[1,2]*, Manon M. H. Huibers[2], Robert J. J. van Es[1,3], Remco de Bree[3] and Stefan M. Willems[2]

Abstract

Background: During posttreatment surveillance of head and neck cancer patients, imaging is insufficiently accurate for the early detection of relapsing disease. Free circulating tumor DNA (ctDNA) may serve as a novel biomarker for monitoring tumor burden during posttreatment surveillance of these patients. In this exploratory study, we investigated whether low level ctDNA in plasma of head and neck cancer patients can be detected using Droplet Digital PCR (ddPCR).

Methods: *TP53* mutations were determined in surgically resected primary tumor samples from six patients with high stage (II-IV), moderate to poorly differentiated head and neck squamous cell carcinoma (HNSCC). Subsequently, mutation specific ddPCR assays were designed. Pretreatment plasma samples from these patients were examined on the presence of ctDNA by ddPCR using the mutation-specific assays. The ddPCR results were evaluated alongside clinicopathological data.

Results: In all cases, plasma samples were found positive for targeted *TP53* mutations in varying degrees (absolute quantification of 2.2–422 mutational copies/ml plasma). Mutations were detected in wild-type *TP53* background templates of 7667–156,667 copies/ml plasma, yielding fractional abundances of down to 0.01%.

Conclusions: Our results show that detection of tumor specific *TP53* mutations in low level ctDNA from HNSCC patients using ddPCR is technically feasible and provide ground for future research on ctDNA quantification for the use of diagnostic biomarkers in the posttreatment surveillance of HNSCC patients.

Keywords: Head and neck cancer, Circulating tumor DNA, Droplet digital PCR, *TP53* mutations, Diagnostic biomarker

Background

Monitoring tumor response during posttreatment surveillance of head and neck cancer patients heavily relies on clinical examination supported by endoscopy and/or imaging (e.g. computerized tomography (CT), magnetic resonance imaging (MRI), or positron emission tomography (PET)). However, early detection of recurrent disease is challenging due to lymph nodal micrometastases and radiation or surgery induced fibrosis and inflammation, obscuring residual or recurrent tumor tissue [1–3]. Accurate and timely detection of locoregional metastases and recurrent disease is pivotal as survival rates rapidly decline with late detection and delayed salvage surgery [4, 5]. With recent developments in molecular diagnostics, the use of (blood-based) genetic biomarkers is growing in a wide variety of cancer types [6]. Cell free circulating tumor DNA (ctDNA), released into the bloodstream by apoptotic and necrotic tumor cells, harbor tumor-specific mutations [7]. These mutations can be detected in blood plasma from cancer patients by blood sampling, also known as "liquid biopsy" [8]. For head and neck cancer, research has been focused mainly on actionable oncogenic mutations such as *PIK3CA* and *HRAS*, hot-spot *TP53* mutations, and

* Correspondence: j.h.vanginkel-2@umcutrecht.nl
[1]Department of Oral and Maxillofacial Surgery, University Medical Center Utrecht, Utrecht, The Netherlands
[2]Department of Pathology, University Medical Center Utrecht, Heidelberglaan 100, 3584 CX Utrecht, The Netherlands
Full list of author information is available at the end of the article

HPV-related biomarkers to use as prognosticators or predictors for establishing and adjusting targeted therapy [9–12]. For similar purposes, transcriptional and epigenetic changes are studied substantially [13–15]. For the early detection of recurrent disease, early driver mutations in HNSCC such as TP53 mutations would be favorable to use as biomarkers, as these are likely to occur consistently throughout clonal evolution [16, 17], and are found to be most frequent and concordant in recurrent and metastatic HPV-negative tumors compared to mutations in other genes [18–22]. By targeting and quantifying early driver mutations in ctDNA, tumor burden could be monitored after treatment, facilitating earlier detection of asymptomatic residual and/or recurrent disease. Previous studies showed correlations between ctDNA levels and tumor dynamics during posttreatment monitoring in patients with various types of cancer [23–26]. However, accurate detection of ctDNA in plasma is challenging, because ctDNA concentrations can be very low. This could greatly impair reliable and valid measurement of tumor dynamics. Highly sensitive Droplet Digital PCR (ddPCR) facilitates detection and quantification of low levels of ctDNA by partitioning DNA samples into 20,000 water-in-oil droplets [27]. In this exploratory study, we investigated whether detection and quantification of ctDNA in plasma from several head and neck squamous cell carcinoma (HNSCC) patients using ddPCR is technically feasible.

Methods

Patients and samples

Six patients (median age 60.5 [42–77] years) with histologically confirmed HPV-negative HNSCC were selected retrospectively for analysis of archived primary tumor samples and presurgically obtained blood samples. Patient selection was based on TNM stage (stage II or higher) and availability of blood plasma samples in our biobank. Additional clinicopathological and radiological data were collected from hospital charts of selected patients (Table 1; Fig. 1).

Sample workup

All primary tumor samples were acquired from formalin fixed paraffin embedded (FFPE) incisional or excisional biopsy specimens, microscopically containing >30% tumor cells. In order to reveal TP53 mutation status of primary tumor samples, targeted next-generation sequencing (NGS) was performed using the Ion Torrent™ PGM platform (Thermo Fisher Scientific, Waltham, MA, USA), as previously described [28]. NGS was based on the Cancer Hotspot Panel v2+ (Thermo Fisher Scientific, Waltham, MA, USA), covering TP53 exons 2–10 [29]. All blood samples were collected in 10 ml K_2EDTA blood collection tubes (BD Vacutainer, Franklin Lakes, NJ, USA). Prior to archiving, centrifugation took place for 10 min at 800 g (Rotina 380, Hettich, Germany), after which supernatant plasma was aliquoted in 1 ml portions and stored at −80 °C until DNA isolation. Storage time of patient FFPE and corresponding plasma samples varied from 4 months to 9 years.

Plasma samples were thawed and DNA was immediately isolated from 2 ml of plasma using QIAamp Circulating Nucleic Acid (NA) kit (Qiagen, Hilden, Germany) according to the manufacturer's instructions. Isolated plasma samples were eluted in 50 μl elution buffer as provided with the kit and stored at 4 °C until ddPCR analysis. Positive control samples, containing both wild-type (WT) and mutant (MT) DNA, were created for all patients by isolating tumor DNA from the primary tumor FFPE samples using COBAS DNA Sample Preparation Kit (Roche, Basel, Switzerland) according to manufacturer's instructions. After quantity measurement of isolated DNA samples with a Qubit fluorometer using the dsDNA HS (High Sensitivity) Assay Kit (Thermo Fisher Scientific), cfDNA was diluted to 10 ng/ul using purified water. For each assay, no template controls (NTC) were used to control for environmental contamination, and wild-type-only (WT-only) samples were used in order to estimate false-positive rates. Five WT-only samples were created by isolating plasma DNA

Table 1 Summary of patient and tumor characteristics

Patient ID	Sex	Smoking (pack years)	Alcohol (units/day)	Biopsy type	TNM-stage	Tumor site[a]	Differentiation grade	Max diameter primary tumor (mm)	Growth type[b]	Vascular invasion
P1	M	0	8	Excisional	T4aN1M0	OSCC	Moderate	40	NS	No
P2	M	0	0	Excisional	T4aN2cM0	OSCC	Poor	72	NS	Yes
P3	F	0	0	Excisional	T2N0Mx	OSCC	Moderate	32	Unknown	Yes
P4	M	Unknown	1	Excisional	T4aN2bM0	OSCC	Moderate	46	S	No
P5	M	49	12	Excisional	T4aN1M0	OSCC	Moderate/poor	37	Unknown	No
P6	F	42	2	Incisional	T3N2cM0	OPSCC	Unknown	13	N/A	No

[a]OSCC Oral Squamous Cell Carcinoma, OPSCC Oropharyngeal Squamous Cell Carcinoma
[b]NS Non Spiculated, S Spiculated

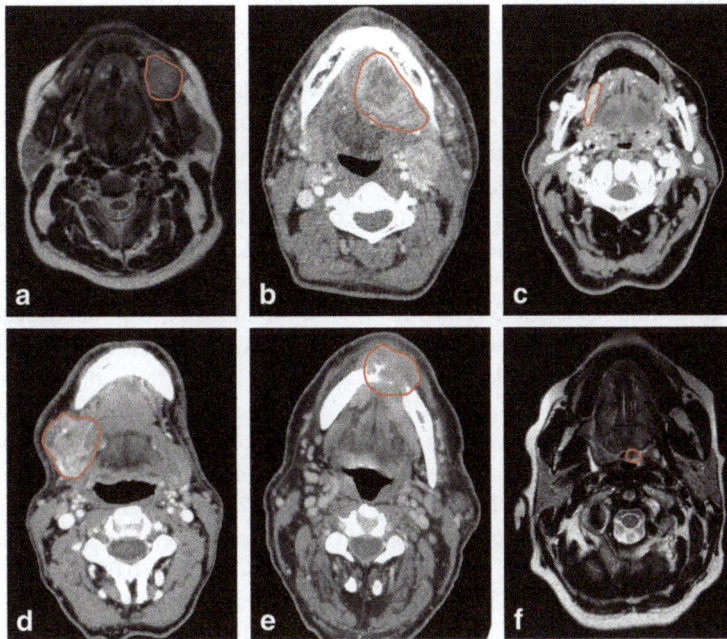

Fig. 1 Primary tumors of six patients encircled in *red*. **a** Axial T1 MRI image of a tumor in the left mandible of patient 1. **b** Axial ceCT image of a tumor in the floor of mouth of patient 2. **c** Axial ceCT image of a tumor in the right lateral tongue of patient 3. **d** Axial ceCT image of a tumor in the right mandible/floor of mouth/tongue of patient 4. **e** Axial ceCT image of a tumor in the floor of mouth in patient 5. **f** Axial T1 MRI image of tumor in left mid tongue base of patient 6. ceCT = contrast enhanced computed tomography

from anonymous healthy individuals using the QIAamp Circulating NA kit.

ddPCR

The plasma samples from all 6 patients were analyzed for *TP53* point mutations, identified in the primary tumor tissue by NGS. MT and WT *TP53* sequences were used as DNA template for designing ddPCR (Bio-Rad Laboratories, Hercules, CA, USA) assays following the MIQE guidelines (Additional file 1: Table S1) [30]. DdPCR reaction volumes of 22 μl were prepared, consisting of 13 μl mastermix (11 μl Supermix for Probes [no deoxyuridine triphosphate], 1 μl of primer/probe mix for both MT and WT *TP53*), and 9 μl cfDNA sample of patient plasma. The NTCs contained 9 μl of purified water instead of cfDNA sample. The WT-only samples contained 1–7 ul of cfDNA. From the PCR reaction mixture, 20 μl was used for droplet generation. Droplet Digital PCR was performed using the QX200 ddPCR system according to manufacturer's instructions (Bio-Rad Laboratories). QuantaSoft v1.7.4.0917 (Bio-Rad Laboratories) software was used for data analysis.

Prior to plasma sample testing, thermal gradient experiments were performed on FFPE samples in order to determine optimal amplification conditions during thermal cycling for each assay independently. Based on clearest separation of negative and positive droplet clusters, thermal cycling conditions for all 6 assays were set at 95 °C for 10 min (1 cycle), 94 °C for 30 s and 55 °C for 60 s (55 cycles), and infinite hold at 12 °C. To ensure experiment quality, wells with total droplet counts of less than 10,000 would be considered invalid and excluded from analysis. The positive control samples were used to verify assay performance and facilitate thresholding in fluorescence values. Additionally, positive control samples were validated by comparing the fractional abundance (FA) in FFPE samples to NGS mutation frequencies. False-positive rate estimation was determined by performing 5 experiments for each assay using the WT-only samples, where total amounts of detected MT-positive droplets determined thresholds above which positive droplets in patient samples were to be considered as true positive.

Post-analysis

For each patient, plasma was analyzed in duplicate. Therefore, PCR results of patients samples were based on the mean of estimated target DNA concentrations (copies/μl) in merged wells, automatically calculated by manufacturer software. Correction for false positivity was performed by virtually subtracting the amount of MT-false-positive droplets from the amount of MT-positive droplets detected in the patients sample with the corresponding assays. Subsequently, absolute sample concentrations were (re)calculated as described in

Additional file 1: Eq. S1. Relative quantification was defined as the FA of MT to total (WT + MT) copies.

Results

Assay validation

In all six patients, *TP53* mutations were detected in FFPE by both NGS and ddPCR (Additional file 1: Table S1 and Additional file 2: Figure S1). FA of MT copies ranged from 6.1–71.7% in positive control samples, compared to NGS mutant percentages of 7–70%. False-positive rate estimation was necessary to determine aspecific MT signal (Additional file 1: Table S2). One MT-false-positive droplet was detected in the WT-only sample control series for assay 1 and 3, establishing a true positivity threshold of >1 MT-positive droplet for these assays (Additional file 3: Figure S2 and Additional file 4: Figure S3). For the remaining assays, no MT-false-positive droplets were detected in the WT-only samples. WT-false-positive droplets for all used assays in NTCs ranged from 0 to 10 droplets. No MT-positive droplets were detected in any of the NTC samples (Additional file 5: Figure S4).

ctDNA quantification

The amount of ctDNA was quantified and analyzed in blood plasma samples from all 6 patients (Table 2). MT copies of *TP53* were detected in plasma samples from all patients (Fig. 2a), ranging from 0.04 to 7.60 copies/µl ddPCR mix and 1–181 MT-positive droplets in merged wells (Fig. 2b). When corrected for MT-false-positive droplets, plasma ctDNA concentrations ranged from 2.2 to 422 copies/ml plasma (Fig. 3a). MT copies were detected in WT backgrounds of 138–2821 copies/µl, yielding FA of MT copies of 0.01–5.2% (Fig. 3b).

Discussion

Our study shows that quantification of rare target mutations in ctDNA in plasma from HNSCC patients using ddPCR is technically feasible. Highly sensitive detection methods like digital PCR are needed in order to detect rare MT targets within high concentrations of WT background [31]. WT background size (i.e. concentration of WT cfDNA) can strongly vary over time for each patient individually, depending on multiple factors. For instance, patient's physical status (e.g. inflammation, post-traumatic, post-exercise, chronic illness), as well as pre-analytical technical procedures (e.g. white blood cell lysis caused by whole blood transportation and processing) appear to affect cfDNA concentrations [32–35]. Increased cfDNA concentration causes dilution of ctDNA, which could lower the accuracy of rare MT fragment detection. Therefore, pre-analytical steps should be most optimally in lowering background DNA; e.g. blood plasma instead of serum is preferred as source for ctDNA, as the amount of cfDNA in serum can be 2–4 times higher than that in plasma [36].

It has been shown for various applications that ddPCR is capable of rare target DNA quantification with higher precision and accuracy compared to quantitative PCR [27, 37–39]. Although we did not perform quantitative PCR we found relative quantification measurements of MT copies down to 0.01%. This falls within the potential dynamic range for absolute quantification of rare target DNA within a 100,000-fold of WT background as previously demonstrated [40, 41]. Similar quantification results were reported in a study where *TP53* mutations were identified in plasma using another PCR-based detection method in 88% of HPV-negative HNSCC patients (*n* = 22) with MT fractions varying between 0.016 and 2.9% [42]. We also found large variability in MT quantification measurements among patient samples. This is consistent with previous mutation analysis of blood samples from HNSCC patients, in which MT *TP53* fragments of 0–1500 per 5 ml plasma were targeted and detected by conventional PCR [43].

Variances in detected MT copies among patients can be the result of various (pre)analytical deficiencies and technical errors like plasma sample contamination from the environment. Furthermore, decreased DNA concentration due to prolonged storage, poor sample quality, subsampling during whole blood retrieval and/or centrifugation, inefficient DNA isolation from plasma samples, poor droplet handling leading to shredding or coalition of droplets, instrument artifacts, intrinsic PCR errors caused by PCR inhibition and/or minor mismatches

Table 2 Absolute and relative quantifications of MT and WT DNA in plasma samples from HNSCC patients

Sample ID	MT DNA concentration			WT DNA concentration		FA_{mut}
	Sample (copies/µl)	Sample$_{corr}$ (copies/µl)	Plasma (copies/ml)	Reaction (copies/µl)	Plasma (copies/ml)	
P1	0.47	0.43	24	315	17,500	0.13%
P2	7.60	7.60	422	138	7667	5.50%
P3	0.17	0.16	8.9	158	8778	0.10%
P4	1.79	1.79	99	2821	156,667	0.06%
P5	0.37	0.37	21	380	21,167	0.10%
P6	0.04	0.04	2.2	397	22,056	0.01%

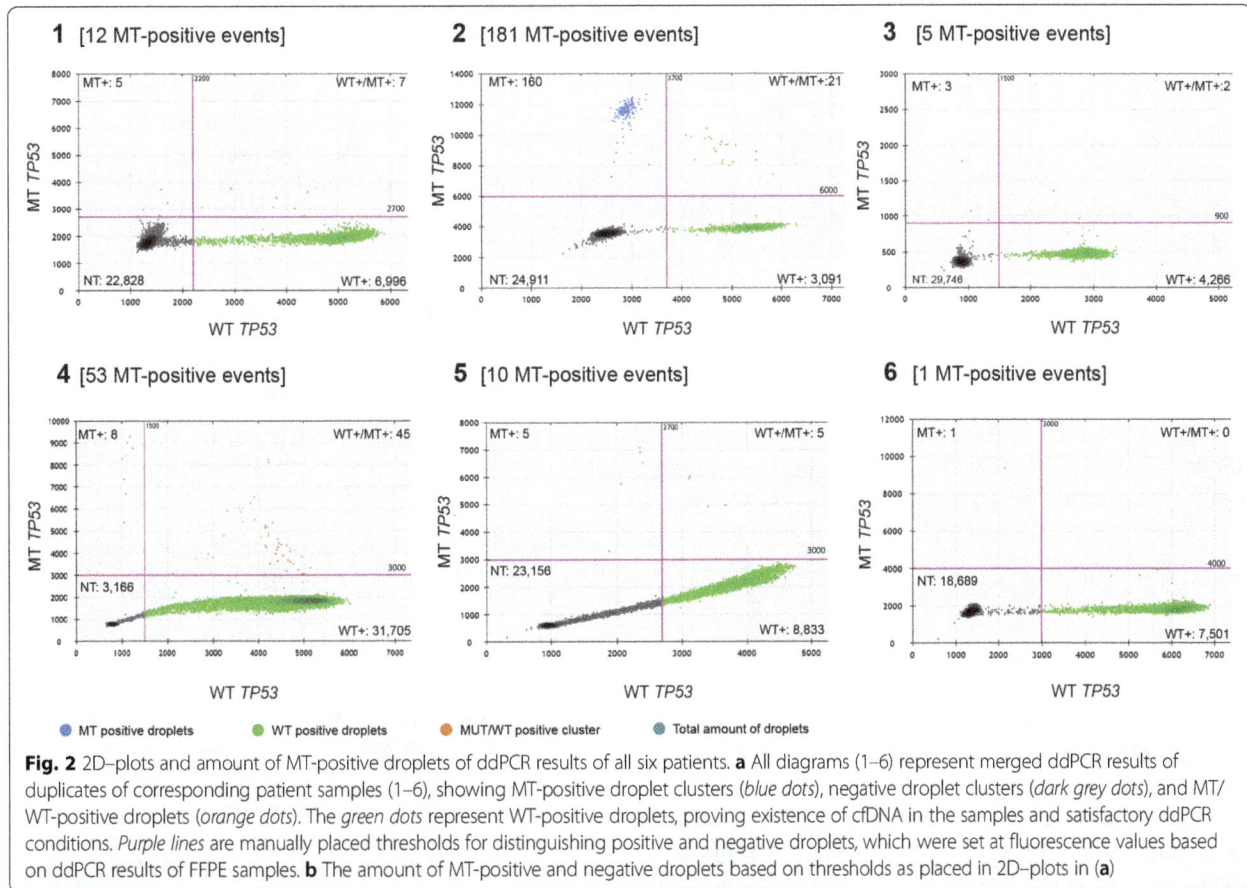

Fig. 2 2D–plots and amount of MT-positive droplets of ddPCR results of all six patients. **a** All diagrams (1–6) represent merged ddPCR results of duplicates of corresponding patient samples (1–6), showing MT-positive droplet clusters (*blue dots*), negative droplet clusters (*dark grey dots*), and MT/WT-positive droplets (*orange dots*). The *green dots* represent WT-positive droplets, proving existence of cfDNA in the samples and satisfactory ddPCR conditions. *Purple lines* are manually placed thresholds for distinguishing positive and negative droplets, which were set at fluorescence values based on ddPCR results of FFPE samples. **b** The amount of MT-positive and negative droplets based on thresholds as placed in 2D–plots in (**a**)

between primer/probes and target molecules can all affect PCR results [44, 45].

During ddPCR post-analysis, manual threshold determination and stochastic sampling errors could directly lead to over- or underestimation of target copies, resulting in inaccurate quantification of results [46]. Furthermore, we know from previous validation experiences that fluorescence values of positive droplet clusters can vary inter-experiment, while assessing DNA samples derived from the same individual and using identical ddPCR assays. The same holds true for ddPCR experiments on DNA samples derived from different plasma matrices and/or volumes, containing different PCR inhibitors [47]. These points concerning post-analysis need to be addressed in order to implement ddPCR for ctDNA quantification into clinical practice. Therefore each assay and each sample should be analyzed individually. Although we used FFPE for positive control samples for threshold placement and plasma from different individuals for false-positive rate estimation, samples were

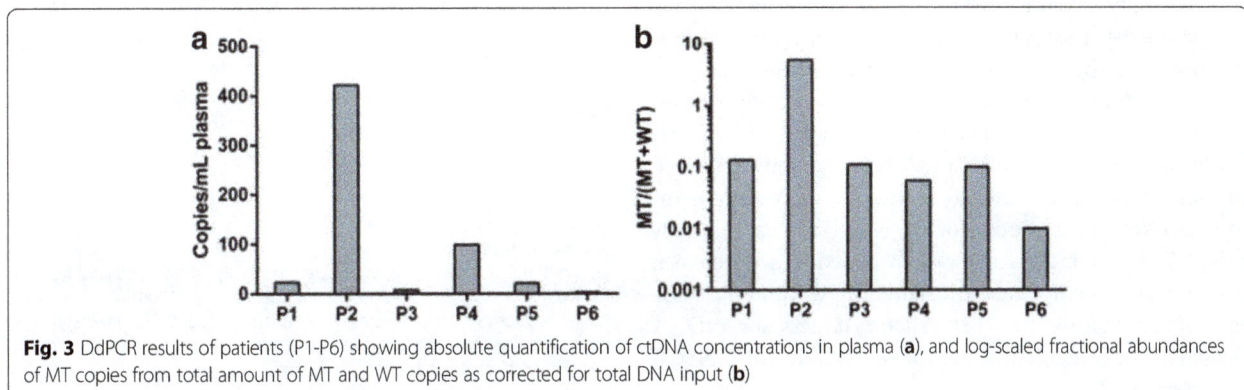

Fig. 3 DdPCR results of patients (P1-P6) showing absolute quantification of ctDNA concentrations in plasma (**a**), and log-scaled fractional abundances of MT copies from total amount of MT and WT copies as corrected for total DNA input (**b**)

patient specific and of similar matrix of DNA source, respectively. In this way, plasma DNA composition from the patients was mimicked most realistically. Moreover, the alternative of using (spiked) series of artificially synthesized DNA oligonucleotides for creating control samples can provoke overestimation of PCR targets due to the high purity of these solutions. Eventually, interpretation of ddPCR results depends on the accuracy of ctDNA quantification which is determined by false positive rate estimation.

Several biological factors could affect ctDNA concentration. Especially tumor volume is of interest as it may reflect tumor burden and actual disease status through correlation with ctDNA concentration. Simultaneously, tumor characteristics such as histological grade, localization, growth pattern, growth rate, and degree of vascularization possibly complicate reliable monitoring of tumor burden by ctDNA quantification, as these factors might affect ctDNA release into the bloodstream all differently [44, 48]. However, in a series of 117 patients with primary HNSCC, no significant correlation was found between gender, tumor stage, site, and plasma ctDNA concentration detected by touchdown PCR [49]. Interestingly, in our study, the highest amount of ctDNA was detected in plasma from the patient that harbored the largest tumor diameter of all six included patients. This tumor also had a poor histological differentiation grade with vascular invasion. At the other end, the lowest amount of ctDNA was detected in plasma from the patient with the smallest tumor diameter and without vascular invasion. However, we studied and compared plasma samples retrieved at one time point from a rather small group of high-stage HNSCC patients with presumably greater tumor burden and plasma ctDNA concentrations.

Therefore, serial ctDNA quantification in clinical patients diagnosed with primary HNSCC of all stages is needed to clarify its significance for posttreatment disease monitoring and the possible advantages of its specific application with respect to early tumor detection in relation to current clinical diagnostics [50]. Tumor heterogeneity could further complicate monitoring tumor burden through ctDNA detection, because intratumoral heterogeneity of the primary tumor induces branched tumor evolution of subclonal populations harboring different molecular alterations [51]. This could lead to increased clonal heterogeneity between primary tumor and matched metastatic or recurrent tumors, risking mistargeting of ctDNA. However, as early driver TP53 mutations show high concordance between primary and recurrent and/or metastatic tumors, these may hold promise as most reliable targets for ctDNA detection and for early tumor detection of HNSCC recurrences [21].

Conclusion

The detection of tumor specific TP53 mutations in ctDNA from HNSCC using a ddPCR is technically feasible and provide ground for further research on ctDNA quantification to be used as a diagnostic biomarker in the posttreatment surveillance of HNSCC patients.

Additional files

Additional file 1: Table S1–2. NGS data, PCR assays, and Assay validation. Eq. S1 Equation used for manual conversion of target copies to plasma concentrations.

Additional file 2: Figure S1. DdPCR results of 6 different MT TP53 assays on positive control (FFPE) samples of all 6 patients are shown. The MT-positive clusters (blue dots) and MT/WT-positive clusters (orange dots) are clearly separated from the negative droplet clusters (dark grey dots) and WT-positive droplet clusters. Thresholds are placed manually.

Additional file 3: Figure S2. 2D–plots with the amounts of droplets of ddPCR results in healthy individuals using assay 1–6. All threshold are placed using exact values as derived from the 2D–plots in Additional file 2: Figure S1. The plots represent merged results of plasma samples from 4 to 5 different healthy individuals for each assay. MT+ MT-positive droplets, WT+ WT-positive droplets, MT+/WT+ MT/WT-positive droplets, NT No template droplets.

Additional file 4: Figure S3. DdPCR results for all 6 patients side-by-side with the WT-only samples from healthy individuals. All patient samples are shown in duplicate. In order to estimate the false positive rate for patient samples, plasma samples from five different healthy individuals were used. In the samples from healthy individuals 3 and 1 used during validation of assay 2 and assay 6, less than 10,000 droplets were detected. Therefore, these results were excluded from false positive estimation for the corresponding assays.

Additional file 5: Figure S4. NTC samples showing minimal environmental contamination with WT-positive droplets. No MT-positive droplets were detected in any of the NTC samples.

Abbreviations

CT: Computer tomography; ctDNA: Circulating tumor DNA; ddPCR: Droplet digital polymerase chain reaction; FA: Fractional abundance; FFPE: Formalin fixed paraffin embedded; HNSCC: Head and neck squamous cell carcinoma; HPV: Human papilloma virus; MRI: Magnetic resonance imaging; MT: Mutant; NGS: Next-generation sequencing; PET: Positron emission tomography; WT: Wild type

Acknowledgements

R. de Weger and J. van Kuik helped establishing ddPCR in our lab. R. Noorlag initiated acquisition of biomaterials.

Funding

Sequencing and ddPCR assays were funded by the Dutch Cancer Society (clinical fellowship: 2011–4964) on behalf of SW.

Authors' contributions

JG, MH and SW conceived and designed the study. MH, SW, RB, and RE were involved in drafting and revising the manuscript critically for important intellectual content. RB and RE collected and provided biomaterials and clinicopathological data. JG and MH carried out the experiments. JG and MH analyzed and interpreted the data. JG wrote the manuscript. All authors read and approved the final manuscript.

Competing interests

The authors declare that they have no competing interests.

Author details

[1]Department of Oral and Maxillofacial Surgery, University Medical Center Utrecht, Utrecht, The Netherlands. [2]Department of Pathology, University Medical Center Utrecht, Heidelberglaan 100, 3584 CX Utrecht, The Netherlands. [3]Department of Head and Neck Surgical Oncology, UMC Utrecht Cancer Center, University Medical Center Utrecht, Utrecht, The Netherlands.

References

1. Ferlito A, Partridge M, Brennan J, Hamakawa H. Lymph node micrometastases in head and neck cancer: a review. Acta Otolaryngol. 2001;121:660–5.
2. de Bree R, van der Putten L, Brouwer J, Castelijns JA, Hoekstra OS, Leemans CR. Detection of locoregional recurrent head and neck cancer after (chemo)radiotherapy using modern imaging. Oral Oncol. 2009;45:386–93.
3. Muller J, Hullner M, Strobel K, Huber GF, Burger IA, Haerle SK. The value of (18) F-FDG-PET/CT imaging in oral cavity cancer patients following surgical reconstruction. Laryngoscope. 2015;125:1861–8.
4. Gleber-Netto FO, Braakhuis BJ, Triantafyllou A, Takes RP, Kelner N, Rodrigo JP, et al. Molecular events in relapsed oral squamous cell carcinoma: Recurrence vs. secondary primary tumor. Oral Oncol. 2015;51:738–44.
5. Yom SS, Machtay M, Biel MA, Sinard RJ, El-Naggar AK, Weber RS, et al. Survival impact of planned restaging and early surgical salvage following definitive chemoradiation for locally advanced squamous cell carcinomas of the oropharynx and hypopharynx. American Journal of Clinical Oncology-Cancer Clinical Trials. 2005;28:385–92.
6. Kalia M. Biomarkers for personalized oncology: recent advances and future challenges. Metabolism. 2015;64:S16–21.
7. Jahr S, Hentze H, Englisch S, Hardt D, Fackelmayer FO, Hesch RD, et al. DNA fragments in the blood plasma of cancer patients: Quantitations and evidence for their origin from apoptotic and necrotic cells. Cancer Res. 2001;61:1659–65.
8. Diaz LA Jr, Bardelli A. Liquid biopsies: genotyping circulating tumor DNA. J Clin Oncol. 2014;32:579–86.
9. Nemunaitis J, Clayman G, Agarwala SS, Hrushesky W, Wells JR, Moore C, et al. Biomarkers predict p53 gene therapy efficacy in recurrent squamous cell carcinoma of the head and neck. Clin Cancer Res. 2009;15:7719–25.
10. Lui VW, Hedberg ML, Li H, Vangara BS, Pendleton K, Zeng Y, et al. Frequent mutation of the PI3K pathway in head and neck cancer defines predictive biomarkers. Cancer Discov. 2013;3:761–9.
11. Ndiaye C, Mena M, Alemany L, Arbyn M, Castellsague X, Laporte L, et al. HPV DNA, E6/E7 mRNA, and p16INK4a detection in head and neck cancers: a systematic review and meta-analysis. Lancet Oncol. 2014;15:1319–31.
12. Koole K, Brunen D, van Kempen PM, Noorlag R, de Bree R, Lieftink C, et al. FGFR1 Is a Potential prognostic biomarker and therapeutic target in head and neck squamous cell carcinoma. Clin Cancer Res. 2016;22:3884–93.
13. Arantes LMRB, de Carvalho AC, Melendez ME, Carvalho AL, Goloni-Bertollo EM. Methylation as a biomarker for head and neck cancer. Oral Oncol. 2014;50:587–92.
14. Noorlag R, van Kempen PMW, Moelans CB, de Jong R, Blok LER, Koole R, et al. Promoter hypermethylation using 24-gene array in early head and neck cancer Better outcome in oral than in oropharyngeal cancer. Epigenetics. 2014;9:1220–7.
15. Zhang M, Zhao LJ, Liang WQ, Mao ZP. Identification of microRNAs as diagnostic biomarkers in screening of head and neck cancer: a meta-analysis. Genet Mol Res. 2015;14:16562–76.
16. Boyle JO, Hakim J, Koch W, van der Riet P, Hruban RH, Roa RA, et al. The incidence of p53 mutations increases with progression of head and neck cancer. Cancer Res. 1993;53:4477–80.
17. Nees M, Homann N, Discher H, Andl T, Enders C, Herold-Mende C, et al. Expression of mutated p53 occurs in tumor-distant epithelia of head and neck cancer patients: a possible molecular basis for the development of multiple tumors. Cancer Res. 1993;53:4189–96.
18. Hedberg ML, Goh G, Chiosea SI, Bauman JE, Freilino ML, Zeng Y, et al. Genetic landscape of metastatic and recurrent head and neck squamous cell carcinoma. J Clin Invest. 2016;126:169–80.
19. Morris LG, Chandramohan R, West L, Zehir A, Chakravarty D, Pfister DG, et al. The Molecular landscape of recurrent and metastatic head and neck cancers: insights from a precision oncology sequencing platform. JAMA Oncol. 2016;
20. Hiley C, de Bruin EC, McGranahan N, Swanton C. Deciphering intratumor heterogeneity and temporal acquisition of driver events to refine precision medicine. Genome Biol. 2014;15:453.
21. van Ginkel JH, de Leng WW, de Bree R, van Es RJ, Willems SM. Targeted sequencing reveals TP53 as a potential diagnostic biomarker in the post-treatment surveillance of head and neck cancer. Oncotarget. 2016;
22. Seiwert TY, Zuo ZX, Keck MK, Khattri A, Pedamallu CS, Stricker T, et al. Integrative and comparative genomic analysis of HPV-positive and HPV-negative head and neck squamous cell carcinomas. Clin Cancer Res. 2015;21:632–41.
23. Diehl F, Schmidt K, Choti MA, Romans K, Goodman S, Li M, et al. Circulating mutant DNA to assess tumor dynamics. Nat Med. 2008;14:985–90.
24. Dawson SJ, Tsui DWY, Murtaza M, Biggs H, Rueda OM, Chin SF, et al. Analysis of circulating tumor DNA to monitor metastatic breast cancer. N Engl J Med. 2013;368:1199–209.
25. Gray ES, Rizos H, Reid AL, Boyd SC, Pereira MR, Lo J, et al. Circulating tumor DNA to monitor treatment response and detect acquired resistance in patients with metastatic melanoma. Oncotarget. 2015;6:42008–18.
26. Reinert T, Scholer LV, Thomsen R, Tobiasen H, Vang S, Nordentoft I, et al. Analysis of circulating tumour DNA to monitor disease burden following colorectal cancer surgery. Gut. 2015;
27. Hindson CM, Chevillet JR, Briggs HA, Gallichotte EN, Ruf IK, Hindson BJ, et al. Absolute quantification by droplet digital PCR versus analog real-time PCR. Nat Methods. 2013;10:1003–5.
28. de Leng WW, Gadellaa-van Hooijdonk CG, Barendregt-Smouter FA, Koudijs MJ, Nijman I, Hinrichs JW, et al. Targeted Next generation sequencing as a reliable diagnostic assay for the detection of somatic mutations in tumours using minimal DNA amounts from formalin fixed paraffin embedded material. PLoS One. 2016;11:e0149405.
29. Hoogstraat M, Hinrichs JW, Besselink NJ, Radersma-van Loon JH, de Voijs CM, Peeters T, et al. Simultaneous detection of clinically relevant mutations and amplifications for routine cancer pathology. J Mol Diagn. 2015;17:10–8.
30. Huggett JF, Foy CA, Benes V, Emslie K, Garson JA, Haynes R, et al. The digital MIQE guidelines: minimum information for publication of quantitative digital PCR experiments. Clin Chem. 2013;59:892–902.
31. Qin Z, Ljubimov VA, Zhou C, Tong Y, Liang J. Cell-free circulating tumor DNA in cancer. Chin J Cancer. 2016;35:36.
32. Fleischhacker M, Schmidt B. Circulating nucleic acids (CNAs) and cancer–a survey. Biochim Biophys Acta. 2007;1775:181–232.
33. Rothwell DG, Smith N, Morris D, Leong HS, Li YY, Hollebecque A, et al. Genetic profiling of tumours using both circulating free DNA and circulating tumour cells isolated from the same preserved whole blood sample. Mol Oncol. 2016;10:566–74.
34. El Messaoudi S, Rolet F, Mouliere F, Thierry AR. Circulating cell free DNA: preanalytical considerations. Clin Chim Acta. 2013;424:222–30.
35. Swarup V, Rajeswari MR. Circulating (cell-free) nucleic acids - a promising, non-invasive tool for early detection of several human diseases. FEBS Lett. 2007;581:795–9.
36. Jung M, Klotzek S, Lewandowski M, Fleischhacker M, Jung K. Changes in concentration of DNA in serum and plasma during storage of blood samples. Clin Chem. 2003;49:1028–9.
37. Wang P, Jing F, Li G, Wu Z, Cheng Z, Zhang J, et al. Absolute quantification of lung cancer related microRNA by droplet digital PCR. Biosens Bioelectron. 2015;74:836–42.
38. Tang H, Cai Q, Li H, Hu P. Comparison of droplet digital PCR to real-time PCR for quantification of hepatitis B virus DNA. Biosci Biotechnol Biochem. 2016:1–6.
39. Ruelle J, Yfantis V, Duquenne A, Goubau P. Validation of an ultrasensitive digital droplet PCR assay for HIV-2 plasma RNA quantification. J Int AIDS Soc. 2014;17:19675.
40. Hindson BJ, Ness KD, Masquelier DA, Belgrader P, Heredia NJ, Makarewicz AJ, et al. High-throughput droplet digital PCR system for absolute quantitation of DNA copy number. Anal Chem. 2011;83:8604–10.
41. Pinheiro LB, Coleman VA, Hindson CM, Herrmann J, Hindson BJ, Bhat S, et al. Evaluation of a droplet digital polymerase chain reaction format for DNA copy number quantification. Anal Chem. 2012;84:1003–11.
42. Wang Y, Springer S, Mulvey CL, Silliman N, Schaefer J, Sausen M, et al. Detection of somatic mutations and HPV in the saliva and plasma of

patients with head and neck squamous cell carcinomas. Sci Transl Med. 2015;7:293ra104.

43. Bettegowda C, Sausen M, Leary RJ, Kinde I, Wang Y, Agrawal N, et al. Detection of circulating tumor DNA in early- and late-stage human malignancies. Sci Transl Med. 2014;6:224ra224.

44. Ignatiadis M, Lee M, Jeffrey SS. Circulating Tumor Cells and Circulating Tumor DNA: Challenges and Opportunities on the Path to Clinical Utility. Clin Cancer Res. 2015;21:4786–800.

45. Sozzi G, Roz L, Conte D, Mariani L, Andriani F, Verderio P, et al. Effects of prolonged storage of whole plasma or isolated plasma DNA on the results of circulating DNA quantification assays. J Natl Cancer Inst. 2005;97:1848–50.

46. Trypsteen W, Vynck M, De Neve J, Bonczkowski P, Kiselinova M, Malatinkova E, et al. ddpcRquant: threshold determination for single channel droplet digital PCR experiments. Anal Bioanal Chem. 2015;407:5827–34.

47. Devonshire AS, Whale AS, Gutteridge A, Jones G, Cowen S, Foy CA, et al. Towards standardisation of cell-free DNA measurement in plasma: controls for extraction efficiency, fragment size bias and quantification. Anal Bioanal Chem. 2014;406:6499–512.

48. Nygaard AD, Holdgaard PC, Spindler KLG, Pallisgaard N, Jakobsen A. The correlation between cell-free DNA and tumour burden was estimated by PET/CT in patients with advanced NSCLC. Br J Cancer. 2014;110:363–8.

49. Coulet F, Blons H, Cabelguenne A, Lecomte T, Lacourreye O, Brasnu D, et al. Detection of plasma tumor DNA in head and neck squamous cell carcinoma by microsatellite typing and p53 mutation analysis. Cancer Res. 2000;60:707–11.

50. Heitzer E, Ulz P, Geigl JB. Circulating tumor DNA as a liquid biopsy for cancer. Clin Chem. 2015;61:112–23.

51. Burrell RA, McGranahan N, Bartek J, Swanton C. The causes and consequences of genetic heterogeneity in cancer evolution. Nature. 2013; 501:338–45.

52. Netherlands. Medical research involving human subjects act. Bull Med Ethics. 1999;No. 152:13–8.

53. van Diest PJ. For and against - No consent should be needed for using leftover body material for scientific purposes - For. Br Med J. 2002;325:648–9.

7

Galectin 3 expression in primary oral squamous cell carcinomas

Manuel Weber[1]*（iD）, Maike Büttner-Herold[2], Luitpold Distel[3], Jutta Ries[1], Patrick Moebius[1], Raimund Preidl[1], Carol I. Geppert[4], Friedrich W. Neukam[1] and Falk Wehrhan[1]

Abstract

Background: Immunologic factors can promote the progression of oral squamous cell carcinomas (oscc). The phylogenetic highly conserved protein Galectin 3 (Gal3) contributes to cell differentiation and immune homeostasis. There is evidence that Gal3 is involved in the progression of oscc and influences the regulation of macrophage polarization. Macrophage polarization (M1 vs. M2) in solid malignancies like oscc contributes to tumor immune-escape. However, the relationship between macrophage polarization and Gal3 expression in oscc is not yet understood. The current study analyzes the association between histomorphologic parameters (T-, N-, L- Pn-status, grading) and Gal3 expression resp. the ratio between Gal3 expressing cells and CD68 positive macrophages in oscc specimens.

Methods: Preoperative diagnostic biopsies ($n = 26$) and tumor resection specimens ($n = 34$) of T1/T2 oscc patients were immunohistochemically analyzed for Gal3 and CD68 expression. The number of Gal3 expressing cells and the ratio between CD68 and Gal3 expressing cells was quantitatively assessed.

Results: In biopsy and tumor resection specimens, the number of Gal3 positive cells as well as the Gal3/CD68 ratio were significantly ($p < 0.05$) higher in T2 oscc compared to T1 cases. In biopsy specimens, a significantly ($p < 0.05$) increased Gal3 expression and Gal3/CD68 ratio was associated with the progression marker lymph vessel infiltration (L1). Tumor resection specimens of cases with lymph node metastases (N+) had a significantly ($p < 0.05$) increased Gal3 expression. Additionally, a high Gal3/CD68 ratio correlated significantly ($p < 0.05$) with higher grading (G3) in tumor resection specimens.

Conclusion: High Gal3 expression in oscc is associated with tumor size (T-status) and parameters of malignancy (N-, L-status, grading). Gal3 might contribute to M2 macrophage mediated local immune tolerance. Gal3 expression shows association with prognosis in oscc and represent a potential therapeutic target.

Keywords: Oral squamous cell carcinoma, Oral cancer, Galectin 3, Gal3, Macrophage polarization, oscc, M1, M2

Background

TNM classification and grading only partially predict the prognosis of patients with oral squamous cell carcinomas (oscc) and cannot explain individual clinical courses of the disease. For the progression of oscc, genetic mutations which lead to dysregulation of embryonic signaling pathways [1, 2] as well as immunologic factors play a significant role [3, 4]. The phylogenetic highly conserved protein Galectin 3 (Gal3) is an important mediator between cell differentiation and tumor immunity [5, 6] and contributes to the regulation of macrophage polarization [7, 8].

Tumors and their precursor lesions often reveal alterations of Gal3 expression. Accordingly, a possible contribution of Gal3 to the pathogenesis of pancreatic, colorectal, liver and esophageal cancer could already be shown [9]. There is evidence that Gal3 overexpression promotes malign transformation and metastatic spread [10]. Cancer patients showed increased serum Gal3 and a correlation of Gal3 levels with prognosis was detectable [10].

Evidence exists that Gal3 is also relevant for the progression of oscc. Some studies analyzed the role of Gal3 as prognostic factor especially in tongue cancer [11–13]. One immunohistochemical study in patients with tongue

* Correspondence: manuel.weber@uk-erlangen.de
[1]Department of Oral and Maxillofacial Surgery, Friedrich-Alexander University Erlangen-Nürnberg, Glueckstrasse 11, 91054 Erlangen, Germany
Full list of author information is available at the end of the article

cancer showed an association of Gal3 expression with dedifferentiation, metastases and poor prognosis [12]. Another report examined the expression of Gal3 in a cohort of exceptionally young patients with oscc in several locations without identifying a correlation with tumor stage or grading [14]. In addition to invasive squamous cell carcinomas, an increased expression of Gal3 could already be shown in precursor lesions of oral cancer [6, 15].

Due to its contribution to the regulation of macrophage polarization (M1 vs. M2), Gal3 is an important immune modulator [7, 8]. Macrophages are highly plastic cells involved in the formation of the tumor microenvironment and relevant for oscc prognosis [16] and therapy response [17, 18]. In this context M2 polarized macrophages contribute to immune tolerance and promote tumor progression and metastatic spread [18, 19]. Gal3 can shift macrophage polarization towards M2 [7].

Most studies analyzing Gal3 expression in oscc patients were performed in tongue cancer specimens and therefore only represent a subgroup of oscc. Gal3 expression in oscc was not yet analyzed in the context of a macrophage mediated immune-tolerant microenvironment in oscc. As an association of macrophage polarization with histomorphologic [3] and prognostic parameters [16] in oscc has already been shown, a comparative analysis of Gal3 and macrophage infiltration in oscc might elucidate an involved mediator.

Galectins like Gal3 are members of the lectins and are characterized by the ability to bind β-galactosides [20]. Galectins have a phylogenetically conserved structure and are involved in cellular proliferation, survival, adhesion and migration [20, 21]. With two functionally relevant protein domains, Gal3 is an unique member of the galectin family [20]. It can interact with a variety of intracellular and extracellular proteins and is involved in the pathogenesis of fibrotic and malign diseases as well as in immune regulation [20]. Gal3 can be detected in several human cells like immune cells and epithelial cells [10].

Because of its high degree of phylogenetic conservation, its properties in carcinogenesis and regulation of macrophage polarization, Gal3 could be a prognosticator in oscc patients [22, 23]. Moreover, as Gal3 inhibitors like citrus pectin are available, Gal3 could also be a target for molecular immune modulatory cancer therapy [22, 23].

The current study aims to answer the question if Gal3 expression and the ratio of Gal3 positive cells vs. CD68 positive macrophages in diagnostic biopsies and tumor resection specimens of oscc is associated with histomorphologic parameters (T-, N-, L-, Pn-status, grading) of tumor progression.

Methods

Patients and tissue harvesting

A consecutively treated oscc patient collective was selected for this retrospective study. The patient selection was described in previous reports [3, 24]. Biopsies and tumor resection specimens from a total of 34 patients histologically diagnosed with primary oscc were analyzed in this study. Tumor resection specimens from 34 patients and biopsies from 26 patients were available. The biopsies from nine cases were not available for analysis or too small for analysis. Because we counted macrophage infiltration in at least 1.1 mm^2 of carcinoma tissue, specimens with smaller carcinoma fractions were excluded. All patients were treated in 2011 at the Department of Oral and Maxillofacial Surgery of the University Hospital Erlangen. The study protocol was approved by the ethical committee of the University of Erlangen-Nuremberg (Ref.-No. 45_12 Bc). The specimens used in this study were obtained from tissue samples collected for routine histopathologic diagnosis. Each included specimen was judged to be a representative squamous cell carcinoma. In addition to the diagnosis of oscc, the following inclusion criteria were defined: pT1 or pT2 tumors, no restrictions in the grading of the tumor, no adjuvant preoperative radio- or chemotherapy and no distant metastasis at the time of diagnosis. Patients with former radio- or chemotherapy and pT3 and pT4 tumors were excluded. No study-related changes in the patients' treatments took place.

The patient cohort ($n = 34$) consisted of 11 tongue oscc, 11 patients with a tumor of the floor of the mouth, 8 with alveolar crest carcinomas, 3 with a tumor of the palate and 1 of the cheek. The average age of the patients (23 males and 11 females) was 63 years. The pathohistological classified N-status was N0 in 19 cases and N+ in 15 cases (including all positive N-states). The histological grading was G1 in 2 cases, G2 in 26 cases and G3 in 6 cases. None of the patients in our cohort had distant metastases.

Immunohistochemical staining and quantitative analysis

The immunohistochemical staining procedure was performed as previously described [3, 24]. The following primary antibodies were used: anti-Galectin 3 (sc-20,157, clone H-160, Santa Cruz, Dallas, Texas, USA) and anti-CD68 (11,081,401, clone KP1, Dako, Hamburg, Germany). An appropriate positive control was included in each series.

The tumor and biopsy sections were completely scanned and digitized using the method of "whole slide imaging". The scanning procedure was performed in cooperation with the Institute of Pathology of the University of Erlangen-Nürnberg using a Panoramic 250 Flash III Scanner (3D Histech, Budapest, Hungary) in 40× magnification. All samples were digitally analyzed (Case viewer, 3D Histech, Budapest, Hungary). Quality controls were performed using a bright-field microscope (Zeiss Axioskop and Axiocam 5, at 100–400 × magnification).

For each sample, three visual fields showing the highest infiltration rate of positive cells were selected (hot spot analysis). The complete area of all three visual fields of one specimen was between 1.1 and 1.5 mm^2 (Case viewer, 3D Histech, Budapest, Hungary).

Micrographs of the selected areas were imported into the Biomas analysis software (modular systems of applied biology, Erlangen, Germany) for cell counting. Two regions of interest were defined in the visual fields using the Biomas software: the epithelial tumor compartment and the stromal compartment.

A quantitative analysis was performed to determine the numbers of Galectin 3- and CD68-positive cells in the epithelial tumor compartment and the surrounding stroma. A Gal3 background staining, as it was visible in the epithelial tumor compartment of all cases, was not counted. Cells with strong Gal3 expression significantly surpassing the background expression of epithelial oscc

tumor cells were counted as positive. Assessment of the cell density per mm^2 was performed as previously described [16, 24].

Statistical analysis

To analyze the immunohistochemical staining, the cell count per mm^2 was determined as the number of positive cells per mm^2 of the specimen. Multiple measurements were pooled for each sample group prior to analysis. The results are expressed as the median and standard deviation (SD) and range. Box plot diagrams represent the median, the interquartile range, minimum (Min) and maximum (Max).

Two-sided, adjusted p-values ≤ 0.05 were considered to be significant. The analyses were performed using an ANOVA test with SPSS 22 for Mac OS (IBM Inc., New York, USA).

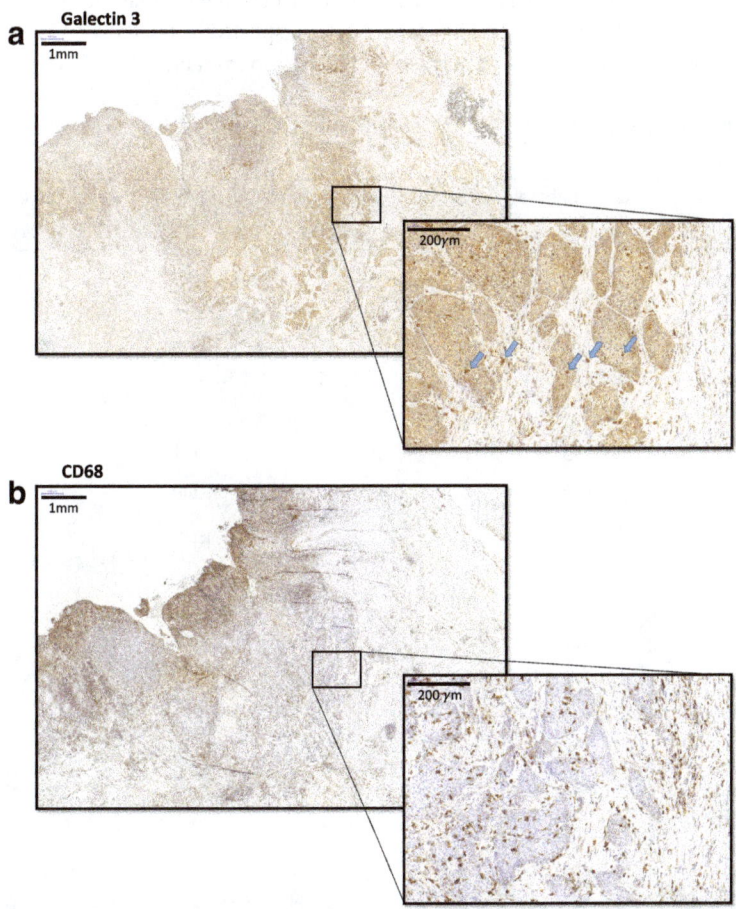

Fig. 1 Typical expression pattern of Galectin 3 and CD68 in a tumor resection specimen. The figure shows the typical expression pattern of Galectin 3 positive cells (**a**) and CD68 positive cells (**b**) in an oscc tumor resection specimen. A panoramic view (2.5× magnification) is given on the left side and a magnification of the indicated region (25× magnification) is displayed on the right side. The epithelial carcinoma cells show a weak expression of Gal3. The Gal3 highly positive cells in the epithelial compartment and the stromal compartment were counted for statistical assessment. Five Gal3 highly positive cells are exemplarily marked with an arrow

Results

General morphologic considerations

Galectin 3 (Gal3) was expressed in all investigated specimens. An expression of Gal3 could be observed in all cellular compartments (Fig. 1a). Oscc tumor cells in all patients showed a low level of Gal3 expression. For statistical analysis, the cells with a Gal3 expression significantly surpassing the background Gal3 staining of epithelial ossc tumor cells were counted. These cells could be found in the epithelial tumor compartment as well as in the tumor stroma. The distribution pattern of these Gal3 highly positive cells was similar to the distribution of CD68 positive macrophages (Fig. 1b). The number of CD68 positive macrophages exceeded the number of Gal3 highly positive cells (except in G3 oscc cases).

Galectin 3 expression in oscc biopsy specimens

Assessing the epithelial compartment of biopsy specimens, the Galectin 3 (Gal3) cell count in T2 oscc cases was significantly higher than in T1 cases (median 256 cells/mm^2 and 103 cells/mm^2, respectively, $p = 0.032$) (Table 1, Fig. 2a). Comparably, Gal3 expression in the whole analyzed specimen area (epithelial + stroma) of biopsies was significantly higher in T2 cases compared to T1 cases (median 293 cells/mm^2 and 101 cells/mm^2, respectively) ($p = 0.024$) (Table 1, Fig. 2b).

The ratio between Gal3-expressing cells and CD68-positive macrophages (Gal3/CD68-ratio) in the epithelial fraction of T2 oscc biopsy samples was significantly higher than in biopsies of T1 cases (median values 0.73 and 0.43, respectively, $p = 0.045$) (Table 1, Fig. 2c). The whole analyzed specimen area (epithelial + stroma) in T2 oscc biopsy specimens revealed a significantly higher Gal3/CD68-ratio than in T1 cases (median value 0.71 and 0.19, respectively, $p = 0.018$) (Table 1, Fig. 2d).

Oscc biopsy specimens in cases with lymph vessel infiltration (L1) showed a significantly higher Gal3 expression compared to L0 cases assessing the whole analyzed specimen area (epithelial + stroma) (median 369 cells/mm^2 and 110 cells/mm^2, respectively, $p = 0.013$) (Table 1, Fig. 2e).

The Gal3/CD68-ratio in the whole analyzed specimen area (epithelial + stroma) of biopsies from L1 oscc cases was significantly higher than in L0 cases (median value 0.95 and 0.31, respectively, $p = 0.008$) (Table 1, Fig. 2f). In the epithelial compartment, the Gal3/CD68-ratio in L1 biopsy

Table 1 Galectin 3 (Gal3) cell count (cells/mm2) and Gal3/CD68 expression ratio in oscc biopsy specimens

Gal3 expression in biopsy specimens									
Marker		Gal3 epithelial		Gal3 epithelial + stroma		Ratio Gal3/CD68 epithelial		Ratio Gal3/CD68 epithelial + stroma	
		Median	SD	Median	SD	Median	SD	Median	SD
T-Status	n								
T1	8	103	72	101	80	0.43	0.23	0.19	0.17
T2	17	256	170	293	162	0.73	0.60	0.71	0.61
p-value		0.032		0.024		0.045		0.018	
N-Status	n								
N0	13	111	174	93	175	0.53	0.61	0.30	0.66
N+	12	290	133	276	125	0.73	0.49	0.68	0.47
p-value		0.143		0.197		0.472		0.511	
L-Status	n								
L0	18	115	132	110	126	0.55	0.41	0.31	0.40
L1	7	323	192	369	169	0.88	0.69	0.95	0.71
p-value		0.054		0.013		0.020		0.008	
Pn-Status	n								
Pn0	13	170	138	124	134	0.58	0.43	0.35	0.43
Pn1	9	256	185	344	178	0.73	0.68	0.66	0.71
p-value		0.295		0.184		0.185		0.129	
Grading	n								
G2	16	170	136	179	130	0.59	0.41	0.57	0.44
G3	6	337	188	369	177	1.00	0.75	1.09	0.79
p-value		0.120		0.083		0.067		0.088	

Table shows the Galectin 3 (Gal3) cell count (positive cells/mm^2) and the ratio of Gal3 positive cells and CD68 positive cells in oscc biopsy specimens in view of histomorphologic parameters (T-, N-, L-, Pn-status, grading). Results for the epithelial tumor compartment and the whole analyzed area (epithelial + stroma) are given. Values represent the median, standard deviation (SD) and *p*-value (ANOVA)

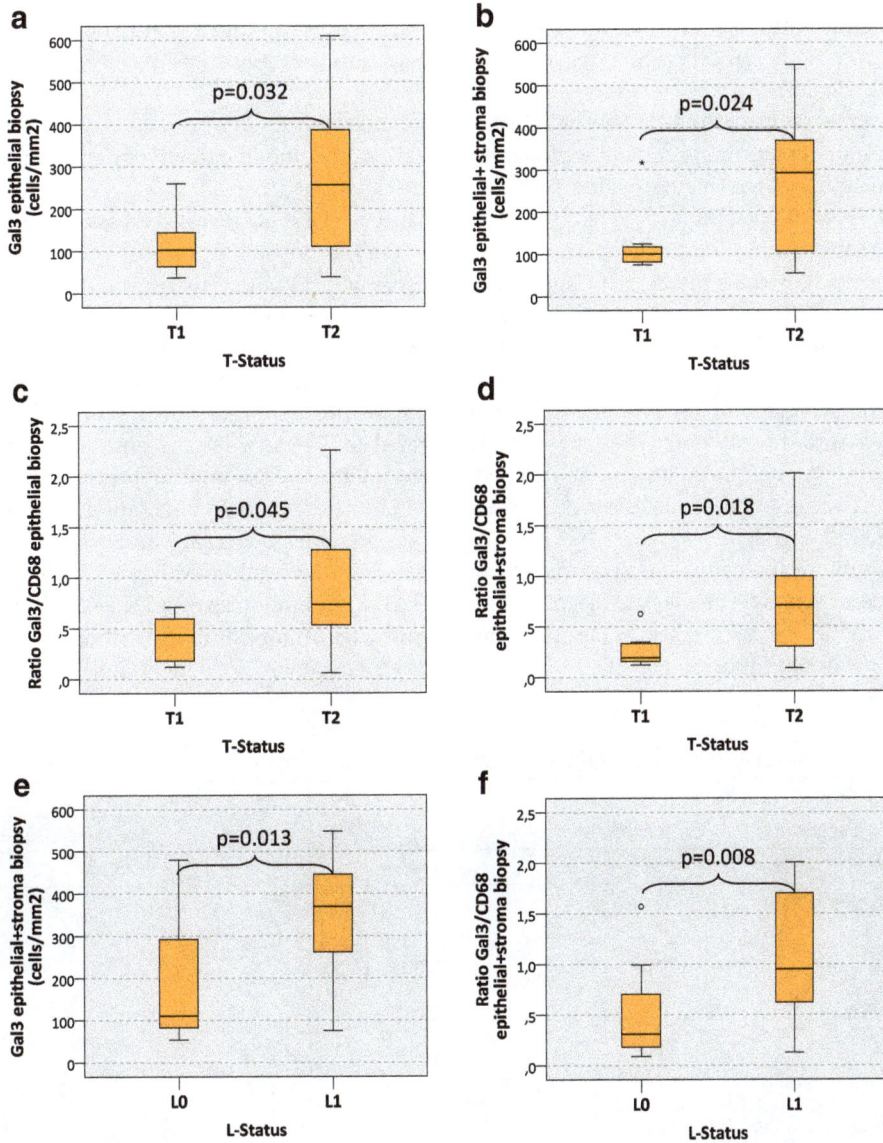

Fig. 2 Galectin 3 expression in biopsy specimens of oral squamous cell carcinomas depending on histomorphologic parameters. The **a** and **b** show the expression of Galectin 3 (Gal3) (cells/mm^2 specimen area) in the epithelial compartment (**a**) and in the whole analyzed specimen area (epithelial + stroma) (**b**) of oscc biopsy specimens depending on the T-status (T1 vs. T2). A significantly increased count of Gal3-positive cells can be found in the epithelial compartment and in the whole analyzed specimen area of T2 oscc biopsy specimens. The **c** and **d** show the ratio between the Gal3 cell count and the CD68 cell count (Gal3/CD68 ratio) in the epithelial compartment (**c**) and in the whole analyzed specimen area (epithelial + stroma) (**d**) of oscc biopsy specimens depending on the T-status (T1 vs. T2). A significantly increased Gal3/CD68 ratio can be found in the epithelial compartment and in the whole analyzed specimen area of T2 oscc biopsy specimens. The **e** and **f** show the expression of Gal3 (cells/mm^2 specimen area) (**e**) and the Gal3/CD68 ratio (**f**) in the whole analyzed specimen area (epithelial + stroma) of oscc biopsy specimens depending on the L-status (L0 vs. L1). A significantly increased count of Gal3-positive cells and a significantly increased Gal3/CD68 ratio can be found in L1 oscc biopsy specimens. *P*-values generated by the ANOVA test are indicated in all boxplots

specimens was also significantly higher than in L0 cases (median value 0.88 and 0.55, respectively, $p = 0.020$) (Table 1).

There was no significant association apparent between Gal3 expression and N-status, Pn-status and tumor grading in oscc biopsy specimens.

Galectin 3 expression in oscc tumor resection specimens

Analyzing the epithelial fraction of tumor resection specimens, the Galectin 3 (Gal3) cell count in T2 cases was significantly higher than in T1 cases (median 241 cells/mm^2 and 97 cells/mm^2, respectively, $p < 0.001$) (Table 2, Fig. 3a). In the whole analyzed specimen area (epithelial + stroma) of tumor resection samples the Gal3 expression in T2 cases was also significantly higher than in T1 cases (median 302 cells/mm^2 and 116 cells/mm^2, respectively, $p = 0.002$) (Table 2, Fig. 3b).

The Gal3/CD68 expression ratio in the epithelial fraction of T2 oscc tumor resection specimens was significantly higher than in T1 cases (median value 0.73 and 0.30, respectively, $p = 0.002$) (Table 2, Fig. 3c). The whole analyzed specimen area (epithelial + stroma) in T2 oscc tumor resection specimens also showed a significantly higher Gal3/CD68-ratio than in T1 cases (median value 0.58 and 0.24, respectively, $p = 0.010$) (Table 2, Fig. 3d).

The epithelial compartment of oscc tumor resection specimens in cases with lymph node metastases (N+) revealed a significantly higher Gal3 cell count than N0 cases (median 234 cells/mm^2 and 126 cells/mm^2, respectively, $p = 0.030$) (Table 2, Fig. 3e).

The Gal3/CD68-ratio in the epithelial compartment of G3 oscc tumor resection specimens was significantly higher compared to G2 cases (median value 1.31 and 0.52, respectively, $p = 0.008$) (Table 2, Fig. 3f).

There was no significant association apparent between Gal3 expression and L-status or Pn-status in oscc tumor resection specimens.

Discussion

Gal3 expression in oscc biopsy and tumor resection specimens

The current study revealed an association between Galectin 3 (Gal3) expression in oral squamous cell carcinoma (oscc) tissue and histomorphologic parameters of tumor progression (T-, N-, L-, Pn-stage, grading). In biopsy and tumor resection specimens, the number of Gal3 positive cells as well as the ratio between Gal3 expressing cells and CD68 positive macrophages was higher in T2 oscc cases compared to T1 cases (Figs. 2 and 3). Considering the tumor promoting and immunosuppressive function of Gal3 [23, 25], this finding could implicate that local immunosuppression promotes increasing tumor growth and consequently size. The correlation between tumor size (T-status) and Gal3 expression resp. Gal3/CD68 ratio was seen in the epithelial tumor compartment as well as the whole analyzed specimen area including stroma and epithelium

Table 2 Galectin 3 (Gal3) cell count (cells/mm2) and Gal3/CD68 expression ratio in oscc tumor resection specimens

Gal3 expression in tumor resection specimens

Marker		Gal3 epithelial		Gal3 epithelial + stroma		Ratio Gal3/CD68 epithelial		Ratio Gal3/CD68 epithelial + stroma	
		Median	SD	Median	SD	Median	SD	Median	SD
T-Status	n								
T1	14	97	48	116	129	0.30	0.29	0.24	0.27
T2	20	241	127	302	169	0.73	0.79	0.58	0.64
p-value		0.000		0.002		0.002		0.010	
N-Status	n								
N0	19	126	89	169	164	0.71	0.71	0.42	0.50
N+	15	234	156	287	182	0.59	0.78	0.57	0.66
p-value		0.030		0.106		0.943		0.337	
L-Status	n								
L0	25	180	138	195	190	0.71	0.74	0.45	0.65
L1	9	203	115	223	143	0.59	0.74	0.46	0.26
p-value		0.892		0.999		0.834		0.595	
Pn-Status	n								
Pn0	21	130	134	191	206	0.48	0.68	0.42	0.67
Pn1	10	199	138	232	134	0.66	0.86	0.56	0.44
p-value		0.452		0.959		0.942		0.679	
Grading	n								
G2	26	155	132	194	169	0.52	0.46	0.45	0.44
G3	6	254	142	232	246	1.31	1.11	0.56	0.96
p-value		0.422		0.528		0.008		0.183	

Table shows the Galectin 3 (Gal3) cell count (positive cells/mm^2) and the ratio of Gal3 positive cells and CD68 positive cells in oscc tumor resection specimens depending on histomorphologic parameters (T-, N-, L-, Pn-status, grading). Results for the epithelial tumor compartment and the whole analyzed area (epithelial + stroma) are given. Values represent the median, standard deviation (SD) and p-value (ANOVA)

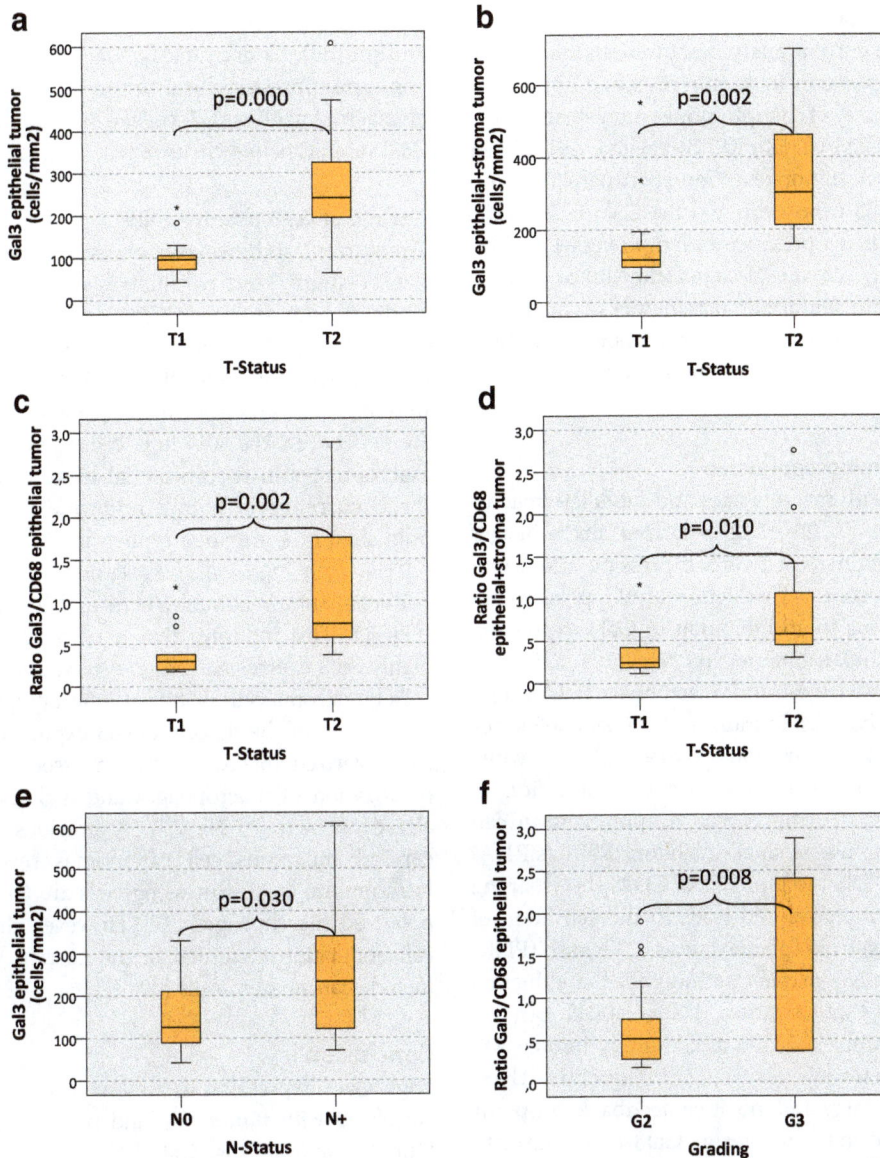

Fig. 3 Galectin 3 expression in tumor resection specimens of oral squamous cell carcinomas depending on histomorphologic parameters. The **a** and **b** show the expression of Galectin 3 (Gal3) (cells/mm² specimen area) in the epithelial compartment (**a**) and in the whole analyzed specimen area (epithelial + stroma) (**b**) of oscc tumor resection specimens depending on the T-status (T1 vs. T2). A significantly increased count of Gal3-positive cells can be found in the epithelial compartment and in the whole analyzed specimen area of T2 oscc tumor resection specimens. The **c** and **d** show the ratio between the Gal3 cell count and the CD68 cell count (Gal3/CD68 ratio) in the epithelial compartment (**c**) and in the whole analyzed specimen area (epithelial + stroma) (**d**) of oscc tumor resection specimens depending on the T-status (T1 vs. T2). A significantly increased Gal3/CD68 ratio can be found in the epithelial compartment and in the whole analyzed specimen area of T2 oscc tumor resection specimens. **e** shows the expression of Gal3 (cells/mm² specimen area) in the epithelial compartment of oscc tumor resection specimens depending on the N-status (N0 vs. N+). A significantly increased count of Gal3-positive cells can be found in N+ oscc tumor resection specimens. **f** shows the Gal3/CD68 ratio in the epithelial compartment of oscc tumor resection specimens depending on the grading (G2 vs. G3). A significantly increased Gal3/CD68 ratio is detected in the epithelial compartment of G3 oscc tumor resection specimens. P-values generated by the ANOVA test are indicated in all boxplots

(Figs. 2a-d and 3a-d). In a previous study in the patient cohort analyzed here, no association was detected between T-status and the density of CD68 positive macrophages [3].

An association between Gal3 expression and T-status was seen in biopsies and in tumor resection specimens. As previously reported, there are immunologic changes

in tumor tissue occurring during the time interval between the diagnostic biopsy and the definitive tumor resection [24]. The association between T-status and Gal3 expression in biopsies and tumor resection samples observed in the current report (Fig. 2a-d and 3a-d) indicates that Gal3 might be a possible robust biologic parameter that is not relevantly influenced by biopsy-derived tissue trauma.

Additionally, the current analysis showed an association of higher Gal3 expression in tumor resection specimens with the occurrence of lymph node metastases (N+) (Fig. 3e). A high Gal3/CD68 ratio correlated with higher grading (G3) in oscc tumor resection specimens (Fig. 3f). In biopsies, the Gal3 expression and the Gal3/CD68 ratio was associated with the presence of lymph vessel infiltration (L1) (Fig. 2e-f). As the N-status, the tumor grading and the L-status are important parameters of malignant behavior, the association of Gal3 expression with these parameters underlines a possible tumor-promoting role of Gal3 in oscc.

Gal3 mediated immunosuppression
Gal3 can interact with macrophages and modulate macrophage polarization [7, 26]. M2 polarized macrophages show a significantly increased Gal3 expression and secretion [7, 26, 27]. In contrast, induction of M1 polarization in macrophages leads to an inhibition of Gal3 expression compared to unstimulated monocytes [7].

Additionally, Gal3 itself can shift macrophage polarization towards M2 polarized cells. In murine cells, Gal3 deficiency prevented the M2 polarization of macrophages while there was no influence observed on the induction of M1 polarization [7]. Furthermore, M2 polarization can be prevented by the use of small inhibitory RNA (siRNA) for Gal3 or for the Gal3 receptor CD98. CD98 shows strong expression on macrophages and leads to the activation of the second messenger phosphatidylinositol 3-kinase (PI3K) [7]. PI3K activation is a relevant pathway for the induction of M2 macrophage polarization. Hence, Gal3 can induce PI3K activation via CD98 and thereby induce M2 polarization of macrophages [7]. Consequently, there might be a Gal3 triggered positive feedback loop for M2 polarization of macrophages as Gal3 contributes to the induction of M2 polarization and M2 macrophages show an increased Gal3 production [7].

This loop could be targeted by pharmacologic inhibition of Gal3 e.g. with citrus pectin [25] or by blocking CD98 [7]. As we detected an association of Gal3 with parameters of malignancy in oscc, targeting the Gal3 – CD98 – PI3K pathway could be a potential immune modulating treatment option for oral cancer patients.

These findings suggest the possibility of an increased Gal3 production in the context of a malign disease leading to an increased degree of M2 polarization of macrophages. On the other hand, it would be conceivable that macrophage-derived Gal3 itself leads to a promotion of malign transformation and metastatic spread of oscc tumor cells. Besides its influence on macrophage polarization, Gal3 can inhibit T-cell activation by destabilizing the immunologic synapse [28]. Additionally, Gal3 can inhibit CD8 positive cytotoxic T-cells in an LAG-3 dependent manner and thereby contribute to local immune tolerance and tumor promotion [29]. Consequently, Gal3 could contribute to an immunosuppressive local tumor environment at the level of macrophages and T-cells which could be targeted by Gal3 inhibitors like citrus pectin [25].

Lineage of Gal3 positive cells
The current study reveals an association between tumor size (T-status) and parameters of malignancy (L-status, grading) with the Gal3/CD68 ratio. In most cases the detected Gal3/CD68 ratio was smaller than 1, meaning that less Gal3-positive cells than CD68-positive macrophages were present in the specimens (Tables 1 and 2). An association between the absolute cell count of CD68-positive macrophages in the epithelial tumor compartment and the occurrence of lymph node metastases was already published in a previous report of our group [3].

Cells with high Gal3 expression were detected in the epithelial tumor compartment and in the tumor stroma (Fig. 1). This indicates that a relevant proportion of the highly Gal3 expressing cells in oscc specimens are no tumor cells but stroma cells or tumor infiltrating immune cells.

One part of the detected Gal3 expressing cells might be M2 polarized macrophages. An association between M2 polarization of macrophages and high Gal3 expression is already shown [7, 26, 27]. A previous report analyzing cervical squamous cell carcinomas revealed that many intratumoral Gal3 expressing cells are CD163 positive M2 polarized macrophages [27]. However, the Gal 3 positive cell population identified in the current study might also include cancer stem cells [30, 31].

Conclusion
High Gal3 expression as well as a high Gal3/CD68 ratio correlated with tumor size and parameters of malignancy. Our data indicate that Gal3 has a negative tumorbiological influence on oral squamous cell carcinomas (oscc) and we hypothesize that it might exert this influence via a modulation of macrophage polarization. Further studies are needed to identify the exact lineage of the Gal3 expressing cells in oscc tumor epithelium and stroma and the mechanisms by which Gal3 influences macrophage polarization and immune surveillance. Gal3 might serve as a target of immune therapy in oscc as Gal3 inhibitors like citrus pectin are available.

Abbreviations
Gal3: Galectin 3; LAG-3: Lymphocyte-activation gene 3; M1: M1 polarized macrophages; M2: M2 polarized macrophages; oscc: Oral squamous cell carcinoma; PI3K: Phosphatidylinositol 3-kinase; SD: Standard deviation; siRNA: Small inhibitory RNA

Acknowledgements
The authors thank Peter Hyckel for his contribution to the discussion and to the interpretation of the findings.

We thank Susanne Schoenherr and Elke Diebel for technical assistance. We also thank the dental students/research fellows Stafanie Queeney and Xiaoquin Lu for processing the tissue specimens, operating the immunohistochemistry autostainer apparatus and performing the cell counting.

Funding
This study was financially supported by the foundation "ELAN Fonds der Universität Erlangen" (grant to Manuel Weber in 2012). The funding body had no role in the design of the study and collection, analysis, and interpretation of data and in writing the manuscript.

Authors' contributions
The authors' initials are used. MW formulated the hypothesis, applied for grant support (ELAN-Fonds, University of Erlangen-Nürnberg), initiated and conducted the study, interpreted the data and wrote the manuscript. FW formulated the hypothesis, interpreted the data and contributed relevantly to the manuscript. MB and JR helped validate the markers, contributed to the discussion and critically reviewed the manuscript. LD helped optimizing the cell counting procedure, contributed to the discussion and critically reviewed the manuscript. PM and CG performed the digitalization of the specimens, helped with cell counting and critically reviewed the manuscript. FN and RP contributed to the discussion and critically reviewed the manuscript. All authors read and approved the final manuscript.

Competing interests
The authors declare that they have no competing interests.

Author details
[1]Department of Oral and Maxillofacial Surgery, Friedrich-Alexander University Erlangen-Nürnberg, Glueckstrasse 11, 91054 Erlangen, Germany. [2]Institute of Pathology, Department of Nephropathology, Friedrich-Alexander University Erlangen-Nürnberg, Erlangen, Germany. [3]Department of Radiation Oncology, Friedrich-Alexander University Erlangen-Nürnberg, Erlangen, Germany. [4]Institute of Pathology, Friedrich-Alexander University Erlangen-Nürnberg, Erlangen, Germany.

References
1. Scanlon CS, Van Tubergen EA, Inglehart RC, D'Silva NJ. Biomarkers of epithelial-mesenchymal transition in squamous cell carcinoma. J Dent Res. 2013;92(2):114–21.
2. Tsantoulis PK, Kastrinakis NG, Tourvas AD, Laskaris G, Gorgoulis VG. Advances in the biology of oral cancer. Oral Oncol. 2007;43(6):523–34.
3. Weber M, Buttner-Herold M, Hyckel P, Moebius P, Distel L, Ries J, Amann K, Neukam FW, Wehrhan F. Small oral squamous cell carcinomas with nodal lymphogenic metastasis show increased infiltration of M2 polarized macrophages–an immunohistochemical analysis. J Craniomaxillofac Surg. 2014;42(7):1087–94.
4. Feller L, Altini M, Lemmer J. Inflammation in the context of oral cancer. Oral Oncol. 2013;49(9):887–92.
5. Wehrhan F, Hyckel P, Guentsch A, Nkenke E, Stockmann P, Schlegel KA, Neukam FW, Amann K. Bisphosphonate-associated osteonecrosis of the jaw is linked to suppressed TGFbeta1-signaling and increased Galectin-3 expression: a histological study on biopsies. J Transl Med. 2011;9:102.
6. Hossaka TA, Focchi GR, Oshima CT, Ribeiro DA. Detection of galectins during malignant transformation of oral cells. Dental Res J. 2013;10(4):428–33.
7. AC MK, Farnworth SL, Hodkinson PS, Henderson NC, Atkinson KM, Leffler H, Nilsson UJ, Haslett C, Forbes SJ, Sethi T. Regulation of alternative macrophage activation by galectin-3. J Immunol. 2008;180(4):2650–8.
8. Jia W, Kidoya H, Yamakawa D, Naito H, Takakura N. Galectin-3 accelerates M2 macrophage infiltration and angiogenesis in tumors. Am J Pathol. 2013; 182(5):1821–31.
9. Song L, Tang JW, Owusu L, Sun MZ, Wu J, Zhang J. Galectin-3 in cancer. Clin Chim Acta. 2014;431:185–91.
10. Newlaczyl AU, Yu LG. Galectin-3–a jack-of-all-trades in cancer. Cancer Lett. 2011;313(2):123–8.
11. Honjo Y, Inohara H, Akahani S, Yoshii T, Takenaka Y, Yoshida J, Hattori K, Tomiyama Y, Raz A, Kubo T. Expression of cytoplasmic galectin-3 as a prognostic marker in tongue carcinoma. Clin Cancer Res. 2000;6(12):4635–40.
12. Alves PM, Godoy GP, Gomes DQ, Medeiros AM, de Souza LB, da Silveira EJ, Vasconcelos MG, Queiroz LM. Significance of galectins-1, −3, −4 and −7 in the progression of squamous cell carcinoma of the tongue. Pathol Res Pract. 2011;207(4):236–40.
13. Wang LP, Chen SW, Zhuang SM, Li H, Song M. Galectin-3 accelerates the progression of oral tongue squamous cell carcinoma via a Wnt/beta-catenin-dependent pathway. Pathol Oncol Res. 2013;19(3):461–74.
14. Mesquita JA, Queiroz LM, Silveira EJ, Gordon-Nunez MA, Godoy GP, Nonaka CF, Alves PM. Association of immunoexpression of the galectins-3 and -7 with histopathological and clinical parameters in oral squamous cell carcinoma in young patients. Eur Arch Otorhinolaryngol. 2016;273(1):237–43.
15. Hossaka TA, Ribeiro DA, Focchi G, Andre S, Fernandes M, Lopes Carapeto FC, Silva MS, Oshima CT. Expression of Galectins 1, 3 and 9 in normal oral epithelium, oral squamous papilloma, and oral squamous cell carcinoma. Dental research journal. 2014;11(4):508–12.
16. Weber M, Iliopoulos C, Moebius P, Buttner-Herold M, Amann K, Ries J, Preidl R, Neukam FW, Wehrhan F. Prognostic significance of macrophage polarization in early stage oral squamous cell carcinomas. Oral Oncol. 2016;52:75–84.
17. Okubo M, Kioi M, Nakashima H, Sugiura K, Mitsudo K, Aoki I, Taniguchi H, Tohnai I. M2-polarized macrophages contribute to neovasculogenesis, leading to relapse of oral cancer following radiation. Sci Rep. 2016;6:27548.
18. Balermpas P, Rodel F, Liberz R, Oppermann J, Wagenblast J, Ghanaati S, Harter PN, Mittelbronn M, Weiss C, Rodel C, et al. Head and neck cancer relapse after chemoradiotherapy correlates with CD163+ macrophages in primary tumour and CD11b+ myeloid cells in recurrences. Br J Cancer. 2014; 111(8):1509–18.
19. Wehrhan F, Buttner-Herold M, Hyckel P, Moebius P, Preidl R, Distel L, Ries J, Amann K, Schmitt C, Neukam FW, et al. Increased malignancy of oral squamous cell carcinomas (oscc) is associated with macrophage polarization in regional lymph nodes - an immunohistochemical study. BMC Cancer. 2014;14:522.
20. Dumic J, Dabelic S, Flogel M. Galectin-3: an open-ended story. Biochim Biophys Acta. 2006;1760(4):616–35.
21. Liu FT. Regulatory roles of galectins in the immune response. Int Arch Allergy Immunol. 2005;136(4):385–400.
22. Nangia-Makker P, Hogan V, Honjo Y, Baccarini S, Tait L, Bresalier R, Raz A. Inhibition of human cancer cell growth and metastasis in nude mice by oral intake of modified citrus pectin. J Natl Cancer Inst. 2002;94(24):1854–62.
23. Ruvolo PP. Galectin 3 as a guardian of the tumor microenvironment. Biochim Biophys Acta. 2016;1863(3):427-37.
24. Weber M, Moebius P, Buttner-Herold M, Amann K, Preidl R, Neukam FW, Wehrhan F. Macrophage polarisation changes within the time between diagnostic biopsy and tumour resection in oral squamous cell carcinomas–an immunohistochemical study. Br J Cancer. 2015;113(3):510–9.
25. Ahmed H, AlSadek DM. Galectin-3 as a potential target to prevent cancer metastasis. Clin Med Insights Oncol. 2015;9:113–21.
26. Novak R, Dabelic S, Dumic J. Galectin-1 and galectin-3 expression profiles in classically and alternatively activated human macrophages. Biochim Biophys Acta. 2012;1820(9):1383–90.
27. Punt S, Thijssen VL, Vrolijk J, de Kroon CD, Gorter A, Jordanova ES. Galectin-1, −3 and −9 expression and clinical significance in Squamous cervical cancer. PLoS One. 2015;10(6):e0129119.
28. Chen HY, Fermin A, Vardhana S, Weng IC, Lo KF, Chang EY, Maverakis E, Yang RY, Hsu DK, Dustin ML, et al. Galectin-3 negatively regulates TCR-mediated CD4+ T-cell activation at the immunological synapse. Proc Natl Acad Sci U S A. 2009;106(34):14496–501.
29. Kouo T, Huang L, Pucsek AB, Cao M, Solt S, Armstrong T, Jaffee E. Galectin-3 shapes antitumor immune responses by suppressing CD8+ T cells via LAG-3 and inhibiting expansion of Plasmacytoid Dendritic cells. Cancer Immunol Res. 2015;3(4):412–23.
30. Ilmer M, Mazurek N, Byrd JC, Ramirez K, Hafley M, Alt E, Vykoukal J, Bresalier RS. Cell surface galectin-3 defines a subset of chemoresistant gastrointestinal tumor-initiating cancer cells with heightened stem cell characteristics. Cell Death Dis. 2016;7(8):e2337.

8

Clinicopathological factors influencing the outcomes of surgical treatment in patients with T4a hypopharyngeal cancer

Sang-Yeon Kim[1], Young-Soo Rho[2], Eun-Chang Choi[3], Min-Sik Kim[1], Joo-Hyun Woo[4], Dong Hoon Lee[5], Eun Jae Chung[6], Min Woo Park[2], Da-Hee Kim[3] and Young-Hoon Joo[1,7]* (iD)

Abstract

Background: The purpose of this study was to determine prognostic factors influencing outcomes of surgical treatment in patients with T4a hypopharyngeal cancer.

Methods: The present study enrolled 93 patients diagnosed with T4a hypopharyngeal cancer who underwent primary surgery between January 2005 and December 2015 at six medical centers in Korea. Primary tumor sites included pyriform sinus in 71 patients, posterior pharyngeal wall in 14 patients, and postcricoid region in 8 patients. Seventy-two patients received postoperative radio(chemo)therapy.

Results: Five-year disease-free survival (DFS) and disease-specific survival (DSS) rates were 38% and 45%, respectively. In univariate analysis, 5-year DFS was found to have significant and positive correlations with margin involvement ($p < 0.001$) and extracapsular spread ($p = 0.025$). Multivariate analysis confirmed that margin involvement (hazard ratio (HR): 2.81; 95% confidence interval (CI): 1.49-5.30; $p = 0.001$) and extracapsular spread (HR: 2.08; 95% CI: 1.08-3.99; $p = 0.028$) were significant factors associated with 5-year DFS. In univariate analysis, cervical lymph node metastasis ($p = 0.048$), lymphovascular invasion ($p = 0.041$), extracapsular spread ($p = 0.015$), and esophageal invasion ($p = 0.033$) were significant factors associated with 5-year DSS. In multivariate analysis, extracapsular spread (HR: 2.98; 95% CI: 1.39-6.42; $p = 0.005$) and esophageal invasion (HR: 2.87; 95% CI: 1.38-5.98; $p = 0.005$) remained significant factors associated with 5-year DSS.

Conclusion: Margin involvement and extracapsular spread are factors influencing recurrence while extracapsular spread and esophageal invasion are factors affecting survival in patients with T4a hypopharyngeal cancer treated by primary surgery.

Keywords: Head and neck neoplasms, Hypopharynx, Squamous cell carcinoma, Surgery, Treatment outcome

Background

Hypopharyngeal cancer represents approximately 7% of all cancers of the upper aerodigestive tract. More than 95% of these cancers are squamous cell carcinomas [1]. Among head and neck cancers, hypopharyngeal squamous cell carcinoma (HPSCC) is known to have the worst prognosis. In one literature, 5-year survival rates for stage III and IV HPSCC have been reported to be 36% and 24%, respectively [2]. A relatively poor prognosis and frequently advanced stage at diagnosis are due to the relative lack of symptoms for early-stage of this disease at this region.

Treatment for HPSCC remains controversial. Some authors advocate for the use of primary radiotherapy alone or in combination with chemotherapy for HPSCC [3–6]. However, treatment of T4a HPSCC continues to fuel debate. Because HPSCC is a relatively rare disease, optimal initial treatment for T4a HPSCC has not been evaluated in any large, prospective, randomized study. Patients exhibiting cartilage invasion have poorer survival

* Correspondence: joodoct@catholic.ac.kr
[1]Department of Otolaryngology-Head and Neck Surgery, College of Medicine, The Catholic University of Korea, Seoul, Republic of Korea
[7]Department of Otolaryngology, Head and Neck Surgery, Bucheon St. Mary's Hospital, College of Medicine, The Catholic University of Korea, 2 Sosa-dong, Wonmi-gu, Bucheon, Kyounggi-do 420-717, Republic of Korea
Full list of author information is available at the end of the article

outcomes after irradiation. Therefore, T4a HPSCC with thyroid cartilage invasion is considered a distinct subcategory [7]. Clinical practice guidelines recommend upfront hypopharyngectomy with adjuvant radiotherapy for T4a HPSCC because rates of successful salvage surgery after failure of nonsurgical treatment are low [8]. The objective of this study was to present treatment results of primary surgery and identify possible prognostic factors affecting treatment outcomes in patients with T4a HPSCC.

Methods

Patients with pathologically confirmed HPSCC were recruited from six general hospitals for this multicenter study organized by a research committee of the Korea Society of Thyroid Head and Neck Surgery. Data for the following clinicopathological parameters in patients with T4a HPSCC who underwent primary surgery between 2005 and 2015 were collected: age, gender, comorbidities, tumor site and stage, postoperative treatment, pathologic specimen analysis, tumor recurrence, death, and cause of death. Tumor stage was determined based on the 2009 American Joint Committee on Cancer TNM classification. Data for a total of 416 patients with T4a HPSCC who underwent primary surgery over the 11-year period (2005 to 2015) were collected from the six centers. Among these patients, 323 were excluded because they received chemoradiotherapy for primary treatment or had recurrence of the primary tumor. Finally, a total of 93 patients were included in the study. Their mean follow-up period was 26.1 months (range, 1–118 months). Those who had positive or close margins and those with advanced T stage, lymphovascular invasion, perineural invasion, multiple nodal metastases, or extracapsular spread received additional treatment.

Statistical analysis

Survival was determined using the Kaplan-Meier method. Relationships between categorical variables were analyzed by Fisher's exact test or Chi-square test. A p-value of less than 0.05 was considered statistically significant. All calculations were performed using SPSS software ver. 16.0 (SPSS, Chicago, IL, USA). Disease-free survival (DFS) was defined as the time from the date of commencement of treatment to tumor recurrence. Disease-specific survival (DSS) was defined as the time from the first day of treatment to the date of death from hypopharyngeal cancer.

Results

Patient demographics

The male to female ratio was 86:7. The median age of all patients was 63.5 years (range, 34–84 years). Primary tumor sites included pyriform sinus in 71 patients, posterior pharyngeal wall in 14 patients, and postcricoid region in 8 patients. Regarding pathologic disease stage of

cervical lymph nodes, 12, 8, 2, 41, 25, and 5 patients were found to have stage N0, N1, N2a, N2b, N2c, and N3, respectively. Detailed patient characteristics are summarized in Table 1.

Regarding surgery types, total laryngectomy with partial pharyngectomy was performed in 41 patients, while

Table 1 Demographic profiles of patients with T4a hypopharyngeal squamous cell carcinoma ($n = 93$)

Parameter	No of patients (%)
Age (years)	
≤ 60	65 (69.9)
> 60	28 (30.1)
Gender	
Male	86 (92.5)
Female	7 (7.5)
Primary tumor site	
Pyriform sinus	71 (76.3)
Posterior pharyngeal wall	14 (15.1)
Postcricoid region	8 (8.6)
N classification	
N0	12 (12.9)
N1	8 (8.6)
N2a	2 (2.2)
N2b	41 (44.1)
N2c	25 (26.9)
N3	5 (5.4)
Adjuvant therapy	
Radiation only	33 (35.5)
Concurrent chemoradiation	39 (41.9)
None	21 (22.6)
Margin involvement	
Yes	27 (29.0)
No	66 (71.0)
Histologic differentiation	
Well differentiated	18 (19.4)
Moderately differentiated	56 (60.2)
Poorly differentiated	11 (11.8)
Unknown	8 (8.6)
Lymphovascular invasion	
Yes	56 (60.2)
No	30 (32.3)
Unknown	7 (7.5)
Extracapsular spread	
Yes	46 (49.5)
No	40 (43.0)
Unknown	7 (7.5)

partial laryngectomy with partial pharyngectomy was performed in 18 patients. Total laryngopharyngectomy with cervical esophagectomy was performed in 12 patients. Total laryngopharyngectomy was performed in 11 patients. Total laryngopharyngoesophagectomy was also performed in 11 patients (Table 2). For reconstruction of hypopharyngeal defects, radial forearm free flap was performed in 34 patients, anterolateral thigh free flap was performed in 11 patients, gastric pull-up was performed in 11 patients, pectoralis major myocutaneous flap was performed in 10 patients, and jejunal free flap was performed in 7 patients. Three kinds of adjuvant chemotherapy regimens were used for these patients: cisplatin, cisplatin plus 5-fluorouracil, and cetuximab. Radiation dose ranged from 4000 cGy to 6640 cGy, with a median dose of 6048 cGy.

Disease-free survival

Recurrences or metastases occurred in 46 patients. Eighteen cases had distant metastasis while 14 cases had both regional recurrence and distant metastasis. Eleven cases had recurrence or metastasis in the neck. One case of recurrence or metastasis was found at the primary site. One case had both local and regional recurrences while one case had both local recurrence and distant metastasis. The recurrence rate was 49.5% (46/93) over a mean observation period of 26.1 months. Five-year DFS was 38%. Five-year survival rates for each contributing clinicopathologic factor analyzed are shown in Table 3. In univariate analysis, resection margin involvement ($p < 0.001$) and extracapsular spread ($p = 0.025$) were significant prognostic factors for DFS (Fig. 1). In multivariate analysis, margin involvement (hazard ratio (HR):

Table 2 Primary surgery and reconstruction types

	No of patients (%)
Primary Surgery	
Partial laryngectomy with partial pharyngectomy	18 (19.4)
Total laryngectomy with partial pharyngectomy	41 (44.1)
Total laryngopharyngectomy	11 (11.8)
Total laryngopharyngectomy with cervical esophagectomy	12 (12.9)
Total laryngopharyngoesophagectomy	11 (11.8)
Reconstruction	
Radial forearm free flap	34 (36.6)
Anterolateral thigh free flap	11 (11.8)
Pectoralis major myocutaneous flap	10 (10.8)
Gastric pull-up	11 (11.8)
Jejunal free flap	7 (7.5)
Primary closure	20 (21.5)

Table 3 Log-Rank test for clinicopathological factors

Parameter	DFS (%)	p value	DSS (%)	p value
Age		0.437		0.216
≥ 60 yrs	38		41	
< 60 yrs	46		57	
Gender		0.437		0.520
Male	37		44	
Female	41		53	
Primary tumor site		0.148		0.554
Pyriform sinus	38		45	
Posterior pharyngeal wall	32		32	
Postcricoid region	50		62	
Cervical metastasis		0.301		0.048*
Yes	34		40	
No	57		78	
Adjuvant therapy		0.316		0.106
Radiation only	39		54	
Concurrent chemoradiation	34		34	
None	59		71	
Margin involvement		<0.001*		0.124
Yes	0		27	
No	48		53	
Histologic differentiation		0.399		0.244
Well differentiated	57		68	
Moderately differentiated	36		43	
Poorly differentiated	32		30	
Lymphovascular invasion		0.426		0.041*
Yes	35		34	
No	41		63	
Extracapsular spread		0.025*		0.015*
Yes	28		34	
No	50		61	
Esophageal invasion		0.197		0.033*
Yes	21		30	
No	43		52	

DFS Disease-free survival, *DSS* disease-specific survival
*Significant at $p < 0.05$

2.81; 95% confidence interval (CI): 1.49-5.30; $p = 0.001$) and extracapsular spread (HR: 2.08; 95% CI: 1.08-3.99; $p = 0.028$) remained significant predictors for unfavorable 5-year DFS. Adjuvant (chemo)radiotherapy rate for patients with margin positive was 77.8% (21 out of 27 patients). It was 82.6% (38 out of 46 patients) for patients with extracapsular spread. However, there was no significant difference in DFS between the group receiving adjuvant (chemo)radiotherapy and those without receiving such therapy ($p = 0.790$ for

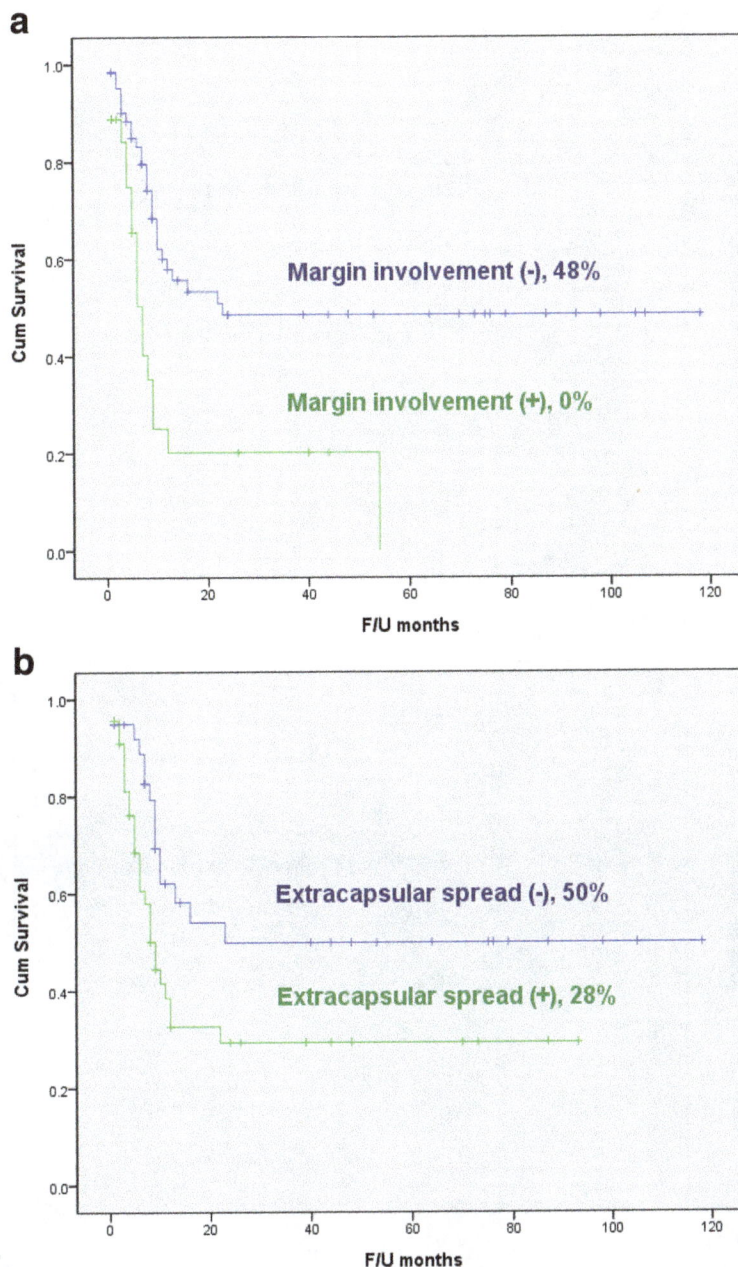

Fig. 1 Kaplan-Meier disease-free survival curves according to resection margin involvement (**a**) and extracapsular spread (**b**). Resection margin involvement ($p < 0.001$) and extracapsular spread ($p = 0.025$) showed significant associations with 5-year disease-free survival

patients with margin positive and $p = 0.180$ for patients with extracapsular spread).

Disease-specific survival

Five-year DSS for all patients who underwent primary surgery were 45%. Thirty-seven patients died, including 35 deaths from HPSCC and two deaths from other diseases. By univariate analysis, extracapsular spread ($p = 0.015$), esophageal invasion ($p = 0.033$), lympho-vascular invasion ($p = 0.041$), and cervical lymph node metastasis ($p = 0.048$) showed significant positive correlations with 5-year DSS (Fig. 2). In multivariate analysis, extracapsular spread (HR: 2.98; 95% CI: 1.39-6.42; $p = 0.005$) and esophageal invasion (HR: 2.87; 95% CI: 1.38-5.98; $p = 0.005$) remained significant factors associated with 5-year DSS.

Discussion

HPSCC is known to have poor prognosis among head and neck cancers. It is mostly found at advanced

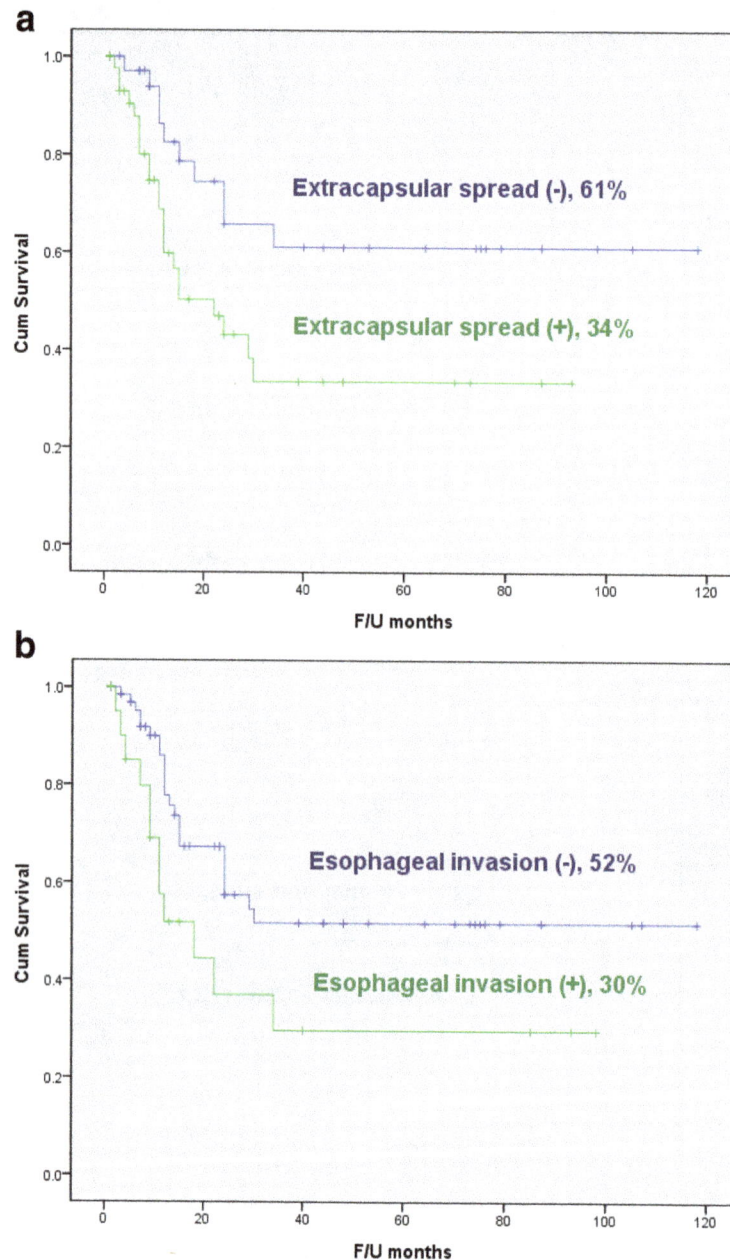

Fig. 2 Kaplan-Meier 5-year disease-specific survival curves according to extracapsular spread (**a**) and esophageal invasion (**b**). Extracapsular spread ($p = 0.015$) and esophageal invasion ($p = 0.033$) showed significant associations with 5-year disease-specific survival

stage [9]. In the past, radical ablative surgery was conducted in hypopharyngeal cancer patients. It resulted in loss of speech and swallowing dysfunction. Total laryngectomy was introduced by Billroth et al. in 1873. It has been used as the main surgical choice for a few decades [3–5]. With development of surgical techniques, many types of conservation surgeries have enabled surgeons to restore the function of the larynx for patients. From 1990s, chemoradiotherapy has been widely used as an alternative option for radical surgery in HPSCC. Some authors have reported

that advanced chemoradiotherapy technique can provide outcome equivalent to primary surgery, even in patients with advanced stage HPSCC [6, 7]. However, for patients with advanced stage HPSCC, oncologic outcomes of chemoradiotherapy are generally inferior to those of primary surgery [4–6]. Especially, patients with cartilage invasion have poor oncologic outcomes when they are treated with radiotherapy [7, 10]. Advanced-stage tumors with bone and cartilage invasion might harbor a hypoxic microenvironment that causes resistance to radiotherapy [11]. Recently, Scherl et al. have reported that prognosis of patients with advanced hypopharyngeal and laryngeal cancer after chemoradiotherapy is worse than that after primary surgery [12]. They concluded that proper selection of treatment modality could increase their survival rate. They also reported that 5-year DSS in the primary surgery group was significant higher than that in the chemoradiotherapy group which showed soft tissue invasion and cartilage invasion (5-year DSS: 51.1% in the primary surgery group vs. 28.5% in the chemoradiotherapy group, $p < 0.05$) [12].

In our series, extracapsular spread was significantly associated with rates of recurrence and survival on multivariate analysis. Many studies have reported that extracapsular spread is an indicator of poor prognosis of patients with HPSCC. Prim et al. have analyzed data of 128 patients with laryngeal and hypopharyngeal cancer and found that 3-year survival rate in patients without extracapsular spread is significantly higher than that in patients with extracapsular spread (73.4% vs. 28.9%, $p < 0.001$) [13]. Brasilino has analyzed data of 170 patients with laryngeal and hypopharyngeal cancer and reported that 5-year DFS of patients without cervical metastases is significantly higher than that in patients with macroscopic extracapsular spread (56.8% vs. 10.2%, $p < 0.0001$) [14]. In the aspect of distant metastasis, extracapsular spread has a negative effect on prognosis. According to Vaidya et al., in patients who underwent surgical resection, majority of them (18 out of 24 patients) showed recurrences for those who had cervical metastases with extracapsular nodal spread involving distant sites, especially to the lung [15].

Another significant indicator of recurrence in this study was margin status. It is known that inadequate resection can lead to increased likelihood of disease recurrence and poorer odds of survival for patients [16–18]. Ravasz has shown that locoregional recurrence observed in 20% of 80 head and neck cancer patients is correlated with tumor positive margins [18]. In our series, involved margins were found in 29% of cases. Five-year DFS of patients with negative margins was 48% and that of patients with positive margins was 0% ($p < 0.001$).

Esophageal invasion was identified as an another negative prognostic factor in our study. It is well-known that patients with advanced cancer simultaneously involving the hypopharynx and cervical esophagus have very poor prognosis. Five-year survival of these patients is approximately 20–30% [19]. Wang et al. have reported about survival and complication rates of patients who have cancer involvement of both hypopharynx and cervical esophagus [3]. They have explained the reason for such difference as follows: (1) Cervical esophagus has abundant lymphatics in the submucosa and the muscularis mucosa; (2) Cervical esophageal cancer is associated with a higher rate of mediastinal lymph node metastasis

than hypopharyngeal cancer [20, 21]; and (3) Carcinoma of the cervical esophagus frequently invades into the posterior membranous portion of the trachea. These reasons and theories could be used to explain results of our study showing that HPSCC with esophageal invasion showed poor outcomes in terms of DSS.

This study has several limitations. First, the number of patients was relatively small. However, HPSCC is quite rare among head and neck cancers and most patients are diagnosed in very advanced stage. Therefore, data collection was the most difficult part of such study. This was why we used a multi-center study design initially. The second limitation of this study was its retrospective nature. Despite these limitations, our study provided an important guide for treatment of T4a HPSCC and suggested prognostic factors for outcomes of surgical treatment. Lastly, patients with HPSCC who were treated by different modalities were not included.

Conclusions

The current study is the largest and the most robust analysis to identify specific prognostic factors in patients with T4a HPSCC treated by primary surgery. Margin involvement and extracapsular spread were significantly related to recurrence. Extracapsular spread and esophageal invasion had negative effects on survival. Such information can be used in patient counseling and appropriate risk stratification. In addition, these factors might be useful as markers to predict recurrence and prognosis of patients with T4a HPSCC.

Abbreviations
CI: Confidence interval; DFS: Disease-free survival; DSS: Disease-specific survival; HPSCC: Hypopharyngeal squamous cell carcinoma; HR: Hazard ratio

Acknowledgments
Not applicable.

Funding
This study was supported by the Research Committee of Korean Society of Thyroid Head and Neck Surgery.

Authors' contributions
YHJ conceptualized the study and critically read the manuscript. SYK, YSR, ECC, MSK, JHW, DHL, EJC, MWP, and DHK performed and/or assisted surgery, managed patients, and participated in data analysis. SYK wrote the manuscript. All authors read and approved the final manuscript.

Competing interests
The authors declare that they have no competing interests.

Author details
[1]Department of Otolaryngology-Head and Neck Surgery, College of Medicine, The Catholic University of Korea, Seoul, Republic of Korea. [2]Department of Otorhinolaryngology-Head and Neck Surgery, Ilsong Memorial Institute of Head and Neck Cancer, Hallym University, College of Medicine, Seoul, Republic of Korea. [3]Department of Otorhinolaryngology, Yonsei University, College of Medicine, Seoul, Republic of Korea. [4]Department of Otolaryngology Head and Neck Surgery, Gachon University Gil Hospital, Incheon, Korea. [5]Department of Otolaryngology-Head and Neck Surgery, Chonnam National University Medical School & Chonnam National University Hwasun Hospital, Hwasun, Korea. [6]Department of Otorhinolaryngology-Head and Neck Surgery, Seoul National University College of Medicine, Seoul, Korea. [7]Department of Otolaryngology, Head and Neck Surgery, Bucheon St. Mary's Hospital, College of Medicine, The Catholic University of Korea, 2 Sosa-dong, Wonmi-gu, Bucheon, Kyounggi-do 420-717, Republic of Korea.

References
1. Muir C, Weiland L. Upper aerodigestive tract cancers. Cancer. 1995;75:147–53.
2. Edge SB, Compton CC. The American joint committee on cancer: the 7th edition of the AJCC cancer staging manual and the future of TNM. Ann Surg Oncol. 2010;17:1471–4.
3. Wang HW, Chu PY, Kuo KT, Yang CH, Chang SY, Hsu WH, et al. A reappraisal of surgical management for squamous cell carcinoma in the pharyngoesophageal junction. J Surg Oncol. 2006;93:468–76.
4. Chu PY, Li WY, Chang SY. Clinical and pathologic predictors of survival in patients with squamous cell carcinoma of the hypopharynx after surgical treatment. Ann Otol Rhinol Laryngol. 2008;117:201–6.
5. Kuo YL, Chang CF, Chang SY, Chu PY. Partial laryngopharyngectomy in the treatment of squamous cell carcinoma of hypopharynx: analysis of the oncologic results and laryngeal preservation rate. Acta Otolaryngol. 2012; 132:1342–6.
6. Harris BN, Biron VL, Donald P, Farwell DG, Luu QC, Bewley AF, et al. Primary surgery vs Chemoradiation treatment of advanced-stage Hypopharyngeal Squamous cell carcinoma. JAMA Otolaryngol Head Neck Surg. 2015;141: 636–40.
7. Lefebvre JL, Chevalier D, Luboinski B, Kirkpatrick A, Collette L, Sahmoud T, EORTC Head and Neck Cancer Cooperative Group. Larynx preservation in pyriform sinus cancer: preliminary results of a European Organization for Research and Treatment of cancer phase III trial. J Natl Cancer Inst. 1996;88:890–9.
8. Pfister DG, Ang KK, Brizel DM, Burtness BA, Busse PM, Caudell JJ, et al. Head and neck cancers, version 2.2013. Featured updates to the NCCN guidelines. J Natl Compr Cancer Netw. 2013;11:917–23.
9. Hussey DH, Latourette HB, Panje WR. Head and neck cancer: an analysis of the incidence, patterns of treatment, and survival at the University of Iowa. Ann Otol Rhinol Laryngol Suppl. 1991;152:2–16.
10. Forastiere AA. Larynx preservation trials: a critical appraisal. Semin Radiat Oncol. 1998;8:254–61.
11. Vaupel P, Mayer A. Hypoxia in cancer: significance and impact on clinical outcome. Cancer Metastasis Rev. 2007;26:225–39.
12. Scherl C, Mantsopoulos K, Semrau S, Fietkau R, Kapsreiter M, Koch M, et al. Management of advanced hypopharyngeal and laryngeal cancer with and without cartilage invasion. Auris Nasus Larynx. 2017;44:333–9.
13. Prim MP, De Diego JI, Hardisson D, Madero R, Nistal M, Gavilán J. Extracapsular spread and desmoplastic pattern in neck lymph nodes: two prognostic factors of laryngeal cancer. Ann Otol Rhinol Laryngol. 1999;108:672–6.
14. Brasilino de Carvalho M. Quantitative analysis of the extent of extracapsular invasion and its prognostic significance: a prospective study of 170 cases of carcinoma of the larynx and hypopharynx. Head Neck. 1998;20:16–21.
15. Vaidya AM, Petruzzelli GJ, Clark J, Emami B. Patterns of spread in recurrent head and neck squamous cell carcinoma. Otolaryngol Head Neck Surg. 2001;125:393–6.
16. Beitler JJ, Smith RV, Silver CE, Quish A, Deore SM, Mullokandov E, et al. Close or positive margins after surgical resection for the head and neck cancer patient: the addition of brachytherapy improves local control. Int J Rad Oncol Phys. 1998;40:313–7.
17. Ravasz LA, Slootweg PJ, Hordijk GJ, Smit F, van der Tweel I. The status of the resection margin as a prognostic factor in the treatment of head and neck carcinoma. J Craniomaxillofac Surg. 1991;19:314–8.
18. Spiro RH, Guillamondegui O Jr, Paulino AF, Huvos AG. Pattern of invasion and margin assessment in patients with oral tongue cancer. Head Neck. 1999;21:408–13.
19. Peracchia A, Bonavina L, Botturi M, Pagani M, Via A, Saino G. Current status of surgery for carcinoma of the hypopharynx and cervical esophagus. Dis Esophagus. 2001;14:95–7.
20. Weber RS, Marvel J, Smith P, Hankins P, Wolf P, Goepfert H. Paratracheal lymph node dissection for carcinoma of the larynx, hypopharynx, and cervical esophagus. Otolaryngol Head Neck Surg. 1993;108:11–7.
21. Riquet M, Saab M, Le Pimpec BF, Hidden G. Lymphatic drainage of the esophagus in the adult. Surg Radiol Anat. 1993;15:209–11.

9

Pretreatment quality of life as a predictor of survival for patients with nasopharyngeal carcinoma treated with IMRT

Shan-Shan Guo[1,2], Wen Hu[1,2], Qiu-Yan Chen[1,2], Jian-Mei Li[1,2], Shi-Heng Zhu[1,2], Yan He[1,2], Jia-Wen Li[1,2], Le Xia[1,2], Lu Ji[1,2], Cui-Ying Lin[1,2], Li-Ting Liu[1,2], Lin-Quan Tang[1,2], Ling Guo[1,2], Hao-Yuan Mo[1,2], Chong Zhao[1,2], Xiang Guo[1,2], Ka-Jia Cao[1,2], Chao-Nan Qian[1,2], Mu-Sheng Zeng[1], Ming-Huang Hong[1,3], Jian-Yong Shao[1,4], Ying Sun[1,5], Jun Ma[1,5], Yu-Ying Fan[1,2] and Hai-Qiang Mai[1,2]*

Abstract

Background: To evaluate the prognostic significance of pretreatment quality of life for patients with nasopharyngeal carcinoma treated with intensity-modulated radiotherapy.

Methods: We performed a prospective, longitudinal study on 554 newly diagnosed patients with NPC from April 2011 to January 2015. A total of 501 consecutive NPC patients were included. Patients were asked to complete the EORTC QLQ-C30 (version 3.0) and QLQ-H&N35 questionnaires before treatment.

Results: Global health status among QLQ-C30 correlates with EBV DNA($P = 0.019$). In addition, pretreatment appetite loss was significantly correlated with EBV DNA($P = 0.02$). Pretreatment teeth, opening mouth, feeding tube was significantly correlated with EBV DNA, with P value of 0.003, < 0.0001, and 0.031, respectively. In multivariate analysis, pretreatment cognitive functioning of QLQ-C30 was significantly associated with LRFS, with HR of 0. 971(95%CI 0.951–0.990), $P = 0.004$. Among scales of QLQ-H&N35 for multivariate analysis, pretreatment teeth ($P = 0.026$) and felt ill ($P = 0.012$) was significantly associated with PFS, with HR of 0.984 (95%CI 0.971–.998) and 1.004 (95%CI 1.001–1.007), respectively. Felt ill of QLQ-H&N35 was significantly associated with DMFS, with HR of 1. 004(95%CI 1.000–1.007), $P = 0.043$. There is no QoL scale significantly associated with OS after multivariate analysis.

Conclusions: In conclusion, our analysis confirms that pretreatment teeth and felt ill was significantly associated with PFS in NPC patients treated with IMRT. In addition, the posttreatment EBV DNA was significantly associated with OS.

Keywords: Nasopharyngeal carcinoma, Quality of life, EBV DNA, Survival, Prognostic factor

Background

Nasopharyngeal carcinoma (NPC) is prevalent in Southern China and Southeast Asia, but rare in the Western world. The annual incidence of NPC is 15–50 cases per 100,000 [1]. NPC differs from other head and neck cancers in its epidemiology, association with Epstein-Barr virus (EBV),

and high risk of distant metastasis [2]. Radiotherapy (RT) is the primary treatment for nonmetastatic disease [3, 4]. Intensity modulated radiation therapy (IMRT) is the most frequently recommended radiation method, if conditions permit, because of excellent local control. Concurrent chemoradiotherapy (CCRT) is recommended as a first line therapy for locally advanced NPC [5, 6]. Induction chemotherapy has been combined in several studies to improve clinical outcomes, but it remains controversial [7–9]. Distant metastasis is the major cause of mortality in NPC patients.

Quality of life (QoL) has been considered to be a prognostic factor for cancer patients, such as for head and neck cancer [10, 11], hepatocellular carcinoma and

* Correspondence: maihq@sysucc.org.cn
Shan-Shan Guo, Wen Hu, Qiu-Yan Chen contributed equally to this article.
Yu-Ying Fan, and Hai-Qiang Mai contributed equally to this article.
[1]State Key Laboratory of Oncology in South China, Collaborative Innovation Center for Cancer Medicine, Sun Yat-Sen University Cancer Center, Guangzhou 510060, People's Republic of China
[2]Department of Nasopharyngeal Carcinoma, Sun Yat-Sen University Cancer Center, 651 Dongfeng Road East, Guangzhou 510060, People's Republic of China
Full list of author information is available at the end of the article

cholangiocarcinoma [12], colorectal cancer [13], liver cancer [14] and lung cancer [15]. Few studies have explored the prognostic significance of pretreatment QoL in NPC [16, 17]. Therefore, we conducted a prospective study using two self-administered questionnaires, the European Oganization for Research and Treatment of Cancer (EORTC) Quality of Life Questionnaire C30 (QLQ-C30) and the EORTC QLQ Head and Neck Cancer–Specific Module (H&N35), to assess the pretreatment QoL scores [18]. We assumed that felt ill among the H&N35 questionnaire was significantly associated with PFS.

Methods
Patients
We performed a prospective, longitudinal study on 554 newly diagnosed patients with NPC in the Sun Yat-Sen University Cancer Center from April 2011 to January 2015. A total of 501 consecutive NPC patients were included in this study. This study was approved by the clinical research ethics committee of the Sun Yat-Sen University Cancer Center, and the participants provided written informed consent. Patients with the following characteristics were excluded: those with distant metastasis at initial diagnosis ($n = 10$), those lost to follow-up posttreatment ($n = 2$), those whose treatment was interrupted ($n = 1$), those who were unable to complete the questionnaire pretreatment ($n = 1$), those who were unable to complete the questionnaire posttreatment ($n = 3$), those who were unable to complete the questionnaire three months posttreatment ($n = 3$), those who did not test for EAIgA and VCAIgA before treatment ($n = 10$), those who did not test for EBV DNA before treatment ($n = 17$), and those who did not test for EBV DNA value posttreatment ($n = 7$). All patients were given a complete physical examination, a fiber-optic nasopharyngoscopy, magnetic resonance imaging (MRI) of the head and neck, chest radiography, abdominal sonography, electrocardiography, bone scan or PET/CT, complete blood count with a differential count, biochemical profile, and Epstein–Barr virus serology.

QoL assessments
The self-administered EORTC QLQ-C30 (version 3.0) and the QLQ-H&N35 questionnaires were prospectively given to the enrolled patients [18–20]. The questionnaires are used by a large number of research groups in cancer clinical trials and have also been used in various other, non-trial studies. The Taiwan Chinese version was available and easily completed by our patients. Patients were asked to complete the Chinese version of the EORTC QLQ-C30 (version 3.0) and QLQ-H&N35 questionnaires before treatment. The QLQ-C30 contains 15 scales: five functional scales (physical, role, emotional, cognitive, and social functioning), three symptom scales

(fatigue, nausea and vomiting, pain), six single-item symptom scales (dyspnea, insomnia, appetite loss, constipation, diarrhea, financial difficulties), and one global health status/QoL scale. The QLQ-H&N35 is meant for use among head and neck cancer patients with varying disease stages and treatment modalities. The QLQ-H&N35 is composed of seven multi-item symptom scales (pain, swallowing, sensation, speech, eating from a social perspective, social interactions, and sexuality) and 11 single-item symptom scales (teeth, opening mouth, dry mouth, sticky saliva, coughing, felt ill, pain medication use, nutritional supplementation, feeding tube requirement, weight loss, and weight gain). All of the scales and items ranged in score from 0 to 100. A high score for a functional or global QoL scale represents a relatively high/healthy level of functional or global QoL, whereas a high score for a symptom scale or item represents a high number of symptoms or problems.

Study treatments
RT techniques
All patients (501 patients) were treated with IMRT. The dose fractionation and total dose of IMRT for NPC patients followed the guidelines of our institute [21, 22], which are in accordance with the International Commission on Radiation Units and Measurements reports 50 and 62. All the target volumes were depicted slice-by-slice on the treatment planning computed tomography scan. The primary nasopharyngeal gross tumor volume (GTVnx) and the involved cervical lymph nodes were determined based on imaging, clinical, and endoscopic findings. The enlarged retropharyngeal nodes together with primary gross tumor volume (GTV) were outlined as the GTVnx on the IMRT plans. The first clinical tumor volume (CTV1) was defined as the area from 0.5–1.0 cm outside the GTV, a site that involves potential sites of local infiltration. The clinical target volume 2 (CTV2) was defined as the margin from 0.5–1.0 cm around CTV1 and the lymph node draining area (Levels II, III, and IV). For stage N1–3 patients, the lower neck area received conventional anterior cervical field radiation with a midline shield to 50 Gy in daily fractions of 2 Gy. For patients with stage N0 disease, RT was not delivered to the lower neck area. The prescribed dose was 66–70 Gy to the planning target volume (PTV), 60 Gy to PTV1, 54 Gy to PTV2, and 60–66 Gy to the PTV of the involved cervical lymph nodes in 30 to 33 fractions. In total, 30–33 fractions were administered at 1 fraction per day, 5 days per week.

Chemotherapy
Patients with clinical stage I were treated with RT alone. Patients with stage II-IVa were treated with CCRT or induction chemotherapy+CCRT. A total of 249 (49.7%)

patients received induction chemotherapy followed by CCRT, the regimen of induction chemotherapy regimens were various regimens of based on cisplatin. Overall, 214 (42.7%) patients received concomitant chemotherapy with cisplatin. Of the 214 patients treated with concomitant chemotherapy of cisplatin regimen, a total of 37 patients received cumulative cisplatin dose of < 100 mg/m^2, 123 patients received cumulative cisplatin dose of 101–200 mg/m^2 and 54 patients received cumulative cisplatin dose of 200–300 mg/m^2. A total of 38 patients (7.6%) were treated with RT alone.

Follow-up and study endpoints
Patients were followed up every 3 months throughout the first 3 years, every 6 months for the next 2 years and annually thereafter. Physical examinations, nasopharyngoscopic examinations, MRIs, chest X-rays, abdominal ultrasounds and EBV DNA tests were performed at each follow-up visit. The follow-up duration was calculated from the first day of treatment to either the day of death or the day of the last examination. The median follow-up duration was 32 months (6–57 months). The primary end point of this study was progression free survival (PFS), and the secondary end points were overall survival (OS), local recurrence-free survival (LRFS) and distant free survival (DMFS). PFS was defined as the time from treatment of NPC to events that included death or disease progression at local, regional, or distant sites or until the date of the last follow-up. OS was defined as the time from treatment of NPC to the date of death or until the date of the last follow-up. LRFS was defined as the time from treatment of NPC to the absence of a primary site or neck lymph node relapse or until the date of the last follow-up. DMFS was defined as the time from treatment of NPC to the date of the first observation of distant metastases or until the date of the last follow-up. The last follow-up date was February 6, 2016.

Statistical methods
All analyses were performed using SPSS version 18.0 (version 18.0; SPSS Inc., Chicago, III). All tests were 2-tailed. The correlation between EBV DNA and QoL scale was analyzed by Spearman's correlation .

Univariate analysis measured by the Cox proportional hazards regression model was used to calculate the P value of each QoL scale from QLQ-C30 and H&N35. When the P value of the QoL scale in univariate analysis was less than 0.05, the scale was separately calculated by multivariate analysis adjusted for age (< 45 vs. ≥ 45), gender (male vs. female), marriage (yes vs. no), education (<high school vs. ≥high school), smoking history (yes vs. no), alcohol history (yes vs. no), T stage (T1,2 vs. T3,4), N stage (N1,2 vs. N3,4), pre-treatment EBV DNA (< 4000 vs. ≥ 4000) and post-treatment EBV DNA (negative vs. positive).

Results
Patient characteristics
In this study population, there were 380 male patients and 121 female patients, with a male: female ratio of 3.14:1. The median age was 44 years (range, 11–72 years). There were 498 (99.4%) of the 501 patients had World Health Organization (WHO) type II or III disease, and 3 (0.6%) had WHO type I disease. There were 9 (1.8%) patients with American Joint of Cancer Committee (AJCC) stage I; 50(10.0%) patients with stage II, 281 (56.1%) patients with stage III, 161 (32.1%) patients with stage IV. A total of 496 (99.0%) patients had an Eastern Cooperative Oncology Group (ECOG) score of 1. More than half of the patients (337, 67.3%) had a history of smoking, and the use of alcohol was not common (53, 10.6%). We represented the characteristics divided by sex in Table 1.

Survival outcomes
There were 16 (3.2%) patients who died, 18 (3.6%) patients who had loco regional recurrence and 42 (8.4%) patients who had distant metastasis. The median follow-up time was 32 months (range, 6–57).

QoL data
Table 2 shows the pretreatment QoL scores of both QLQ-C30 and QLQ-H&N35 for NPC patients.

Correlation between EBV DNA and QoL
We analyzed correlation between each scale among the QLQ-C30 questionnaire and pretreatment EBV DNA, found that global health status correlates with pretreatment EBV DNA($P = 0.019$). In addition, pretreatment appetite loss was significantly correlated with pretreatment EBV DNA($P = 0.02$). We also analyzed the correlation between each scale among the QLQ-H&N35 questionnaire and pretreatment EBV DNA. We found that pretreatment teeth, opening mouth, feeding tube was significantly correlated with pretreatment EBV DNA, with P value of 0.003, < 0.0001, and 0.031, respectively. Appendix: Tables 7 and 8 represented the correlation between EBV DNA and QLQ-C30 or QLQ-H&N35.

Univariate analysis pretreatment
In QLQ-C30, there was no functional scale or symptom scale that was significantly associated with OS, PFS and DMFS in QLQ-C30 pretreatment. Only pretreatment cognitive functioning was significantly associated with LRFS in QLQ-C30 (Fig. 1).

In QLQ-H&N35, were pain and swallowing significantly associated with OS. There were three scales significantly associated with PFS: pain, teeth (Fig. 2) and felt ill (Fig. 3). There were six scales in QLQ-H&N35 that were significantly associated with LRFS: pain, swallowing, speech, social eating and teeth. There were two scales in QLQ-

Table 1 Patient characteristics (n=501)

Variable	Male	Female	P
Median age, years			
Range			
< 45	177(46.6%)	75(62.0%)	0.003
≥45	203(53.4%)	46(38.0%)	
Marital status			
Married	17(4.5%)	6(5.0%)	0.833
Single	363(95.3%)	115(95.0%)	
Education years			
No formal education	6(1.6%)	7(5.8%)	0.065
Primary level	49(12.9%)	20(16.5%)	
Secondary level	99(26.1%)	24(19.8%)	
High school	112(29.5%)	37(30.6%)	
University	114(30.0%)	33(27.3%)	
Smoking history			
Ever	159(41.8%)	116(4.1%)	<0.0001
Never	221(58.2%)	5(95.9%)	
Alcohol history			<0.0001
Ever	53(13.9%)	0(0)	
Never	327(86.1%)	121(100.0%)	
ECOG score			0.174
0	378(99.7%)	118(99.2%)	
1	0(0)	1(0.8)	
2	1(0.3%)	0(0)	
WHO type			0.862
1	2(0.5%)	1(0.8%)	
2	2(0.5%)	1(0.8%)	
3	375(98.9%)	117(98.3%)	
T stage			0.521
1	19(5.0%)	3(2.5%)	
2	67(17.6%)	18(14.9%)	
3	202(53.2%)	71(58.7%)	
4	92(24.2%)	29(24.0%)	
N stage			0.641
0	50(13.2%)	11(9.1%)	
1	144(37.9%)	51(42.1%)	
2	146(38.4%)	45(37.2%)	
3	40(10.5%)	14(11.6%)	
AJCC stage			0.322
1	7(1.8%)	2(1.7%)	
2	44(11.6%)	7(5.8%)	
3	207(54.5%)	72(59.5%)	
4	122(32.1%)	40(33.1%)	

Table 1 Patient characteristics (n=501) (Continued)

Variable	Male	Female	P
Treatment modality			
RT	27(7.1%)	9(7.4%)	
IC + CCRT	194(51.1%)	60(49.6%)	
CCRT	159(41.8%)	52(43.0%)	
Median RT dose, Gy			
VCA IgA			0.188
< 1:80	151(39.7%)	40(33.1%)	
≥ 1:80	229(60.3%)	81(66.9%)	
EA IgA			0.138
< 1:10	199(52.4%)	54(44.6%)	
≥ 1:10	181(47.6%)	67(55.4%)	
Pre-EBV DNA			0.526
≤ 4000	201 (52.9%)	60(49.6%)	
> 4000	179 (47.1%)	61(50.4%)	
Post-EBV DNA			0.780
negative	136(35.8%)	45(37.2%)	
positive	244(64.2%)	76(62.8%)	
Family history of NPC			0.252
yes	18(4.7%)	9(7.4%)	
no	362 (95.3%)	112(92.6%)	

Abbrevations. *No* Number, *ECOG* Eastern Cooperative Oncology Group, *WHO* World Health Organization, *AJCC* American Joint Committee on Cancer, *RT* Radiotherapy, *IC* Induction chemotherapy, *CCRT* Concurrent chemoradiotherapy, *EBV DNA* Epstein-Barr virus deoxyribonucleic acid, *NPC* Nasopharyngeal carcinoma

H&N35 that were significantly associated with DMFS: pain and felt ill (Fig. 4). (Appendix: Table 7).

Multivariate analysis

The scales which were significantly associated with clinical outcomes were included in Cox proportional hazards regression model (Tables 3, 4, 5 and 6). In multivariate analysis, pretreatment cognitive functioning of QLQ-C30 was significantly associated with LRFS, with HR of 0.971 (95%CI 0.951–0.990), P = 0.004. Among scales of QLQ-H&N35 for multivariate analysis, pretreatment teeth (P = 0.026) and felt ill (P = 0.012) was significantly associated with PFS, with HR of 0.984 (95%CI 0.971–0.998) and 1.004 (95%CI 1.001–1.007), respectively. Besides, posttreatment EBV DNA (P = 0.001) and N stage (P = 0.013) was significantly associated with PFS, with HR of 3.130 (95%CI 1.563–6.267) and 1.979 (95%CI 1.156–3.388), respectively. Felt ill of QLQ-H&N35 was significantly associated with DMFS, with HR of 1.004 (95%CI 1.000–1.007), P = 0.043. Besides, post-treatment EBV DNA (P = 0.007) and N stage (P = 0.010) was significantly

Table 2 Pretreatment quality of life scores for 501 patients with nasopharyngeal carcinoma

EORTC scale	Mean	SD
QLQ-C30		
Global health status/QoL	69.84	22.47
Physical functioning	94.07	9.22
Role functioning	93.88	14.73
Emotional functioning	84.21	16.56
Cognitive functioning	88.39	16.02
Social functioning	75.82	25.88
Fatigue	17.25	17.27
Nausea and vomiting	3.46	10.39
Pain	12.28	18.43
Dyspnoea	6.72	15.10
Insomnia	15.77	23.52
Appetite loss	7.12	16.74
Constipation	6.65	15.78
Diarrhea	3.53	10.49
Financial difficulties	31.27	31.45
QLQ-H&N35		
Pain	8.13	11.20
Swallowing	3.71	9.16
Senses	5.76	12.72
Speech	5.26	12.72
Social eating	4.14	9.39
Social contact	3.97	8.75
Sexuality	16.43	20.42
Teeth	15.90	21.45
Opening mouth	6.59	16.16
Dry mouth	17.22	19.72
Sticky saliva	11.50	17.96
Coughing	9.51	17.14
Felt ill	24.42	26.59
Pain killers	20.96	40.74
Nutrition supplements	20.96	40.74
Feeding tube	1.20	10.89
Weight loss	34.53	47.59
Weight gain	7.19	25.85

Abbreviations. *EORTC* European Organisation for Research and Treatment of Cancer, *SD* Standard deviation

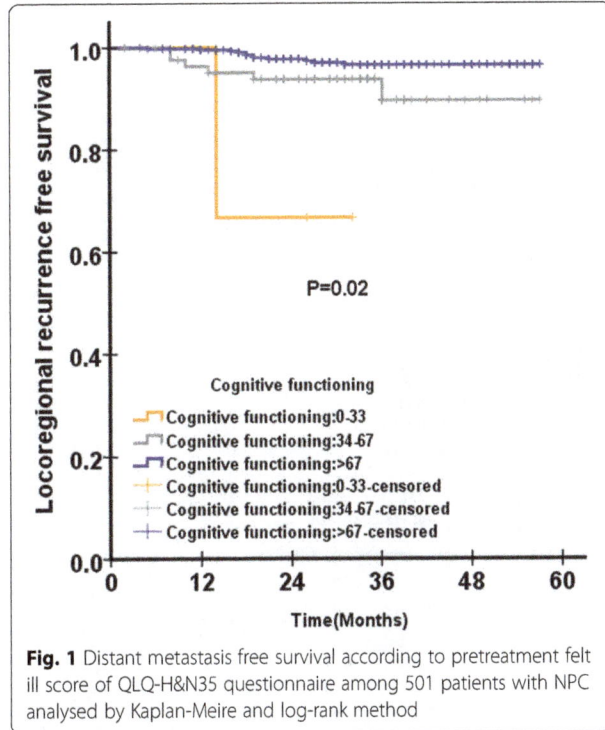

Fig. 1 Distant metastasis free survival according to pretreatment felt ill score of QLQ-H&N35 questionnaire among 501 patients with NPC analysed by Kaplan-Meire and log-rank method

Discussion

There have been previous studies regarding quality of life on NPC patients and head and neck cancer. Until now, only one study had explored the prognostic significance of QoL in QLQ-C30 questionnaires by assessing

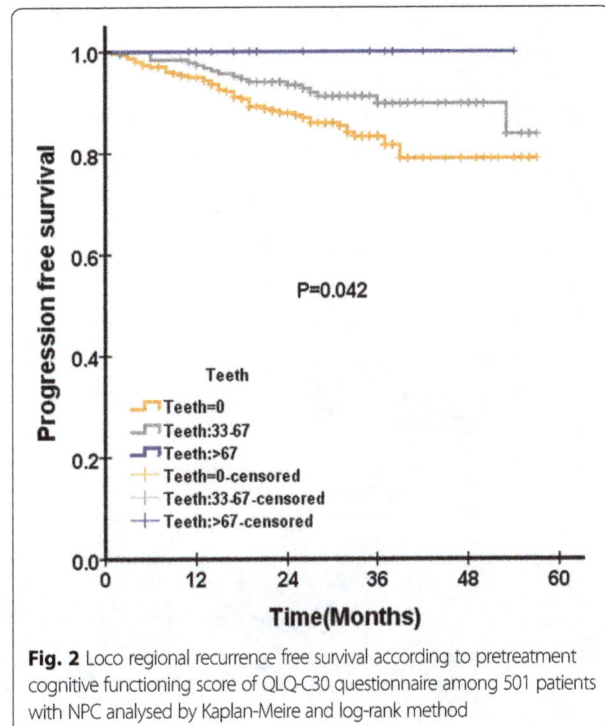

Fig. 2 Loco regional recurrence free survival according to pretreatment cognitive functioning score of QLQ-C30 questionnaire among 501 patients with NPC analysed by Kaplan-Meire and log-rank method

associated with DMFS, with HR of 2.915 (95%CI 1.338–6.350) and 2.251 (95%CI 1.212–4.179). There is no QoL scale significantly associated with OS after multivariate analysis. In addition, the posttreatment EBV DNA was significantly associated with OS ($P = 0.020$), with HR of 11.202 (95%CI 1.473–85.184).

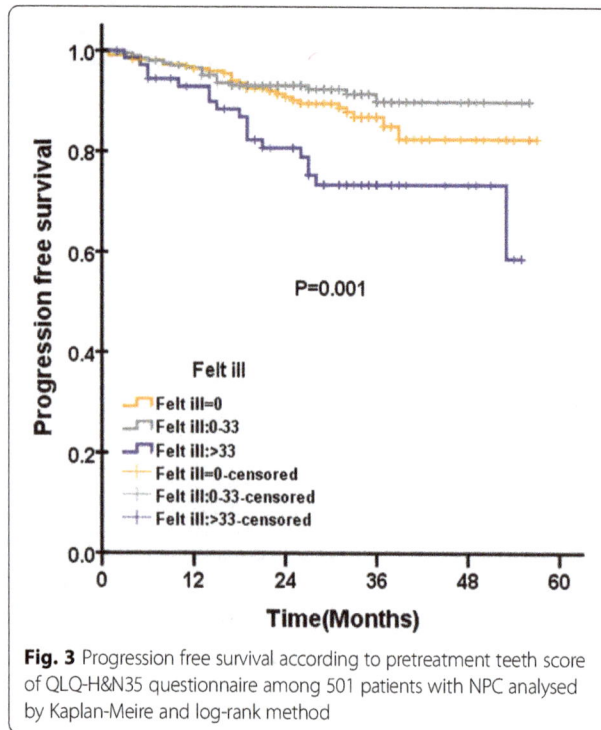

Fig. 3 Progression free survival according to pretreatment teeth score of QLQ-H&N35 questionnaire among 501 patients with NPC analysed by Kaplan-Meire and log-rank method

254 NPC patients who received IMRT and 93 patients who received 3DCRT [17]. To our knowledge, this is the first large scale study of NPC patients in the IMRT era that prospectively explored functional scales and symptom scales in both QLQ-30 and H&N35.

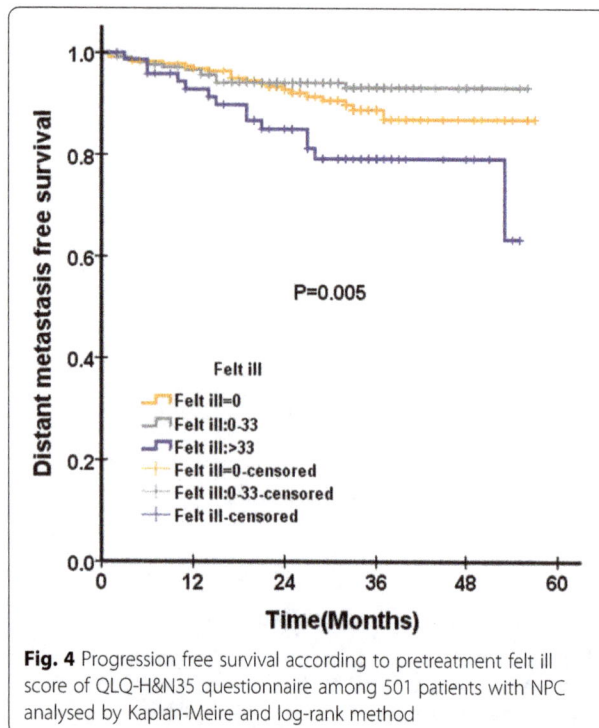

Fig. 4 Progression free survival according to pretreatment felt ill score of QLQ-H&N35 questionnaire among 501 patients with NPC analysed by Kaplan-Meire and log-rank method

Table 3 Multivariate analysis of PFS on pretreatment quality of life of QLQ-C30 among 501 patients with nasopharyngeal carcinoma

	HR	95%CI	P
Age	1.200	0.692–2.079	0.516
Gender	0.772	0.395–1.510	0.450
Marriage	1.470	0.458–4.719	0.517
Education	1.197	0.940–1.525	0.145
Smoking history	0.951	0.518–1.747	0.872
Alcohol history	0.787	0.324–1.910	0.596
T stage	1.383	0.684–2.794	0.367
N stage	1.979	1.156–3.388	0.013
Pre-treatment EBV DNA	1.451	0.866–2.431	0.157
Post-treatment EBV DNA	3.130	1.563–6.267	0.001
Pain	1.015	0.995–1.035	0.146
Teeth	0.984	0.971–0.998	0.026
Felt ill	1.004	1.001–1.007	0.012

Abbreviations: *PFS* Progression free survival, *HR* Harsard ratio

We found that global health status significantly correlates with EBV DNA. High pretreatment EBV DNA level always associates with large tumor or multiple lymph nodes which represents advanced stage. Patients with advanced stage represents poor quality of life scores. This may be the possible explanation for global health status significantly correlates with EBV DNA. In addition, pretreatment appetite loss was significantly correlated with EBV DNA. We found that pretreatment teeth, opening mouth, feeding tube was significantly correlated with EBV DNA. This is the first time that the correlation between quality of life and EBV DNA is reported. The exact mechanism remains unknown. More studies about the correlation between quality of life and EBV DNA is expected to do in the future.

Table 4 Multivariate analysis of LRFS on quality of life of QLQ-C30 among 501 patients with nasopharyngeal carcinoma

	HR	95%CI	P
Age	1.583	0.582–4.302	0.368
Gender	1.017	0.300–3.450	0.978
Marriage	0.479	0.099–2.320	0.360
Education	1.337	0.852–2.098	0.206
Smoking history	1.455	0.512–4.139	0.482
Alcohol history	1.086	0.480–2.458	0.843
T stage	1.267	0.361–4.449	0.712
N stage	1.604	0.616–4.172	0.333
Pre-treatment EBV DNA	1.221	0.491–3.035	0.667
Post-treatment EBV DNA	3.093	0.881–10.857	0.078
Cognitive functioning	0.971	0.951–0.990	0.004

Abbreviations: *LRFS* Loco regional recurrent free survival, *HR* Harsard ratio

Table 5 Multivariate analysis of DMFS on pretreatment quality of life of QLQ-C30 among 501 patients with nasopharyngeal carcinoma

	HR	95%CI	P
Age	1.039	0.560–1.927	0.904
Gender	0.527	0.235–1.183	0.121
Marriage	3.217	0.669–15.479	0.145
Education	1.278	0.967–1.689	0.085
Smoking history	0.731	0.362–1.477	0.383
Alcohol history	0.882	0.342–2.271	0.794
T stage	1.305	0.611–2.787	0.491
N stage	2.251	1.212–4.179	0.010
Pre-treatment EBV DNA	1.730	0.963–3.109	0.067
Post-treatment EBV DNA	2.915	1.338–6.350	0.007
Pain	1.015	0.994–1.038	0.169
Felt ill	1.004	1.000–1.007	0.043

Abbreviations: *DMFS* Distant metastasis free suvival, *HR* Harsard ratio

In the present study, pretreatment teeth in QLQ-H&N35 predicted longer PFS. This result may be explained by a sensitivity to radiotherapy resulting in uncomfortable sensation in the teeth. The exact mechanism is unknown. Interestingly, felt ill pretreatment in QLQ-H&N35 predicted shorter DMFS in multivariate analysis. The possible explanation would be as follows. At the beginning of treatment, pain mostly comes from large tumor region, probably because of invasion along the cranial nerve. Large tumors of head and neck cancers or NPC are significantly associated with distant metastasis. A previous study found that pretreatment pain

Table 6 Multivariate analysis of OS on pretreatment quality of life of QLQ-C30 among 501 patients with nasopharyngeal carcinoma

	HR	95%CI	P
Age	1.329	0.516–3.427	0.556
Gender	0.493	0.136–1.795	0.284
Marriage	1.524	0.226–10.298	0.665
Education	1.145	0.763–1.720	0.513
Smoking history	1.246	0.483–3.216	0.650
Alcohol history	0.268	0.034–2.125	0.213
T stage	2.353	0.539–10.275	0.255
N stage	1.675	0.686–4.090	0.257
Pre-treatment EBV DNA	0.816	0.342–1.946	0.646
Post-treatment EBV DNA	11.202	1.473–85.184	0.020
Pain	1.028	0.996–1.061	0.091
Swallowing	1.014	0.978–1.050	0.458

Abbreviations: *OS* Overall sruvival, *HR* Harsard ratio

influences OS in 2340 newly diagnosed patients with head and neck squamous cancer [23]. We found that a high cognitive functioning score pretreatment in QLQ-C30 predicted longer LRFS. This finding is consistent with previous studies in head and neck cancer [24] and NPC [17]. The exact mechanism of why cognitive function correlates with survival is unknown. The causative relationship between cognitive functioning and survival is indeterminate. Cognitive functioning might be a surrogate for the QoL scales that were potentially prognostic, and we speculate that it may display as a physiological appearance for some undetected predictive factors.

In this study, post treatment EBV DNA predicted OS better than pretreatment EBV DNA. Using multivariate analysis, posttreatment EBV DNA significantly predicted OS for NPC patients in this study. Pretreatment EBV DNA did not show predict value of OS in this study in multivariate analysis, revealed that the prognostic value of pretreatment EBV DNA was covered up by posttreatment EBV DNA in this study. This finding is consistent with previous studies. A recent study explored EBV DNA loading of 273 NPC patients at different time points and found that post treatment EBV DNA was significantly associated with PFS, DMFS and OS [25]. Several studies in Taiwan concluded that post treatment EBV DNA was an important independent prognostic factor for clinical outcomes [26, 27].

Our results revealed that QoL and post treatment EBV DNA can effectively predict survival for NPC patients. The results provide a promising way to guide treatment strategy for NPC patients. Our study has several strengths. First, the present study has the longest longitudinal collection of QoL data that has been used to examine prognostic value during the initial management of patients with NPC. Second, this is the first time that QoL scores in QLQ-H&N35 were found to predict survival for NPC patients. Our study evaluated the prognostic significance of QoL using both the QLQ-C30 questionnaire and QLQ-H&N35 questionnaire.

There were some limitations in the present study. First, this is a single center study in a high incidence area in Southern China. Future studies are needed to calculate the prognostic significance of QoL in NPC patients in other areas in the world. Second, the median follow-up time of this study was 32 months; a longer follow-up time is needed to further validate our results.

Conclusions

In conclusion, our analysis confirms that pretreatment teeth and felt ill was significantly associated with PFS in NPC patients treated with IMRT. In addition, the posttreatment EBV DNA was significantly associated with OS.

Appendix

Table 7 The correlation between quality of life scales among EORTC QLQ-C30 and EBV DNA

Scale	B	P
Global health status/QoL	0.105	0.019
Physical functioning	0.001	0.983
Role functioning	0.082	0.066
Emotional functioning	0.081	0.071
Cognitive functioning	0.059	0.184
Social functioning	0.056	0.208
Fatigue	−0.080	0.071
Nausea and vomiting	−0.057	0.203
Pain	−0.048	0.280
Dyspnoea	−0.080	0.074
Insomnia	−0.081	0.069
Appetite loss	−0.104	0.020
Constipation	−0.042	0.351
Diarrhea	−0.059	0.184
Financial difficulties	−0.057	0.203

Abbrevations. *EORTC* European Organisation for Research and Treatment of Cancer, *QoL* Qualtiy of life

Table 8 The correlation between quality of life scales among EORTC H&N35 and EBV DNA

Scale	B	P
Pain	−0.060	0.178
Swallowing	−0.052	0.244
Senses	−0.038	0.397
Speech	−0.042	0.343
Social eating	−0.031	0.488
Social contact	−0.003	0.950
Sexuality	−0.042	0.343
Teeth	−0.134	0.003
Opening mouth	−0.156	< 0.0001
Dry mouth	−0.025	0.583
Sticky saliva	−0.076	0.089
Coughing	−0.042	0.351
Felt ill	−0.030	0.497
Pain killers	−0.065	0.147
Nutrition supplements	−0.068	0.126
Feeding tube	0.096	0.031
Weight loss	−0.007	0.880
Weight gain	0.015	0.739

Abbrevations. *EORTC* European Organisation for Research and Treatment of Cancer, *QoL* Qualtiy of life

Abbreviations
CCRT: Concurrent chemoradiotherapy; DMFS: Distant free survival; EBV: Epstein-Barr virus; EORTC: European Organization for Research and Treatment of Cancer; H&N35: Head and Neck Cancer–Specific Module; IMRT: Intensity modulated radiation therapy; LRFS: Local regional recurrence-free survival; MRI: Magnetic resonance imaging; NPC: Nasopharyngeal carcinoma; OS: Overall survival; PFS: Progression free survival; QLQ-C30: Quality of Life Questionnaire C30; QoL: Quality of life; RT: Radiotherapy

Acknowledgements
We thank for Professor Qing Liu for his help during this study.

Funding
This work was supported by grants from the National Natural Science Foundation of China (No. 81425018, No. 81072226, No. 81201629), the 863 Project (No. 2012AA02A501), the National Key Basic Research Program of China (No.2013CB910304), the Special Support Plan of Guangdong Province (No.2014TX01R145), the Sci-Tech Project Foundation of Guangdong Province (No.2014A020212103, No.2011B080701034, No.2011B031800161), the Health & Medical Collaborative Innovation Project of Guangzhou City (No. 201400000001),the National Science & Technology Pillar Program during the Twelfth Five-year Plan Period (No.2014BAI09B10), the Sun Yat-Sen University Clinical Research 5010 Program, the Sun Yat-Sen University Cancer Center Clinical Research 308 Program, the Fundamental Research Funds for the Central Universities, and the Medical Research Foundation of Guangdong Province (No: A2014252). The funding body had no role in the design of the study and collection, analysis, and interpretation of data and in writing the manuscript.

Authors' contributions
All authors read and approved the final manuscript. Study concepts: H-QM, Y-YF, S-SG, Q-YC. Study design: H-QM, Q-YC, S-SG, WH, Y-YF. Data acquisition: J-ML, S-HZ, Y H, J-WL, L X. Quality control of data and algorithms: LJ, C-YL, L-TL, L-QT, LG. Data analysis and interpretation: S-SG, H-QM, WH, Q-YC, Y-YF. Statistical analysis: S-SG, H-QM, Y-YF. Manuscript preparation: H-YM, CZ, XG, K-JC, C-NQ. Manuscript editing: M-SZ, M-HH, J-YS, YS. Manuscript review: JM, H-QM, S-SG, Q-YC.

Competing interests
The authors declare that they have no competing interests.

Author details
[1]State Key Laboratory of Oncology in South China, Collaborative Innovation Center for Cancer Medicine, Sun Yat-Sen University Cancer Center, Guangzhou 510060, People's Republic of China. [2]Department of Nasopharyngeal Carcinoma, Sun Yat-Sen University Cancer Center, 651 Dongfeng Road East, Guangzhou 510060, People's Republic of China. [3]Good Clinical Practice center, Sun Yat-Sen University Cancer Center, 651 Dongfeng Road East, Guangzhou 510060, People's Republic of China. [4]Department of Molecular Diagnostics, Sun Yat-Sen University Cancer Center, 651 Dongfeng Road East, Guangzhou 510060, People's Republic of China. [5]Department of Radiation Oncology, Sun Yat-Sen University Cancer Center, Guangzhou 510060, People's Republic of China.

References
1. Wee JT, Ha TC, Loong SL, Qian CN. Is nasopharyngeal cancer really a "Cantonese cancer"? Chin J Cancer. 2010;29(5):517–26.
2. Lee AW, Lin JC, Ng WT. Current management of nasopharyngeal cancer. Semin Radiat Oncol. 2012;22(3):233–44.
3. Chen JL, Huang YS, Kuo SH, Chen YF, Hong RL, Ko JY, Lou PJ, Tsai CL, Chen WY, Wang CW. Intensity-modulated radiation therapy for T4 nasopharyngeal carcinoma. Treatment results and locoregional recurrence. Strahlenther Onkol. 2013;189(12):1001–8.

Pretreatment quality of life as a predictor of survival for patients with nasopharyngeal carcinoma treated...

73

4.   Wang R, Wu F, Lu H, Wei B, Feng G, Li G, Liu M, Yan H, Zhu J, Zhang Y, et al. Definitive intensity-modulated radiation therapy for nasopharyngeal carcinoma: long-term outcome of a multicenter prospective study. J Cancer Res Clin Oncol. 2013;139(1):139–45.

5.   Chen L, Hu CS, Chen XZ, Hu GQ, Cheng ZB, Sun Y, Li WX, Chen YY, Xie FY, Liang SB, et al. Concurrent chemoradiotherapy plus adjuvant chemotherapy versus concurrent chemoradiotherapy alone in patients with locoregionally advanced nasopharyngeal carcinoma: a phase 3 multicentre randomised controlled trial. Lancet Oncol. 2012;13(2):163–71.

6.   Blanchard P, Lee A, Marguet S, Leclercq J, Ng WT, Ma J, Chan AT, Huang PY, Benhamou E, Zhu G, et al. Chemotherapy and radiotherapy in nasopharyngeal carcinoma: an update of the MAC-NPC meta-analysis. Lancet Oncol. 2015;16(6):645–55.

7.   Fountzilas G, Ciuleanu E, Bobos M, Kalogera-Fountzila A, Eleftheraki AG, Karayannopoulou G, Zaramboukas T, Nikolaou A, Markou K, Resiga L, et al. Induction chemotherapy followed by concomitant radiotherapy and weekly cisplatin versus the same concomitant chemoradiotherapy in patients with nasopharyngeal carcinoma: a randomized phase II study conducted by the Hellenic cooperative oncology group (HeCOG) with biomarker evaluation. Ann Oncol. 2012;23(2):427–35.

8.   Tan T, Lim WT, Fong KW, Cheah SL, Soong YL, Ang MK, Ng QS, Tan D, Ong WS, Tan SH, et al. Concurrent chemo-radiation with or without induction gemcitabine, carboplatin, and paclitaxel: a randomized, phase 2/3 trial in locally advanced nasopharyngeal carcinoma. Int J Radiat Oncol Biol Phys. 2015;91(5):952–60.

9.   Hui EP, Ma BB, Leung SF, King AD, Mo F, Kam MK, Yu BK, Chiu SK, Kwan WH, Ho R, et al. Randomized phase II trial of concurrent cisplatin-radiotherapy with or without neoadjuvant docetaxel and cisplatin in advanced nasopharyngeal carcinoma. J Clin Oncol. 2009;27(2):242–9.

10. Siddiqui F, Pajak TF, Watkins-Bruner D, Konski AA, Coyne JC, Gwede CK, Garden AS, Spencer SA, Jones C, Movsas B. Pretreatment quality of life predicts for locoregional control in head and neck cancer patients: a radiation therapy oncology group analysis. Int J Radiat Oncol Biol Phys. 2008;70(2):353–60.

11. Karvonen-Gutierrez CA, Ronis DL, Fowler KE, Terrell JE, Gruber SB, Duffy SA. Quality of life scores predict survival among patients with head and neck cancer. J Clin Oncol. 2008;26(16):2754–60.

12. Steel JL, Geller DA, Robinson TL, Savkova AY, Brower DS, Marsh JW, Tsung A. Health-related quality of life as a prognostic factor in patients with advanced cancer. Cancer. 2014;120(23):3717–21.

13. Fournier E, Jooste V, Woronoff AS, Quipourt V, Bouvier AM, Mercier M. Health-related quality of life is a prognostic factor for survival in older patients after colorectal cancer diagnosis: a population-based study. Dig Liver Dis. 2016;48(1):87–93.

14. Klein J, Dawson LA, Jiang H, Kim J, Dinniwell R, Brierley J, Wong R, Lockwood G, Ringash J. Prospective longitudinal assessment of quality of life for liver cancer patients treated with stereotactic body radiation therapy. Int J Radiat Oncol Biol Phys. 2015;93(1):16–25.

15. Fiteni F, Vernerey D, Bonnetain F, Vaylet F, Sennelart H, Tredaniel J, Moro-Sibilot D, Herman D, Laize H, Masson P, et al. Prognostic value of health-related quality of life for overall survival in elderly non-small-cell lung cancer patients. Eur J Cancer. 2016;52:120–8.

16. Fang FM, Chiu HC, Kuo WR, Wang CJ, Leung SW, Chen HC, Sun LM, Hsu HC. Health-related quality of life for nasopharyngeal carcinoma patients with cancer-free survival after treatment. Int J Radiat Oncol Biol Phys. 2002;53(4):959–68.

17. Fang FM, Tsai WL, Chien CY, Chen HC, Hsu HC, Huang TL, Lee TF, Huang HY, Lee CH. Pretreatment quality of life as a predictor of distant metastasis and survival for patients with nasopharyngeal carcinoma. J Clin Oncol. 2010; 28(28):4384–9.

18. Bjordal K, de Graeff A, Fayers PM, Hammerlid E, van Pottelsberghe C, Curran D, Ahlner-Elmqvist M, Maher EJ, Meyza JW, Bredart A, et al. A 12 country field study of the EORTC QLQ-C30 (version 3.0) and the head and neck cancer specific module (EORTC QLQ-H&N35) in head and neck patients. EORTC Quality of Life Group. Eur J Cancer. 2000;36(14):1796–807.

19. Efficace F, Therasse P, Piccart MJ, Coens C, van Steen K, Welnicka-Jaskiewicz M, Cufer T, Dyczka J, Lichinitser M, Shepherd L, et al. Health-related quality of life parameters as prognostic factors in a nonmetastatic breast cancer population: an international multicenter study. J Clin Oncol. 2004;22(16):3381–8.

20. Aaronson NK, Ahmedzai S, Bergman B, Bullinger M, Cull A, Duez NJ, Filiberti A, Flechtner H, Fleishman SB, de Haes JC, et al. The European Organization for Research and Treatment of cancer QLQ-C30: a quality-of-life instrument for use in international clinical trials in oncology. J Natl Cancer Inst. 1993;85(5):365–76.

21. Zhao C, Han F, Lu LX, Huang SM, Lin CG, Deng XW, Lu TX, Cui NJ. Intensity modulated radiotherapy for local-regional advanced nasopharyngeal carcinoma. Ai Zheng. 2004;23(11 Suppl):1532–7.

22. Sun X, Su S, Chen C, Han F, Zhao C, Xiao W, Deng X, Huang S, Lin C, Lu T. Long-term outcomes of intensity-modulated radiotherapy for 868 patients with nasopharyngeal carcinoma: an analysis of survival and treatment toxicities. Radiother Oncol. 2014;110(3):398–403.

23. Reyes-Gibby CC, Anderson KO, Merriman KW, Todd KH, Shete SS, Hanna EY. Survival patterns in squamous cell carcinoma of the head and neck: pain as an independent prognostic factor for survival. J Pain. 2014;15(10):1015–22.

24. Meyer F, Fortin A, Gelinas M, Nabid A, Brochet F, Tetu B, Bairati I. Health-related quality of life as a survival predictor for patients with localized head and neck cancer treated with radiation therapy. J Clin Oncol. 2009;27(18):2970–6.

25. Zhang Y, Li WF, Mao YP, Guo R, Tang LL, Peng H, Sun Y, Liu Q, Chen L, Ma J. Risk stratification based on change in plasma Epstein-Barr virus DNA load after treatment in nasopharyngeal carcinoma. Oncotarget. 2016;7(8):9576–85.

26. Wang WY, Lin TY, Twu CW, Tsou HH, Lin PJ, Liu YC, Huang JW, Hsieh HY, Lin JC. Long-term clinical outcome in nasopharyngeal carcinoma patients with post-radiation persistently detectable plasma EBV DNA. Oncotarget; 2016;7(27): 42608–42616.

27. Lin JC, Wang WY, Chen KY, Wei YH, Liang WM, Jan JS, Jiang RS. Quantification of plasma Epstein-Barr virus DNA in patients with advanced nasopharyngeal carcinoma. N Engl J Med. 2004;350(24):2461–70.

10

A change in the study evaluation paradigm reveals that larynx preservation compromises survival in T4 laryngeal cancer patients

Gerhard Dyckhoff[1]* (iD), Peter K. Plinkert[1] and Heribert Ramroth[2]

Abstract

Background: Larynx preservation (LP) is recommended for up to low-volume T4 laryngeal cancer as an evidence-based treatment option that does not compromise survival. However, a reevaluation of the current literature raises questions regarding whether there is indeed reliable evidence to support larynx preservation for T4 tumor patients.

Methods: In an observational cohort study of 810 laryngeal cancer patients, we evaluated the outcomes of all T4 tumor patients treated with primary chemo-radiotherapy (CRT) or primary radiotherapy alone (RT) compared with upfront total laryngectomy followed by adjuvant (chemo)radiotherapy (TL + a[C]RT). Additionally, we reevaluated the studies that form the evidence base for the recommendation of LP for patients with up to T4 tumors (Pfister et al., J Clin Oncol 24:3693–704, 2006).

Results: The evaluation of all 288 stage III and IV patients together did not show a significant difference in overall survival (OS) between CRT-LP and TL + a(C)RT (hazard ratio (HR) 1.23; 95% confidence interval (CI): 0.82–1.86; $p = 0.31$) using a multivariate proportional hazard model. However, a subgroup analysis of T4 tumor patients alone ($N = 107$; 13.9%) revealed significantly worse OS after CRT compared with TL + a(C)RT (HR 2.0; 95% CI: 1.04–3.7; $p = 0.0369$). A reevaluation of the subgroup of T4 patients in the 5 LP studies that led to the ASCO clinical practice guidelines revealed that only 21–45 T4 patients had differential data on survival outcome. These data, however, showed a markedly worse outcome for T4 patients after LP.

Conclusions: T4 laryngeal cancer patients who reject TL as a treatment option should be informed that their chance of organ preservation with primary conservative treatment is likely to result in a significantly worse outcome in terms of OS. Significant loss of survival in T4 patients after LP is also confirmed in recent literature.

Keywords: Laryngeal cancer, Advanced stage, Larynx preservation, Laryngectomy, Outcome

Background

In the landmark larynx preservation (LP) studies [1–3], common practice has been to investigate and evaluate locally advanced stage III and IV cancers of the larynx or hypopharynx together. These groups comprise T4 carcinoma as well as T2 and T3 cancers. The results of these studies led to the American Society of Clinical Oncology (ASCO) 2006 clinical practice guidelines for the use of larynx preservation strategies [4]. These guidelines recommend that "for most patients with T3 or T4 disease without tumor invasion through cartilage into soft tissues, a larynx preservation approach is an appropriate, standard treatment option, and concurrent chemo-radiotherapy is the most widely applicable approach." [4] Furthermore, they state that with "further surgery reserved for salvage, survival is not compromised." [4] These guidelines are currently the official standard for avoiding total laryngectomy, particularly in

* Correspondence: Gerhard.Dyckhoff@med.uni-heidelberg.de
[1]Department of Otorhinolaryngology, Head and Neck Surgery, University of Heidelberg, Im Neuenheimer Feld 400, 69120 Heidelberg, Germany
Full list of author information is available at the end of the article

the United States [5], as recent reviews have reconfirmed [6–9]. Thus, in patients with early T4 disease, LP is explicitly recommended. According to the current National Comprehensive Cancer Network (NCCN) treatment guidelines, concurrent chemoradiation should be considered only for "selected T4a patients who decline surgery" [10]. As a result, one might expect that only a minority of carefully selected T4a laryngeal cancer patients are treated using primary conservative treatment. However, nearly two-thirds of patients with T4a disease undergo LP chemo-radiation [11].

We evaluated the outcomes of all T4 laryngeal cancer patients between 1998 and 2004 in a study region covering a population of approximately 2.7 million people with a follow-up of up to 17 years.

Motivated by the poor outcome after LP in this subgroup, we reevaluated the literature cited in the ASCO 2006 guidelines to investigate whether there is indeed reliable evidence of equal survival in T4 laryngeal cancer patients who receive primary chemo-radiotherapy (CRT) or radiation therapy alone (RT) compared with those who undergo upfront total laryngectomy (TL).

Furthermore, we searched the literature for studies published since 2006 providing evidence of the outcomes of T4 laryngeal cancer patients after LP compared with primary surgical treatment.

Methods

From 1998 to 2004, all laryngeal cancer patients ($N = 810$) treated in the Southwestern region of Germany (covering a population of 2.7 million people) were identified as part of an observational cohort study and followed for at least 10 years. In this region, laryngeal cancer is exclusively treated in the clinics from which the cases were obtained. Local practitioners were also contacted to identify possible cases sent to more distant clinics and to verify complete case ascertainment.

Demographic data and clinical information were extracted from hospital medical records using a standardized form. Vital status and date and cause of death were requested from local registries.

Overall survival (OS) rates were calculated using the Kaplan–Meier method. Regression analysis was performed using multivariate proportional hazards models. The overall survival rates of CRT and RT, both with the option of salvage TL, were compared with those of surgery (i.e., upfront TL in T4 cases) with adjuvant radiotherapy or adjuvant chemo-radiotherapy, as indicated by stage (TL+/-a[C]RT). Survival time was measured as the time from the first diagnosis until death or until 21 March 2015. For the analysis, patients who migrated out of Germany were censored after 1 month of emigration. Only OS estimates are presented. P-values below 0.05 were considered statistically significant.

The following variables, which showed an effect in the univariate analysis ($p < 0.20$), were included in the multivariate analysis as explanatory variables: age at first diagnosis (continuous), tumor location, TNM classification, comorbidities, recurrences and second primary carcinomas and therapy approach. Backward selection was used to obtain a final model. Proportional hazards assumption was checked by adding a time-dependent version of all the variables in the model [12]. The assumption was met for all variables. The metastatic status could not be evaluated as M1 status could be clearly determined for only 5 patients. Comorbidity conditions were determined using the Charlson comorbidity index (CCI), which summarizes 18 different comorbidities, weighted by severity, in a single score [13]. For this analysis, we considered the binary form of the variable, which is set to one for CCI values of two or higher. The development of local or regional recurrence or a second primary carcinoma (SPC) was included in the model as a time-dependent covariate. For the date of diagnosis of a recurrence or an SPC, the corresponding variable was set to one. SAS 9.4 statistical software was used for all analyses.

Additionally, the literature quoted in the ASCO 2006 guidelines as the evidence base for recommending LP for patients with up to T4 cancer was reevaluated. According to the classical meaning, LP studies were defined as those that included either advanced-stage laryngeal or hypopharyngeal cancers that require or are amenable to laryngectomy and are treated with LP as an alternative to TL. To the extent that the available data permitted, we checked i.) the number of T4 patients who eventually received primary conservative treatment compared with those who had been assigned to the conservative treatment arm and ii.) the outcomes of this subgroup. A further literature search was conducted to identify the studies that have investigated the treatment of T4 laryngeal patients to date.

Results

During the seven-year recruitment period, 810 laryngeal cancer patients were identified. For the current analyses, 41 patients were excluded as they either received no treatment with curative intent ($n = 28$) or their tumor stage was unknown ($n = 13$).

The median follow-up time for the remaining 769 patients was 8.3 years, with a range from 14 days to 16.8 years.

A subgroup of 288 patients (37.5%) was classified as advanced stage and received treatment with curative intent. The subgroup included 119 stage III (15.5%) and 169 stage IV (22.0%) patients. Most of those patients were treated with surgery ($n = 238$); 30 (10.4%) were treated with CRT, and 20 (6.9%) were treated with RT alone. Additional information regarding the demographic and clinical characteristics of the three treatment groups is provided in Table 1.

Our evaluation revealed that when the stage III and stage IV patients were considered together, the patients who received CRT had a non-significantly worse outcome

Table 1 Demographic and clinical characteristics of the three treatment groups

Characteristic	Category	OP+/−a(C)RT N (%)	CRT N (%)	RT N (%)
Total		684 (100)	40 (100)	45 (100)
Age (continuous)[a]		61.9 (9.7)	61.2 (11.1)	64.6 (9.8)
Sex	Males	626 (91.5)	33 (82.5)	36 (80.0)
	Females	58 (8.5)	7 (17.5)	9 (20.0)
CCI	0	494 (72.2)	33 (82.5)	22 (48.9)
	1	100 (14.6)	1 (2.5)	15 (33.3)
	2	63 (9.2)	5 (12.5)	6 (13.3)
	3+	27 (3.9)	1 (2.5)	2 (4.4)
Tumour location	glottic	435 (63.6)	8 (20.0)	23 (51.1)
	supraglottic	168 (24.6)	22 (55.0)	14 (31.1)
	subglottic	13 (1.9)	1 (2.5)	1 (2.2)
	transglottic	42 (6.1)	6 (15.0)	3 (6.7)
	unknown	26 (3.8)	3 (7.5)	4 (8.9)
Stage	I	304 (44.4)	3 (7.5)	10 (22.2)
	II	142 (20.8)	7 (17.5)	15 (33.3)
	III	103 (15.1)	10 (25.0)	6 (13.3)
	IV	135 (19.7)	20 (50.0)	14 (31.1)
T stage	1	319 (46.6)	5 (12.5)	12 (26.7)
	2	176 (25.7)	11 (27.5)	18 (40.0)
	3	103 (15.1)	11 (27.5)	7 (15.6)
	4	86 (12.6)	13 (32.5)	8 (17.8)
N stage	0	528 (77.2)	20 (50.0)	30 (66.7)
	1	40 (5.8)	3 (7.5)	4 (8.9)
	2	75 (11.0)	12 (30.0)	8 (17.8)
	3	3 (0.4)	3 (7.5)	2 (4.4)
	unknown	38 (5.6)	2 (5.0)	1 (2.2)
Grading	1	47 (6.9)	1 (2.5)	3 (6.7)
	2	420 (61.4)	16 (40.0)	16 (35.6)
	3,4	118 (17.3)	5 (12.5)	7 (15.6)
	0, x	99 (14.5)	18 (45.0)	19 (42.2)
Laser		452 (66.1)	–	–
Partial resection		59 (8.6)	–	–
TL		173 (25.3)	–	–
RT	Primary	–	–	45 (100)
	Adjuvant	145 (21.2)	–	–
RCT	Primary	–	40 (100)	–
	Adjuvant	22 (3.2)		–

[a]Mean (Std.Dev)

in terms of OS than those who underwent upfront TL (Fig. 1a). The corresponding multivariate Cox proportional hazard analysis showed a difference in OS between the RT and the surgery group (HR 1.92; 95% CI: 1.16–3.19; $p = 0.0117$) but no significant difference in survival between the CRT and the immediate surgery group (HR 1.23; 95% CI: 0.82–1.86; $p = 0.31$).

However, the Kaplan Meier curve for the subgroup of T4 carcinoma patients ($N = 107$; 13.9%) revealed severely compromised survival after conservative LP (log-rank test: p-value < 0.0001, Fig. 1b). This was confirmed with the multivariate Cox proportional hazard analysis: Not only was OS worse after RT compared with the immediate surgery group (HR 4.6; 95% CI: 2.1–9.8; $p = 0.0001$), but more importantly, survival was also worse after CRT (HR 2.0; 95% CI: 1.04–3.7; $p = 0.0369$) (Table 2). Approximately 90% of the T4 patients died within 1 year after RT and within 2.5 years after CRT. Not a single T4 patient survived 7 years after primary conservative therapy, whereas the 10-year OS was 20% after TL + aR(C)T (95% CI: 9%–28%).

In the 179 references cited as evidence in the ASCO guidelines, five classical LP studies were found. Four of these five studies included T4 cancer patients. Differential outcome data on treated T4 tumor patients were presented in three of these four studies. In one of these three studies, the number of patients who did not respond to induction chemotherapy was not given. These patients were part of the conservative treatment arm but received upfront TL + adjuvant radiotherapy. Thus, the exact number of T4 patients in the conservative treatment arm of that study who eventually received conservative treatment was unclear. Thus, differential outcome data were presented for only 21–45 T4 tumor patients. These data, however, show a markedly worse outcome for the T4 subgroup (Table 3).

Discussion

In the observational study, survival among T4 patients was significantly worse when their larynx was not removed as part of the primary treatment regimen. This result contrasts with the 2006 ASCO clinical guidelines' statement that LP methods result in equal survival compared with primary surgery. Although the number of T4 patients in the CRT and RT groups was small, the data present the outcome of a representative cohort of all laryngeal cancer patients within a population of 2.7 million inhabitants.

Hospital records were used to extract data on disease-specific characteristics, socio-demographic variables of the study population and any events after diagnosis. The presence of comorbidities in 28.6% of the patients is likely to be an underestimation as information about comorbidities might be collected differently by physicians

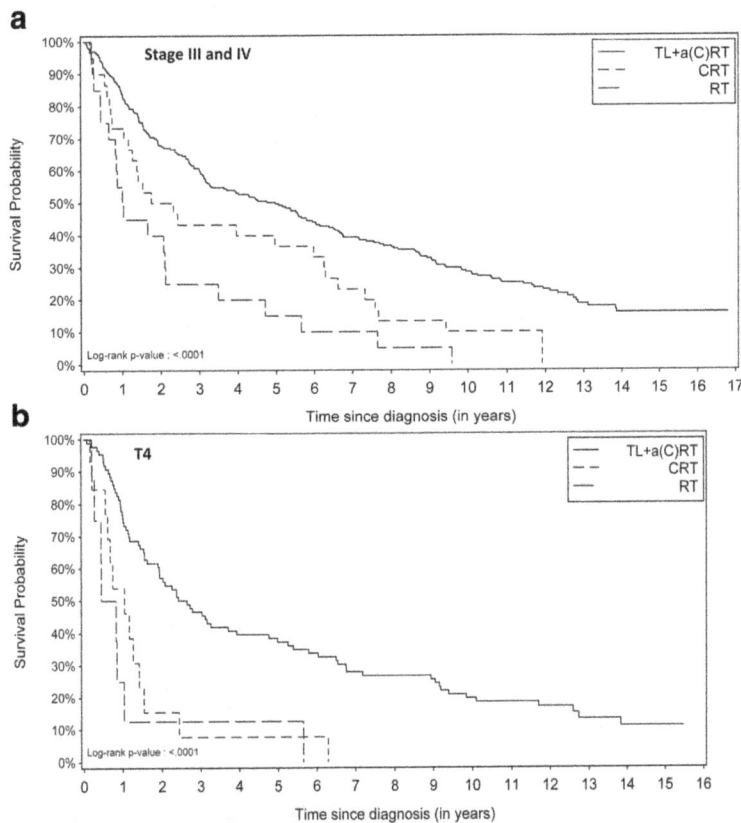

Fig. 1 a Kaplan Meier curves of stage III and stage IV patients by therapy group (OS); **b** Kaplan Meier curve for T4 carcinoma patients by therapy group (OS)

in different hospitals. Although validity could not be verified, the comorbidities recorded at the time of diagnosis should present a non-differential bias at the most and therefore should not have led to an overestimation of the real effect or interfered with the other variables in our analysis.

The Veterans Affairs Laryngeal Cancer Study Group (VALCSG) and the European Organization for Research and Treatment of Cancer (EORTC) trials proved that LP with induction chemotherapy followed by radiotherapy (ICRT) was feasible for advanced laryngeal and hypopharyngeal cancer patients without jeopardizing survival [1, 2]. However, the question is whether these large, randomized trials yielding level I evidence [9] provide sufficient evidence that LP is as appropriate for early T4 patients as for T3 patients, as stated in the 2006 ASCO guidelines. In the EORTC hypopharyngeal trial, [2] induction chemotherapy (ICT) served as stratifier for patients who might profit from mere conservative treatment. Not a single T4 disease patient responded to ICT with complete remission. Thus, no T4 patient in this study received primary RT, but all of them were treated with upfront TL and aRT. The VALCSG laryngeal cancer study [1] is the largest prospective randomized controlled trial to date of laryngeal cancer

patients; it included 332 stage III and IV patients, with 42 and 43 T4 patients in the two treatment arms. In total, 59 of the 116 patients in the conservative arm underwent TL: 30 before and 29 after RT. "Salvage laryngectomy was required, however (...) in 56 percent of the patients with T4 cancers compared with 29% of patients with smaller primary tumors (p=0.0001)." [1]. Further multivariable analysis in 1999 revealed that T4 tumors had a 5.6-fold lower likelihood of responding to chemotherapy than T1–3 tumors (95% CI, 1.5–20.8; $p = 0.0108$) [14]. The full multivariate model for predicting LP in patients treated with ICRT showed that T4 patients had a 7.1-fold worse organ preservation rate than T1–3 patients (95% CI, 1.7–29.5; $p = 0.0070$) [14]. In other words, T4 tumor patients had a markedly higher risk of failure after ICRT.

The Groupe d'Etude des Tumeurs de la Tête et du Cou (GETTEC) study [15] included only T3 laryngeal carcinoma patients. Although these patients' tumors were less advanced than T4, 21 of the 36 patients in the ICT group were treated with TL (58%), and despite salvage TL, "survival and disease-free survival were significantly worse in the induction chemotherapy group than in the no chemotherapy group (p=0.006 and p=0.02, respectively)" [15]. Richard concluded that "larynx

Table 2 Univariate and multivariate Cox proportional hazard analysis results for all T4 patients (N = 107), 1998–2015

Characteristic	Category	Deceased	Survived	HR (crude)[a,b]	95%-CI (crude)[a,b]	p-value[b]	HR (adjusted)[a,c]	95%-CI (adjusted)[a,c]	p-value[c]
Therapy	TL + a(C)RT	74 (77.9)	12 (100)	1	-	-	1	-	-
	CRT	13 (13.7)	0 (0.0)	3.0	(1.6, 5.6)	0.0004	2.0	(1.04, 3.7)	0.0369
	RT	8 (8.4)	0 (0.0)	4.2	(2.0, 8.9)	0.0002	4.6	(2.1, 9.8)	0.0001
Age[d]	(10 year units)			1.3	(1.1, 1.6)	0.0085	1.4	(1.1, 1.7)	0.0014
Recurrences	No	74 (77.9)	12 (100)	1	-	-	1	-	-
	Yes	21 (22.1)	0 (0.0)	8.5	(5.1, 14.7)	<.0001	7.3	(4.1, 12.9)	<.0001
N-stage	N0,N1	56 (58.9)	10 (83.3)	1	-	-	1	-	-
	N2,N3	39 (41.1)	2 (16.7)	2.2	(1.5, 3.4)	0.0002	1.6	(1.0, 2.5)	0.0489
Tumour location	glottic	18 (18.9)	0 (0.0)	1	-	-			
	supraglottic	34 (35.8)	4 (33.3)	0.75	(0.42, 1.3)	0.3282			
	subglottic	6 (6.3)	2 (16.7)	0.62	(0.24, 1.6)	0.3067			
	transglottic	26 (27.4)	3 (25.0)	0.74	(0.40, 1.4)	0.3300			
	Unknown	11 (11.6)	3 (25.0)	0.71	(0.33, 1.5)	0.3706			
CCI[e]	None	56 (58.9)	11 (91.7)	1	-	-			
	One and more	39 (41.1)	1 (8.3)	1.8	(1.2, 2.7)	0.0061			
2nd primary carcinoma	None	88 (92.6)	11 (91.7)	1	-	-			
	Yes	7 (7.4)	1 (8.3)	1.3	(0.60, 2.9)	0.4857			

[a]HR: Hazard Ratio; CI: Confidence interval; [b]Results from univariate analysis; [c]Results from multivariate analysis using backward selection; [d]continuous, [e]CCI: Charlson Comorbidity Index

preservation for patients selected on the basis of having responded to ICT cannot be considered a standard treatment at the present time." [15] Consistently, the GET-TEC study was stopped because of these poor results for patients with fixed cord cancer [16]. Although fixation of the vocal cord does not surpass the T3 criteria, Horn interpreted the poor results as a logical consequence of tumors with a worse prognosis per se [6]. These results suggest that LP might reach its limits of efficacy even in less advanced stages than T4.

In the Bhalavat study [17], there were only two patients with a T4 tumor in the radiotherapy arm

Table 3 Summary of patient outcomes in 5 studies comparing LP and TL in advanced laryngeal tumors

Study	T4 patients assigned to conservative treatment arm	T4 patients eventually treated by primary CRT or RT	Comments
VALCSG [4, 14]	43	Unclear, 19 < N < 43	59 TL in 116 T1-T4 patients in the conservative treatment arm, 30 upfront 24 TL (upfront + salvage) in 43 T4 patients TL in T4: 56% TL in T1–3: 29% T4 had 5.6-fold lower probability to achieve response to ICT T4 had 7.1-fold poorer organ preservation rate than T1–3
EORTC [1]	4	0	No T4 patient in the chemo arm eventually received conservative treatment, i.e. upfront TL followed by RT was the treatment for all T4 patients in the surgery as well as in the chemo arm
GETTEC [15]	0	0	Only T3 patients were included TL in 58% of patients of ICT arm OS after CRT significantly poorer than after surgery (p = 0.006)
Bhalavat [16]	2	2	1 local recurrence after partial remission 1 survived for 5 years
RTOG 91–11 [2, 8, 17, 18]	18 ICRT 17 CCRT 16 RT	Unclear	No T4 tumor with penetration through the cartilage, cartilage at the most minimally eroded 7 upfront TL in ICRT No data given about T category No differential data given for T4

compared with seven T4 patients in the primary surgery arm. One of the two patients treated with RT relapsed after a moderate response, while the other one survived for 5 years. In contrast, the T4 patients treated with primary TL had a 5-year OS of 75%. However, it is impossible to draw any reliable conclusions from these results.

The Intergroup RTOG 91–11 study was supposed to show the non-inferiority of concomitant chemoradiotherapy (CCRT) compared with the VALCSG induction chemotherapy regimen (ICRT) [3]. Provided that the OS outcome after ICRT was superior to that after CCRT, non-responsiveness to induction chemotherapy might identify the patients who require a more radical treatment strategy than primary CRT alone (as was the case for all the T4 patients in the EORTC study). The non-responders in the ICRT arm received primary TL followed by RT and thus were likely to have outcomes comparable to those of the patients in the surgical arm of the VALCSG study; however, this stratification was missing in the CCRT arm. In the RTOG study, CCRT was superior to ICRT and RT alone in terms of larynx preservation, and the five-year OS estimates did not differ significantly. However, the recently published long-term results showed 10-year OS rates of 38.8% and 27.5% in the ICRT and the CCRT groups, respectively. Although it was not statistically significant ($p = 0.08$; HR 1.25; 95% CI 0.98–1.61) [18], this strong effect cannot be ignored [8]. The RTOG study cohort contained a mix of approximately 10% T2 patients, 30% T3 patients without cord involvement, 50% T3 patients with fixed cord involvement, and only 10% T4 patients in each group. Nonetheless, earlier-stage tumors have a much better responsiveness to chemo-RT. Thus, a marked statistically significant difference could be anticipated if a T4 subgroup analysis were performed. However, a statistical comparison among the T4 patients in the three treatment arms was precluded, according to Forastière, as "only 10% of patients enrolled in RTOG 91-11 had T4 cancers" [19]. There were 18, 17, and 16 T4 tumor patients in each arm of the study and a huge number of other stage III and IV patients with T2 and T3 tumors. Desirably, within the same treatment arm, the outcome of this relatively small number of T4 patients could be compared with those of the large number of T2 and T3 patients. This subgroup analysis might provide revealing level I evidence of the outcome of T4 laryngeal cancer patients compared with lower T stage patients after different types of LP.

In the RTOG 91–11 trial, the reported successful salvage TL rates after CCRT and ICRT were 69% and 71%, respectively [20]. The salvage TL success rate, however, depends on the T category. Johansen reported a salvage TL success rate of 79% for T1a, 68% for T2, 60% for T3 and only 44% for T4 glottic carcinoma [21]. Parsons reported a success rate of 25% for T4 tumors compared with 50% successful salvage TL for other T categories

[22]. Thus, the salvage TL success rate for T4 larynx carcinoma is not as favorable as the overall success rate of approximately 70% reported for all T categories in the RTOG 91–11 trial; instead, it is 25–50%.

In summary, the RTOG 91–11 does not prove the non-inferiority of CCRT compared with ICRT in T4 larynx carcinoma in the absence of differential data for T4 patients. In the long run, the survival outcome after CCRT was increasingly worse than after ICRT. After 10 years, the difference reached almost statistical significance for the whole treatment arm, which comprised T2, T3, and T4 tumors. This effect is probably more pronounced in the subgroup of T4 tumor patients, who were less responsive to CRT and had a worse outcome with salvage surgery. Forastière stated in 2015 that in her study, "no level I evidence supports a non-operative organ preservation strategy for patients with T4a disease and penetration through cartilage". These patients were not eligible for the RTOG 91–11 study; "only patients with minimal cartilage erosion" were included [7], and mere cartilage erosion is a notable criterion for a T3 disease in laryngeal cancer. In the other LP studies cited in the ASCO guideline, a total of 21 to 45 T4 patients eventually received primary conservative LP treatment (see Table 2). Thus, the grade I evidence for LP in T4 in these studies is based on a rather low number of patients. Additionally, in terms of differential results, the T4 patients showed a markedly worse outcome after LP compared with the other stage III and IV patients.

Shortly after the establishment of the ASCO guidelines in 2006, some studies were published that supported our finding that a conservative LP approach compromises survival in T4 laryngeal cancer patients. Chen [23] evaluated the outcome of 10,590 patients with advanced laryngeal cancer registered in a national hospital-based cancer registry. Over 900 T4 tumor patients were treated using a primary conservative approach (CRT, $n = 358$; RT, $n = 566$), and 1690 patients were treated with upfront TL + aRT. Among patients with stage IV disease, TL was associated with significantly greater survival than CRT or RT ($p < 0.001$) [23]. "Because the choice between chemo-RT and TL as optimal treatment for patients with T3 primary cancers is a matter of debate" [23], Chen performed a separate proportional hazards (PH) analysis for patients with T3 primary laryngeal cancers. T3 patients treated with CRT had a significantly increased risk of death compared with those treated with TL (HR = 1.18; $p = 0.03$). The effect was even more pronounced for those treated with RT (HR = 1.59; $p = 0.001$). Separate analyses of T4 patients were not performed. In a large monocentric retrospective case series of 451 patients, Gourin collected 50 primarily non-surgically treated T4 patients compared with 77 surgically treated T4 patients over 17 years [24]. After controlling for nodal status, the authors found an increased HR of death for patients treated with CRT (HR 2.0) or RT (HR 7.2) compared with TL + aRT. The 5-year OS of these T4 tumor patients was significantly better after TL + aRT (55%) than after CRT (25%) or RT (0%; $p < 0.0001$) [24].

Accordingly, Olsen pronounced severe concern regarding the actual treatment of T4 laryngeal carcinoma [16]. He especially stated that the distinction of "low-volume T4 tumors from T4 tumors" based on examination or imaging "has not worked and is unproved" [16]. "Tumors that extend through the laryngeal cartilage should be treated with total laryngectomy" [16].

Five recent database studies corroborate the finding of a significant loss of survival after LP in T4 patients. Grover investigated the outcome of 969 T4a laryngeal cancer patients, most (64%) of whom were treated with LP-CRT [11]. He reported a markedly worse outcome for patients treated with LP-CRT compared with patients treated with upfront TL. "Median survival for TL versus LP was 61 versus 39 months (p<0.001)" [11]. CRT showed an inferior OS compared with TL (HR, 1.31; 95% CI 1.10–1.57) after potential confounders were controlled [11]. Megwalu reported 5394 advanced-stage laryngeal carcinoma that were treated between 1992 and 2009. During this period, the rate of non-surgical treatment increased from 32% to 62%. The subgroup of T4 N0 patients who received surgical treatment had a better 5-year OS (56% vs. 38%; $p < 0.001$) than patients who underwent non-surgical treatment, and this effect was markedly more pronounced than that for T3 N0 patients (59% vs. 48%; $p < 0.001$) [25]. In multivariable analysis controlling for potential confounders, non-surgical patients had worse OS (HR, 1.32; 95% CI, 1.22–1.43) than surgically treated patients.

Evaluating 258 laryngeal cancer patients in a prospective longitudinal population-based cohort study, Dziegielewski reported 5-year OS rates for T4a cancers of 70% for TL + a(C)RT, 52% for CRT and 18% for RT. [26] The HRs for RT and CRT compared with TL + a(C)RT were 4.9 ($p < 0.001$) and 2.3 ($p = 0.04$), respectively. It is worth noting that in terms of tumor site, the patients were "balanced with nearly a 50/50 glottic/supraglottic split", while in the VA and RTOG trials, there was a heavy bias toward supraglottic tumors, which are well known to respond better to CRT. Furthermore, patients with increasingly advanced disease were treated with TL + a(C)RT. Nevertheless, the surgically treated patients had a much better outcome. Moreover, Dziegielewski called attention to the fact that the pivotal LP trials were performed when the AJCC (5th edition until 2002) classified minor cartilage invasion tumors as T4 lesions. "These patients would be downstaged to T3 lesions by today's standard" [26]. The exclusion of patients

with a low Karnofsky index, the inclusion of more supraglottic tumors, and the consequent restriction to T4 tumors, e.g., those with "minimal thyroid cartilage invasion or suspicion of invasion on imaging" per protocol in RCTs constitute "selection bias" [27]. Sanabria critically states that the results of the randomized controlled LP studies are more favorable than those of observational cohort studies and may not generally be extrapolated to standard practice [27].

Timmermans reported the outcome of 1722 T4 laryngeal cancer patients treated in The Netherlands between 1991 and 2010 [28]. The difference in survival outcome compared with the other three recent population-based studies [11, 25, 26] was less marked but was statistically significant: The 5-year OS after TL + a(C)RT, CRT and RT was 48%, 42%, and 34%, respectively (overall $p < 0.0001$) [28]. It is worth noting that the cohort comprised a considerable number of tumors that would be classified as T3 according to today's standard.

In a long-term retrospective analysis of 221 T4 patients (TL + a(C)RT; $n = 161$, CRT; $n = 51$, and RT; $n = 9$), Rosenthal reported an initially superior locoregional control with upfront TL compared with LP (log-rank $p < 0.007$) [29]. However, successful salvage surgery resulted in an equal median survival time of 64 months in the TL+(C)RT group as well as the LP groups. However, the preponderance of nodal positivity in the surgery group must be taken in consideration (35.5% N2/3 in the TL + aR(C) group vs. 11.5% in the LP group) as the study revealed that node positivity represented the "primary determinant of mortality" ($p < 0.0001$) [29].

A recent database analysis presented the results of 3682 T4 M0 laryngeal cancer patients diagnosed from 2004 through 2012 [30]. Stokes divided the LP cohort into ICRT and CCRT groups (TL + a(C)RT, $n = 1599$ compared with CCRT, $n = 1597$, and ICRT, $n = 386$). The comparison between TL + a(C)RT and CCRT strongly confirms the superiority of surgery over conservative LP in T4 patients in terms of OS (HR, 1.55; 95% CI 1.41–1.70, $p < 0.01$). The ICRT cohort was defined as "undergoing RT plus multi-agent chemotherapy with chemotherapy starting 43 to 98 days before RT" [30]. According to this definition, non-responders to IC and patients discontinuing therapy due to death or no lethal toxicity during the induction period were not included in the ICRT cohort. As it is difficult to identify intention-to-treat ICRT patients in a database analysis, there is no evidence to date that ICRT might yield OS results comparable to those of TL + a(C)RT.

In a systematic review, Francis retrieved 24 retrospective studies reporting survival outcomes in T4 laryngeal cancer patients. The 5-year OS outcome ranged from 10% to 80.9% for surgery, 16% to 50.4% for CRT, and 0% to 75% for RT. However, due to major heterogeneity among the studies in terms of inclusion/exclusion criteria, laryngeal subsite, neck staging and treatment protocols, no clear conclusions can be drawn from these trials [31].

A multidisciplinary international consensus panel developed recommendations for conducting phase III clinical trials of LP in patients with locally advanced laryngeal and hypopharyngeal cancer. The panel explicitly considered whether patients with T4 disease should be eligible for future organ preservation trials "because these patients may suffer worse outcomes with this approach" [32]. This statement was supported by substantial literature. According to the consensus panel, the inclusion criteria for further LP studies are "T2 or T3 laryngeal or hypopharyngeal SCC not considered for partial laryngectomy" but not T4 carcinoma [32]. However, the NCCN treatment guidelines state that while the first recommendation for T4a tumor patients is laryngectomy, concurrent chemoradiation should be considered for "selected T4a patients who decline surgery" [10]. This recommendation is difficult for two reasons: 1.) Almost every patient will naturally reject laryngectomy if offered possible organ preservation as an alternative, especially when preservation is mentioned in current guidelines. 2.) The term "selected" implies that there might be T4a tumors for which a conservative, larynx-preserving treatment might be an appropriate approach. Forastière claimed as recently as 2015 that "selected low-volume T4 tumors endorse concomitant cisplatin and RT on the basis of level I randomized controlled trial data" [7]. As evidence, she quotes the 2006 ASCO clinical practice guidelines for LP [4]. However, our re-evaluation of the differential data from the T4 laryngeal cancer patients in precisely these cited studies shows a strong indication that this subgroup has a significantly worse outcome when treated non-surgically. A meta-analysis of the updated data of all T4 patients treated with primary conservative LP in the cited studies compared with the T2 and T3 patients in the same treatment arms could further substantiate this finding.

In summary, the evaluation of the differential data published in the large randomized controlled LP trials for the subgroup of T4 tumor patients revealed that CRT compromises survival in T4 laryngeal cancer patients. Until now, this effect was blurred by the evaluation of all stage III and IV patients together in a group that comprised T2, T3, and T4 patients. Recent large retrospective database studies, a large series with contemporaneous controls, and our own observational cohort study have shown a statistically significant loss of survival in T4 patients treated with conservative LP.

Conclusions

CRT and RT should no longer be recommended as equivalent treatment options for T4 laryngeal cancer patients, even in selected cases. T4 tumor patients who definitively reject laryngectomy should be informed that the possibility of larynx preservation with primary conservative treatment will likely result in a significantly worse outcome in terms of overall survival. A statement to this effect should be added to the NCCN guidelines.

Abbreviations
ASCO: American Society of Clinical Oncology; CCI: Charlson comorbidity index; CCRT: Concurrent chemo-radiotherapy; CI: Confidence interval; CRT: Primary chemo-radiotherapy; EORTC: European Organization for Research and Treatment of Cancer; GETTEC: Groupe d'Etude des Tumeurs de la Tête et du Cou; HR: Hazard ratio; ICRT: Induction chemo-radiotherapy; ICT: Induction chemotherapy; LP: Larynx preservation; NCCN: National Comprehensive Cancer Network; OP+/−a(C)RT: Radical surgery with or without adjuvant radiotherapy or adjuvant chemo-radiotherapy, as indicated by stage; OS: Overall survival; PH: Proportional hazards; RCT: Randomized controlled trial; RT: Primary radiotherapy alone; SPC: Second primary carcinoma; TL + a(C)RT: Upfront total laryngectomy followed by adjuvant radiotherapy or chemo-radiotherapy; TL: Total laryngectomy; VALCSG: Veterans Affairs Laryngeal Cancer Study Group

Acknowledgements
Not applicable.

Funding
Data collection of this study was supported by Dietmar Hopp Stiftung GmbH; St. Leon-Rot (grant number: 23,011,184).
We also acknowledge financial support from Deutsche Forschungsgemeinschaft and Ruprecht-Karls-Universität Heidelberg within the Open Access Publishing funding program (award number: IN-1150438).

Authors' contributions
GD and HR conducted the study, where HR conducted the data analyses and GD drafted the manuscript. HR, PP, and GD interpreted the results of the study. All authors participated in writing the manuscript and read and approved the final version.

Competing interests
The authors declare that they have no competing interests.

Author details
Department of Otorhinolaryngology, Head and Neck Surgery, University of Heidelberg, Im Neuenheimer Feld 400, 69120 Heidelberg, Germany. ²Institute of Public Health, University of Heidelberg, INF 324, 69120 Heidelberg, Germany.

References
1. Wolf G. Induction chemotherapy plus radiation compared with surgery plus radiation in patients with advanced laryngeal cancer. The Department of Veterans Affairs Laryngeal Cancer Study Group. N Engl J Med. 1991;324(24):1685–90.
2. Lefebvre JL, Chevalier D, Luboinski B, Kirkpatrick A, Collette L, Sahmoud T. Larynx preservation in pyriform sinus cancer: preliminary results of a European Organization for Research and Treatment of cancer phase III trial. EORTC head and neck cancer cooperative group. J Natl Cancer Inst. 1996; 88(13):890–9.
3. Forastiere AA, Goepfert H, Maor M, Pajak TF, Weber R, Morrison W, et al. Concurrent chemotherapy and radiotherapy for organ preservation in advanced laryngeal cancer. N Engl J Med. 2003;349(22):2091–8.
4. Pfister DG, Laurie SA, Weinstein GS, Mendenhall WM, Adelstein DJ, Ang KK, et al. American Society of Clinical Oncology clinical practice guideline for the use of larynx-preservation strategies in the treatment of laryngeal cancer. J Clin Oncol. 2006;24(22):3693–704.

5.   Lefebvre JL, Pointreau Y, Rolland F, Alfonsi M, Baudoux A, Sire C, et al. Induction chemotherapy followed by either chemoradiotherapy or bioradiotherapy for larynx preservation: the TREMPLIN randomized phase II study. J Clin Oncol. 2013;31(7):853–9.

6.   Horn S, Ozsahin M, Lefebvre JL, Horiot JC, Lartigau E, Association of R, et al. Larynx preservation: what is the standard treatment? Crit Rev Oncol Hematol. 2012;84(Suppl 1):e97–e105.

7.   Forastiere AA, Weber RS, Trotti A. Organ preservation for advanced larynx cancer: issues and outcomes. J Clin Oncol. 2015;33(29):3262–8.

8.   Corry J, Peters L, Kleid S, Rischin D. Larynx preservation for patients with locally advanced laryngeal cancer. J Clin Oncol. 2013;31(7):840–4.

9.   Hartl DM, Ferlito A, Brasnu DF, Langendijk JA, Rinaldo A, Silver CE, et al. Evidence-based review of treatment options for patients with glottic cancer. Head Neck. 2011;33(11):1638–48.

10. Pfister DG, Spencer S, Brizel DM, Burtness B, Busse PM, Caudell JJ, et al. Head and neck cancers, version 2.2014. Clinical practice guidelines in oncology. J Natl Compr Cancer Netw. 2014;12(10):1454–87.

11. Grover S, Swisher-McClure S, Mitra N, Li J, Cohen RB, Ahn PH, et al. Total Laryngectomy versus larynx preservation for T4a larynx cancer: patterns of care and survival outcomes. Int J Radiat Oncol Biol Phys. 2015;92(3):594–601.

12. Allison P. Survival Analysis using SAS - a practical guide. 2nd ed. SAS Institute Inc.2010.

13. Charlson ME, Pompei P, Ales KL, MacKenzie CR. A new method of classifying prognostic comorbidity in longitudinal studies: development and validation. J Chronic Dis. 1987;40(5):373–83.

14. Bradford CR. Predictive factors in head and neck cancer. Hematol Oncol Clin North Am. 1999;13(4):777–85.

15. Richard JM, Sancho-Garnier H, Pessey JJ, Luboinski B, Lefebvre JL, Dehesdin D, et al. Randomized trial of induction chemotherapy in larynx carcinoma. Oral Oncol. 1998;34(3):224–8.

16. Olsen KD. Reexamining the treatment of advanced laryngeal cancer. Head Neck. 2010;32(1):1–7.

17. Bhalavat RL, Fakih AR, Mistry RC, Mahantshetty U. Radical radiation vs surgery plus post-operative radiation in advanced (resectable) supraglottic larynx and pyriform sinus cancers: a prospective randomized study. Eur J Surg Oncol. 2003;29(9):750–6.

18. Forastiere AA, Zhang Q, Weber RS, Maor MH, Goepfert H, Pajak TF, et al. Long-term results of RTOG 91-11: a comparison of three nonsurgical treatment strategies to preserve the larynx in patients with locally advanced larynx cancer. J Clin Oncol. 2013;31(7):845–52.

19. Forastiere AA. Larynx preservation and survival trends: should there be concern? Head Neck. 2010;32(1):14–7.

20. Weber RS, Berkey BA, Forastiere A, Cooper J, Maor M, Goepfert H, et al. Outcome of salvage total laryngectomy following organ preservation therapy: the radiation therapy oncology group trial 91-11. Arch Otolaryngol Head Neck Surg. 2003;129(1):44–9.

21. Johansen LV, Grau C, Overgaard J. Glottic carcinoma–patterns of failure and salvage treatment after curative radiotherapy in 861 consecutive patients. Radiother Oncol. 2002;63(3):257–67.

22. Parsons JT, Mendenhall WM, Stringer SP, Cassisi NJ, Million RR. Salvage surgery following radiation failure in squamous cell carcinoma of the supraglottic larynx. Int J Radiat Oncol Biol Phys. 1995;32(3):605–9.

23. Chen AY, Halpern M. Factors predictive of survival in advanced laryngeal cancer. Arch Otolaryngol Head Neck Surg. 2007;133(12):1270–6.

24. Gourin CG, Conger BT, Sheils WC, Bilodeau PA, Coleman TA, Porubsky ES. The effect of treatment on survival in patients with advanced laryngeal carcinoma. Laryngoscope. 2009;119(7):1312–7.

25. Megwalu UC, Sikora AG. Survival outcomes in advanced laryngeal cancer. JAMA Otolaryngol Head Neck Surg. 2014;140(9):855–60.

26. Dziegielewski PT, O'Connell DA, Klein M, Fung C, Singh P, Alex Mlynarek M, et al. Primary total laryngectomy versus organ preservation for T3/T4a laryngeal cancer: a population-based analysis of survival. J Otolaryngol. 2012;41(Suppl 1):S56–64.

27. Sanabria A, Chaves AL, Kowalski LP, Wolf GT, Saba NF, Forastiere AA, et al. Organ preservation with chemoradiation in advanced laryngeal cancer: the problem of generalizing results from randomized controlled trials. Auris Nasus Larynx. 2017;44(1):18–25.

28. Timmermans AJ, van Dijk BA, Overbeek LI, van Velthuysen ML, van Tinteren H, Hilgers FJ, et al. Trends in treatment and survival for advanced laryngeal cancer: a 20-year population-based study in The Netherlands. Head Neck. 2016;38(Suppl 1):E1247–55.

29. Rosenthal DI, Mohamed AS, Weber RS, Garden AS, Sevak PR, Kies MS, et al. Long-term outcomes after surgical or nonsurgical initial therapy for patients with T4 squamous cell carcinoma of the larynx: a 3-decade survey. Cancer. 2015;121(10):1608–19.

30. Stokes WA, Jones BL, Bhatia S, Oweida AJ, Bowles DW, Raben D, et al. A comparison of overall survival for patients with T4 larynx cancer treated with surgical versus organ-preservation approaches: a National Cancer Data Base analysis. Cancer. 2017;123(4):600–8.

31. Francis E, Matar N, Khoueir N, Nassif C, Farah C, Haddad A. T4a laryngeal cancer survival: retrospective institutional analysis and systematic review. Laryngoscope. 2014;124(7):1618–23.

32. Ang KK. Larynx preservation clinical trial design: summary of key recommendations of a consensus panel. Oncologist. 2010;15(Suppl 3):25–9.

11

PD-L1 expressing circulating tumour cells in head and neck cancers

Arutha Kulasinghe[1,2], Chris Perry[3], Liz Kenny[4,5,6], Majid E. Warkiani[7,8,9], Colleen Nelson[10] and Chamindie Punyadeera[1,2*] (iD)

Abstract

Background: Blockade of the PD-1/PD-L1 immune checkpoint pathway is emerging as a promising immunotherapeutic approach for the management and treatment of head and neck cancer patients who do not respond to 1st/2nd line therapy. However, as checkpoint inhibitors are cost intensive, identifying patients who would most likely benefit from anti PD-L1 therapy is required. Developing a non-invasive technique would be of major benefit to the patient and to the health care system.

Case presentation: We report the case of a 56 year old man affected by a supraglottic squamous cell carcinoma (SCC). A CT scan showed a 20 mm right jugulodigastric node and suspicious lung lesions. The lung lesion was biopsied and confirmed to be consistent with SCC. The patient was offered palliative chemotherapy. At the time of presentation, a blood sample was taken for circulating tumour cell (CTC) analysis. The dissemination of cancer was confirmed by the detection of CTCs in the peripheral blood of the patient, measured by the CellSearch System (Janssen Diagnostics). Using marker-independent, low-shear spiral microfluidic technology combined with immunocytochemistry, CTC clusters were found in this patient at the same time point, expressing PD-L1.

Conclusion: This report highlights the potential use of CTCs to identify patients which might respond to anti PD-L1 therapy.

Keywords: PD-L1, Head and neck cancers, Circulating tumour cells, Non-invasive tools, Liquid biopsy

Background

Head and neck cancer (HNC) patients often present with advanced metastatic disease. Whilst there have been improvements in the management of locoregional disease, distant metastatic spread remains a challenge in the field [1–3]. Palliative chemotherapy is platinum based and for patients who progress after first line treatment or are refractory, therapeutic options are limited. Numerous agents including cetuximab, paclitaxel, gemcitabine and docetaxel have been assessed prospectively in the treatment of platinum refractory patients and the time to progression ranged from 2 to 6 months [4]. These systemic treatments produce a significant degree of morbidity and new therapeutic options are therefore a

need in these patients. Once there is an established role in metastatic disease, translation into the curative setting is appropriate.

The programmed cell death-1/programmed cell death-1 ligand (PD-1/PD-L1) pathway has shown to play a crucial role in tumour immune invasion. Recent literature suggests that PD-L1 over expression in solid tumour types has shown direct tumour protection. Recent studies have shown that antibodies targeting PD-1/PD-L1 have significant anti-tumour activity with a much lower toxicity profile and are currently being investigated in a number of tumour types [5, 6]. Pembrolizumab (previously MK-3475) is a highly selective, humanized igG4 (kappa) isotype monoclonal antibody designed to block PD-1 interacting with ligands, PD-L1 and PD-L2, thereby allowing the immune system to target and destroy the tumour. Pembrolizumab was the first anti PD-1 antibody to be approved by the FDA [6].

In the 2014, American Society of Clinical Oncology (ASCO) meeting, it was reported that in a majority

* Correspondence: chamindie.punyadeera@qut.edu.au
[1]The School of Biomedical Sciences, Institute of Health and Biomedical Innovation, Queensland University of Technology, Kelvin Grove, QLD, Australia
[2]Translational Research Institute, Brisbane, Australia
Full list of author information is available at the end of the article

(77.9%) of pre-treated HNSCC patients, PD-L1 is expressed in the tumour, defined by ≥1% stained cells in the tumour microenvironment [7]. In the Keynote 012 trial presented at ASCO 2015, tumour shrinkage was found in 57% of patients, and overall response of 24.8%, comprised of 26.3% in HPV-negative and 20.6% HPV-positive patients [5, 8]. The Keynote 012 study indicated that Pembrolizumab was twice as effective as cetuximab with durable responses in patients which has not been seen previously in HNC. Pembrolizumab was also well tolerated in these patients with low rates of adverse effects. 86% of the responsive patients enrolled in the Keynote 012 study continued to receive treatment highlighting the acceptable safety profile [7, 8].

Metastatic sites have shown unique genomic alterations, which can be quite different from the primary site [9, 10]. Invasive procedures are currently required to biopsy these metastatic sites, some of which may be inaccessible. Other studies have shown that these biopsies may not be representative of all of the metastatic disease [11]. An alternative approach used in other cancer types is the analysis of blood samples for circulating tumour cells (CTCs) as a form of "liquid biopsy" [12–14]. These rare tumour cells in circulation represent the "transient" cancer cell population that have the propensity to metastasize to distant sites. Recent reports have shown how CTCs may provide complementary information to identify candidate therapeutic targets and drug resistance mechanisms [9, 12, 15]. Moreover, CTCs represent cells from the primary and metastatic sites, thereby possibly providing a more comprehensive overview of the tumour burden of an individual patient. CTCs in the blood of HNC patients provide an opportunity to identify patients "at-risk" of developing overt metastasis in due course. More importantly, the analysis of these metastatic seeds in circulation may reveal important information for systemic therapy targeting metastatic disease [9]. CTCs are currently being investigated as predictive biomarkers for HER-2 targeted therapies [16]. A similar strategy could be used for immune checkpoint blockade therapies such as PD-L1.

We report the case study of a 56 year old man who had been diagnosed with a supraglottic SCC and treated with chemoradiotherapy. The patient was assessed for CTCs by the FDA-approved CellSearch (Janssen Diagnostics) and spiral microfluidics platform. Single CTCs were detected by both platforms. Using the spiral approach, CTC clusters were identified expressing PD-L1. We propose the notion that CTC PD-L1 assessment may be an avenue to identify patients who would be suitable candidates for anti-PDL1 therapy.

Case presentation

A 56 year old Caucasian male with a background history of Crohn's disease, treated with azathioprine, presented at the end of 2013 with a supraglottic T3N2b squamous cell carcinoma which was treated with upfront chemoradiotherapy, utilising Cisplatin. In October 2014, a CT scan showed a 20 mm right jugulodigastric node. Lung lesions were observed which were queried to be fungal/distant metastasis by the MDT clinic. Biopsied specimen of the lung lesions confirmed moderately differentiated SCC. Progressive disease to the lungs and pelvic bone were observed whilst on Taxol and Carboplatin, given weekly. Having limited options, a trial of infusional 5-FU (fluorouracil) was given at the end of 2015. The patient died in February 2016.

Chest X-ray

Nodules were projected over the left infrahilar region and within the right upper lobe suspicious for SCC metastasis (Fig. 1).

CTC assessment by CellSearch

The Patient presented with CellSearch-positive CTCs (2CTCs/7.5 ml) in circulation at time of presentation to clinic (Fig. 2).

CTC assessment by spiral technology

The Patient presented with 4 single CTCs (EGFR + CK + DAPI + CD45-) (Fig. 3) and 2 CTC clusters (EGFR + PDL1 + DAPI+) (Fig. 4). The CTC clusters showed a PD-L1 mean intensity in the mid to high

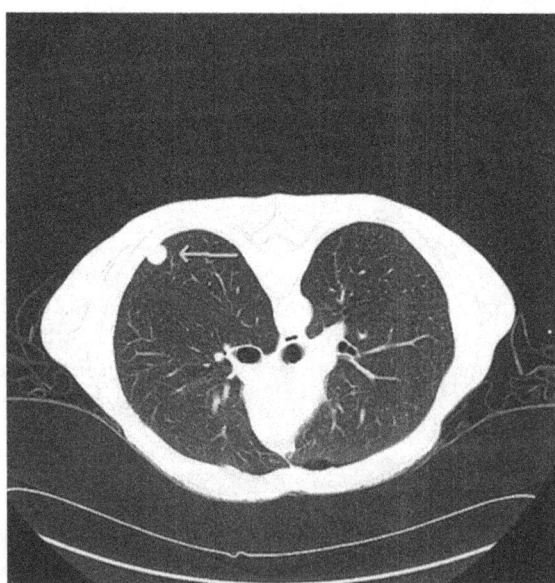

Fig. 1 Chest CT scan of Patient showing lung lesion indicated by arrow. The lung biopsy was consistent with moderately differentiated SCC

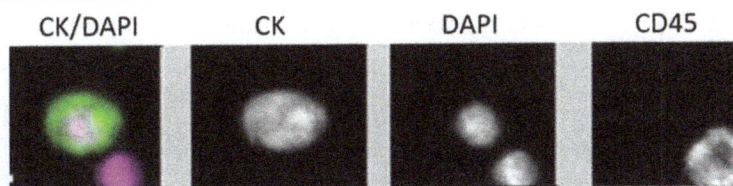

Fig. 2 Patient presented with CellSearch-positive CTCs in circulation at time of presentation to clinic. CTCs: EpCAM + CK + DAPI + CD45-, Leukocytes: CD45 + DAPI+

dynamic range, determined using a panel of known HNC cell lines (Fig. 5).

Immunoassay

The antibody against PD-L1 showed a relatively high mean intensity for (FaDu-Additional file 1: Fig. S1), medium (SCC25, CAL27), low (SCC15, 93-VU-147 T) and a negative control (K562 – Additional file 1: Fig. S2). PD-L1 staining of the CTC channel with spiked SCC-15 cells (Additional file 1: Fig. S3) and waste channel showing the bulk of leukocytes (Additional file 1: Fig. S4).

Isolation of CTCs by CellSearch

7.5 mL of whole blood collected in CellSave blood collection tubes (Janssen Diagnostics) was mixed with 6.5 ml of CellTracks™ buffer and centrifuged at 800 x g for 10 mins. The sample was placed on the AutoPrep™ system and the protocol followed as per manufacturer's instructions. The system uses a positive selection enrichment based on EpCAM antibodies and characterizes the selected cells for pan-cytokeratin (pan-CK), CD45 and DAPI staining. A CTC was determined based on the following parameters: positive for EpCAM, pan-CK, DAPI, at least a diameter of 4x4μm and negative for CD45 (common leukocyte marker). The results were reported as the number of CTCs/7.5 ml whole blood.

Enrichment of CTCs by spiral microfluidics technology

8 mL of whole blood was collected in EDTA tubes (BD-Plymouth, UK). To reduce the cellular components passing through the spiral chip, a red blood cell (RBC) lysis

was performed. Briefly, post RBC lysis (Astral Scientifix), the sample was centrifuged and the pellet resuspended in 10 mL of sheath buffer (1xPBS, 2 mM EDTA, 0.5% BSA). Tygon® tubing was inserted into the inlet/outlets of the spiral chip, and the inlet tubing connected to a syringe pump. The spiral chip was fixed into position on a phase contrast microscope (Olympus, IX71). The outlet tubing was connected to sterile 15 mL BD falcon collection tubes. To run the patient sample, the sample was carefully loaded into a 10 ml syringe and pumped through the spiral chip at a flow rate of 1.7 ml/min [17]. The outputs were collected and spun down at 300 x g for 5 mins. The enriched cell suspension was cytospun onto 2 glass slides using the Cytospin™ 4 Cytocentrifuge (ThermoScientific, USA). The presence of CTCs was determined by immunofluorescent staining.

Development of an immunoassay for PD-L1

Five head and neck cell lines were used to develop a dynamic range of PD-L1 expression. FaDu (ATCC®HTB43™), CAL27 (ATCC®CRL2095™), SCC25 (ATCC®CRL-1628™) were from the American Type Culture Collection (ATCC™). SCC15 (ATCC®CRL-1623™) a generous gift from Dr. Glen Boyle (QIMR, Brisbane) and 93-VU-147 T (CVCL_L895) (HPV-positive) cell line from Dr. Johan de Winter (VU Medical Center, Netherlands). The human chronic myelogenous leukemia K562 (ATCC®CCL-243) cells were used as a negative control (gift from Prof Maher Gandhi, UQDI, Brisbane). Briefly, cytospins (Cytospin™ Cytocentrifuge, USA) were prepared using aliquots of 1000 cells/slide by centrifugation at 300 x g for 5 mins.

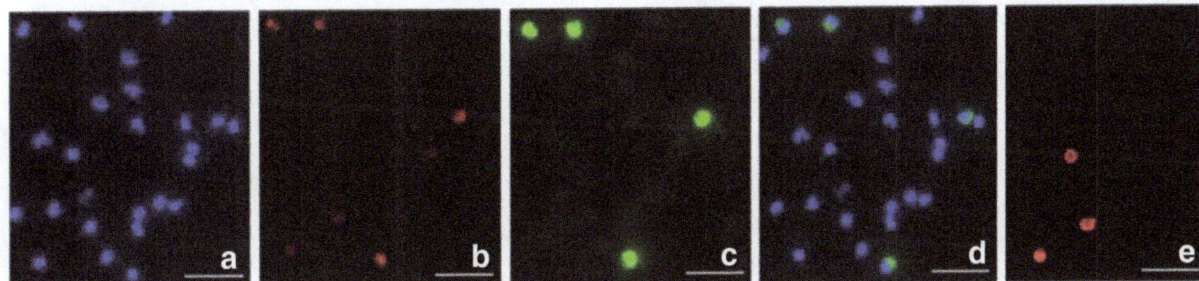

Fig. 3 Single CTCs detected after enrichment using spiral microfluidics. Immunofluorescent staining for (**a**) DAPI (**b**) Cytokeratin (**c**) EGFR (**d**) Composite EGFR/DAPI (**e**) CD45. CTCs: EGFR + CK + DAPI + CD45-. White blood cells: CD45 + DAPI+. Scale bar represents 50 μm

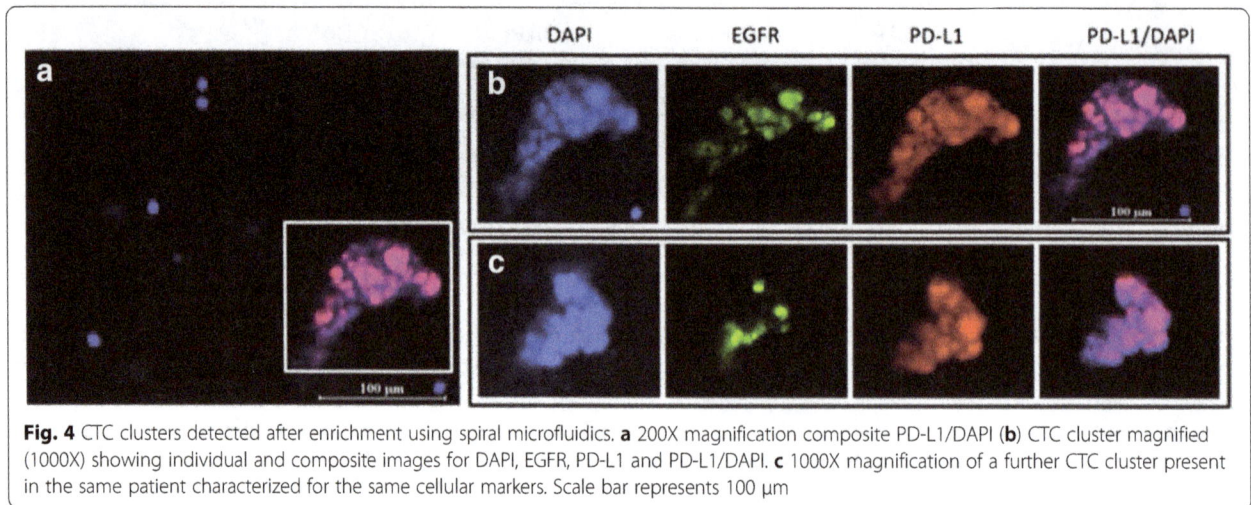

Fig. 4 CTC clusters detected after enrichment using spiral microfluidics. **a** 200X magnification composite PD-L1/DAPI (**b**) CTC cluster magnified (1000X) showing individual and composite images for DAPI, EGFR, PD-L1 and PD-L1/DAPI. **c** 1000X magnification of a further CTC cluster present in the same patient characterized for the same cellular markers. Scale bar represents 100 μm

The slides were stained with PD-L1 as per the immuno-cytochemistry protocol below.

Immunocytochemistry

Briefly, the initial sample was stained using the Cell-Search antibody cocktail (Janssen Diagnostics) and anti-EGFR antibody (AY13, Biolegend, San Diego) as previously described [18–20]. A further slide was fixed with 4% formaldehyde for 10 mins, permeabilized with 0.2% Triton X-100 for 5 mins and blocked with 10% fetal-bovine serum in 0.1% PBS-Tween for 1 h at room temperature. The cells were incubated overnight at 4 °C with anti-EGFR antibody and anti-PD-L1 antibody [28-8] (Alexa Fluor® 647) (Abcam ab209960) 1/100 dilution. Nuclear DNA was visualized with DAPI. Rabbit IgG

monoclonal isotype control (Alexa Fluor®647) (ab199093) was used to identify nonspecific binding. Cells were imaged on the Olympus IX3 inverted microscope.

Discussion and conclusions

The predictive value of PD-L1 expression in primary tissues is limited [9]. Furthermore, there is weak correlation between matched primary tumour and distant metastasis, suggesting that primary tumour is not an adequate surrogate for determining PD-L1 expression at metastatic sites [21]. Importantly, this highlights the fact that a single core biopsy may not suffice to determine tumour PD-L1 expression [9]. The FDA-approved Cell-Search technology has shown clinical significance of

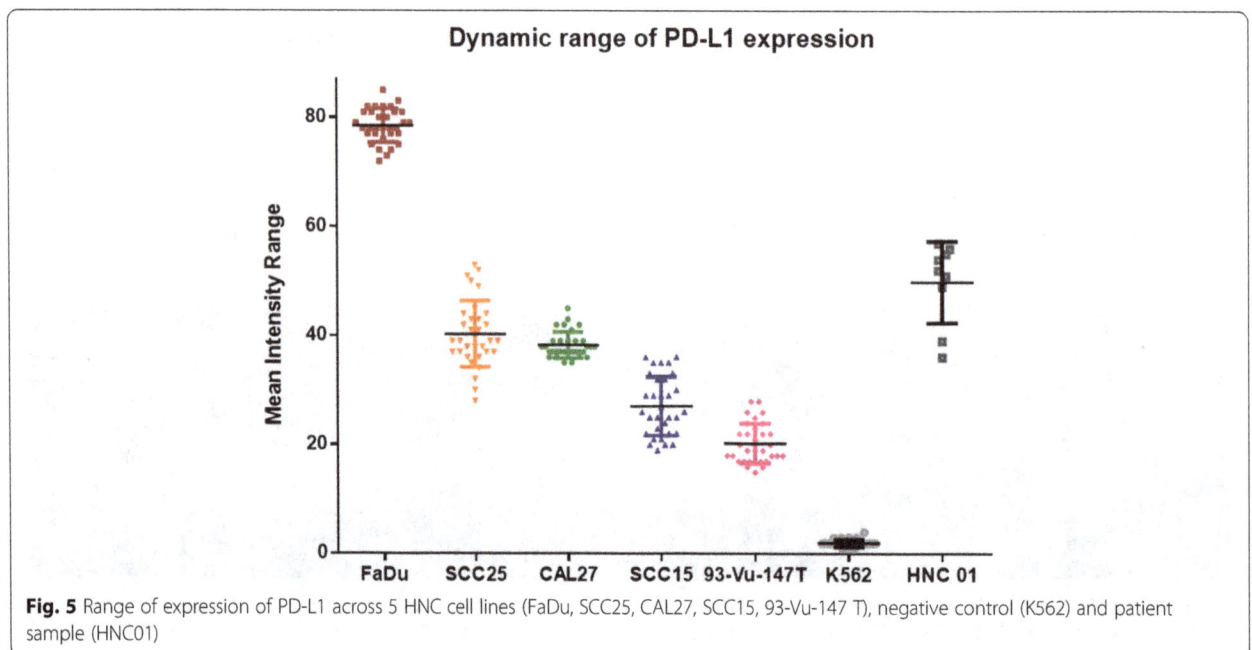

Fig. 5 Range of expression of PD-L1 across 5 HNC cell lines (FaDu, SCC25, CAL27, SCC15, 93-Vu-147 T), negative control (K562) and patient sample (HNC01)

EpCAM-positive CTCs [22]. However, there has been a shift in the field to maker-independent technologies to capture a greater proportion of CTCs in circulation in an unbiased fashion [18, 23]. By the use of established [9, 22] and spiral microfluidics technology [17, 24] this study aimed to capture the tumour cells in circulation of this patient and characterize the PD-L1 expression.

The patient presented with CTCs by enrichment using both CellSearch and spiral technologies. Importantly, the spiral technology was able to enrich for CTC clusters which are rarely detectable by CellSearch [25]. These microemboli/tumour cell clusters have shown an increased metastatic potential compared to single cells [26, 27]. Moreover, the cluster had a mid-high PD-L1 expression compared to the panel of known head and neck cancer cell lines. The PD-L1 + CTCs indicate that the patient had tumour cells in circulation with the capacity to block the immune system. These could be a potential targets for PD-L1 therapies [9]. The development of an immune-score is desirable for metastatic HNC patients.

In the 2016 AACR meeting, in locally advanced HNC patients, PD-L1+ CTCs were associated with shorter progression free survival (PFS) and overall survival (OS), and were proposed to "select and monitor patients for PD-1 checkpoint inhibitors" [28, 29]. These studies as well as this study, demonstrate that PD-L1 is expressed in HNSCC tumours and CTCs and may contribute to the tumours ability to evade the immune system. Moreover, that PD-L1 may be used as a biomarker for predicting responders from non-responders in lieu of the cost burden of such therapies.

This case report highlights the potential of using of CTCs to (i) identify patients 'at-risk' of developing metastasis (ii) identifying HNC patients that are likely to benefit from anti PD-L1 therapy and (iii) the development of a CTC PD-L1 immune-score for HNC. Further studies are warranted comparing patient tumour and CTC PD-L1 expression to develop predictive biomarkers.

Additional file

Additional file 1: Fig. S1. HNSCC cell lines (FaDu) immunofluorescent staining with DAPI (Blue), PD-L1 (Red). Scale bar represents 10 μm. Fig. S2 Rabbit IgG monoclonal Isotype control (AlexaFluor 647) (ab199093). Scale bar represents 10 μm. Fig. S3 DAPI and PD-L1 staining on HNSCC cell line (SCC15) spiked into Normal healthy blood and sorted on the spiral chip (CTC outlet). White arrows indicate leukocytes in the background of spiked tumour cells. Scale bar represents 10 μm. Fig. S4 PD-L1 staining of white blood cells in the waste channel of the spiral chip. Scale bar represents 10 μm.

Abbreviations
5-FU: 5-fluorouracil; BSA: Bovine serum albumin; CK: cytokeratin; CTC: circulating tumour cells; DAPI: 4',6-diamudubi-2-phenylindole; EGFR: epidermal growth factor recptor; FDA: Food and Drug Administration; HNC: Head and neck cancer; NHMRC: National Health and Medical Research Council; OS: Overall Survival; PAH: Princess Alexandra Hospital;

PBS: Phosphate buffered saline; PD-L: Programmed cell death ligand; PD-L1: Programmed cell death ligand one; PFS: Progression free surivival; SCC: squamous cell carcinoma; UQ: University of Queensland

Acknowledgements
The authors would like to thank Prof William B Coman (Brisbane, Australia) for clinical guidance, Dr. Mitesh Gandhi (Radiologist, Queensland Health, PAH), Ms. Dana Middleton (Clinical Trials Coordinator, PAH) and Dr. Christin Gasch for editorial assistance.

Funding
The study was supported by the Queensland Centre for Head and Neck funded by Atlantic Philanthropies and the Queensland Government in the design of the study. CP: QUT VC Fellowship. AK: QUT Postgraduate research scholarship.

Authors' contributions
Study concept and design: AK, CN, CP, MEW. Acquisition of data: AK, CP1. Analysis and interpretation of data: AK, CN, CP, LK, CP1, MEW. Drafting of manuscript: AK, MEW, CP, LK. Critical revision: AK, MEW, CP1, CP, LK. CP1: Chris Perry, CP: Chamindie Punyadeera. All authors have read and approved and manuscript.

Competing interests
The authors declare that they have no competing interests.

Author details
[1]The School of Biomedical Sciences, Institute of Health and Biomedical Innovation, Queensland University of Technology, Kelvin Grove, QLD, Australia. [2]Translational Research Institute, Brisbane, Australia. [3]Department of Otolaryngology, Princess Alexandra Hospital, QLD, Woolloongabba, Australia. [4]School of Medicine, University of Queensland, Brisbane, QLD, Australia. [5]Royal Brisbane and Women's Hospital, Brisbane, QLD, Australia. [6]Central Integrated Regional Cancer Service, Queensland Health, Brisbane, QLD, Australia. [7]School of Mechanical and Manufacturing Engineering, Australian Centre for NanoMedicine, University of New South Wales, Sydney, Australia. [8]Garvan Institute for Biomedical Research, Sydney, Australia. [9]School of Medical Sciences, Edith Cowan University, Joondalup, Perth, WA 6027, Australia. [10]Australian Prostate Cancer Research Centre - Queensland, Institute of Health and Biomedical Innovation, Queensland University of Technology, Princess Alexandra Hospital, Translational Research Institute Brisbane, Brisbane, Australia.

References
1. Kulasinghe A, Perry C, Jovanovic L, Nelson C, Punyadeera C. Circulating tumour cells in metastatic head and neck cancers. Int J Cancer. 2015;136: 2515–23.
2. Schmidt H, Kulasinghe A, Kenny L, Punyadeera C. The development of a liquid biopsy for head and neck cancers. Oral Oncol. 2016;61:8–11.
3. Chai RC, Lim Y, Frazer IH, Wan Y, Perry C, Jones L, Lambie D, Punyadeera C. A pilot study to compare the detection of HPV-16 biomarkers in salivary oral rinses with tumour p16(INK4a) expression in head and neck squamous cell carcinoma patients. BMC Cancer. 2016;16:178.
4. Zandberg DP, Strome SE. The role of the PD-L1:PD-1 pathway in squamous cell carcinoma of the head and neck. Oral Oncol. 2014;50:627–32.
5. Shin DS, Ribas A. The evolution of checkpoint blockade as a cancer therapy: what's here, what's next? Curr Opin Immunol. 2015;33:23–35.
6. Khoja L, Butler MO, Kang SP, Ebbinghaus S, Joshua AM. Pembrolizumab. J Immunother Cancer. 2015;3:36.
7. T S, Burtness B, J W, al e: A phase 1b study of MK-3475 in patients with human papillomavirus (HPV)-associated and non-HPV-associated head and neck (H/N) cancer. Journal of Clinical Oncology 2014;32:5s.
8. Starr P. Encouraging results for Pembrolizumab in head and neck cancer. American Health & Drug Benefits. 2015;8:16–6.

9. Mazel M, Jacot W, Pantel K, Bartkowiak K, Topart D, Cayrefourcq L, Rossille D, Maudelonde T, Fest T, Alix-Panabieres C. Frequent expression of PD-L1 on circulating breast cancer cells. Mol Oncol. 2015;9:1773–82.

10. Kang Y, Pantel K. Tumor cell dissemination: emerging biological insights from animal models and cancer patients. Cancer Cell. 2013;23:573–81.

11. Gerlinger M, Rowan AJ, Horswell S, Larkin J, Endesfelder D, Gronroos E, Martinez P, Matthews N, Stewart A, Tarpey P, et al. Intratumor heterogeneity and branched evolution revealed by multiregion sequencing. N Engl J Med. 2012;366:883–92.

12. Alix-Panabieres C, Pantel K. Clinical applications of circulating tumor cells and circulating tumor DNA as liquid biopsy. Cancer Discov. 2016;6:479–91.

13. Gasch C, Oldopp T, Mauermann O, Gorges TM, Andreas A, Coith C, Muller V, Fehm T, Janni W, Pantel K, Riethdorf S. Frequent detection of PIK3CA mutations in single circulating tumor cells of patients suffering from HER2-negative metastatic breast cancer. Mol Oncol. 2016;

14. Gasch C, Bauernhofer T, Pichler M, Langer-Freitag S, Reeh M, Seifert AM, Mauermann O, Izbicki JR, Pantel K, Riethdorf S. Heterogeneity of epidermal growth factor receptor status and mutations of KRAS/PIK3CA in circulating tumor cells of patients with colorectal cancer. Clin Chem. 2013;59:252–60.

15. Schmidt H, Kulasinghe A, Perry C, Nelson C, Punyadeera C. A liquid biopsy for head and neck cancers. Expert Rev Mol Diagn. 2016;16:165–72.

16. Bidard FC, Fehm T, Ignatiadis M, Smerage JB, Alix-Panabieres C, Janni W, Messina C, Paoletti C, Muller V, Hayes DF, et al. Clinical application of circulating tumor cells in breast cancer: overview of the current interventional trials. Cancer Metastasis Rev. 2013;32:179–88.

17. Warkiani ME, Guan G, Luan KB, Lee WC, Bhagat AA, Chaudhuri PK, Tan DS, Lim WT, Lee SC, Chen PC, et al. Slanted spiral microfluidics for the ultra-fast, label-free isolation of circulating tumor cells. Lab Chip. 2014;14:128–37.

18. Kulasinghe A, Perry C, Warkiani ME, Blick T, Davies A, O'Byrne K, Thompson EW, Nelson CC, Vela I, Punyadeera C. Short term ex-vivo expansion of circulating head and neck tumour cells. Oncotarget. 2016;

19. Kulasinghe A, Kenny L, Perry C, Thiery J-P, Jovanovic L, Vela I, Nelson C, Punyadeera C. Impact of label-free technologies in head and neck cancer circulating tumour cells. Oncotarget. 2016;7:71223–34.

20. Kulasinghe A TT, Blick T, O'Byrne K, Thompson EW, Warkiani ME, Nelson C, Kenny L, Punyadeera C.: Enrichment of circulating head and neck tumour cells using spiral microfluidic technology *Scientific Reports* 2017, in press.

21. Jilaveanu LB, Shuch B, Zito CR, Parisi F, Barr M, Kluger Y, Chen L, Kluger HM. PD-L1 expression in clear cell renal cell carcinoma: an analysis of nephrectomy and sites of metastases. J Cancer. 2014;5:166–72.

22. Allard WJ, Matera J, Miller MC, Repollet M, Connelly MC, Rao C, Tibbe AG, Uhr JW, Terstappen LW. Tumor cells circulate in the peripheral blood of all major carcinomas but not in healthy subjects or patients with nonmalignant diseases. Clin Cancer Res. 2004;10:6897–904.

23. Warkiani ME, Khoo BL, Wu L, Tay AK, Bhagat AA, Han J, Lim CT. Ultra-fast, label-free isolation of circulating tumor cells from blood using spiral microfluidics. Nat Protoc. 2016;11:134–48.

24. Khoo BL, Warkiani ME, Tan DS, Bhagat AA, Irwin D, Lau DP, Lim AS, Lim KH, Krisna SS, Lim WT, et al. Clinical validation of an ultra high-throughput spiral microfluidics for the detection and enrichment of viable circulating tumor cells. PLoS One. 2014;9:e99409.

25. Farace F, Massard C, Vimond N, Drusch F, Jacques N, Billiot F, Laplanche A, Chauchereau A, Lacroix L, Planchard D, et al: A direct comparison of CellSearch and ISET for circulating tumour-cell detection in patients with metastatic carcinomas. Br J Cancer 2011;105:847–853.

26. Aceto N, Bardia A, Miyamoto DT, Donaldson MC, Wittner BS, Spencer JA, Yu M, Pely A, Engstrom A, Zhu H, et al. Circulating tumor cell clusters are oligoclonal precursors of breast cancer metastasis. Cell. 2014;158:1110–22.

27. Au SH, Storey BD, Moore JC, Tang Q, Chen Y-L, Javaid S, Sarioglu AF, Sullivan R, Madden MW, O'Keefe R, et al. Clusters of circulating tumor cells traverse capillary-sized vessels. Proc Natl Acad Sci. 2016;113:4947–52.

28. G K, Strati A, A M, al e: PDL1-expressing circulating tumor cells (CTCs) in head and neck squamous cell carcinoma (HNSCC). J Clin Oncol 2015;33.

29. Strati A, Koutsodontis G, Angelidis I, Sasaki C, Avgeris M, Psyrri A, Lianidou ES. Abstract 3108: PD-L1 expressing circulating tumor cells (CTCs) in patients with head and neck squamous cell carcinoma (HNSCC). Cancer Res. 2016; 76:3108–8.

12

New paste for severe stomatitis in patients undergoing head-and-neck cancer radiotherapy and/or chemotherapy with oral appliance

Ayumi Sakuramoto[1†], Yoko Hasegawa[1*†] (iD), Kazuma Sugahara[1], Yoshiyuki Komoda[2], Kana Hasegawa[1], Shinichi Hikasa[3], Mai Kurashita[1], Junya Sakai[1], Masahiro Arita[4], Kazuhiro Yasukawa[5] and Hiromitsu Kishimoto[1]

Abstract

Background: The aim of the present study was to evaluate the physical properties of "admixture paste", which is a commercially available gel containing hinokitiol for use against severe stomatitis, and its characteristics as a moisturizing gel and denture adhesive.

Methods: The admixture paste, which contained dexamethasone (Dexaltin®), gel for oral care (Refrecare H®) and petrolatum, and its 3 components, either alone or in different combinations, were subjected to viscosity, adhesiveness and elution testing to compare their physical properties. Viscosity was measured with a stress-controlled rheometer. Adhesive force was measured by tension test. Elution under a simulated oral environment was evaluated by monitoring with a fixed-point camera and absorbance. Both adhesiveness and elution were evaluated every hour for 6 h. A linear mixed-effects model was used to assess differences in the time course of elution between samples. In 3 og-rank test was used to compare time to elution into saliva among samples.

Results: The results of viscosity testing demonstrated that the admixture paste had similar viscosity to cream-type denture adhesives and this was temperature independent. In the adhesiveness tests, the admixture paste showed stronger adhesiveness than that of cream-type denture adhesives. In the elution test, the admixture paste demonstrated gradual dissolution and apparent temporal changes for 6 h in a simulated oral environment.

Conclusions: The results of the present study demonstrated that the admixture paste has adhesive force similar to those of denture adhesives and good local retention in saliva, and that it might be suitable for therapeutic use in patients with severe stomatitis derived from radiotherapy and/or chemotherapy for cancer.

Keywords: Stomatitis, Head-and-neck cancer, Treatment paste, Denture adhesives, Radiotherapy and/or chemotherapy

Background

Multidisciplinary treatments consisting of surgery, radiotherapy and chemotherapy are performed for patients with malignancy [1]. However, these treatments can induce severe oral stomatitis, thus interfering with oral ingestion. In our daily clinical practice, we frequently encounter patients undergoing treatment by radiotherapy and/or chemotherapy (hereinafter referred to as "CRT") for cancer in the head and neck region with severe oral stomatitis. Radiotherapy for head and neck cancer has a nearly 100% risk of causing oral stomatitis in the irradiated area [2, 3]. Chemotherapy is also associated with a 1–10% risk of causing severe oral stomatitis [4, 5]. However, there is no established pre-treatment management practice for preventing stomatitis, as the method of treatment for stomatitis varies between institutions [6].

* Correspondence: cem17150@hyo-med.ac.jp
†Equal contributors
[1]Department of Dentistry and Oral Surgery, Hyogo College of Medicine, 1-1 Mukogawa-cho, Nishinomiya, Hyogo 663-8501, Japan
Full list of author information is available at the end of the article

At the Department of Dentistry and Oral Surgery in the College of Medicine, we provide pre-operative oral management for almost all patients with head and neck cancer among those who are hospitalized. For stomatitis occurring in these patients after CRT, we perform oral management practices, such as oral cleaning, application of gel for oral care, laser treatment and use of mouthwash containing local anesthetic. Many of the patients with head and neck cancer are elderly and have postoperative defects of teeth, jaw bone and oral tissue, which is necessary for the use of oral appliances such as removable dentures and palatal augmentation prosthesis (PAP) [7]. Thus, there are many patients who experience severe stomatitis including mucositis, which interferes with the use of dentures during CRT. The interruption of oral appliance use significantly affects quality of life (QOL) by preventing patients from talking and eating [8–10]. Severe stomatitis may result in interruption or even discontinuation of cancer treatment [11] by infections derived from severe oral stomatitis, neutropenia and/or uncontrollable pain. Nevertheless, no established treatment is currently available for severe stomatitis in patients undergoing head-and-neck cancer CRT with oral appliances. Dexamethasone ointment and other steroid ointments are often prescribed for the purpose of pain relief, but indiscriminate use of these agents may induce microbial substitution with *Candida* and other fungi [12, 13]. Furthermore, steroid ointments are effective against oral stomatitis caused by head-and-neck cancer treatments such as CRT [14]. Gel for oral care is often prescribed for pain relief and to moisten the oral cavity. In general treatment, all of these components are used separately, but not simultaneously.

In our clinical practice, we found that dexamethasone and oral gel with hinokitiol are effective when mixed together because the viscosity is increased. Vaseline is added to further adjust the viscosity, which improves the handling. Subsequently, we mixed various ointments and oral gels for use against oral stomatitis with the aim of finding a paste having an appropriate coefficient of viscosity. As a consequence, we developed an "admixture paste" formulated from equal amounts of dexamethasone ointment (Dexaltin® Oral Ointment, Nippon Kayaku Co., Ltd., Tokyo, Japan; hereinafter referred to as "Dexi"), gel for oral care (Refrecare® H, Nippon Zettoc Co., Ltd., Tokyo, Japan; "Moist") and petrolatum (Kenei Seiyaku, Osaka, Japan; "Vase") for infection prevention and symptom relief of severe stomatitis in patients with head and neck cancer. With this paste, we expect good local retention and lasting drug/gel efficacy regardless of the flow of saliva.

For clinical use of "admixture paste", we obtained approval from the Hyogo College of Medicine Ethics Committee regarding the safety and approach used. Subsequently, the admixture paste was available for short-term (maximal 3 weeks) treatment of severe stomatitis in patients undergoing head-and-neck cancer CRT and using oral appliances (dentures and PAP). Short-term use of the admixture paste for head and neck cancer with severe stomatitis resulted in symptom relief of severe stomatitis and appeared to provide stability of oral appliances. We have not yet performed quantitative assessment of the physical properties (viscosity and elution characteristics to saliva) of this admixture paste.

The aim of the study was to evaluate the physical properties and moisturizing characteristics of "admixture paste" (containing dexamethasone, gel for oral care and petrolatum), which has a viscosity and adhesiveness equivalent to that of denture adhesive.

Methods
Preparation of mixed paste
The components of the admixture paste and their compositions are shown in Table 1. The admixture paste was prepared by mixing equal volumes of Dexi, Moist and Vase in a rubber cup for dental use (28 mm in inner diameter and 33 mm in height; Tokuyama Dental, Osaka, Japan) using a metal spatula (YDM Corporation, Tokyo, Japan) for 30 s until a homogeneous knead was obtained. Kneading was performed by either a dentist or a dental hygienist. The obtained admixture paste was stored in an airtight container at room temperature for up to 24 h before use. An additional movie file shows the paste preparation in more detail (see Additional file 1).

Physical property evaluation
Viscosity measurement
Viscosity was measured with a stress-controlled rheometer (Anton-Paar Japan, Tokyo, Japan) on the following 8 materials: Dexi+Moist+Vase (DMV; i.e., admixture paste), Dexi, Dexi+Moist (DM), Moist, Moist+Vase (MV), Vase, cream-type denture adhesive New Poligrip® (GlaxoSmithKline K.K., Tokyo, Japan; hereinafter referred to as "Poli") and cushion-type denture adhesive Toughgrip (Kobayashi Pharmaceutical Co., Ltd., Osaka, Japan; "Tough"). We prepared fresh DMV for each experiment. Viscosity η [Pa·s] and shear stress σ [Pa] were measured at two temperatures (25 °C and 37 °C to mimic room and oral temperatures, respectively) at shear rates (dγ/dt) varying from 0 to 30 s^{-1}. Originally, the method for viscosity measurement basically followed Japanese Industrial Standards (JISK7117–2). However, the aim of rheological measurement in the present study was to describe how the newly proposed material deforms with the application of force and to compare this

Table 1 Composition of each material

Dexi		Moist		Vase	
Active component	Dexamethasone	Active component	Hinokitiol Dipotassium glycyrrhizinate	Active component	White vaseline
Additive	Liquid paraffin Sodium polyacrylate Plastibase	Sweetener	Xylitol		
		Solubilizing agent	Polyoxyethylene hydrogenated castor oil		
		Preservative	Sodium benzoate		
		Preservative	A hydrogenphosphate melanian snail thorium Citric acid Humecant sodium hyaluronate (2) Concentrated glycerin A propylene glycol		
		Solvent	Purified water Ethanol		
		Binding agent	Sodium polyacrylate A carrageenan		
		Stabilizer	An edetic acid melanian snail thorium		
		Flavor	Rifrecare H and menthol		

Dexi: dexamethasone ointment (Dexaltin® Oral Ointment); Moist: gel for oral care (Refrecare H®); Vase: petrolatum

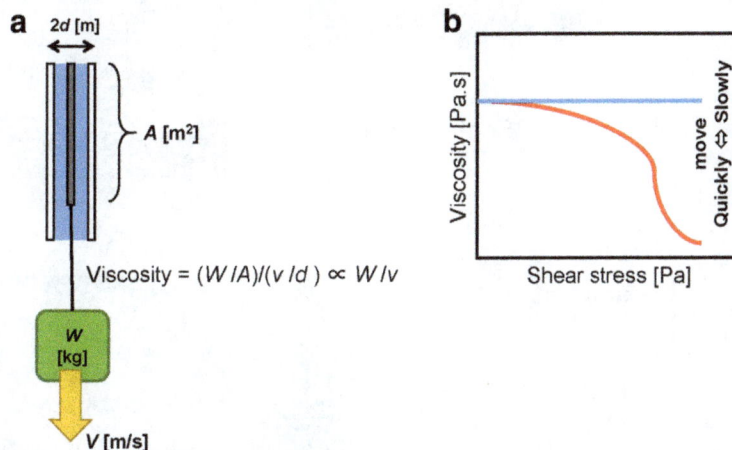

Fig. 1 Meaning of viscosity. **a** Suppose that a thin plate (zero thickness) having an area A [m2] is sandwiched between the material of interest and large plates. They are aligned vertically, and a paper weight having a weight W [kg] is suspended from the thin plate. The paper weight falls at a speed v [m/s] when the distance between plates is 2d [m]. Viscosity is defined as follows: Viscosity = $(Wg/2A)/(v/d) \propto W/v$ (e.g., water has viscosity of 0.001 Pa·s). This equation indicates that the falling speed of the paper weight is proportional to the weight under constant viscosity. A heavier paper weight falls at a higher speed, and a lighter one falls more slowly. **b** If the viscosity is decreased with increasing shear stress, as expressed by the red curve, how does the paper weight falls? If the paper weight is sufficiently light, the falling speed is roughly same as that in the case of constant viscosity, blue line, because they have almost the same viscosity in the small shear stress region. In contrast, when a heavy paper weight is suspended, the paper weight must fall down quickly in the case of non-constant viscosity, because the falling speed is inversely proportional to viscosity. Therefore, a higher viscosity at a larger shear stress means that an obstacle stuck to the material moves more slowly. In other words, the obstacle feels a larger resistance in a more viscous material, and is difficult to move, which is characterized as being "more sticky"

with other well-known materials. In this research, we therefore measured viscosity at exponentially increasing shear stress levels. Figure 1 shows an explanation of viscosity and how it is plotted on a graph.

Adhesive force measurement

The measurement of adhesive force was performed on three types of sample, i.e., Poli, Tough and DMV, which were stored for up to 6 h in a simulated oral environment. Figure 2 shows the experimental procedure. Each sample having a roughly constant volume of 0.024 ml is squeezed between two stainless steel disks (SUS304; diameter, 35 mm; thickness, 1 mm). As two pieces of scotch tape are superposed on the bottom disk, the gap between the disks should be constant at 0.12 mm for all experiments. Subsequently, the cross-sectional area of the squeezed sample was constant at 200 mm^2. The disks were then immersed in artificial saliva (Saliveht; Teijin Pharma Ltd., Tokyo, Japan) and incubated in an FMS-1000 thermostatic chamber (Tokyo Rikakikai Co., Ltd., Tokyo, Japan) at 37 °C while shaking at 37 rpm (MMS-3010; Tokyo Rikakikai Co., Ltd., Tokyo, Japan). Saliveht, which can only be prescribed in Japan, was used as artificial saliva throughout all experiments, and

was treated with a Vacuum mixer (J. Morita Corporation, Tokyo, Japan) in order to remove CO_2.

The bottom disk was firmly fixed onto a fixed glass disk using glue, while a hook was fixed on the top disk using strong double-side tape. A hanging weight scale (Electronic Portable Luggage Digital Scale, accuracy, 5 g; Weiheng, Shenzhen, China) was hitched to the hook attached to the top disk in order to measure the changes in normal force as a weight change. The normal force increased gradually as the top disk was stuck to the sample. However, the normal force instantaneously decreased when the top disk was separated from the sample. The hanging scale was manually pulled at a sufficiently slow and constant speed, such that the digits of the scale changed slowly to clearly see the maximum, and that the effect of acceleration on the measured value is negligible. The maximum normal force was determined from digit changes while pulling the scale. The adhesive force was divided by the cross-sectional area of the sample in order to account for the effects of variations in sample volume.

An additional movie file shows this experimental procedure in more detail (see Additional File 2).

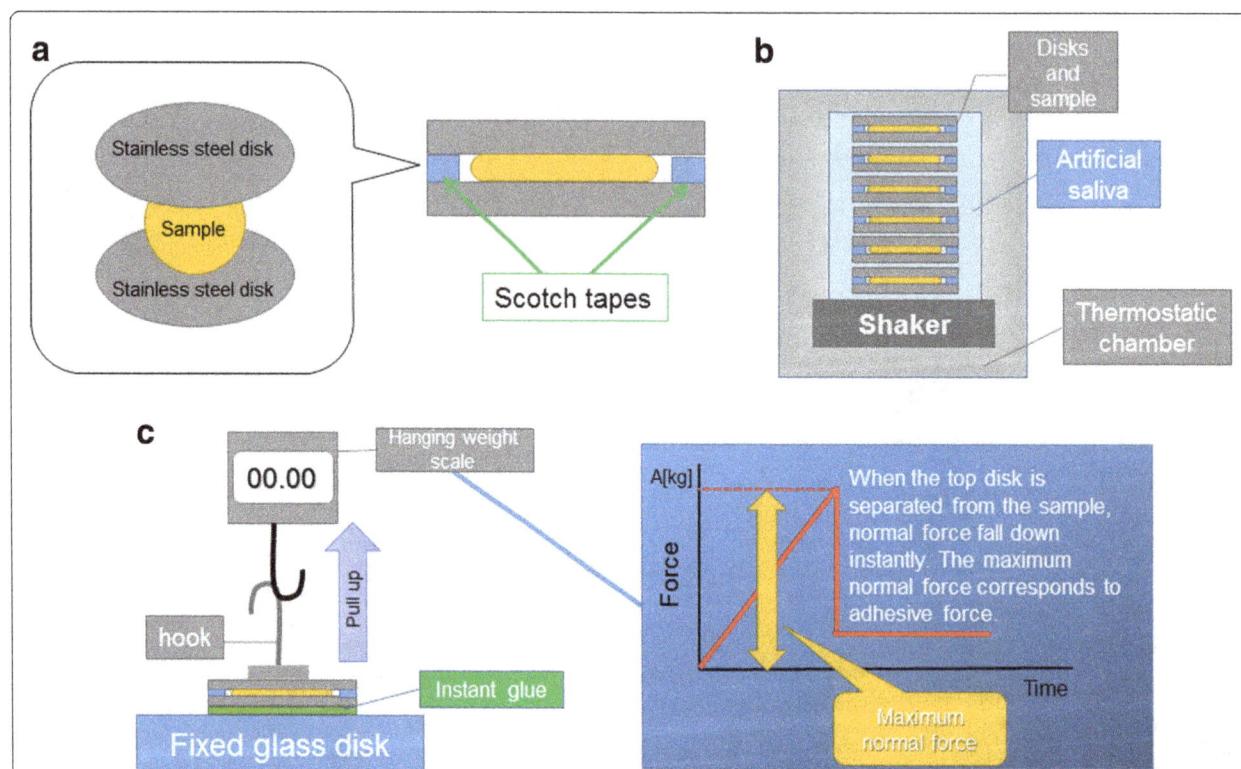

Fig. 2 Adhesive force measurement **a**; Sample having a constant volume of 0.1 ml is squeezed between two stainless steel disks (diameter, 35 mm; thickness, 1 mm). Thickness of the sample between disks is maintained by 2 layers of scotch tape stuck on the bottom disk. **b**; Sample is immersed in artificial saliva, and shaken at 37 °C at 37 rpm (1, 2, 3, 4, 5 or 6 h). **c**; Bottom disk is firmly fixed to a glass disk, while a hook is fixed to the top plate using glue. A portable hanging weight scale is hitched to the hook on the top plate, and the hanging scale (see Additional File 2.) is pulled. Normal force caused by sample adhesiveness is measured

$$\text{Adhesive stress [Pa]} = \frac{\text{Adhesive force [kgf]} \cdot \text{Gratational acceleration } (= 9.801^2/s)}{\text{Cross-sectional area of sample [m}^2\text{]}}$$

In order to ensure the reproducibility of the adhesive force measurement, we prepared DMV samples three times, and repeated the measurement 15 times per each. The result indicates that we could prepare DMV with experimental error less than 10%, and the variation between samples was 50% of mean values. Since the variation was smaller than the difference of mean value between other two samples. Thus in this experiment, one sample was measured per condition.

Elution tests under simulated oral environment

Each material was mixed with a blue water-soluble ink (THC-7C4N; Elecom, Osaka, Japan), kneaded and placed in a well of a 96-well tissue culture microplate (Iwaki, Tokyo, Japan) filled to a level that ensured all samples were at an equal volume. Each of the paste-filled wells was transferred to the wells of a 12-well tissue culture microplate (Iwaki), to which 5 ml of artificial saliva (Saliveht) was added. The above-mentioned micro-plate was used to prepare 6 sets, and was then placed on a PSU-2 T shaker (Waken B Tech Co., Ltd., Kyoto, Japan) and incubated in an FMS-1000 thermostatic chamber (Tokyo Rikakikai Co., Ltd., Tokyo, Japan) at 37 °C for 1–6 h while shaking at 37 rpm to test for elution of each material under conditions similar to the oral environment. Elution monitoring with a fixed-point camera was started immediately after addition of artificial saliva, and images were obtained after every hour.

Every hour, supernatant was collected from each well, and was transferred to a 96-well multiplate (200 μL per well). Absorbance at 535 nm was measured in triplicate for each sample in a SPECTRAmax (A) microplate reader (Molecular Devices Japan K.K., Tokyo, Japan). We performed measurements three times for each sample. Differences in the time course of elution between samples were assessed using a linear mixed-effects model with the main effects of time and group, and their interaction effect, as fixed effects, followed by post-hoc analyses to examine time course changes and sample differences. The time effect was treated as categorical. In addition, time to elution into saliva was compared among the samples using a log-rank test. Elution of the sample into saliva was defined as absorbance being more than 0.02, which was determined based on the absorbance of water-insoluble materials (cushion-type denture adhesive (Tough) and petrolatum (Vase)). All statistical analyses were performed using SPSS statistics version 22.0 software (IBM, Armonk, NY).

Results

Viscosity measurement

The results of viscosity measurement are shown in Fig. 3. This graph shows the change of the relative difficulty of altering the shape of the sample with increasing force applied to each sample; viscosity increases with the values on the vertical axis.

DMV maintained a constant level of viscosity up to a certain level of stress, showing a stress-dependent pattern similar to that of Poli. However, both DMV and Poli showed marked decreases in viscosity under extreme stress. DMV showed a consistent level of viscosity at varying temperatures, as observed with Dexi, Moist and Tough, demonstrating its temperature independence. Tough showed neither stress nor temperature dependence, with its level of viscosity being slightly lower than those of the other materials and comparable to that of DMV under extreme stress. These findings indicate that DMV has combined properties of Poli and Tough. Furthermore, none of the components of DMV alone showed such properties. The timing of fluidity increases in DMV was almost the same as that in Poli.

Adhesive force measurement

The results of adhesiveness tests are shown in Fig. 4. With regard to the 6 h temporal change, the temporal adhesion force changes for every sample were different, but the adhesive force maintained the same order of Tough>DMV > Poli. This suggests that the DMV showed stronger adhesiveness when compared with cream-type denture adhesives and weaker adhesiveness when compared with cushion-type denture adhesive in the oral environment. In the oral environment, we found that the adhesive stress of DMV falls between that of Poli and that of Tough, and this rank order (Tough>DMV > Poli) did not change after 6 h.

Elution tests

The results of the elution tests using the microplate setting are shown in Figs. 5 and 6. Linear mixed-effect model analysis demonstrated a significant difference in the time course of elution between the samples (p-value< 0.001 for interaction between time and group), the elution being increased in four samples (DM, Poli, Moist and Dexi), but not in the other four samples. The highest elution rate was observed for DM, followed in descending order by Poli, Moist, Dexi, MV, DMV, Vase and Tough. The elution of DMV was relatively stable. DMV showed similar

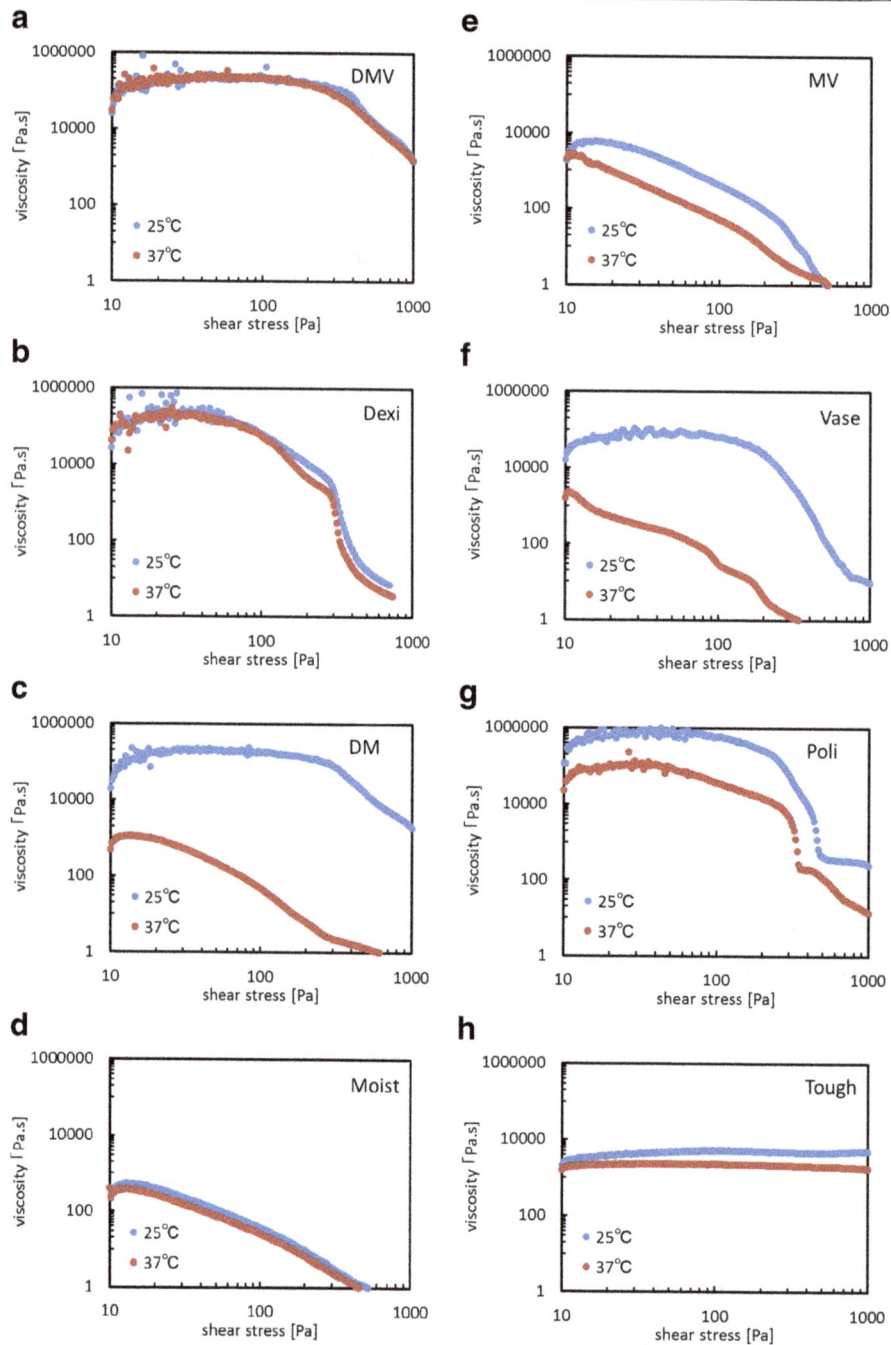

Fig. 3 Viscosity of each material Horizontal and vertical axes represent shear stress [Pa] and shear viscosity [Pa·s], respectively, both on a logarithmic scale. Red and Blue dots represent data measured at 37 °C and 25 °C, respectively. Viscosity measurement was carried out using one sample of each substance. Figure 1 provides background information for the interpretation of this Fig. **a**) DMV: Mixed paste consisting of dexamethasone, gel for oral care and petrolatum. **b**) Dexi: Dexamethasone. **c**) DM: Mixed paste consisting of dexamethasone and gel for oral care. **d**) Moist: Gel for oral care. **e**) MV: Mixed paste consisting of gel for oral care and petrolatum. **f**) Vase: Petrolatum. **g**) Poli: Cream-type denture adhesive: New Poligrip®. **h**) Tough: Cushion-type denture adhesive: Toughgrip. This figure shows changes in the viscosity of each material when an increasing force was applied to them. All materials showed increasing fluidity with increasing force applied. More specifically, viscosity of "Tough" was small but constant while that of "Poli" was the highest and decreased with increasing stress and tempereature. "DMV" falls between them, showing relatively large viscosity even at the highest stresses, as well as no temperature dependence

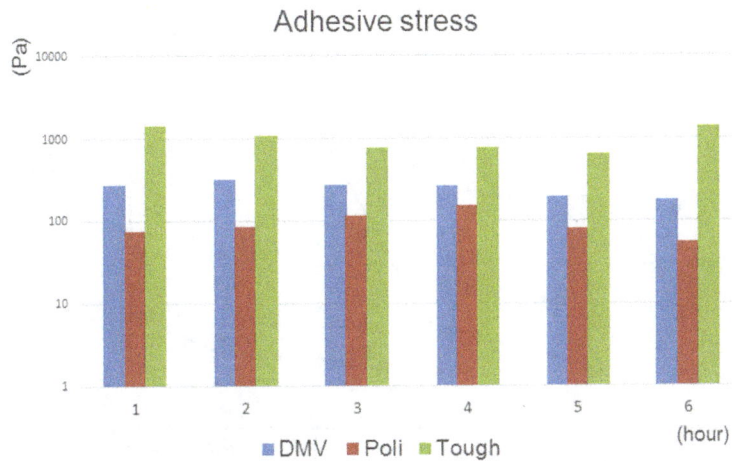

Fig. 4 Adhesiveness force test. The results of measurement of adhesive force was performed on three kinds of samples, i.e., Poli, Tough and DMV, which are stored for up to 6 h in a simulated oral environment. Each bar expresses one sample ($n = 1$)

temporal changes in elution as Vase (without significant differences between DMV and Vase). The log-rank test showed that there was a significant difference among the samples ($p < .0001$). This suggests that DMV gradually dissolves and remains firm for 6 h in the oral environment, and is comparable to paste with a greasy base. While no elution was observed with Tough, DMV maintained slight elution in artificial saliva for 6 h, suggesting that DMV has good moisture retention while maintaining the long-term

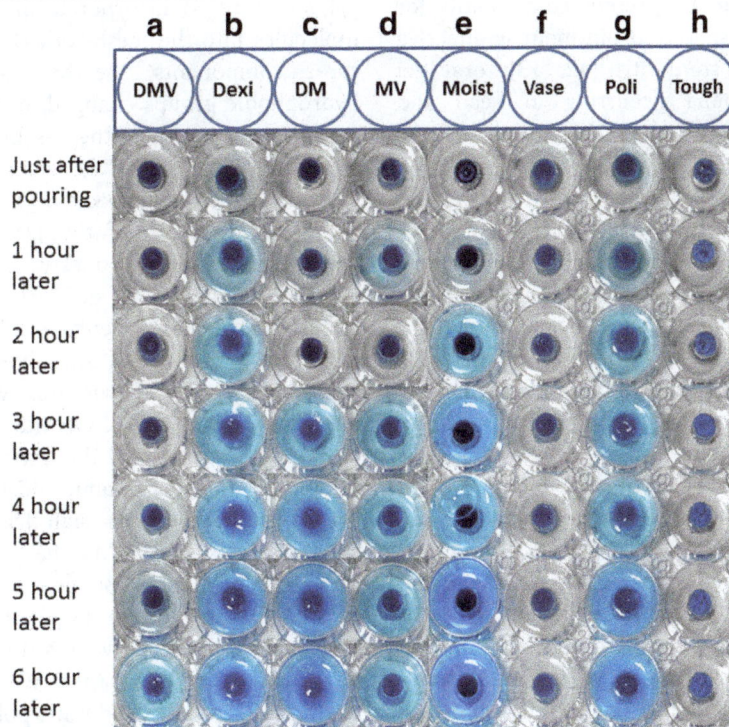

Fig. 5 Elution monitoring. Elution monitoring immediately after the addition of distilled water, and at 1h, 2 , 3 , 4 , 5 or 6 h later. **a**) DMV: Mixed paste consisting of dexamethasone, gel for oral care and petrolatum. **b**) Dexi: Dexamethasone. **c**) DM: Mixed paste consisting of dexamethasone and gel for oral care. **d**) MV: Mixed paste consisting of gel for oral care and petrolatum. **e**) Moist: Gel for oral care. **f**) Vase: Petrolatum. **g**) Poli: Cream-type denture adhesive: New Poligrip® . **h**) Tough: Cushion-type denture adhesive: Toughgrip. Elution monitoring with a fixed-point camera was started immediately after the addition of artificial saliva. The figure shows elution monitoring immediately after the addition of artificial saliva, and at 1 h, 2 h, 3 h, 4 h, 5 h or 6 h later

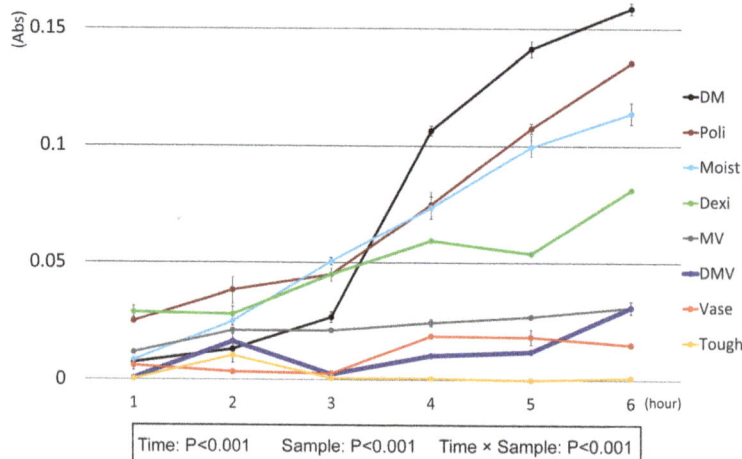

Fig. 6 Absorbance measurement in paste elution test. Vertical axis represents absorbance measurements obtained with a spectrometer for each of the test materials arranged along the horizontal axis. Lower box shows the results for the linear mixed-effects model. Data are expressed as means ± S.D. ($n = 3$). Comparative materials are the same as those in Figs. 3 and 5

steroid elution and helping to protect the affected area.

Discussion

Methodological considerations

The reasons for selecting the present components for the paste were as follows: steroid ointment is effective for pain relief in oral stomatitis [12, 13]; oral gel ameliorates the xerostomia occurring in head and neck cancer CRT [15, 16]; and Vaseline is a safe modifier for viscosity [17].

Admixture of the three agents (Dexi/Moist/Vase) yielded a mixed paste that was stickier than any single component or 2-component mixtures (Fig. 3), and this property did not show temperature dependence. These results may be explained as follows. Plastibase (Table 1), which is present in Dexi, is used to decrease temperature dependence ("Dexi"; Fig. 3B). On the other hand, although Dexi and Moist alone show temperature independence (Fig. 3B,D), temperature dependence was observed when mixing these two components ("DM"; Fig. 3C). It is possible that the sodium polyacrylate (superabsorbent polymer) present in Moist leads to temperature dependence, as it possesses hydrophilic and hydrophobic groups, causing it to desorb at high temperatures, thereby inducing viscosity changes [18].

The reason for the temporal change at 6 h is as follows: the interval between meals is about 6 h at most, as the majority of patients using an oral appliance would clean the oral appliance after each meal. As the mixed paste (DM, DV, MV and DMV) components were not quantitatively analyzed for subsidiary ingredients, we are uncertain whether such components exhibited effects on temperature dependence. However, the sodium polyacrylate present in Moist is associated with temperature changes, and when it was mixed with Dexi, viscosity might have changed with temperature.

Sodium polyacrylate is a type of superabsorbent polymer having a hydrophilic carboxyl group, and it forms a gel structure to incorporate a large number of water molecules into the meshwork [19, 20]. After mixing the three components, the balance of hydrophilic and hydrophobic groups changed, particularly due to the oil and fat components of the Vaseline, forming a gelatinous structure, which may have increased viscosity to a greater degree than expected.

The adhesiveness of the DMV was as stable as a commercial denture adhesive for 6 h. Based on the results in Fig. 4, we show that DMV has sufficient adhesive stress as a denture adhesive, and that DMV would be a useful denture adhesive. The DM samples mixed with gel-like structures were easily dissolved in artificial saliva (Fig. 6). On the other hand, when DM and Vase were mixed, the action of Vaseline's hydrophobic groups was potent, and elution to artificial saliva of the DMV was significantly lower than DM. This suggests that DMV has long-term steroid efficacy and local retention in the oral environment. We cannot explain the reasons for the poor dissolution and persistent adhesiveness under a simulated oral environment in this paper. We believe that both the characteristics of sodium polyacrylate (containing Moist) and the osmotic pressure of artificial saliva (including NaCl) influenced our results. Miwa et al. reported that in artificial saliva, samples with a Vaseline base did not elute to saliva [21]. In addition, because the suction force of sodium polyacrylate, the gelling agent, included in Moist decreases on mixing with Dexi, temporal changes may have occurred. However, these physical properties require further investigation.

Clinical application of admixture paste

In this paper, for a small number of patients, we applied admixture paste for the treatment of stomatitis. Subjective pain in DMV-treated patients was improved or unchanged, and slight macroscopic changes in stomatitis were seen. In addition, we have no data on a control group (patients without DMV-use) at this time, or sufficient data on the clinical use of DMV to confirm its clinical benefit. In Additional File 3, we show our clinical trial results to date, and we will present further results in the future.

Dexamethasone ointment is indicated for refractory stomatitis according to the package insert. In fact, steroid application is not typically the first-choice treatment for stomatitis. However, this admixture paste contains hinokitiol, the active ingredient in Refrecare H®, which has been shown to exert antimicrobial activity against *Candida* and to inhibit biofilm formation [22, 23].

The admixture paste has physical properties similar to those of denture adhesives and was developed with the intention of using it in denture-wearing patients. In patients with head and neck cancer, severe stomatitis may occur in both the oral cavity and in the pharynx. The latter often causes contact/swallowing pain and thereby prevents oral food intake [6, 24]. Denture use has been shown to be effective in improving mastication/swallowing disorder, increasing chewing-stimulated salivary secretion [25, 26] and preventing disuse atrophy of surrounding tissue in the head and neck [27]. The present admixture paste may therefore contribute to the maintenance of patient QOL by treating severe stomatitis and allowing them to use their oral appliances.

Meanwhile, the admixture paste contains dexamethasone, a steroid, and thus has a risk of inducing microbial substitution on long-term use. Its use should therefore be limited in patients with immune systems that have been compromised by CRT [12, 28]. At the same time, it has been shown to be highly effective in treating oral mucosal lesions, particularly for the relief of pain [29]. Dexamethasone is a steroidal agent and is generally recommended for use in aphthae or refractory stomatitis. Frequent monitoring of adverse reactions and worsening of symptoms by an oral surgeon is therefore recommended. As a future clinical theme, we believe that we need to examine the efficacy and safety of this admixture paste.

Study limitations

There are some limitations in our research: an elution of admixture paste was exploratorily evaluated with no sample size calculation in advance; the adhesive force evaluation was performed with a single sample, which did not allow to make statistical comparisons and therefore compare differences. Thus, in the future, to demonstrate the hypothesis that admixture paste has an adhesiveness similar to that of denture adhesive and has gradual solubility, a behavioral study should be carried out over time, with a planned sample size.

Conclusion

The application of admixture paste (mixture of dexamethasone, gel for oral care and petrolatum) for severe stomatitis in patients with head and neck cancer may facilitate oral food intake while using an oral appliance through its high levels of local retention, adhesiveness and gradual solubility in oral environment, which are not achieved with any of the 3 components alone.

Abbreviations
CRT: Radiotherapy and/or chemotherapy; Dexi: Dexamethasone; DM: Mixed paste consisting of dexamethasone and gel for oral care; DMV: Mixed paste consisting of dexamethasone, gel for oral care and petrolatum; Moist: Gel for oral care; MV: Mixed paste consisting of gel for oral care and petrolatum; PAP: Palatal augmentation prosthesis; Poli: Cream-type denture adhesive: New Poligrip®; QOL: Quality of life; Tough: Cushion-type denture adhesive: Toughgrip; Vase: Petrolatum

Acknowledgements
The authors would like to express their sincere appreciation to K. Yoshikiyo, M. Shiramizu, and K. Yasukawa for their tremendous support.

Funding
None.

Authors' contributions
YH, MA, SH and HK made substantial contributions in the conception and design of the study. KS, KH, MK, YK, JS and KY participated in data collection and analysis for experimental records. AS, YK and SH were involved in drafting the manuscript. YH and HK helped to draft and carefully revise the manuscript. All authors have read and approved the final manuscript.

Competing interests
The authors declare that they have no competing interests.

Author details
[1]Department of Dentistry and Oral Surgery, Hyogo College of Medicine, 1-1 Mukogawa-cho, Nishinomiya, Hyogo 663-8501, Japan. [2]Department of Chemical Science and Engineering, Graduate School of Engineering, Kobe University, Kobe, Hyogo 657-8501, Japan. [3]Department of Pharmacy, Hyogo College of Medicine, 1-1 Mukogawa-cho, Nishinomiya, Hyogo 663-8501, Japan. [4]Division of Occlusion & Maxillofacial Reconstruction, Department of Oral Function, School of Dentistry, Kyushu Dental University, Kitakyushu, Fukuoka 803-8580, Japan. [5]Medical Research Group, Development Department. Takiron Co., Ltd., Osaka, Japan.

References

1. Beck TN, Golemis EA. Genomic insights into head and neck cancer. Cancers of the Head & Neck. 2016;1(1)

2. Sonis ST, Elting LS, Keefe D, Peterson DE, Schubert M, Hauer-Jensen M, et al. Perspectives on cancer therapy-induced mucosal injury: pathogenesis, measurement, epidemiology, and consequences for patients. Cancer. 2004; 100(Suppl 9):1995–2025.

3. Keefe DM, Schubert MM, Elting LS, Sonis ST, Epstein JB, Raber-Durlacher JE, et al. Updated clinical practice guidelines for the prevention and treatment of mucositis. Cancer. 2007;109:820–31.

4. Lalla RV, Sonis ST, Peterson DE. Management of oral mucositis in patients who have cancer. Dent Clin N Am. 2008;52:61–77.

5. Kishimoto H. The oral management in the cancer medical care; we prevent complications and aim at the improvement of a treatment outcome and the quality of life. Journal of Hyogo college of. Medicine. 2014;39:25–9.

6. Katou K. Nutrition support and oral Care for Head and Neck Cancer Patients Undergoing Chemoradiotherapy. Head and Neck Cancer Frontier. 2014;2: 48–51.

7. Valente VB, Takamiya AS, Ferreira LL, Felipini RC, Biasoli ÉR, Miyahara GI, et al. Oral squamous cell carcinoma misdiagnosed as a denture-related traumatic ulcer: a clinical report. J Prosthet Dent. 2016;115:259–62.

8. Elting LS, Keefe DM, Sonis ST, Garden AS, Spijkervet FK, Barasch A, et al. Patient-reported measurements of oral mucositis in head and neck cancer patients treated with radiotherapy with or without chemotherapy: demonstration of increased frequency, severity, resistance to palliation, and impact on quality of life. Cancer. 2008;113:2704–13.

9. Elting LS, Cooksley C, Chambers M, Cantor SB, Manzullo E, Rubenstein EB. The burdens of cancer therapy. Clinical and economic outcomes of chemotherapy-induced mucositis. Cancer. 2003;98:1531–9.

10. Raber-Durlacher JE, Elad S, Barasch A. Oral mucositis. Oral Oncol. 2010;46(6): 452.

11. Mizukami N, Ymauchi M, Watanabe A, Danzuka K, Sato T, Oomori K, et al. Satisfaction survey of pain management for severe mucositis caused by cancer therapy for head and neck cancer. Palliative Care Res. 2012;7:408–14.

12. Arizumi M, Ikemura Y, Tanabe K. Clinical Evaluation of new-type Aphtasolon (dexamethasone) on stomatitis. Oral therapeutics and. Pharmacology. 1985; 4:28–40.

13. Takeuchi-Igarashi H, Ito H, Numabe Y. A case report of moderate periodontitis with chronic desquamative gingivitis. Journal of the Japanese Society of Periodontology. 2012;54:183–92.

14. Teshima A, Tyatani M, Inoue T. Effectiveness of Kenarogu ointment to radiation stomatitis of head and neck cancer patients, study of safety. Japanese Pharmacology & Therapeutics. 1986;14:7163–6.

15. Watanabe T. Perioperative Oral care in cancer patient. The bulletin of Tsurumi college Pt 3, studies in infant education and. dental hygiene. 2013;50:49–52.

16. Kishimoto H. Oral Management for cancer patients undergoing chemotherapy and/or radiotherapy. Journal of. Clin Exp Med. 2012;243:657–62.

17. Fukami T, Yamamoto Y, Nakamura Y, Kamano M, Umeda Y, Makimura M, et al. Quality testing of steroidal ointment mixed with white petrolatum : rheological properties and stability testing. Jpn J Pharm Health Care Sci. 2006;32(9):964.

18. Aoyama M. Adsorption behavior during the clay suspension of the acrylic acid-based polymer. Trend. 1999:20–6.

19. Harada M. Japanese Standard of Food Additives explanatory note. vol. 3th. Kinpara publication;1974.p.805.

20. Masuda F. Some Charactors of hydrogel from super absorbent polymer. J Jpn Soc Colour Mater. 1986;59:221–6.

21. Miwa Y, Yamaji A, Miki Y, Kimura S, Okada H. The basic study on dissolution behavior of dental drugs. Oral therapeutics and. Pharmacology. 1991;10: 127–32.

22. Nakamura M, Fujibayashi T, Tominaga A, Satoh N, Kawarai T, Shinozuka O, et al. Hinokitiol inhibits Candida Albicans adherence to oral epithelial cells. J Oral Biosci. 2010;52:42–50.

23. Sato N, Nakamura M, Senpuku H, Yamazaki T. The antibacterial action of the oral care blend hinokitiol. DENTAL. DIAMOND. 2008;33:164–8.

24. Tosaka C, Tajima H, Inoue T, Omoya M, Kobayashi M, Miura H, et al. Investigation of how to prevent mucositis induced by chemoradiotherapy. Japanese journal of cancer and. Chemotherapy. 2011;38:1647–51.

25. Yamamoto T, Yoshimuta Y, Nokubi T, Yasui S, Kusunoki C, Nokubi H, et al. Clinical study of the relationship between different methods of masticatory function measurement and intraoral factors. The Japanese journal of mastication science and. Health Promotion. 2013;23:30–8.

26. Hurukawa Y, Takita M, Takahashi S, Okada Y, Ikeda J, Setogawa K, et al. Relief of oral complaint on cancer patient : practice of taste and oral function. The Japanese journal of taste and smell research. 2011;18:491–4.27.

27. Takagi N. Rehabilitation of disuse atrophy; we think about correspondence of dentistry in accord with needs of the aged society denture, oral care, oral rehabilitation. The Journal of Ibaraki synthesis rehabilitation care. 2012;21:7–11.

28. Ohashi Y, Abe M, Ueda N. Use experience of the dexamethasone paste for the stomatitis radiation of patients with oral cancer. Journal of New Remedies & Clinics. 1981;30:832–8.

29. Agarie Y. The regimen method; digestive disease Inraoral inflammation. Clinic All-Round. 2008;57:947–9.

13

Patient- and treatment-related risk factors associated with neck muscle spasm in nasopharyngeal carcinoma patients after intensity-modulated radiotherapy

Lu-Lu Zhang[1†], Guan-Qun Zhou[1†], Zhen-Yu Qi[1], Xiao-Jun He[2], Jia-Xiang Li[3], Ling-Long Tang[1], Yan-Ping Mao[1], Ai-Hua Lin[3,4], Jun Ma[1,4] and Ying Sun[1*]

Abstract

Background: To evaluate the incidence of neck muscle spasm in nasopharyngeal carcinoma (NPC) patients that received intensity-modulated radiotherapy (IMRT), and to analyse the patient- and treatment-related risk factors associated with neck muscle spasm.

Methods: A sample of 152 IMRT-treated, biopsy-proven, nondisseminated NPC patients were retrospectively analysed. All had documented IMRT treatment plans and had returned for follow-up review at 4 years post-radiotherapy. Spasm of the sternocleidomastoid (SCM) muscle was graded from 0 to 3 (absent to severe) and this grade served as the clinical endpoint. Risk factors were identified using logistic regression analysis.

Results: Within 4 years of radiotherapy, neck muscle spasm developed in 23.68% of the patients; Grades 0, 1, 2 and 3 were respectively assigned to 83.55, 7.57, 6.58 and 2.30% of assessed SCMs. Multivariate analysis indicated that gender, N stage, V60 (percentage of SCM volume that received >60 Gy) were independent prognostic variables, and that the optimal threshold for using V60 to predict neck muscle spasm was 61.92% (sensitivity = 0.900, specificity = 0.953).

Conclusions: Gender, N stage and V60 were independent predictive factors for post-radiotherapy neck muscle spasm, and a V60 of ≤61.92% in the SCM was relatively safe.

Keywords: Nasopharyngeal carcinoma, Neck muscle spasm, Intensity-modulated radiotherapy, Dose tolerance

Background

Nasopharyngeal carcinoma (NPC) represents the most common malignant tumour of the nasopharyngeal epithelium. While relatively rare in western countries, it is more frequently diagnosed in Southeast Asia. The highest incidence is found in Southern China, where the incidence in males can reach 20–50 per thousand. [1]. NPC is one of the most radiosensitive cancers, and radiation therapy (RT) is usually the definitive treatment [2].

In recent years, intensity-modulated radiotherapy (IMRT) has become accepted as a more advanced radiation technique for treatment of NPC [3–5]. With the 5-year overall survival rate for NPC patients treated with IMRT increasing to 79.6% [6], focus has shifted to improving the quality of life of these survivors, who can experience late adverse events such as cervical subcutaneous fibrosis, hearing loss and skin dystrophy [7].

Having the neck muscles present within or adjacent to the high-dose radiation fields is unavoidable for NPC patients. High-dose-radiation induced neck muscle spasm, which has received little attention until recently, is a sudden and involuntary 'Charlie-horse-like' contraction of the neck muscles with or without pain. It lasts for seconds to minutes and is concentrated in the

* Correspondence: sunying@sysucc.org.cn
†Equal contributors
[1]Department of Radiation Oncology, Sun Yat-sen University Cancer Center, State Key Laboratory of Oncology in South China, Collaborative Innovation Center for Cancer Medicine, 651 Dongfeng Road East, Guangzhou 510060, People's Republic of China
Full list of author information is available at the end of the article

sternocleidomastoid (SCM) muscles of head and neck cancer (HNC) patients [8]. It may be triggered by head turning, lifting and yawning, and it can be alleviated by neck stretching or massage. In some HNC patients, the spasm-induced pain is sufficient to require additional interventions such as physical therapy, medication or injection of botulinum-A toxin [8–10]. However, these interventions can only relieve the neck spasms temporarily; therefore, investigating risk factors and developing preventative measures seems a better focus for research.

Previous research has demonstrated a strong dose-response relationship between neck muscle spasm and the radiation dose received by the SCM of HNC patients [9]. However, the independent prognostic variables for post-radiotherapy neck muscle spasm remain unclear; moreover, of the few published studies on the topic, none examined patients with NPC [8–10]. Hence, we carried out this retrospective study to investigate the incidence of post-radiotherapy neck muscle spasm in NPC patients, and to analyse potential clinical and treatment-related risk factors.

Methods
Patient selection
This was a retrospective longitudinal cohort study performed at our cancer centre. Between July and September 2011, 267 newly diagnosed, nondisseminated, biopsy-proven NPC patients were treated using IMRT with or without chemotherapy. Patients returned to the hospital for follow-up review at least every 3 months for the first 2 years, and then every 6 months until death. During each follow-up, a detailed history was taken and a thorough physical examination was performed, along with chest radiography and abdominal ultrasonography. Magnetic resonance imaging (MRI) of the neck and nasopharynx was performed every 6 to 12 months.

Of the 267 NPC patients, 37 were excluded owing to the loss of 4-year follow-up results, and 78 were excluded because their IMRT treatment-plan documents were unavailable. In the 152 remaining subjects, the occurrence and severity of neck muscle spasm was ascertained via a phone-based following-up at 4 years post-radiotherapy. This retrospective study was approved by the institutional ethics committee and the need for informed consent was waived.

Treatment methods
Before treatment, all patients underwent a baseline evaluation, including a thorough history and physical examination, haematology and biochemistry profiles, MRI of the nasopharynx and neck, chest radiography, abdominal ultrasonography, and bone scan emission computed tomography. All patients were staged according to the 7th edition of the AJCC staging system [11].

All patients underwent definitive IMRT with or without chemotherapy. Details concerning the implementation of IMRT at our cancer centre, which complies with reports 50 and 62 of the International Commission on Radiation Units and Measurements, have been reported previously [12–15]. The total radiation doses (delivered in 28–33 fractions) were 66–72 Gy for the primary tumour, 64–70 Gy for the cervical lymph nodes, 60–63 Gy for the high-risk region, and 54–56 Gy for the low-risk and neck nodal regions.

During the study, institutional guidelines recommended only IMRT for stage I and concurrent chemoradiotherapy with or without neoadjuvant/adjuvant chemotherapy for stages II to IVB. Concurrent chemotherapy consisted of cisplatin every one or 3 weeks, and neoadjuvant or adjuvant chemotherapy consisted of three cycles of cisplatin with 5-fluorouracil, or cisplatin with taxanes every 3 weeks. Patients exhibiting persistent disease or relapse underwent salvage treatment procedures such as surgery, chemotherapy and afterloading.

Data collection
Patient- and treatment-related factors
The medical records of the sample group were retrospectively reviewed to collect data concerning potential patient- and disease-related risk factors (gender, age, T stage, N stage, smoking status, drinking status), as well as treatment-related risk factors (dosimetric parameters for the SCM, use of chemotherapy and/or neck surgery). The dosimetric parameters were obtained from dose volume histograms (DVHs) of the SCM. We re-delineated bilateral SCMs according to our previously proposed methods [16] to generate the bilateral neck DVHs for each patient using the CERR DICOM-RT toolbox (version 3.0 beta 3; School of Medicine, Washington University, St. Louis, USA). The following dosimetric parameters were collected: mean dose (Dmean), maximum dose (Dmax), minimum dose (Dmin), percentage of the SCM volume that received more than X Gy (VX), the dose received by X% of the SCM volume (DX); values of X were 20, 25, 30, 35, 40, 45, 50, 55, 60, 65, 70, 75 and 80.

Grading of neck muscle spasm to yield study endpoints
Owing to the lack of a universally recognized classification system, we proposed a 4-point scale to score SCM muscle spasm according to the most serious degree of neck muscle spasm in the 4 years post-treatment, as follows: grade 1 for mild SCM spasm occurring infrequently, without pain and/or impaired neck mobility; grade 2 for moderate SCM spasm occurring frequently with contractile pain, but without impaired neck mobility; and grade 3 for severe SCM spasm occurring

daily with pain and occasionally also with impaired neck mobility. This grade served as the clinical endpoint.

Statistical analysis

All statistical analyses were performed using SPSS 13.0 (Chicago, IL, USA) and a two-tailed P value of <0.05 was considered statistically significant. For analysis of differences between SCMs without neck muscle spasm and those with it, a χ^2 test was used for categorical variables and a Wilcoxon rank-sum test was used for continuous variables. Binary logistic regression was used for univariate analyses. Receiver operating characteristic (ROC) curves were generated to estimate the cut-off points for all significant dosimetric parameters in the univariate logistic regression analysis and to create a dose-volume histogram (DVH) for neck muscle spasm. All factors that had a P value of <0.05 after univariate logistic regression analysis were included in a multivariate logistic regression analysis to determine the independent factors associated with neck muscle spasm. Receiver operating characteristic (ROC) curve analysis was adopted for selecting optimal cut-off points for independent dosimetric factors that were predictive of neck muscle spasm.

Results

Pre-treatment (baseline) characteristics of patients and incidence of neck muscle spasms

Of the 152 NPC patients included in the final study, 114 were men and 38 were woman. Their ages ranged from 14 to 71 years, with the median being 41. The proportion with stage-I, –II, –III and -IV disease were 3/152 (1.97%), 16/152 (10.53%), 67/152 (44.08%) and 66/152 (43.42%), respectively.

Almost all the patients (151/152, 99.34%) were diagnosed with undifferentiated squamous-cell carcinoma (type II) according to the World Health Organization (WHO) classification, and 1 (0.66%) patient was diagnosed with squamous-cell carcinoma (type I). Radiotherapy (RT) alone was used to treat 14 patients (9.21%), while the remaining 137 (90.13%) were treated using chemo-radiotherapy. One patient (0.66%) underwent bilateral neck dissection and 9 (5.92%) underwent unilateral neck dissection after completion of RT.

By 4 years post-IMRT, 36 patients (23.68%) had developed SCM muscle spasms, and among these, there were 22 cases of unilateral spasm and 14 cases of bilateral spasm. Owing to the fact that both right and left SCM muscles were evaluated, a total of 304 (2 × 152) SCMs were included in the study. Most (254; 83.55%) exhibited no spasms, while 23 (7.57%) showed mild spasms, 20 (6.58%) showed moderate spasms and 7 (2.30%) exhibited severe spasms. Of the 36 patients in the current study who developed SCM muscle spasms, no patient underwent medication, and only two patients underwent

physiotherapy. Most patients relieved symptoms temporarily by neck stretching or massage.

Comparison of baseline characteristics of SCMs with spasms to those of SCMs without spasms

A more detailed list of the comparisons is given in Table 1, but the following parameters were found to be significantly different between SCMs with and without spasms: gender, N stage, Dmean, Dmin, Dmax, V20–75 and D20–80. Difference in age, T stage, smoking status, drinking status, induction chemotherapy, concurrent chemotherapy, neck dissection and V80 ($P = 0.537$) were not found to be significant.

Univariate analysis and dose-volume histogram

The univariate logistic regression analysis is described in Table 2 and it showed that gender, N stage, Dmean, Dmin, Dmax, V20–65 and D20–80 were significantly associated with post-radiotherapy SCM spasm. In contrast, there was no significant association with age, T stage, smoking status, drinking status, induction chemotherapy, concurrent chemotherapy, neck dissection, V75 and V80.

The significant dosimetric parameters from the regression analysis were included in the ROC curve analysis to identify the dose tolerance cut-off points for SCM spasm. The cut-off points were selected using the Youden index at the level of $P < 0.05$, and were as follows (Table 3): V20 (99.99%), V25 (99.99%), V30 (99.94%), V35 (98.94%), V40 (97.58%), V45 (94.72%), V50 (90.02%), V55 (65.78%), V60 (61.92%), V65 (28.94%) and V70 (0.57%).

A DVH was established using the above cut-off points (Fig. 1). The area under the DVH curve represented tolerable doses for the SCM with respect to neck muscle spasm, and the area above the curve represented intolerable doses. As the dose and percentage volume of the SCM increased, the tolerable area gradually reduced, indicating that the probability of neck muscle spasm increased gradually with radiation dose.

Multivariate analysis

After multivariate logistic regression analysis, differences in gender ($P = 0.024$, $\beta = 1.113$, $SE = 0.494$, *odds ratio [OR]* = 3.044, 95% *CI* = 1.157 to 8.012), N stage ($P = 0.035$, $\beta = 1.038$, $SE = 0.491$, $OR = 2.823$, 95% $CI = 1.078$ to 7.398) and V60 ($P < 0.001$, $\beta = 0.169$, $SE = 0.026$, $OR = 1.185$, *95% CI* = 1.126 to 1.246) were found to be significant (Table 2). Female gender and an advanced N stage were patient-related risk factors for neck muscle spasm. The ROC curve for V60 is shown in Fig. 2, and the area under the curve was 0.934. The optimal threshold for V60 to predict neck muscle spasm was 61.92% (sensitivity = 0.900 and specificity = 0.953). Among the SCMs without neck muscle spasm, 4.7% received a radiation dose where V60

Table 1 Baseline (pre-treatment) characteristics of SCMs without neck muscle spasm and those with neck muscle spasm

Variables	SCMs without neck muscles spasm	SCMs with neck muscles spasm	P value
Group number	254	50	
Sex			0.003
Male	199 (78.35%)	29 (58.00%)	
Female	55 (21.65%)	21 (42.00%)	
Age (years)			0.471
≤ 41	131 (51.57%)	23 (46.00%)	
> 41	123 (48.43%)	27 (54.00%)	
T stage			0.356
T1–2	61 (24.02%)	9 (18.00%)	
T3–4	193 (75.98%)	41 (82.00%)	
N stage			0.002
N0–1	127 (50.00%)	13 (26.00%)	
N2–3	127 (50.00%)	37 (74.00%)	
Smoking status			0.799
Yes	86 (33.86%)	16 (32.00%)	
No	168 (66.14%)	34 (68.00%)	
Drinking status			0.851
Yes	38 (14.96%)	8 (16.00%)	
No	216 (85.04%)	42 (84.00%)	
Induction chemotherapy			0.839
Yes	123 (48.43%)	25 (50.00%)	
No	131 (50.57%)	25 (50.00%)	
Concurrent chemotherapy			0.851
Yes	216 (85.04%)	42 (84.00%)	
No	38 (14.96%)	8 16.00%)	
Neck dissection			0.324
Yes	8 (3.15%)	3 (6.00%)	
No	246 (96.85%)	47 (94.00%)	
D mean	50.54 Gy (38.04 Gy – 58.91 Gy)	62.05 Gy (61.22 Gy – 62.35 Gy)	< 0.001
D min	2.68 Gy (1.04 Gy – 29.44 Gy)	35.88 Gy (30.35 Gy – 39.58 Gy)	< 0.001
D max	68.82 Gy (66.24 Gy – 71.46 Gy)	70.80 Gy (68.58 Gy –72.51 Gy)	0.048
V20[a]	84.94% (61.87% – 100%)	100% (100% – 100%)	< 0.001
V25	81.70% (59.84% – 100%)	100% (100% – 100%)	< 0.001
V30	79.52% (57.88% – 99.99%)	100% (100% – 100%)	< 0.001
V35	77.57% (56.23% – 99.76%)	100% (99.88% – 100%)	< 0.001
V40	75.57% (54.40% – 98.99%)	99.89% (99.22% – 100.00%)	< 0.001
V45	74.00% (52.43% – 96.44%)	99.07% (97.67% – 99.70%)	< 0.001
V50	70.87% (47.81% – 90.72%)	96.32% (93.59% – 98.32%)	< 0.001
V55	64.00% (41.94% – 78.86%)	87.74% (84.56% – 91.79%)	< 0.001
V60	39.02% (23.11% – 52.10%)	68.33% 64.01% – 72.25%)	< 0.001
V65	8.16% (0.97% – 20.59%)	35.01% (23.10% – 41.22%)	< 0.001
V70	0.00% (0.00% – 0.76%)	1.66% (0.00% – 13.78%)	< 0.001
V75	0.00% (0.00% – 0.00%)	0.00% (0.00% – 0.00%)	0.010
V80	0.00% (0.00% – 0.00%)	0.00% (0.00% – 0.00%)	0.537

Table 1 Baseline (pre-treatment) characteristics of SCMs without neck muscle spasm and those with neck muscle spasm *(Continued)*

Variables	SCMs without neck muscles spasm	SCMs with neck muscles spasm	P value
D20[b]	63.12 Gy (60.59 Gy – 65.28 Gy)	66.74 Gy (64.93 Gy – 68.01 Gy)	< 0.001
D25	62.39 Gy (59.74 Gy – 64.31 Gy)	66.04 Gy (64.30 Gy – 67.35 Gy)	< 0.001
D30	61.69 Gy (58.95 Gy – 63.39 Gy)	65.27 Gy (63.61 Gy – 66.61 Gy)	< 0.001
D35	60.76 Gy (57.74 Gy – 62.53 Gy)	64.76 Gy (63.05 Gy – 65.92 Gy)	< 0.001
D40	59.79 Gy (55.88 Gy – 61.70 Gy)	63.97 Gy (62.68 Gy – 64.85 Gy)	< 0.001
D45	59.06 Gy (53.84 Gy – 61.01 Gy)	63.23 Gy (62.31 Gy – 64.05 Gy)	< 0.001
D50	58.17 Gy (49.85 Gy – 60.38 Gy)	62.48 Gy (61.59 Gy – 63.14Gy)	< 0.001
D55	57.52 Gy (38.66 Gy – 59.55 Gy)	61.75 Gy (61.01 Gy – 62.44 Gy)	< 0.001
D60	56.26 Gy (27.73 Gy – 58.83 Gy)	61.10 Gy (60.35 Gy – 61.67 Gy)	< 0.001
D65	54.85 Gy (16.57 Gy – 58.14 Gy)	60.22 Gy (59.61 Gy – 60.86 Gy)	< 0.001
D70	51.52 Gy (9.49 Gy – 57.19 Gy)	59.80 Gy (58.47 Gy – 57.81 Gy)	< 0.001
D75	43.68 Gy (5.57 Gy – 56.15 Gy)	58.42 Gy (57.51 Gy – 59.37 Gy)	< 0.001
D80	35.34 Gy (3.21 Gy – 54.78 Gy)	57.21 Gy (56.01 Gy – 58.29 Gy)	< 0.001

Abbreviations: *SCM* sternocleidomastoid muscle, *Dmean* Mean dose to the sternocleidomastoid muscle, *Dmax* Maximum dose to the sternocleidomastoid muscle; V20[a] is the percentage of the sternocleidomastoid muscle volume that received more than 20 Gy; D20[b] is the dose to 20% of the sternocleidomastoid muscle volume; the other dosimetric parameters are reported in a similar manner

was >61.92%, while for those with spasm, V60 was >61.92% in 90.0% of cases (*P* < 0.001).

Discussion

This is the first and largest retrospective study to date to identify the incidence and risk factors for neck muscle spasm in NPC patients treated with IMRT. Analysis of the results identified gender, N stage and V60 as independent risk factors and these findings could be used to aid IMRT planning in NPC patients.

NPC patients suffered a high incidence of post-radiotherapy neck muscle spasm

Post-radiotherapy neck muscle spasm among HNC patients began to receive attention about two decades ago, however, to date, only three papers have been published regarding this adverse effect in HNC patients. Van Daele et al. first reported the condition in 2002, finding that after RT in the neck area, 9 HNC patients suffered neck muscle spasm, concentrated in the SCM [9]. Then in 2011, Gelblum et al. reported that 14 HNC patients developed severe neck spasm after undergoing IMRT ± chemotherapy [10]. Finally, in 2013, Hunter et al. observed that 9.7% (34/352) of HNC patients complained of radiation-induced bilateral or unilateral neck spasm during follow-up (median, 51 months; range, 30–90 months); with the spasms being especially pronounced in the SCM [8]. The mechanism of postradiation muscle spasm is not clear, but it is likely related to high-dose-radiation-induced and progressive fibrosis-induced ischemia.

In the present study, the occurrence rate of neck muscle spasm among patients with NPC 48 months after RT was 23.68% (36/152); this is more than double the

incidence of neck muscle spasm among patients with other types of HNC, as reported by Hunter et al. The discrepancy may be explained as follows: on account of the rich lymphatic network in the nasopharynx, the incidence of cervical-lymph-node metastasis is higher for NPC than for other HNCs [17]. Therefore, irradiation of the neck nodes, along with the entire region of lymphatic drainage, is the standard treatment method [2]. However, neck dissection is the standard procedure for HNC patients with clinically positive neck lymph node metastases [18]. Above all, the radiation dose to the SCM region is higher in NPC patients versus those with other HNCs, and this leads to a higher incidence of post-radiotherapy neck muscle spasm.

Advanced N stage and female gender were patient-related independent risk factors

We found that being at the advanced N stage was a negative risk factor for neck muscle spasm. This may be due to the fact that advanced N-stage NPC merits an increased dose of radiation to the positive cervical lymph nodes and the region of lymphatic drainage. Therefore, the volume of the SCM and peripheral nerve receiving high-dose radiation is necessarily higher, and this increases the probability of muscle and nerve injury [19].

Studies regarding the relationship between gender and RT-induced late complications in NPC patients remain controversial [20, 21]. Lee et al. found that male gender was a negative risk factor for temporal lobe necrosis, cranial nerve neuropathy, radiation myelitis, osteoradionecrosis and dysphagia in NPC patients [20]. In contrast, Yeh et al. found that female gender was a negative independent predictor of hearing deficits, tinnitus and

Table 2 Univariate and multivariate analysis of patient- and treatment-related risk factors for neck muscle spasm

	P value	OR (95% CI)
Univariate analysis		
Sex		
Male		Ref
Female	0.003	2.620 (1.387, 4.949)
Age (years)		
≤ 41		Ref
> 41	0.472	1.250 (0.681, 2.297)
T stage		
T1–2		Ref
T3–4	0.358	1.440 (0.662, 3.131)
N stage		
N0–1		Ref
N2–3	0.002	2.846 (1.445, 5.607)
Smoking status		
Yes	0.799	0.919 (0.481, 1.758)
No		Ref
Drinking status		
Yes	0.851	1.083 (0.472, 2.485)
No		Ref
Induction chemotherapy		
Yes	0.839	1.065 (0.581, 1.953)
No		Ref
Concurrent chemotherapy		
Yes	0.851	0.924 (0.402, 2.120)
No		Ref
Neck dissection		
Yes	0.332	1.963 (0.502, 7.671)
No		Ref
D mean	< 0.001	1.002 (1.001, 1.003)
D min	< 0.001	1.001 (1.001, 1.001)
D max	0.007	1.001 (1.000, 1.002)
V20[a]	< 0.001	1.085 (1.045, 1.127)
V25	< 0.001	1.085 (1.046, 1.125)
V30	< 0.001	1.083 (1.046, 1.121)
V35	< 0.001	1.081 (1.045, 1.118)
V40	< 0.001	1.082 (1.046, 1.120)
V45	< 0.001	1.085 (1.048, 1.122)
V50	< 0.001	1.118 (1.068, 1.171)
V55	< 0.001	1.148 (1.096, 1.202)
V60	< 0.001	1.192 (1.133, 1.255)
V65	< 0.001	1.106 (1.076, 1.136)
V70	< 0.001	1.126 (1.072, 1.183)
V75	0.653	1.173 (0.585, 2.349)

Table 2 Univariate and multivariate analysis of patient- and treatment-related risk factors for neck muscle spasm *(Continued)*

	P value	OR (95% CI)
V80	0.999	0.000 (0.000, 0.000)
D20[b]	< 0.001	1.004 (1.003, 1.005)
D25	< 0.001	1.005 (1.003, 1.006)
D30	< 0.001	1.005 (1.003, 1.006)
D35	< 0.001	1.005 (1.004, 1.007)
D40	< 0.001	1.005 (1.004, 1.007)
D45	< 0.001	1.005 (1.004, 1.007)
D50	< 0.001	1.005 (1.003, 1.007)
D55	< 0.001	1.003 (1.002, 1.005)
D60	0.001	1.002 (1.001, 1.003)
D65	0.001	1.001 (1.000, 1.002)
D70	< 0.001	1.001 (1.000, 1.001)
D75	< 0.001	1.001 (1.000, 1.001)
D80	< 0.001	1.001 (1.000, 1.001)
Multivariate analysis		
Sex		
Male		Ref
Female	0.024	3.044 (1.157, 8.012)
N stage		
N0–1		Ref
N2–3	0.035	2.823 (1.078, 7.398)
V60	< 0.001	1.185 (1.126, 1.246)

Abbreviations: *Dmean* mean dose to the sternocleidomastoid muscle, *Dmax* maximum dose to the sternocleidomastoid muscle, *V20*[a] percentage of the sternocleidomastoid muscle volume that received >20 Gy, *D20*[b] dose to 20% of the sternocleidomastoid muscle volume; other dosimetric parameters are reported in a similar manner

otorrhea in NPC patients [21]. Our results indicate that female gender is a negative independent risk factor for neck muscle spasm. Although the mechanism of these gender-related differences remains unclear, we speculate that differences in gene expression and hormone secretion between males and females may play an important role.

These findings should prompt us to pay more attention to female patients and advanced N-stage patients during follow-up on account of the higher probability of neck muscle spasm.

Chemotherapy and neck dissection had no effect on neck muscle spasm

Several studies have shown that combining chemotherapy with RT does not seem to sensitize soft tissue to radiation injury [16, 19, 22]. Consistent with these studies, our results suggest that chemotherapy does not increase the incidence of neck muscle spasm when compared with RT alone.

Table 3 Radiation dose tolerances for the SCM with respect to neck muscle spasm, as determined using ROC curve analysis

	Area under ROC curve	Standard error	P	Lower limit	Upper limit	Cut-off point	Sensitivity	Specificity
V20[a]	0.795	0.030	<0.001	0.737	0.853	99.99%	0.920	0.673
V25	0.810	0.029	<0.001	0.752	0.867	99.99%	0.900	0.713
V30	0.815	0.029	<0.001	0.758	0.872	99.94%	0.900	0.709
V35	0.834	0.029	<0.001	0.777	0.892	98.94%	0.920	0.665
V40	0.834	0.029	<0.001	0.777	0.891	97.58%	0.920	0.685
V45	0.826	0.029	<0.001	0.769	0.883	94.72%	0.900	0.689
V50	0.860	0.025	<0.001	0.810	0.910	90.02%	0.900	0.732
V55	0.895	0.023	<0.001	0.849	0.941	65.78%	0.940	0.524
V60	0.934	0.024	<0.001	0.887	0.981	61.92%	0.900	0.953
V65	0.848	0.303	<0.001	0.784	0.912	28.94%	0.680	0.902
V70	0.675	0.046	<0.001	0.584	0.766	0.57%	0.600	0.744

Abbreviations: *SCM* sternocleidomastoid muscle, *ROC* receiver operating characteristic, *V20*[a] percentage of the sternocleidomastoid muscle volume that received >20 Gy; other dosimetric parameters are reported in a similar manner

The findings of earlier studies concerning the association between neck dissection and the development of post-radiotherapy neck muscle spasm have been inconsistent. Hunter et al. found that neck dissection did not increase the risk of post-radiotherapy neck muscle spasm in patients with oropharyngeal cancer [8]. On the other hand, Gelblum et al. reported that neck surgery may increase the incidence of neck muscle spasm for HNC patients following IMRT; however, the study only included a small number of patients, so this conclusion needs to be verified [10]. In our study, we did not observe an effect of neck dissection on muscle spasm. This may be explained by the fact that neck dissection can cause serious damage to SCM muscle innervation, thus hindering the associated neural activity, including the abnormal spontaneous variety.

V60 was an independent risk factor

Until to now, only Hunter et al. had investigated the association between dose and neck muscle spasm. By comparing (*t*-test) dosimetric parameters between SCMs with and without neck muscle spasm, the authors found that the differences between spasm groups were significant for all such parameters (univariate analysis). Owing to the authors' belief that Dmean was the most convenient dosimetric parameter to use, they put forward its use in formulating the cut-off points for predicting the occurrence of neck muscle spasm. However, in the current study, Dmean was only significant in the univariate analysis, not in the multivariate analysis. Our study

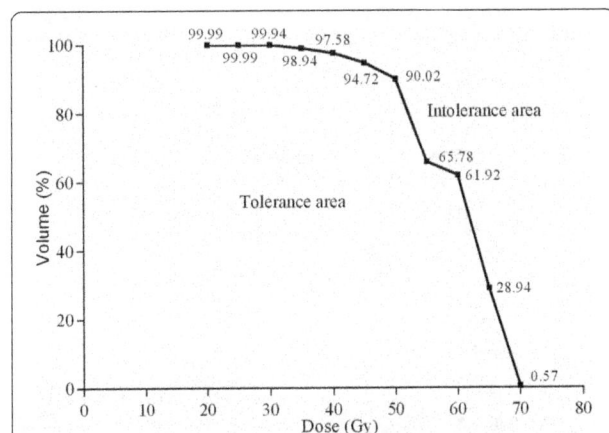

Fig. 1 Dose tolerance curves for post-radiotherapy neck muscle spasm in the sternocleidomastoid muscle (SCM). Dose-volume histograms was created using the cut-off points in Table 3. The area under the DVH curve represented tolerable doses for the SCM with respect to post-radiotherapy neck muscle spasm

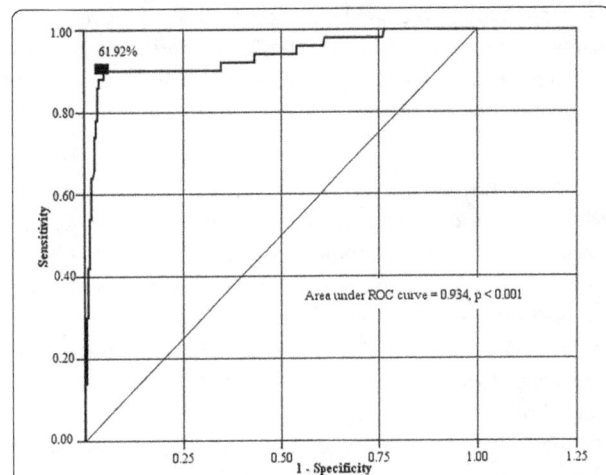

Fig. 2 Receiver operating characteristic (ROC) curve for the V60 (percentage of the sternocleidomastoid muscle volume that received more than 60 Gy). A ROC curve was generated to determine the dose tolerance for moderate/severe neck muscle spasm. A V60 of 61.92% had a sensitivity of 0.900 and a specificity of 0.953 and was considered the tolerance dose of the sternocleidomastoid (SCM) muscle with respect to post-radiotherapy spasms. The area under the ROC curve for a V60 of 61.92% was 0.934

indicated V60 to be the independent dosimetric risk factor. Moreover, our results showed that keeping the SCM's V60 below 61.92% makes post-radiotherapy neck muscle spasm relatively unlikely.

Currently, the Radiation Therapy Oncology Group (RTOG) protocol recommends 70 Gy to the cervical lymph nodes and 54 Gy to the lymphatic drainage regions [23]. SCMs that were located near to drainage regions, may have suffered a high dose of radiation. However, IMRT provides the ability to deliver excellent target-volume coverage while protecting adjacent normal tissues. Therefore, it may be possible for radiation oncologists to design IMRT plans that keep V60 below 61.92% for the SCM. Of course, the true clinical utility of applying a V60 of 61.92% as the cut-off value for predicting post-radiotherapy neck muscle spasm requires more evidence.

Limitations

It is worth noting two limitations of the current study. Firstly, the its retrospective nature was unavoidable, but it means that a prospective study will be necessary to validate the findings. Secondly, a longer follow-up period may yield additional conclusions: 4 years may not be long enough. However, in previous studies, the median latency for occurrence of neck muscle spasm ranged from 23 to 37 months, implying that 4 years (48 months) is a reasonable choice. Thirdly, due to the lack of a universally recognized classification system, we proposed a four-point scale to score SCM muscle spasm, which was not previously validated. Evaluation bias may exist due to using such an unvalidated clinician-graded measure as the primary endpoint. Prospective design of studies of patient-reported neck spasm may be required in future research to increase the reliability of the evaluation.

Conclusions

NPC patients exhibited a high frequency of neck muscle spasm at 4 years post-radiotherapy. The patient-related factors, gender and N stage, and the treatment-related factor, V60, were independent predictors of neck muscle spasm. Moreover, a V60 of 61.92% may represent the tolerance dose for this late post-radiotherapy complication. These findings may help improve risk assessment for neck muscle spasm, and aid the optimization of IMRT treatment plans in NPC patients.

Abbreviations

Dmax: Maximum dose; Dmean: Mean dose; Dmin: Minimum dose; DVH: Dose-volume histogram; DVHs: Dose volume histograms; DX: the Dose received by X% of the sternocleidomastoid volume; HNC: Head and neck cancer; IMRT: Intensity-modulated radiotherapy; MRI: Magnetic resonance imaging; NPC: Nasopharyngeal carcinoma; OR: Odds ratio; ROC: Receiver operating characteristic; RT: Radiation therapy; RTOG: Radiation Therapy Oncology Group; SCM: Sternocleidomastoid; VX: Percentage of the sternocleidomastoid volume that received more than X Gy; WHO: World Health Organization

Acknowledgements
Not applicable.

Funding
This work was supported by grants from the National Natural Science Foundation of China (No. 81372409), the Science and Technology Project of Guangzhou City, China (No.132000507), the Sun Yat-Sen University Clinical Research 5010 Program (No.2012011), and the National Natural Science Foundation of China (No. 81402532). The funders had no role in study design, data collection and analysis, decision to publish, or preparation of the manuscript.

Authors' contributions
ZL and ZG conducted data collection and drafted the manuscript. QZ, HX, LJ and LA helped to perform the statistical analysis. TL, MY, MJ and SY participated in the design of the study. ZL and SY conceived of the study, and participated in its design. All authors read and approved the final manuscript.

Competing interests
The authors declare that they have no competing interests.

Author details
[1]Department of Radiation Oncology, Sun Yat-sen University Cancer Center, State Key Laboratory of Oncology in South China, Collaborative Innovation Center for Cancer Medicine, 651 Dongfeng Road East, Guangzhou 510060, People's Republic of China. [2]Department of Clinical Medicine, School of Public Health, Sun Yat-sen University, Guangzhou, People's Republic of China. [3]Department of Oncology, First People's Hospital of Zhaoqing City, Guangdong, People's Republic of China. [4]Department of Medical Statistics and Epidemiology, School of Public Health, Sun Yat-sen University, Guangzhou, People's Republic of China.

References
1. Jemal A, Bray F, Center MM, Ferlay J, Ward E, Forman D. Global cancer statistics. CA Cancer J Clin. 2011;61:69–90.
2. Wei WI, Sham JS. Nasopharyngeal carcinoma. Lancet. 2005;365:2041–54.
3. Tham IW, Hee SW, Yeo RM, et al. Treatment of nasopharyngeal carcinoma using intensity-modulated radiotherapy—the National Cancer Centre Singapore experience. Int J Radiat Oncol Biol Phys. 2009;75:1481–6.
4. Lee N, Xia P, Quivey JM, et al. Intensity-modulated radiotherapy in the treatment of nasopharyngeal carcinoma: an update of the UCSF experience. Int J Radiat Oncol Biol Phys. 2002;53:12–22.
5. Kam MK, Teo PM, Chau RM, et al. Treatment of nasopharyngeal carcinoma with intensity-modulated radiotherapy: the Hong Kong experience. Int J Radiat Oncol Biol Phys. 2004;60:1440–50.
6. Peng G, Wang T, Yang KY, et al. A prospective, randomized study comparing outcomes and toxicities of intensity-modulated radiotherapy vs conventional two-dimensional radiotherapy for the treatment of nasopharyngeal carcinoma. Radiother Oncol. 2012;104:286–93.
7. Zheng Y, Han F, Xiao W, et al. Analysis of late toxicity in nasopharyngeal carcinoma patients treated with intensity modulated radiation therapy. Radiat Oncol. 2015;10:17.
8. Hunter KU, Worden F, Bradford C, et al. Neck spasm after chemoradiotherapy for head and neck cancer: natural history anddosimetric correlates. Head Neck. 2014;36:176–80.
9. Van Daele DJ, Finnegan EM, Rodnitzky RL, Zhen W, McCulloch TM, Hoffman HT. Head and neck muscle spasm after radiotherapy: management with botulinum toxin A injection. Arch Otolaryngol Head Neck Surg. 2002;128:956–9.
10. Gelblum D, Wolden S, Schupak K, Lee N. Neck spasms as a late effect of intensity modulated radiation therapy (IMRT) for head and neck cancer. Available at: http://astro2011.abstractsnet.com/pdfs/2708.pdf. Accessed 2 Feb 2013.
11. Edge SB, et al. AJCC cancer staging manual. New York: Springer; 2010.

Patient- and treatment-related risk factors associated with neck muscle spasm in nasopharyngeal carcinoma...

107

12. Zhao C, Han F, Lu LX, et al. Intensity modulated radiotherapy for local-regional advanced nasopharyngeal carcinoma [in Chinese]. Ai Zheng. 2004; 23:1532–7.

13. Luo W, Deng XW, Lu TX. Dosimetric evaluation for three dimensional conformal, conventional, and traditional radiotherapy plans for patients with early nasopharyngeal carcinoma [in Chinese]. Ai Zheng. 2004;23:605–8.

14. Ma J, Liu L, Tang L, et al. Retropharyngeal lymph node metastasis in nasopharyngeal carcinoma: prognostic value and staging categories. Clin

15. Li WF, Sun Y, Chen M, et al. Locoregional extension patterns of nasopharyngeal carcinoma and suggestions for clinical target volume delineation. Chin J Cancer. 2012;31:579–87.

16. Zhang LL, Mao YP, Zhou GQ, et al. The evolution of and risk factors for neck muscle atrophy and weakness in nasopharyngeal carcinoma treated with intensity-modulated radiotherapy: a retrospective study in an endemic area. Medicine. 2015;94:e1294.

17. Sham JS, Choy D, Wei WI. Nasopharyngeal carcinoma: orderly neck node spread. Int J Radiat Oncol Biol Phys. 1990;19:929–33.

18. Liao LJ, Lo WC, Hsu WL, Wang CT, Lai MS. Detection of cervical lymph node metastasis in head and neck cancer patients withclinically N0 neck-a meta-analysis comparing different imaging modalities. BMC Cancer. 2012;12:236.

19. Gillette EL, Mahler PA, Powers BE, Gillette SM, Vujaskovic Z. Late radiation injury to muscle and peripheral nerves. Int J Radiat Oncol Biol Phys. 1995;31:1309–18.

20. Yeh SA, Tang Y, Lui CC, Huang YJ, Huang EY. Treatment outcomes and late complications of 849 patients with nasopharyngeal carcinoma treated with radiotherapy alone. Int J Radiat Oncol Biol Phys. 2005;62:672–9.

21. Lee CC, Ho CY. Post-treatment late complications of nasopharyngeal carcinoma. Eur Arch Otorhinolaryngol. 2012;269:2401–9.

22. Peters LJ, Harrison ML, Dimery IW, Fields R, Goepfert H, Oswald MJ. Acute and late toxicity associated with sequential bleomycin-containing chemotherapy regimens and radiation therapy in the treatment of carcinoma of the nasopharynx. Int J Radiat Oncol Biol Phys. 1988;14:623–33.

23. Lee NY, Zhang Q, Pfister DG, et al. Addition of bevacizumab to standard chemoradiation for locoregionally advanced nasopharyngeal carcinoma (RTOG 0615): a phase 2 multi-institutional trial. Lancet Oncol. 2012;13:172–80.

14

E3 ubiquitin ligase, RNF139, inhibits the progression of tongue cancer

Lina Wang[1,2], Wei Yin[1*] and Chun Shi[2]

Abstract

Background: Tongue cancer is still one of the leading causes of mortality around the world. Recently, the ubiquitin system has been established as a critical modulator of tumors. In order to find the oral cancer related E3 ubiquitin ligases, we screened the human E3 ubiquitin ligase library and found that RING finger protein 139 (RNF139) regulated the biological behavior of tongue cancer cells.

Methods: MTT assay was used to analyze the cell viability changes of tongue cancer SCC9 and SCC25 cells caused by RNF139. The invasion ability of SCC9 and SCC25 cells with or without the knockdown of RNF139 was evaluated through transwell assay. The immunoblotting was recruited to determine the expression level of RNF139 in human tongue cancer tissues and para-carcinoma tissues. The effect of RNF139 on tumorigenicity of tongue cancer cells was analyzed by xenograft model on immunodeficient Balb/c nude mice.

Results: Overexpression of RNF139 inhibits the viability of tongue cancer cells since day 2. The colony formation ability of SCC9 and SCC25 cells was also decreased with the overexpression of RNF139. Knockdown of RNF139 significantly promoted the invasion ability of SCC9 and SCC25 cells. Furthermore, knockdown of RNF139 also induced the activation of AKT signaling pathway. While human tongue cancer tissues had low expression of RNF139. In nude mice, knockdown of RNF139 promoted the tumorigenicity of the SCC25 cells.

Conclusions: Our data establish a role for RNF139 in regulating the progression of tongue cancer.

Keywords: RNF139, Cell viability, Invasion, Tongue cancer, SCC25 cells

Background

Tongue cancer is one of the leading cancers in prevalence and around 16,400 new American cases are estimated in 2017 [1]. The dysfunction of P53 signaling pathway, phospho-inositide-3-kinase (PI3K)/v-akt murine thymoma viral oncogene homolog (AKT) signaling pathway as well as transforming growth factor-β (TGFβ) signaling pathway plays a critical role in the carcinogenesis of tongue cancer. The activity of these signaling pathways is regulated by post-translational modification.

Ubiquitination is one of the post-translational modification which involves in several cellular activity, including gene transcription, cell-cycle control, DNA repair and protein degradation [2–5]. It is mediated by the sequential participated enzymes, E1 ubiquitin activating enzymes, E2 ubiquitin conjugating enzymes, and E3 ubiquitin ligases [6, 7]. Several E3 ubiquitin ligases have been confirmed to participate in the pathogenesis of cancers [8–11]. Although the role of E3 ubiquitin ligases is still not well-understood, it is continuously being discovered [12–14].

In order to find the oral cancer related E3 ubiquitin ligases, we screened the human E3 ubiquitin ligase library [12] and found that RING finger protein 139 (RNF139) regulated the proliferation of tongue cancer cells. In this study, we further analyzed the role of RNF139 on the development of tongue cancer.

* Correspondence: tjzbyw2007@163.com
[1]The State Key Laboratory Breeding Base of Basic Science of Stomatology (Hubei-MOST) & Key Laboratory of Oral Biomedicine Ministry of Education, School & Hospital of Stomatology, Wuhan University, 237 Luoyu road, Wuhan 430079, China
Full list of author information is available at the end of the article

Methods

Reagents and antibodies

Lipofectamine 2000 (Life Technologies), 3-(4,5-dimethyl-thiazol-2-yl)-2,5-diphenyltetrazolium bromide (MTT) (Antgene), mouse antibodies against β-actin (Sigma) and

RNF139 (Santa Cruz); rabbit polyclonal antibodies against AKT (CST), phospho-AKT (308 and 473) (CST), phospho-FoxO1 (CST), phospho-GSK3β (CST), and phospho-mTOR (CST) were purchased from the indicated manufacturers. SCC9 (CRL 1629™), SCC25 (CRL 1628™) and HEK293 (CRL 1573™) cells were obtained from ATCC.

Cell culture, plasmid and RNAi construction

Human tongue cancer SCC9 and SCC25 cells were maintained in DMEM medium with the supplement of 10% FBS and 1% Penicillin-Streptomycin. Mammalian expression plasmids for the RNF139 and RNF139-RNAi were constructed according to the instructions of molecular cloning: a laboratory manual.

The stable RNF139 overexpression/knockdown SCC9 and SCC25 cells

The protocol was the same with our previous report [11]. In brief, the RNF139 or RNF139-RNAi retrovirus was packaged in the HEK293T cells and incubated with SCC9 and SCC25 cells. The retrovirus infected SCC9 and SCC25 cells were treated with puromycin (0.5 mg/ml) for 7 days before the following experiments.

Cell viability assay

The stable RNF139 overexpression/knockdown SCC9 and SCC25 cells (2×10^3) were seeded on the 96 well plates. MTT (5 μg/ml) was used and incubated at 37 °C for 4 h. Then the cells were incubated with Dimethyl sulfoxide (DMSO) for 30 min. The cell viability was determined by microplate reader at day 2, 4 and 6.

Cell invasion assay

The cell invasion assay was performed with the same procedure [11]. Briefly, after coating with the matrigel basement membrane matrix, the upper chamber of the transwell plate was seeded with the stable RNF139 overexpression/knockdown SCC9 and SCC25 cells with serum-free DMEM medium. The complete DMEM medium was added into the bottom chamber. They were incubated at 37 °C for 24 h. After fixing and staining, the transwell membrane was graphed by Olympus IX71 light microscope.

Colony formation assay

The stable RNF139 overexpression SCC9 and SCC25 cells were cultured in 10-cm cell dishes for 18 days. The cell culture medium was changed every other two days. The cell colonies were stained with crystal violet and quantified with ImageJ software.

Immunoblotting analysis

Cells were lysed with the lysis buffer (Nonidet P-40 buffer). Protein were seperated with the polyacrylamide

gel electrophoresis and transferred into polyvinylidene membrane. The membrane was immunoblotted with the correspondent antibodies and developed with the ECL reagent.

Xenograft model

Eight-week-old male athymic immunodeficient Balb/c nude mice were purchased from Shanghai Laboratory Animal Center. The stable RNF139-knockdown SCC25 (5×10^7) cells were injected subcutaneously into the flank. Tumor diameters were recorded every 4 days. Specimens were harvested at 40 days.

Patients and specimen collection

The tumor tissues of tongue cancer patients were collected from Jan. 2016 to Sep. 2016. None of them received any anticancer therapies before surgery. The diagnosis was based on the pathologically analysis. The total protein was extracted with the Minute TM Total Protein Extraction Kit (Inventbiotech).

Statistics

The tumor volume of mice xenograft was analyzed by two-way ANOVA. One-way ANOVA was used to analyze the results of cell viability assay, cell invasion assays and colony formation assays. All data were analyzed by the SPSS package for Windows (Version 18.0, Chicago, IL). The statistically significant refers to the P value <0.05.

Results

RNF139 inhibits the viability of tongue cancer cells

In order to elaborate the role of RNF139 in regulating the biological behavior of tongue cancer, we analyzed the viability changes of tongue cancer cells, SCC9 and SCC25 cells, induced by RNF139. The results suggested that overexpression of RNF139 significantly inhibited the viability of SCC9 and SCC25 cells (Fig. 1a). While knockdown RNF139 had the opposite effects (Fig. 1b). Then we further analyzed the effect of RNF139 on colony formation ability of SCC9 and SCC25 cells. As shown in Fig. 1c, the number of cell colony was also decreased with the overexpression of RNF139.

RNF139 regulates the invasion of tongue cancer cells

We next investigated the functions of RNF139 on cell invasion. The transwell assay was used to analyze the invasion changes of tongue cancer cells. Knockdown of RNF139 significantly promoted the invasion ability of SCC9 and SCC25 cells (Fig. 1d). Taken together, these data suggest that RNF139 inhibits cell viability and invasion of tongue cancer SCC9 and SCC25 cells.

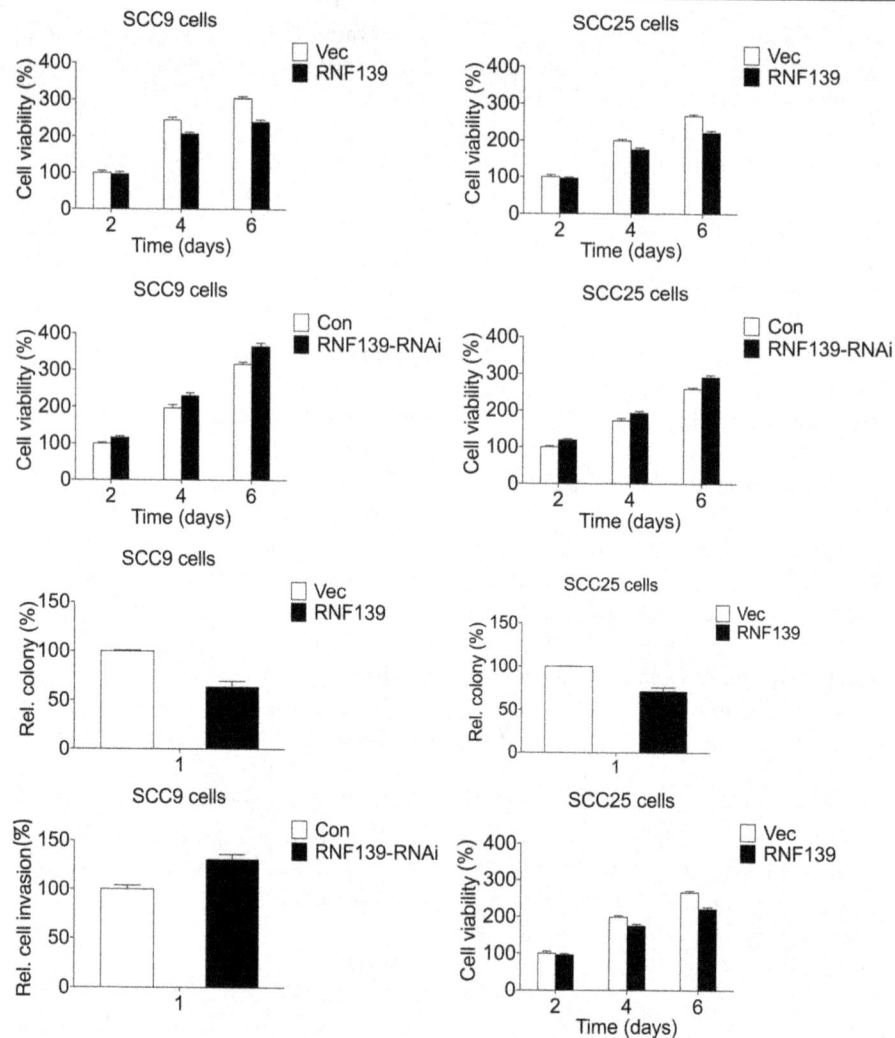

Fig. 1 RNF139 regulates the viability, colony formation and invasion of tongue cancer SCC9 and SCC25 cells. **a** Overexpression of RNF139 inhibits the viability of SCC9 and SCC25 cells. $N = 6$. **b** Knockdown of RNF139 promotes the viability of SCC9 and SCC25 cells. $N = 6$. **c** Overexpression of RNF139 inhibited the colony formation ability of SCC9 and SCC25 cells. $N = 3$. **d** Knockdown of RNF139 promoted the invasion of SCC9 and SCC25 cells. The gel/blots which indicates the efficiency of RNF139 overexpression were the same gel/blots in (**a**) and (**c**). The gel/blots which indicates the efficiency of RNF139 knockdown were the same gel/blots in (**b**) and (**d**). $N = 3$. *:$P < 0.05$, **:$P < 0.01$

Human tongue cancer tissues had low expression of RNF139

To analyze the role of RNF139 in human lung cancers, we detected the protein level of RNF139 in 23 tongue cancer patients' tumor tissues through western blotting. Most of these patients were 51–70 years old. Squamous cell carcinoma accounted for 91.30% (21 out of 23). The protein level of RNF139 was significantly decreased in the tongue cancer tissues in comparison to paracarcinoma tissues (Fig. 2a&b).

RNF139 promotes activation of AKT1

After determining the correlation between RNF139 and tongue cancer, we further analyze the regulating mechanism of RNF139 on tongue cancer. We screened the

expression changes of critical components in PI3K-AKT, JAK-STAT, p53 and MAPK signaling pathway. The AKT signaling pathway had evident changes with the knockdown of RNF139. As shown in Fig. 3, knockdown of RNF139 significantly potentiated the phosphorylation of AKT1 at Ser308 and Ser473, which is the hall mark of AKT1 activation [28]. Meanwhile, knockdown of RNF139 also induced the activation of downstream molecules of AKT1, such as mTOR, FoxO1 and GSK3β in SCC9 and SCC25 cells.

Knockdown of RNF139 promoted the growth of the tumor xenografts

Next, we performed in vivo xenograft analysis by subcutaneously injecting stable RNF139 knockdown SCC25

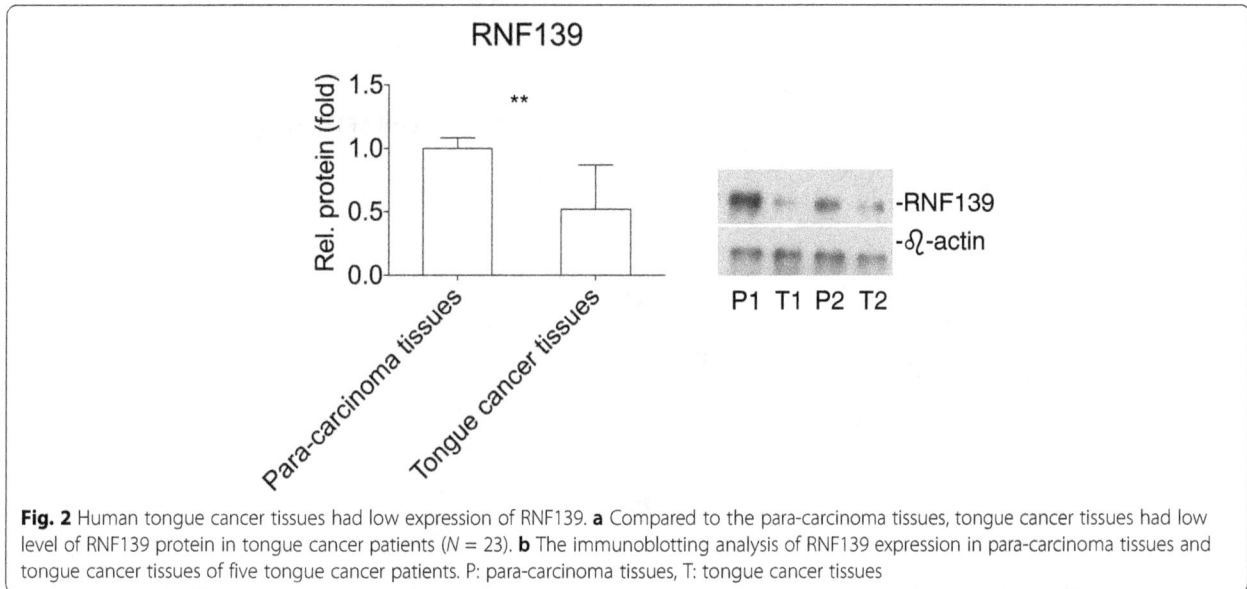

Fig. 2 Human tongue cancer tissues had low expression of RNF139. **a** Compared to the para-carcinoma tissues, tongue cancer tissues had low level of RNF139 protein in tongue cancer patients ($N = 23$). **b** The immunoblotting analysis of RNF139 expression in para-carcinoma tissues and tongue cancer tissues of five tongue cancer patients. P: para-carcinoma tissues, T: tongue cancer tissues

cells into nude mice to further analyze the function of RNF139. As shown in Fig. 4a, knockdown of RNF139 markedly promoted the volumes of the tumor xenografts. The histological analysis indicated that the expression of pAKT1 was strongly increased in the SCC25 cells induced xenografts with the knockdown of RNF139 (Fig. 4b).

Discussion

Despite advances made in detection and diagnosis as well as treatments in the past ten years, tongue cancer is still one of the leading causes of mortality around the world [12]. The body of the tongue has abundant

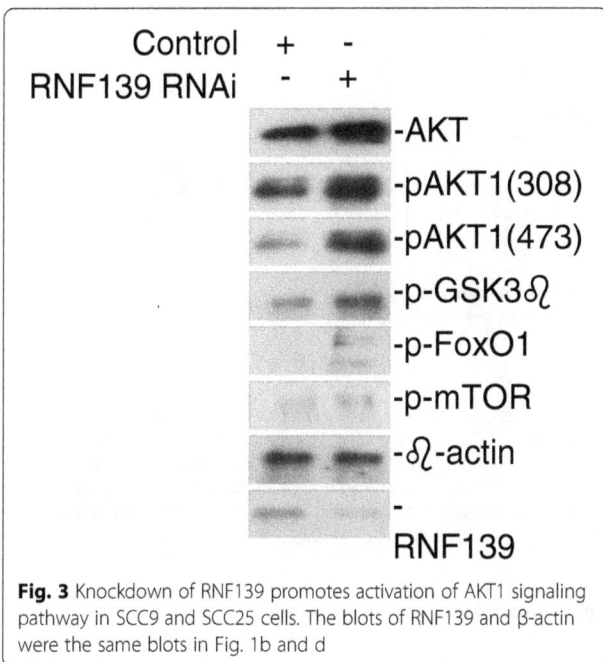

Fig. 3 Knockdown of RNF139 promotes activation of AKT1 signaling pathway in SCC9 and SCC25 cells. The blots of RNF139 and β-actin were the same blots in Fig. 1b and d

lymphatic and blood vessel and frequent movement which promotes the metastasis of tongue cancer. The impressive progresses achieved in tumor biology make us realize that each tumor has unique character and should receive corresponding precision treatment. In the past decades, patients with breast and lung cancer already benefited from the personalized treatment which aimed to treat patients according to their own molecular characteristics [15, 16]. In order to search the candidate treatment target for tongue cancer, we focused on the E3 ubiquitin ligase and screened the human E3 ubiquitin ligase library. RNF139 as was one of the candidates.

Ubiquitin is a widely existed protein which can be found in all eukaryotic cells. It consists of 76 amino acids with an exposed C-terminal. The isopeptide bond connection between the carboxyl-terminal glycine residue of ubiquitin and an internal K residue or the amino-terminal methionine (M1) of another ubiquitin forms the polyubiquitin chains. Ubiquitination is indispensable for several biological processes. Several E3 ubiquitin ligases have been confirmed to be related with initiation and progression of tumor [12, 13].

E3 ubiquitin ligases mainly include RING and HECT type E3 ubiquitin ligases. The multimembrane-spanning protein RNF139 belongs to the RING type E3 ubiquitin ligases and has a RING-H2 domain with E3 ubiquitin ligase activity at the COOH-terminal. It locates in the endoplasmic reticulum (ER) and transfers the ubiquitin from the E2 ubiquitin conjugating enzymes to substrate. Previous study suggested that RNF139 could utilize several E2 ubiquitin conjugating enzymes for ubiquitylation. RNF139 ubiquitinated and degraded the antioxidant enzyme heme oxygenase-1 (HO-1) and suppressed HO-1-induced cancer cell growth, migration and invasion [17].

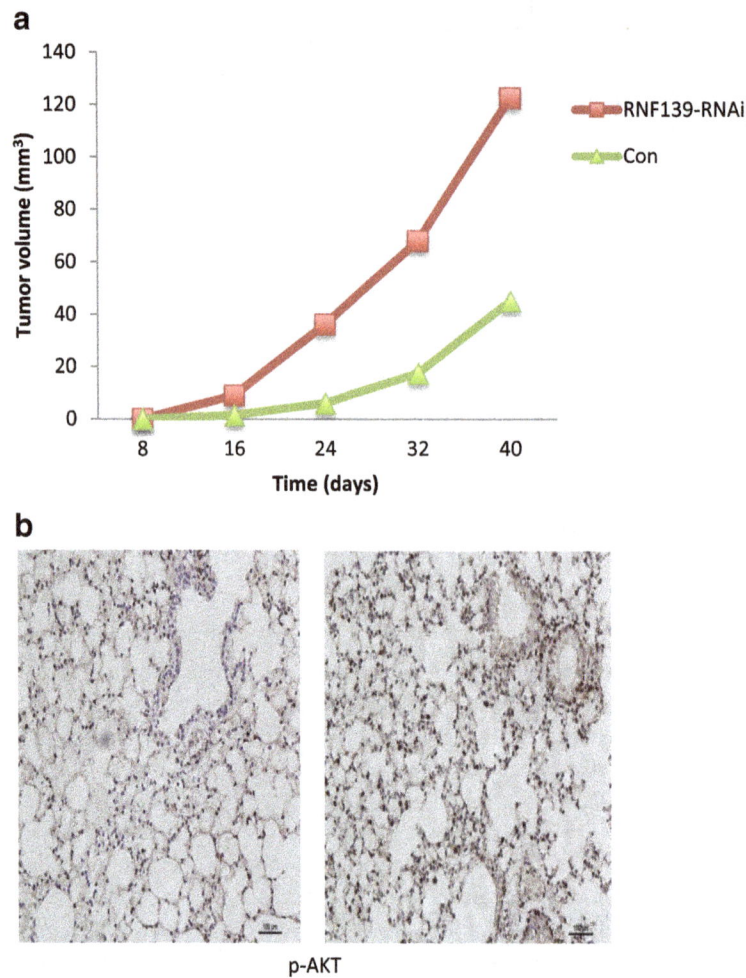

Fig. 4 Knockdown of promoted the tumorigenicity of the SCC25 cells. **a** The growth curve of xenograft tumor model of nude mice which was originated from the SCC25 cells with or without knockdown of RNF139. **b** The expression of pAKT1 was increased in the xenografts which was originated from with the RNF139 stable knockdown SCC25 cells

In this study, we contributed to add another evidence that RNF139 was a antioncogene protein. We demonstrated that RNF139 was a suppressor of tongue cancer SCC9 and SCC25 cells growth and invasion. Knockdown of RNF139 promoted the tumorigenicity of the SCC25 cells. Although we did not find the direct substrate of it, we observed the significant changes in AKT signaling pathway which was induced by RNF139. Furthermore, we determined the low expression of RNF139 in human tongue cancer tissues. These results support a tumor suppressor role for RNF139 in tongue cancer.

Conclusions
Our data clearly establish a correlation between RNF139 and tongue cancer. Of clinical relevance is the fact that our results contribute to the new molecule treatment targets for tongue cancer.

Abbreviations
AKT: v-akt murine thymoma viral oncogene homolog; DMSO: Dimethyl sulfoxide; ER: Endoplasmic reticulum; HO-1: Heme oxygenase-1; PI3K: Phospho-inositide-3-kinase; RNF139: RING finger protein 139; TGFβ: Transforming growth factor-β

Acknowledgements
We appreciate the patients and their families for participating in this study.

Funding
This study was supported by the National Natural Science Foundation of China (81501750), the open research fund program of Hubei-MOST KLOS & KLOBME (201601) and and the Natural Scientific Foundation of Liaoning (2014023037). The foundation had no role in the design of the study and collection, analysis, and interpretation of data and in writing the manuscript.

Authors' contributions
LNW, CS and WY designed the study, performed the study and analyzed the data. WY wrote the main manuscript. All authors read and approved the final

manuscript. WY is accountable for all aspects of the work in ensuring that questions related to the accuracy or integrity of any part of the work are appropriately investigated and resolved.

Competing interests
The authors declare that they have no competing interests.

Author details
[1]The State Key Laboratory Breeding Base of Basic Science of Stomatology (Hubei-MOST) & Key Laboratory of Oral Biomedicine Ministry of Education, School & Hospital of Stomatology, Wuhan University, 237 Luoyu road, Wuhan 430079, China. [2]Department of Endodontics, College of Stomatology, Dalian Medical University, Dalian 116044, China.

References
1. Siegel RL, Miller KD, Jemal A. Cancer statistics, 2017. CA Cancer J Clin. 2017;67(1):7–30.
2. Lan X, Atanassov BS, Li W, Zhang Y, Florens L, Mohan RD, et al. USP44 is an integral component of N-CoR that contributes to Gene repression by deubiquitinating histone H2B. Cell Rep. 2016;17:2382–93.
3. Lim KH, Song MH, Baek KH. Decision for cell fate: deubiquitinating enzymes in cell cycle checkpoint. Cell Mol Life Sci. 2016;73:1439–55.
4. Wang Y, Zhang N, Zhang L, Li R, Fu W, Ma K, et al. Autophagy regulates chromatin ubiquitination in DNA damage response through elimination of SQSTM1/p62. Mol Cell. 2016;63:34–48.
5. Bhogaraju S, Kalayil S, Liu Y, Bonn F, Colby T, Matic I, et al. Phosphoribosylation of ubiquitin promotes serine ubiquitination and impairs conventional ubiquitination. Cell. 2016;167:1636–49.
6. Li J, Chai QY, Liu CH. The ubiquitin system: a critical regulator of innate immunity and pathogen-host interactions. Cell Mol Immunol. 2016;13(5):560–76.
7. Xu D, Wang H, You G. Posttranslational regulation of organic anion transporters by ubiquitination: known and novel. Med Res Rev. 2016;36:964–79.
8. Ji W, Rivero F. Atypical Rho GTPases of the RhoBTB Subfamily: Roles in Vesicle Trafficking and Tumorigenesis. Cells. 2016;5 pii: E28.
9. Lazzari E, Meroni G. TRIM32 ubiquitin E3 ligase, one enzyme for several pathologies: from muscular dystrophy to tumours. Int J Biochem Cell Biol. 2016;79:469–77.
10. Dallavalle C, Albino D, Civenni G, Merulla J, Ostano P, Mello-Grand M, et al. MicroRNA-424 impairs ubiquitination to activate STAT3 and promote prostate tumor progression. J Clin Invest. 2016;126:4585–602.
11. Zhang X, Li CF, Zhang L, Wu CY, Han L, Jin G, et al. TRAF6 restricts p53 mitochondrial translocation, apoptosis, and tumor suppression. Mol Cell. 2016;64:803–14.
12. Wang L, Wang X, Zhao Y, Niu W, Ma G, Yin W, et al. E3 ubiquitin ligase RNF126 regulates the progression of tongue cancer. Cancer Med. 2016;5:2043–7.
13. Jin J, Zhao L, Li Z. The E3 ubiquitin ligase RNF135 regulates the tumorigenesis activity of tongue cancer SCC25 cells. Cancer Med. 2016;5:3140–6.
14. Voutsadakis IA. Ubiquitination and the ubiquitin - proteasome system in the pathogenesis and treatment of squamous head and neck carcinoma. Anticancer Res. 2013;33(9):3527–41.
15. Yang Y, Yin W, He W, Jiang C, Zhou X, Song X, et al. Phenotype-genotype correlation in multiple primary lung cancer patients in China. Sci Rep. 2016;6:36177.
16. Yang Y, Shi C, Sun H, Yin W, Zhou X, Zhang L, et al. Elderly male smokers with right lung tumors are viable candidates for KRAS mutation screening. Sci Rep. 2016;6:18566.
17. Lin PH, Lan WM, Chau LY. TRC8 suppresses tumorigenesis through targeting heme oxygenase-1 for ubiquitination and degradation. Oncogene. 2013;32:2325–34.

15

The prognostic value of *TP53* mutations in hypopharyngeal squamous cell carcinoma

Go Omura[1,2], Mizuo Ando[1*] ⓘ, Yasuhiro Ebihara[1,3], Yuki Saito[1], Kenya Kobayashi[1,2], Osamu Fukuoka[1], Ken Akashi[1], Masafumi Yoshida[1], Takahiro Asakage[1,4] and Tatsuya Yamasoba[1]

Abstract

Background: *TP53* is the most frequently mutated gene in human cancers. Previous studies reported that *TP53* mutations correlated with poor prognoses in patients with head and neck squamous cell carcinoma (HNSCC). However, the relationship between *TP53* mutations and hypopharyngeal squamous cell carcinoma (HPSCC) is not known. The current study aimed to evaluate *TP53* mutation status as a predictive biomarker in patients with HPSCC.

Methods: We retrospectively reviewed the clinical charts of 57 HPSCC patients treated with initial surgery between 2008 and 2014. *TP53* mutation status was determined by Sanger sequencing, and patients were classified into wild-type, missense mutation, and truncating mutation groups. Additionally, p53 expression was determined using immunohistochemistry in surgical specimens.

Results: *TP53* mutations were identified in 39 (68%) patients. The 3-year disease-specific survival (DSS) rate of wild-type, missense mutation, and truncating mutation group were 94%, 61%, and 43%, respectively. The *TP53* mutation group displayed significantly worse DSS and overall survival rates than the wild-type group ($P = 0.01$ and $P = 0.007$, respectively). Multivariate analyses revealed that the presence of *TP53* mutations and ≥ 4 metastatic lymph nodes were independent adverse prognostic factors for HPSCC. p53 immunopositivity was detected in 22 patients, including 5 (28%) and 17 (71%) patients in the wild-type and missense mutation groups, whereas none of the patients with truncating mutation exhibited p53 immunopositivity ($P = 0.0001$).

Conclusion: The *TP53* mutation status correlated with poor prognosis in surgically treated HPSCC patients. Specifically, truncating mutations which were not detected by p53 immunohistochemistry were predictive of worst survival.

Keywords: *TP53* mutation, Hypopharyngeal squamous cell carcinoma, Truncating mutation, Prognosis, Pharyngectomy

Background

Among squamous cell carcinomas (SCC) originating in the upper aerodigestive tract, the management of hypopharyngeal squamous cell carcinoma (HPSCC) remains to be one of the most challenging and controversial topics, due to the poor survival rate and potentially devastating effects on speech and swallowing [1]. Alcohol consumption and acetaldehyde, a toxic product of ethanol metabolism, are widely known as carcinogen of head and neck SCC (HNSCC) and esophageal SCC (ESCC). The activity of *aldehyde dehydrogenase 2*, a key enzyme in the elimination of aldehyde, is reduced by the germline polymorphism

Glu504Lys (previously described as Glu487Lys), which is prevalent in Mongoloid but not in Caucasoid or Negroid populations [2]. Therefore, this different genetic background is considered as a major reason of high HPSCC and ESCC incidence rates in East Asia [3, 4].

Tumor suppressor gene *TP53* is the most frequently mutated gene in human cancers: more than 50% of human cancers contain somatic mutations in this gene [5, 6]. Tumor suppressor p53, encoded by the *TP53* gene, is a key protein involved in many cellular anticarcinogenic processes such as apoptosis and cell-cycle control [7]; therefore, p53 is widely known as the guardian of the genome [8]. Molecular alterations in carcinogenesis of HNSCC include loss of p53 function, which is mediated by genetic mechanisms such as *TP53* mutations [9] and loss

* Correspondence: andom-tky@umin.ac.jp
[1]Department of Otolaryngology-Head and Neck Surgery, Faculty of Medicine, The University of Tokyo, 7-3-1 Hongo, Bunkyo-ku, Tokyo 113-8655, Japan
Full list of author information is available at the end of the article

of heterozygosity [10], or degradation of p53 meditated by the human papillomavirus (HPV) oncoprotein E6 [11].

Two studies previously demonstrated the association between *TP53* mutations and prognosis in surgically treated HNSCC patients. [12, 13] However, these studies did not examine these associations based on the anatomical location of the HNSCCs. Moreover, patients with oropharyngeal SCC (OPSCC) comprised the majority of the cases, and there were a total of only two patients with HPSCC in the two studies. HPV-related OPSCCs commonly express wild type *TP53* [14], creating a potential confounder as HPV-related tumors have a generally favorable prognosis. In contrast, HPV-driven HPSCC is considered rare [15] and the prognostic significance of *TP53* mutation status in HPSCC has not yet been investigated. The aim of this study was to evaluate the prognostic significance of *TP53* mutation status among surgically treated HPSCC patients in Japan, where the HPSCC incidence rate is high.

Methods

We retrospectively reviewed the clinical charts of HPSCC patients, who had been surgically treated between 2008 and 2014 at the University of Tokyo Hospital. We excluded patients, who underwent salvage surgery after the definitive radiotherapy (RT) or chemoradiotherapy (CRT), and those who received preoperative chemotherapy. We identified 57 HPSCC patients (55 men and 2 women; age range: 46–84 years, median age: 68 years) who underwent initial surgery of primary lesions. Subsites of primary tumor were the pyriform sinus, posterior wall, and postcricoid region, in 37 (65%), 15 (26%), and 5 (9%) patients, respectively. TNM staging was done according to the 7th edition of the Union for International Cancer Control (2009) staging guidelines. The indication for postoperative RT/CRT was comprehensively determined on the basis of the clinicopathological status of the patients including impaired performance status, inadequate surgical margin, ≥4 metastatic LNs, presence of extranodal extension (ENE), and postoperative complications as well as the consent of patient. The Institutional Review Board of the University of Tokyo Hospital approved this study (#2487 and #2904).

Determination of human papillomavirus status

In OPSCC, p16 immunopositivity is commonly used as a surrogate marker for HPV determination [16]. Therefore, the p16 status was evaluated in surgically excised specimens using immunohistochemistry (IHC) according to the standard techniques as previously described [17]. A mouse p16 monoclonal antibody (1:100 dilution; Santa Cruz Biotechnology, CA, USA) was used as the primary antibody, and immunostained samples were blindly reviewed and scored independently by two investigators (M. A and Y. S). In

accordance with previous studies, p16 positivity by IHC was defined as strong and diffuse nuclear and cytoplasmic staining in ≥70% of the tumor cells [16, 17].

However, p16 expression does not always indicate the presence of HPV DNA, and the combination of p16 expression determined by IHC with HPV DNA determination by polymerase chain reaction (PCR) or in situ hybridization (ISH) is considered to provide the almost perfect sensitivity and specificity [18, 19]. Therefore, p16-immunopositive specimens were also tested for HPV DNA by HPV-ISH, as previously described [19, 20]. Briefly, HPV DNA was detected using an ISH method with catalyzed signal amplification (GenPoint signal amplification system; Dako, Kyoto, Japan), in accordance with the manufacturer's instructions. Slides were hybridized using a biotinylated GenPoint HPV probe (This probe has been found to react with HPV types 16, 18, 31, 33, 35, 39, 45, 51, 52, 56, 58, 59, and 68 on FFPE tissues and/or cells by ISH, Dako). Slides were scored as positive for HPV if a punctate signal pattern was observed in almost all tumor nuclei.

Genomic DNA extraction

Tumor tissue specimens were collected during surgery, and snap-frozen in liquid nitrogen and stored at −80 °C. Genomic DNA was extracted using the QIAamp DNA Mini Kit (Qiagen, Hilden, Germany), in accordance with the manufacturer's protocol. In specimens where the harvest of frozen sections appeared to interfere with the pathological margins, DNA was isolated from formalin-fixed, paraffin-embedded (FFPE) tissue blocks. Briefly, the tumor lesions on hematoxylin and eosin-stained slides were marked, and the corresponding areas were identified on unstained tissue sections. Each selected area was carefully dissected under microscopic observation. Genomic DNA was then extracted using the QIAamp DNA FFPE Tissue Kit (Qiagen).

Detection of *TP53* mutations

PCR amplification and Sanger sequencing were performed to detect *TP53* mutations in exons 2–9, containing 98% of all mutations described in HNSCC cases [21]. A total of 20 ng/μl genomic DNA per sample was used for PCR amplification using PrimeSTAR HS DNA Polymerase(Takara Bio, Shiga, Japan). Amplification conditions included two-step cycle of 98 °C for 15 s and 68 °C for 90 s, for a total of 44 cycles, except for the amplification of exon 2–3 fragments harvested from frozen and FFPE specimens and exon 6 fragments harvested from FFPE specimens, which were amplified by nested PCR (25 cycles each) using two primer pairs. Subsequently, PCR products harvested from FFPE tissue were purified using the QIAquick PCR Purification Kit (Qiagen), in accordance with the manufacturer's protocol. Mutations were confirmed by Sanger sequencing using the Big Dye Terminator v3.1 Cycle Sequencing Kit and 3130xL Genetic Analyzer (Applied Biosystems, CA, USA). In this study, nonsense mutations, splice variants, and frameshifts were defined as truncating mutations, that lead to non-functional p53, based on previous studies [13, 22]. All samples were sequenced twice with independent PCR using forward and reverse primers.

Immunohistochemistry for p53 expression

IHC for p53 expression was performed according to standard IHC techniques. A mouse p53 monoclonal antibody clone DO-7 (1:100 dilution; Leica Biosystems, Nussloch, Germany) was used as the primary antibody. In accordance with a previous study, a sample was determined as p53-immunopositive when ≥10% of tumor nuclei were immunostained [23].

Statistical analyses

Primary endpoint was disease-specific survival (DSS) and secondary endpoint was overall survival (OS). Potential correlations between the treatment method and several clinical features were evaluated using the chi-square test; for analyses in which there were <4 patients, the Fisher's exact test was used. Survival was analyzed using the Kaplan–Meier method and the log-rank test. Variables were also analyzed by multivariate survival analysis using the Cox proportional hazards model. Hazard ratios (HR) and 95% confidence intervals (CI) were calculated to determine the effect of each variable on outcomes. P values <0.05 were considered statistically significant. GraphPad Prism software version 5 (Graph-Pad Software, CA, USA) was used for the chi-square, Fisher's exact, Mann-Whitney's U, and log-rank tests. Mac Tahenryo-Kaiseki version 2.0 (ESUMI, Tokyo, Japan) was used for multivariate Cox regression models.

Results

Human papillomavirus status of patients with hypopharyngeal squamous cell carcinoma

In this cohort of 57 HPSCC patients, 3 (5%) patients were immunopositive for p16; however, none of these three patients had detectable HPV DNA by HPV-ISH. Therefore, HPSCC was confirmed to be unrelated to HPV in all patients in this study (Fig. 1).

Distribution of TP53 mutations

TP53 mutations were detected in 39 (68%) patients. Missense mutations, nonsense mutations, splicing variants, and frameshift mutations were found in 24 (42%), 9 (16%), 4 (7%), and 2 (3%) patients, respectively. *TP53* mutations in exon 2, 3, 4, 5, 6, 7, 8, and 9 were found in 1, 0, 3, 11, 9, 4, 8, and 3 patients, respectively (Fig. 2).

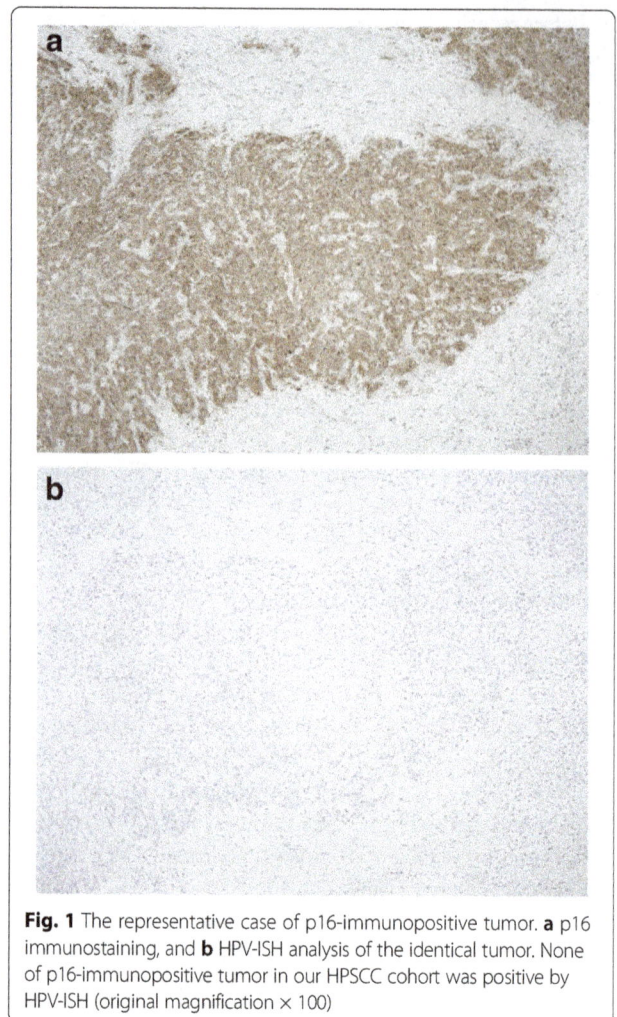

Fig. 1 The representative case of p16-immunopositive tumor. **a** p16 immunostaining, and **b** HPV-ISH analysis of the identical tumor. None of p16-immunopositive tumor in our HPSCC cohort was positive by HPV-ISH (original magnification × 100)

Clinicopathological features and *TP53* mutation status

Table 1 summarizes the clinical data and *TP53* status. Table 2 shows the clinicopathological features according to *TP53* mutation status. Histopathological analysis revealed positive surgical margins in 11 (19%) patients, ≥4 metastatic LNs in 14 (25%) patients, and ENE in 15 (26%) patients. Postoperative RT/CRT was administered to 16 (28%) patients. Of note, all of stage I/II patients (5 patients) had wild-type *TP53*, and patients with a past history of HNSCC or ESCC were significantly greater in the *TP53* mutation groups than in the wild-type groups ($P = 0.02$). Administration of postoperative RT/CRT did not correlate with *TP53* mutation status ($P = 0.25$).

Association between *TP53* mutation and p53 expression

Representative images of specimens exhibiting p53 immunopositivity are presented in Fig. 3. p53 immunopositivity was detected in 22 patients, including 5 (28%) and 17 (71%) patients in the wild-type and missense mutation groups, whereas there were no patients with p53

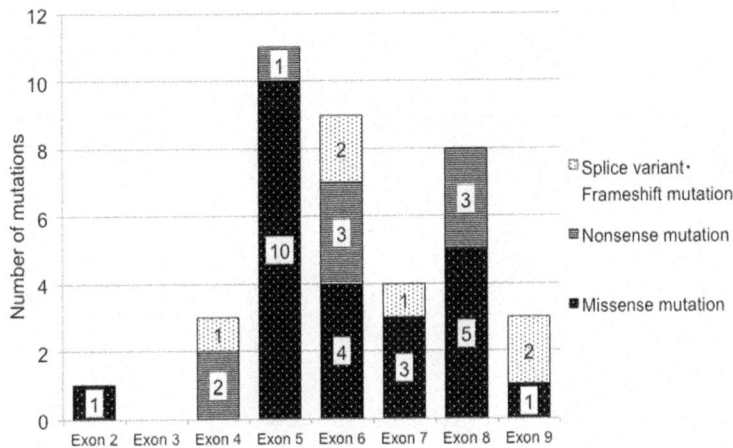

Fig. 2 Distribution of *TP53* mutations according to the affected exons. Exon 2, 3, 4, 5, 6, 7, 8, and 9 of *TP53* mutations were found in 1, 0, 3, 11, 9, 4, 8, and 3 patients, respectively

immunopositivity in the truncating mutation group ($P = 0.0001$, chi-square test).

Correlation between *TP53* mutation status and prognosis
Eighteen (32%) patients died from HPSCC, whereas 8 (14%) patients died from other causes. The remaining 31 (54%) patients were alive and disease-free on last follow-up date. The median follow-up period for the entire co-hort was 29 months (range: 3.5–101 months), whereas 45 months (range: 24–101 months) for patients who survived ($n = 31$) and 16 months (range: 3.5–85 months) for those who died ($n = 26$). The 3-year DSS of the wild-type group was significantly longer than that of the *TP53* mu-tation group (94% vs 55%; $P = 0.01$, Fig. 4). Furthermore, patients with wild-type/missense mutations had signifi-cantly better 3-year DSS than those with truncating mu-tations (76% vs 43%; $P = 0.03$). The 3-year DSS rate of wild-type, missense mutation, and truncating mutation groups were 94%, 61%, and 43%, respectively (Fig. 5). The 3-year OS of the wild-type group was significantly longer than that of the *TP53* mutation group (89% vs 42%; $P = 0.007$). The 3-year OS rate of wild-type/mis-sense mutation group was not significantly different than that of the truncating mutation group (66% vs 40%; $P = 0.14$). The 3-year OS rate of the wild-type, missense mutation, and truncating mutation group were 89%, 43%, and 40%, respectively. In contrast, p53 immunopo-sitivity did not correlate with DSS ($P = 0.77$). In the subgroup analyses of 52 stage III/IV patients, the 3-year DSS of the wild-type group was significantly longer than that of the *TP53* mutation group (92% vs 55%; $P = 0.02$). The 3-year OS of the wild-type group was significantly longer than that of the *TP53* mutation group (92% vs 42%; $P = 0.006$).

Table 3 shows the associations between the clinico-pathological factors and DSS in univariate analysis. The

presence of ≥ 4 metastatic LNs ($P = 0.04$) and ENE ($P = 0.03$) were poor prognostic factors. In contrast, tumor differentiation grade, T classification, stage, surgical mar-gin, and postoperative RT/CRT did not correlate with DSS.

Multivariate Cox proportional hazard analysis using variables based on univariate analyses was conducted to determine independent prognostic factors for DSS and OS. The presence of *TP53* mutations ($P = 0.04$; HR, 4.96; 95% CI, 1.08–22.8, and $P = 0.02$; HR, 4.75; 95% CI, 1.35–16.7, respectively) and ≥ 4 metastatic LNs ($P = 0.03$; HR, 3.00; 95% CI, 1.12–8.04, and $P = 0.02$; HR, 2.89; 95% CI, 1.22–6.86, respectively) have significant adverse effects on both DSS and OS. In the subgroup analyses of 52 stage III/IV patients, the presence of *TP53* mutations was a significant adverse prognostic factor on OS, and nearly reached significance on DSS. (Table 4).

Discussion
In this retrospective study, we demonstrated that the *TP53* mutation status significantly correlated with poor prognosis in surgically treated HPSCC patients. Specific-ally, patients with truncating mutations exhibited the worst prognosis. To the best of our knowledge, this is the first study focusing on the association between *TP53* mutation status and prognosis of HPV-unrelated HPSCC. The result of the current study was consistent with the previous studies investigating all HNSCC sub-sites [12, 13], which included patients with HPV-driven OPSCC.

HPSCC is rarely caused by HPV-driven carcinogenesis as we confirmed in the current study and occurs more frequently in East Asian population than in other re-gions of the world. Survival of patients with HPSCC has not markedly improved in recent decades. In the last two-decades, CRT and induction chemotherapy followed

Table 1 Clinical data and *TP53* status

Age, gender	TN	*TP53*	p53-IHC	No. of LNs	Tumor differentiation	Margins	ENE	Follow-up periods (months)	
62 M	T3N2b	truncating	–	2	M	+	–	101	NED
73 M	T3N2b	wt	+	9	M	+	–	85	DOC
78 M	T3 N0	truncating	–	0	M	–	–	11	DOD
49 M	T2 N0	wt	+	0	W	–	–	94	NED
72 M	T3 N1	missense	+	2	W	–	–	36	DOC
65 M	T3N2b	missense	+	3	M	–	+	27	NED
68 M	T2N2b	wt	–	11	W	–	–	92	NED
67 M	T3N2b	truncating	–	5	M	+	–	11	DOD
81 M	T3 N1	wt	–	3	W	–	–	66	NED
80 M	T3N2b	truncating	–	3	M	–	+	17	DOD
64 M	T1N2b	truncating	–	2	W	–	+	82	NED
79 M	T3 N0	missense	–	0	M	–	–	66	NED
81 M	T3N2b	truncating	–	2	M	–	+	24	DOD
66 M	T4aN0	truncating	–	0	M	–	–	76	NED
81 M	T3 N0	missense	+	0	W	–	–	4	DOC
62 M	T2 N0	wt	–	1	P	–	–	75	NED
83 M	T1 N0	wt	–	0	P	+	–	41	DOD
70 M	T3N2b	truncating	–	14	M	–	+	11	DOD
75 M	T2N2b	wt	+	2	M	+	–	55	NED
55 M	T4aN2b	missense	+	4	W	–	+	24	DOD
46 M	T4aN0	missense	+	0	M	–	–	66	DOC
55 M	T4aN2b	missense	–	6	W	–	–	12	NED
71 M	T3N2c	missense	+	25	M	–	+	17	DOD
79 M	T4aN0	missense	+	1	M	–	–	7	DOD
63 M	T3 N0	missense	–	2	M	–	–	29	DOD
67 M	T2 N0	wt	–	0	W	–	–	60	NED
61 M	T4aN2b	missense	+	4	W	+	+	5	DOD
84 M	T4aN0	truncating	–	0	M	–	–	8	DOD
60 M	T4aN2c	truncating	–	12	P	–	–	9.2	DOC
68 M	T3 N0	truncating	–	0	M	–	–	55	NED
60 M	T1 N0	wt	–	0	M	–	–	53	NED
67 M	T4aN0	wt	–	4	W	–	–	50	NED
72F	T3 N0	missense	+	0	M	–	–	27	NED
72 M	T3 N0	missense	–	0	M	–	–	49	NED
81 M	T3 N1	wt	–	3	W	–	–	17	DOD
72 M	T3 N1	missense	+	1	M	–	–	49	NED
84 M	T3 N0	missense	+	2	M	+	–	5	DOD
47 M	T3 N0	wt	–	0	W	–	–	23	DOC
69 M	T1N2a	missense	–	2	W	+	+	6	DOD
64F	T3N2c	missense	+	3	M	–	–	14	DOD
69 M	T3 N1	missense	–	2	W	–	+	45	NED
64 M	T3 N0	missense	+	0	M	+	–	43	NED
63 M	T3 N1	truncating	–	3	M	–	–	41	NED

Table 1 Clinical data and *TP53* status *(Continued)*

Age, gender	TN	TP53	p53-IHC	No. of LNs	Tumor differentiation	Margins	ENE	Follow-up periods (months)	
76 M	T3 N0	wt	+	1	M	–	+	37	NED
71 M	T4aN2b	missense	+	1	M	–	+	16	DOC
75 M	T3N2b	missense	–	3	M	–	+	37	NED
67 M	T4aN2b	wt	–	4	M	–	–	36	NED
74 M	T3 N0	wt	–	3	P	–	–	42	NED
82 M	T4aN2b	missense	+	1	M	–	–	32	NED
52 M	T3N2c	wt	+	3	M	–	+	32	NED
64 M	T4aN0	missense	+	0	P	–	–	24	DOC
48 M	T4aN2b	truncating	–	4	W	–	–	30	NED
71 M	T4aN0	wt	–	3	M	+	–	28	NED
64 M	T4aN2b	truncating	–	2	M	–	+	17	DOD
84 M	T3N2b	truncating	–	14	M	–	–	16	DOD
64 M	T3 N1	missense	+	1	M	+	–	25	NED
79 M	T4aN1	wt	–	1	W	–	–	24	NED

IHC immunohistochemistory, *No. LNs* the number of metastatic lymph nodes, *ENE* extranodal extension, *M* male, *F* female, *W* well differentiated, *M* moderately differentiated, *P* poorly differentiated, *NED* no evidence of disease, *DOD* died of the disease, *DOC* died of other cause

Table 2 Clinicopathological parameters according to *TP53* mutation status

Clinicopathological features		Total (n = 57)	TP53 status		P value
			Wild-type (n = 18)	Mutation (n = 39)	
Age	Range (median)		47–83 (70)	46–84 (68)	0.45**
Subsites	PS	27	12	15	0.25
	PC	5	0	5	
	PW	15	6	9	
T	T1–3	40	14	26	0.30*
	T4	17	4	13	
N	N0/1	32	13	19	0.15
	N2/3	25	5	20	
Stage	I/II	5	5	0	0.002*
	III/IV	52	13	39	
Tumor differentiation	W./M. SCC	52	15	37	0.31*
	P. SCC	5	3	2	
Margin	Negative	46	14	32	0.73
	Positive	11	4	7	
No. of metastatic LNs	≤3	43	14	29	1.00
	≥4	14	4	10	
ENE	Absent	42	16	26	0.11*
	Present	15	2	13	
PORT/CRT	Absent	41	14	27	0.25
	Present	16	4	12	
Anamnestic SCC	Absent	42	17	25	0.02*
	Present	15	1	14	

PS pyriform sinus, *PC* postcricoid, *PW* posterior wall, *T* tumor classification, *N* nodal classification, *Stage* stage classification, *W* well differentiated, *M* moderately differentiated, *P* poorly differentiated, *SCC* squamous cell carcinoma, *No* number, *LN* lymph node, *ENE* extranodal extension, *PORT/CRT* postoperative radiotherapy/chemoradiotherapy, *Anamnestic SCC* anamnestic squamous cell carcinoma arising from esophagus and head and neck region, *: Fisher's exact tests were used. **: Mann-Whitney's U test was used

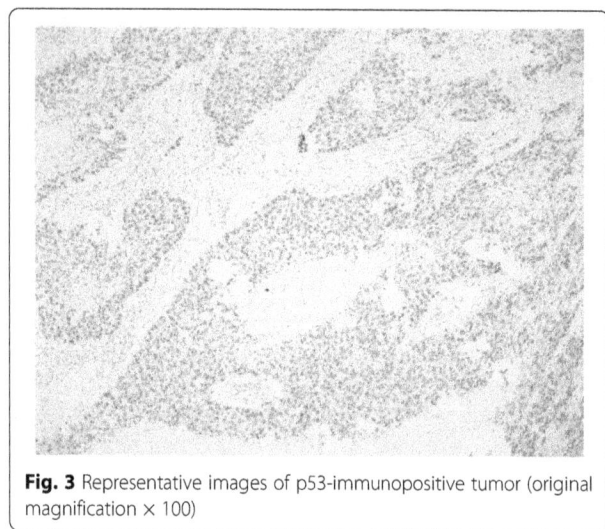

Fig. 3 Representative images of p53-immunopositive tumor (original magnification × 100)

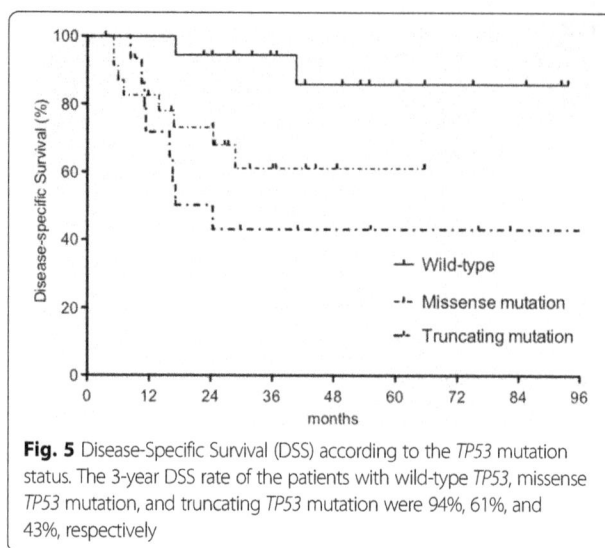

Fig. 5 Disease-Specific Survival (DSS) according to the *TP53* mutation status. The 3-year DSS rate of the patients with wild-type *TP53*, missense *TP53* mutation, and truncating *TP53* mutation were 94%, 61%, and 43%, respectively

by RT have become the option for advanced HNSCC patients who prefer nonsurgical organ preservation [24–26]. However, RT-induced late toxicity, such as dysphasia and osteonecrosis distresses emerging issues for cancer survivors. The recent development of minimally invasive surgical procedures, such as transoral robotic surgery (TORS) and transoral videolaryngoscopic surgery (TOVS) techniques, has broadened surgical indications and appeared to result in better outcomes with respect to the postoperative speech and swallowing function [27, 28]. Therefore, surgery remains the main treatment modality for HPSCC patients. Our multivariate analyses revealed that both the *TP53* mutation status and the presence of ≥4 metastatic LNs were independent adverse prognostic factors for surgically treated HPSCC patients. In the previous study, we demonstrated that the presence of multiple metastatic LNs was significantly associated with the poor prognosis and the incidence of distant metastases in

advanced HPSCC patients treated with total pharyngolaryngectomy [29]. Collectively, *TP53* mutations can be a useful biomarker for HPSCC patients, in addition to the traditional metastatic LN number.

Interestingly, the past history of HNSCC or ESCC was significantly higher in the *TP53* mutation group than in the wild-type group in the present study. HNSCC and ESCC have been known to occur synchronously or metachronously, which might be explained by the concept of "field cancerization" first introduced by Slaughter et al. in 1953 [30]. Currently, repetitive exposure to acetaldehyde is considered to play a key role in field cancerization of the squamous epithelium in the head and neck region and the esophagus [31]. Moreover, Waridel et al. reported that mutations in *TP53* were

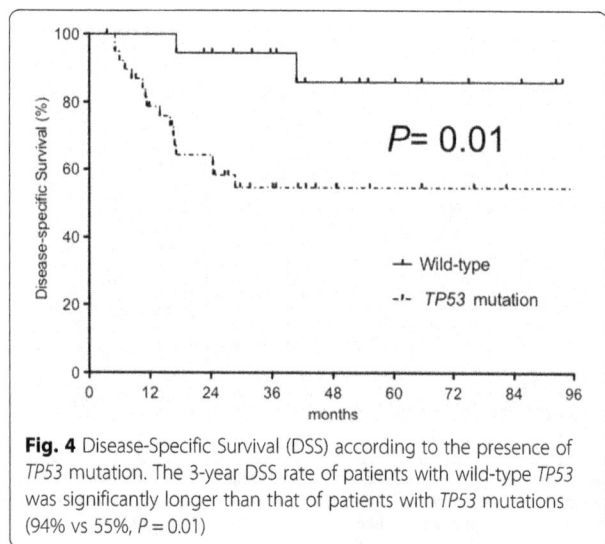

Fig. 4 Disease-Specific Survival (DSS) according to the presence of *TP53* mutation. The 3-year DSS rate of patients with wild-type *TP53* was significantly longer than that of patients with *TP53* mutations (94% vs 55%, $P = 0.01$)

Table 3 Univariate analyses for disease-specific survival

Variables		HR (95% CI)	P value
Tumor differentiation	W./M. vs. P.SCC	0.63 [0.13–3.09]	0.57
T classification	T1–3 vs. T4	1.12 [0.39–3.25]	0.83
Stage	Stage I/II vs. III/IV	2.30 [0.55–9.56]	0.25
Margin	Negative vs. Positive	2.08 [0.61–7.07]	0.24
No. of metastatic LNs	≤3 vs. ≥4	3.34 [1.04–10.7]	0.04
ENE	Absent vs. Present	3.34 [1.11–10.1]	0.03
PORT/CRT	Performed vs. Not performed	0.91 [0.33–2.53]	0.86
TP53 mutation	Wild-type vs. Mutation	3.32 [1.28–8.60]	0.01
p53 immunopositivity	Negative vs. Positive	0.87 [0.33–2.27]	0.77

HR hazard ratio, *95% CI* 95% confidence interval, *W* well differentiated, *M* moderately differentiated, *P* poorly differentiated, *SCC* squamous cell carcinoma, *T* tumor classification, *No* number, *LN* lymph node, *ENE* extranodal extension, *PORT/CRT* postoperative radiotherapy/chemoradiotherapy

Table 4 Multivariate analyses for disease-specific and overall survival

Variables		Overall (n = 57)				Stage III/IV (n = 52)			
		DSS		OS		DSS		OS	
		HR [95% CI]	P value	HR [95% CI]	P value	HR [95% CI]	P value	HR [95% CI]	P value
TP53	Wild-type vs. Mutation	4.96 [1.08–22.8]	0.04	4.75 [1.35–16.7]	0.02	7.72 [0.98–60.7]	0.05	5.51 [1.24–24.5]	0.03
No. of metastatic LNs	≤3 vs. ≥4	3.00 [1.12–8.04]	0.03	2.89 [1.22–6.86]	0.02	3.07 [1.13–8.35]	0.03	2.89 [1.20–6.94]	0.02
ENE	Absence vs. Presence	1.85 [0.70–4.86]	0.21	1.39 [0.59–3.27]	0.45	1.81 [0.68–4.80]	0.23	1.36 [0.58–3.21]	0.48

DSS disease-specific survival, OS overall survival, HR hazard ratio, 95% CI 95% confidence interval, No the number, ENE extranodal extensio

frequent and early events in the pathogenesis of HNSCC and identified the expansion of multiple clones of mutant p53-containing cells as an important biological step in field cancerization [32]. Our findings in the current study led further support to these observations. Future studies with larger sample size and longitudinal evaluations, supported with basic research, are necessary to confirm this hypothesis.

In the current study, we demonstrated that p53 immunopositivity was observed most frequently in the presence of missense mutations. Wild-type p53 protein is rapidly degraded via the ubiquitin-proteasome system, resulting in low p53 protein expression. Conversely, the nonsense-mediated RNA decay and the resultant decreased amount of the protein considered to be the reason why truncating p53 proteins cannot be detected by IHC [33]. Some missense mutations, that result in increased p53 immunopositivity can lead to a dominant-negative or a gain-of-function phenotype [34, 35], Our observations in the current study support these biological mechanisms; therefore, the distinction between missense and truncating mutations is reasonable for the clinical categorization of the TP53 mutation status.

The Cancer Genome Atlas (TCGA) reported that TP53 mutations were detected in 84% of HPV-unrelated HNSCC cases using whole-exome sequencing analysis [14]. In comparison, the frequency of TP53 mutations was lower in the HPSCC cohort of the current study, which might be partially due to differences in racial composition and tumor subsites. The HNSCC cohort of TCGA consisted almost entirely of Caucasoid and Negroid populations, with only two HPSCC patients. Additionally, it is possible that mutation detection sensitivity of whole-exome sequencing was superior to that of Sanger sequencing.

To improve the prognoses of HPSCC patients with TP53 mutations, adjuvant therapy should be selectively administered to these patients. TP53 mutation, however, is also known as a predictive marker for chemo- and radioresistance in HNSCCs. [36, 37] Therefore, it might be unreasonable to use TP53 mutation status as a therapeutic biomarker for existing postoperative treatments including RT/CRT. Although most of the current targeted therapies are inhibitors of oncogenic pathways, development of p53-targeted therapy is warranted.

One of the limitations of our study was a lack of detailed comparison and functional study of each TP53 mutations, due to the small sample size. In line with previous reports on HNSCC [13], various mutation types were detected in various regions of TP53 genes. Further investigation with larger sample size is required to elucidate the potential associations between the mutations with respect to functional and biological effects and prognosis. Furthermore, the number of T1–2 tumors was small in this study. Recently, TORS and TOVS techniques for T1–2 tumors to which RT/CRT was previously preferable were broadened. Therefore, further accumulation of T1–2 patients is also required.

Conclusions

We demonstrated that TP53 mutations had a significant impact on prognosis, in surgically treated HPSCC patients. In particular, truncating mutations which were not detected by p53 IHC were shown to have predictive value for a worst survival. Further confirmation from prospective studies with larger sample size including more T1–2 patients is warranted.

Abbreviations
CRT: Chemoradiotherapy; ENE: Extranodal extension; ESCC: Esophageal squamous cell carcinoma; FFPE: Formalin-fixed, paraffin-embedded; HNSCC: Head and neck squamous cell carcinoma; HPSCC: Hypopharyngeal squamous cell carcinoma; HPV: Human papillomavirus; IHC: Immunohistochemistry; ISH: In situ hybridization; LN: Lymph node; ND: Neck dissection; OPSCC: Oropharyngeal squamous cell carcinoma; PCR: Polymerase chain reaction; RT: Radiotherapy; SCC: Squamous cell carcinoma; TCGA: The Cancer Genome Atlas; TORS: Transoral robotic surgery; TOVS: Transoral videolaryngoscopic surgery

Acknowledgements
We thank Ms. A. Tsuyuzaki for her excellent technical assistance.

Funding
This study was supported by JSPS KAKENHI Grant Number 15 K20184 and 26,893,058.

Authors' contributions

Conceptualization: GO, MA, Methodology: GO, TA, Validation: MA, YS, Formal analysis: GO, YS, Investigation: GO, MA, YE, Resources: KK, OF, KA, MY, Data curation: OF, Writing – original draft: GO, Writing – review and editing: MA, Visualization: GO, Supervision: TA, TY, Project administration: MA, TA, Funding acquisition: GO, MA. All authors read and approved the final manuscript.

Competing interests

The authors declare that they have no competing interests.

Author details

[1]Department of Otolaryngology-Head and Neck Surgery, Faculty of Medicine, The University of Tokyo, 7-3-1 Hongo, Bunkyo-ku, Tokyo 113-8655, Japan. [2]Department of Head and Neck Surgery, National Cancer Center Hospital, Tokyo, Japan. [3]Department of Head and Neck Surgery, Saitama Medical University International Medical Center, Saitama, Japan. [4]Department of Head and Neck Surgery, Faculty of Medicine, Tokyo Medical and Dental University, Tokyo, Japan.

References

1. Montgomery PQ, Phys Evan PH, Gullane PJ. Principles and practice of head and neck surgery and oncology. 2nd ed. Informa Healthcare: Colchester; 2009. p. 233.
2. Goedde HW, Agarwal DP, Fritze G, Meier-Tackmann D, Singh S, Beckmann G, et al. Distribution of ADH2 and ALDH2 genotypes in different populations. Hum Genet. 1992;88:344–6.
3. Hamajima N, Takezaki T, Tajima K. Allele frequencies of 25 polymorphisms pertaining to cancer risk for Japanese, Koreans and Chinese. Asian Pac J Cancer Prev. 2002;3:197–206.
4. Asakage T, Yokoyama A, Haneda T, Yamazaki M, Muto M, Yokoyama T, et al. Genetic polymorphisms of alcohol and aldehyde dehydrogenases, and drinking, smoking and diet in Japanese men with oral and pharyngeal squamous cell carcinoma. Carcinogenesis. 2007;28:865–74.
5. Levine AJ. p53, the cellular gatekeeper for growth and division. Cell. 1997;88:323–31.
6. Toledo F, Wahl GM. Regulating the p53 pathway: in vitro hypotheses, in vivo veritas. Nat Rev Cancer. 2006;6:909–23.
7. Vogelstein B, Lane D, Levine AJ. Surfing the p53 network. Nature. 2000;408: 307–10.
8. Efeyan A, Serrano M. p53: guardian of the genome and policeman of the oncogenes. Cell Cycle. 2007;6:1006–10.
9. Olshan AF, Weissler MC, Pei H, Conway K. p53 mutations in head and neck cancer: new data and evaluation of mutational spectra. Cancer Epidemiol Biomark Prev. 1997;6:499–504.
10. Gonzalez MV, Pello MF, Lopez-Larrea C, Suarez C, Menendez MJ, Coto E. Loss of heterozygosity and mutation analysis of the p16 (9p21) and p53 (17p13) genes in squamous cell carcinoma of the head and neck. Clin Cancer Res. 1995;1:1043–9.
11. Scheffner M, Werness BA, Huibregtse JM, Levine AJ, Howley PM. The E6 oncoprotein encoded by human papillomavirus types 16 and 18 promotes the degradation of p53. Cell. 1990;63:1129–36.
12. Poeta ML, Manola J, Goldwasser MA, Forastiere A, Benoit N, Califano JA, et al. TP53 mutations and survival in squamous-cell carcinoma of the head and neck. N Engl J Med. 2007;357:2552–61.
13. Lindenbergh-van der Plas M, Brakenhoff RH, Kuik DJ, Buijze M, Bloemena E, Snijders PJ, et al. Prognostic significance of truncating TP53 mutations in head and neck squamous cell carcinoma. Clin Cancer Res. 2011;17:3733–41.
14. The Cancer Genome Atlas Network. Comprehensive genomic characterization of head and neck squamous cell carcinomas. Nature. 2015;517:576–82.
15. Ang KK, Harris J, Wheeler R, Weber R, Rosenthal DI, Nguyen-Tân PF, et al. Human papillomavirus and survival of patients with oropharyngeal cancer. N Engl J Med. 2010;363:24–35.
16. Gillison ML, Zhang Q, Jordan R, Xiao W, Westra WH, Trotti A, et al. Tobacco smoking and increased risk of death and progression for patients with p16-positive and p16-negative oropharyngeal cancer. J Clin Oncol. 2012;30:2102–11.
17. Saito Y, Yoshida M, Ushiku T, Omura G, Ebihara Y, Shimono T, et al. Prognostic value of p16 expression and alcohol consumption in Japanese patients with oropharyngeal squamous cell carcinoma. Cancer. 2013;119:2005–11.
18. Thavaraj S, Stokes A, Guerra E, Bible J, Halligan E, Long A, et al. Evaluation of human papillomavirus testing for squamous cell carcinoma of the tonsil in clinical practice. J Clin Pathol. 2011;64:308–12.
19. Saito Y, Yoshida M, Omura G, Kobayashi K, Fujimoto C, Ando M, et al. Prognostic value of p16 expression irrespective of human papillomavirus status in patients with oropharyngeal carcinoma. Jpn J Clin Oncol. 2015;45:828–36.
20. Saito Y, Ebihara Y, Ushiku T, Omura G, Kobayashi K, Ando M, et al. Negative human papillomavirus status and excessive alcohol consumption are significant risk factors for second primary malignancies in Japanese patients with oropharyngeal carcinoma. Jpn J Clin Oncol. 2014;44:564–9.
21. Bouaoun L, Sonkin D, Ardin M, Hollstein M, Byrnes G, Zavadil J, Olivier M. TP53 Variations in Human Cancers: New Lessons from the IARC TP53 Database and Genomics Data. Hum Mutat. 2016;37(9):865–76.
22. Oliver M, Langer A, Carrieri P, Bergh J, Klaar S, Eyfjord J, et al. The clinical value of somatic TP53 gene mutations in 1,794 patients with breast cancer. Clin Cancer Res. 2006;12:1157–67.
23. Rodrigo JP, Martínez P, Allonca E, Alonso-Durán L, Suárez C, Astudillo A, et al. Immunohistochemical markers of distant metastasis in laryngeal and hypopharyngeal squamous cell carcinomas. Clin Exp Metastasis. 2014;31:317–25.
24. Pignon JP, Bourhis J, Domenge C, Designe L. Chemotherapy added to locoregional treatment for head and neck squamous-cell carcinoma: three meta-analyses of updated individual data. MACH-NC collaborative group. Meta-analysis of chemotherapy on head and neck cancer. Lancet. 2000;355:949–55.
25. Posner MR, Hershock DM, Blajman CR, Mickiewicz E, Winquist E, Gorbounova V, et al. Cisplatin and fluorouracil alone or with docetaxel in head and neck cancer. N Engl J Med. 2007;357:1705–15.
26. Posner MR, Norris CM, Wirth LJ, Shin DM, Cullen KJ, Winquist EW, et al. Sequential therapy for the locally advanced larynx and hypopharynx cancer subgroup in TAX 324: survival, surgery, and organ preservation. Ann Oncol. 2009;20:921–7.
27. Park YM, Kim YS, De Virgilio A, Lee SY, Seol JH, Kim SH. Transoral robotic surgery for hypopharyngeal squamous cell carcinoma: 3-year oncologic and functional analysis. Oral Oncol. 2012;48:560–6.
28. Tomifuji M, Araki K, Yamashita T, Shiotani A. Transoral videolaryngscopic surgery for oropharyngeal, hypopharyngeal, and supraglottic cancer. Eur Arch Otorhinolaryngol. 2014;271:589–97.
29. Omura G, Ando M, Saito Y, Kobayashi K, Yamasoba T, Asakage T. Disease control and clinicopathological prongostic factors of total pharyngolaryngectomy for hypopharyngeal cancer: a single-center study. Int J Clin Oncol. 2015;20:290–7.
30. Slaughter DP, Southwick HW, Smejkal W. Field cancerization in oral stratified squamous epithelium; clinical implications of multicentric origin. Cancer. 1953;6:963–8.
31. Ohashi S, Miyamoto S, Kikuchi O, Goto T, Amanuma Y, Muto M. Recent advances from basic and clinical studies of esophageal squamous cell carcinoma. Gastroenterology. 2015;149:1700–15.
32. Waridel F, Estreicher A, Bron L, Flaman JM, Fontolliet C, Monnier P, et al. Field cancerisation and polyclonal p53 mutation in the upper aero-digestive tract. Oncogene. 1997;14:163–9.
33. Ebihara Y, Iwai K, Akashi K, Ito T, Omura G, Saito Y, et al. High incidence of null-type mutations of the TP53 gene in Japanese patients with head and neck squamous cell carcinoma. J Cancer Ther. 2014;5:664–71.
34. Petitjean A, Achatz MIW, Borresen-Dale AL, Hainaut P, Olivier M. TP53 mutations in human cancers: functional selection and impact on cancer prognosis and outcomes. Oncogene. 2007;26:2157–65.
35. Xu Y. Induction of genetic instability by gain-of-function p53 cancer mutants. Oncogene. 2008;27:3501–7.
36. Perrone F, Bossi P, Cortelazzi B, Locati L, Quattrone P, Pierotti MA, et al. TP53 mutations and pathologic complete response to neoadjuvant cisplatin and fluorouracil chemotherapy in resected oral cavity squamous cell carcinoma. J Clin Oncol. 2010;28:761–6.
37. Skinner HD, Sandulache VC, Ow TJ, Meyn RE, Yordy JS, Beadle BM, et al. TP53 disruptive mutations lead to head and neck cancer treatment failure through inhibition of radiation-induced senescence. Clin Cancer Res. 2012;18:290–300.

16

JMJD2A promotes the Warburg effect and nasopharyngeal carcinoma progression by transactivating LDHA expression

Yi Su[1][*][†], Qiu-hong Yu[1][†], Xiang-yun Wang[1], Li-ping Yu[2], Zong-feng Wang[1], Ying-chun Cao[1] and Jian-dong Li[1]

Abstract

Background: Jumonji C domain 2A (JMJD2A), as a histone demethylases, plays a vital role in tumorigenesis and progression. But, its functions and underlying mechanisms of JMJD2A in nasopharyngeal carcinoma (NPC) metabolism are remained to be clarified. In this study, we investigated glycolysis regulation by JMJD2A in NPC and the possible mechanism.

Methods: JMJD2A expression was detected by Western blotting and Reverse transcription quantitative real-time PCR analysis. Then, we knocked down and ectopically expressed JMJD2A to detect changes in glycolytic enzymes. We also evaluated the impacts of JMJD2A-lactate dehydrogenase A (LDHA) signaling on NPC cell proliferation, migration and invasion. ChIP assays were used to test whether JMJD2A bound to the LDHA promoter. Finally, IHC was used to verify JMJD2A and LDHA expression in NPC tissue samples and analyze their correlation between expression and clinical features.

Results: JMJD2A was expressed at high levels in NPC tumor tissues and cell lines. Both JMJD2A and LDHA expression were positively correlated with the tumor stage, metastasis and clinical stage. Additionally, the level of JMJD2A was positively correlated with LDHA expression in NPC patients, and higher JMJD2A and LDHA expression predicted a worse prognosis. JMJD2A alteration did not influence most of glycolytic enzymes expression, with the exception of PFK-L, PGAM-1, LDHB and LDHA, and LDHA exhibited the greatest decrease in expression. JMJD2A silencing decreased LDHA expression and the intracellular ATP level and increased LDH activity, lactate production and glucose utilization, while JMJD2A overexpression produced the opposite results. Furthermore, JMJD2A could combine to LDHA promoter region and regulate LDHA expression at the level of transcription. Activated JMJD2A-LDHA signaling pathway promoted NPC cell proliferation, migration and invasion.

Conclusions: JMJD2A regulated aerobic glycolysis by regulating LDHA expression. Therefore, the novel JMJD2A-LDHA signaling pathway could contribute to the Warburg effects in NPC progression.

Keywords: Nasopharyngeal carcinoma, Jumonji C domain 2A, LDHA, Glycolysis

Background

Nasopharyngeal carcinoma (NPC) is arising from the nasopharynx epithelium. Although NPC has a low morbidity worldwide, its geographical distribution pattern is very unique. Though the incidence of NPC in all cancers are only 0.6% diagnosed in one year, yet 71% of new patients appeared in the east and southeast of Asia [1, 2].

Although a decrease in the incidence and a substantial reduction in mortality have been observed due to the early diagnosis of NPC and advanced radiotherapy and chemotherapy, unsatisfactory outcomes remain for patients with locally advanced and metastatic NPC. Therefore, studies identifying novel and specific biomarkers for NPC are critically important and urgently needed, with the hope of improving NPC patient's prognosis. In addition to regular genetic regulation, epigenetic modification plays a vital role in NPC, particularly in gene methylation [3] and histone methylation [4]. However, histone demethylation,

---

* Correspondence: suent2016@163.com
[†]Equal contributors
[1]Department of E.N.T., Dongying People's Hospital, Shandong 257091, China
Full list of author information is available at the end of the article

have been remained immensely uncovered in NPC mechanisms.

The majority of histone demethylases belong to the Jumonji C domain-containing (JMJD) proteins family [5]. JMJD2A belongs to this family and is capable of demethylating H3K9 and H3K36 [6]. It is overexpressed in many types of cancers, such as prostate [7], breast [8–10] and lung [11] cancers, promoting tumor progression. Dependency on aerobic glycolysis, is a highlighting hallmark of cancers, as known as the Warburg effects [12]. Abnormal glycolysis was recently observed in NPC cells and was associated with a poor prognosis for NPC patients [13, 14]. Additionally, metabolic reprogramming orchestrates cancer stem cell properties, promoting NPC development and progression [15].

Here, we show how JMJD2A exerted its cellular functions through the Warburg effect by interacting with a key element of glycolysis, lactate dehydrogenase A (LDHA). To our knowledge, we are also the first to report that high levels of JMJD2A expression may be a possible cause of NPC tumorigenesis and might be a prognostic marker for patients with NPC. Therefore, JMJD2A should be highlighted as a valid anticancer drug target.

Methods

Human tissue specimens

Fifty cases of NPC samples and 20 normal controls were collected from the E.N.T. Department, Dongying People's Hospital, Shandong Province, from July 2002 to December 2012. All the patients were diagnosed and verified of NPC by histology, without receiving radiotherapy or chemotherapy. We collected the clinicopathological features of patients with NPC, and the follow-up concluded in January 2017. The research was approved and supervised by the Research Ethics Committee of Dongying People's Hospital, Shandong Province, China, and the written consent had been obtained from all the NPC patients.

We used xylene to deparaffinize the tissue samples and then rehydrated then in a series of graded alcohol solutions. Endogenous peroxidases were blocked with 3% H_2O_2, and antigens were retrieved by heating the samples in citrate buffer. We then incubated the tissue samples with a rabbit antibody against JMJD2A (dilution 1:100; CST, Cambridge, UK) or LDHA (dilution 1:400; CST, Cambridge, UK) overnight at 4 °C followed by horseradish peroxidase (Gene Tech GTVision III Detection Kit, Shanghai, China) for 40 min at room-temperature. Then washing the sections with PBS buffer for 3 times, and testing the signal by a DAB solution.

Scoring of the immunohistochemistry (IHC)

A double-blind method was used to analyze the IHC results: two pathologists without access to the patients' clinical and pathological characteristics independently evaluated the results. Five different areas of visual fields selected from each specimen were randomly chosen for the immunohistochemical evaluation. JMJD2A and LDHA expression were scored by the percentage of positive cells as well as the staining intensity as previously described [16, 17]. The IHC scorings were as follows: 0, no positive cells; 1, ≤10% positive cells; 2, 10–50% positive cells; and 3, >50% positive cells; 0, no staining; 1, faint staining; 2, moderate staining; and 3, dark staining. Comprehensive scores = staining percentage × intensity. JMJD2A and LDHA expression were classified as follows: ≤2 low expression or >2 high expressions.

Cell lines and reagents

The nasopharyngeal epithelial cell lines NP69 (ATCC-5859) and NPC cell lines CNE2 (ATCC-1434), CNE1(ATCC-0364), HONE1(ATCC-0369), HNE1(ATCC-0366), 5-8F (ATCC-2496) and 6-10B (ATCC-6605) were obtained from Jennio-bio (Guangzhou, China). NP69 cells were cultivated in keratinocyte/serum-free medium (Invitrogen, Carlsbad, CA, USA) supplemented with EGF (epidermal growth factor, Invitrogen). All NPC cell lines were cultured in RPMI 1640 medium ((Gibco, Rockville, MD, USA)) supplemented with 10% FBS (HyClone, Logan, UT, USA). All the cell lines were incubated at 37 °C with the humidity of 5% CO_2 atmosphere. Oxamate (Oxa) sodium was bought from Sigma-Aldrich Corp. (St. Louis, MO, USA). Oxa was dissolved and diluted in the sterile water, and the final concentration was achieved by diluting Oxa in culture medium, which was phenol-red-free RPMI with 1% FBS.

Plasmids construction and small interfering RNAs

The control vector pcDNA3.1 and plasmids pcDNA3.1-JMJD2A (pJMJD2A) was described previously [18]. A small interfering RNA (siRNA) targeting JMJD2A (siJMJD2A) (GenePharma, Shanghai, China) was used to decrease its expression. The sequences were as follows: Sense: 5′ GUA UGAUCUUCCAGACUUA 3′ and Antisense: 5′ UAAGU CUGGAAGAUCAUAC 3′.

Transient transfection

We used Lipofectamine 2000 and Lipofectamine RNAi-MAX (Invitrogen, Grand Island, NY, USA) to transfect plasmids and siRNAs into NPC cells lines, respectively. For transient transfections, NPC cells were transfected with the indicated plasmids or siRNAs for 24 or 48 h prior to the functional assays or WB assays, respectively. NPC cells transfected with empty vectors were defined as control groups, and untreated cells were defined as mock groups.

RNA extraction and Reverse transcription quantitative real-time PCR analysis

We used TRIzol reagent (Invitrogen; Thermo Fisher Scientific, Inc.) to extract total RNA from tissue samples and cells lines, according to the manufacturers' protocol. The extracted RNA was tested and quantified by ultraviolet spectrophotometry. Then the quantified RNA was reversely transcribed into cDNAs by ExScript RT-PCR kit (TaKaRa Bio, Inc., Otsu, Japan). Then, quantitative real-time PCR analysis was used to detect the targeted genes expression. GAPDH was used as an internal control. The primer sequences are listed in Table 1. Comparative threshold cycle (Ct) ($2^{-\Delta\Delta Ct}$) method was used to calculate the gene relative mRNA expression.

Western blotting analysis

Standard Western blotting was conducted using proteins from whole cells lysed in RIPA buffer, and using primary antibodies against JMJD2A, LDHA and GAPDH, and indicated secondary antibody.

Table 1 The primer sequences of glycolytic enzyme

Name	Abbreviation	Primers
Jumonji domain containing 2A	JMJD2A	Sense: 5'-ATCCCAGTGCTAGGATAATGACC-3'
		Anti-sense: 5'-ACTCTTTTGGAGGAACCCTTG-3'
Glucose transporter-1	GLUT-1	Sense: 5'-CTTTGTGGCCTTCTTTGAAGT-3'
		Anti-sense: 5'-CCACACAGTTGCTCCACAT-3'
Glucose transporter-4	GLUT-4	Sense: 5'-CTTCATCATTGGCATGGGTTT-3'
		Anti-sense: 5'-CGGGTTTCAGGCACTTTTAGG-3'
Hexokinase-II	HK-II	Sense: 5'-GATTTCACCAAGCGTGGACT-3'
		Anti-sense: 5'-CCACACCCACTGTCACTTTG-3'
Glucose-6-phosphate isomerase	G6PI	Sense: 5'-AGGCTGCTGCCACATAAGGT-3'
		Anti-sense: 5'-AGCGTCGTGAGAGGTCACTTG-3'
Muscle-type phosphofructokinase	PFK-M	Sense: 5'-ATTCGGGCTGTGTTCTGG-3'
		Anti-sense: 5'-TGGCTAGGATTTTGAGGATGG-3'
Liver-type phosphofructokinase	PFK-L	Sense: 5'-GGACAGGAAAGAGGAAGTGAC-3'
		Anti-sense: 5'-CGTAGATGAGGAAGACTTTGGC-3'
Platelet isoform of phosphofructokinase	PFK-P	Sense: 5'-CATCGACAATGATTTCTGCGG-3'
		Anti-sense: 5'-CCATCACCTCCAGAACGAAG-3'
Aldolase B	AldoB	Sense: 5'-ATGCCACTCTCAACCTCAATGCTATC-3'
		Anti-sense: 5'-TTATTTTCTTGGGTGGGTATTCTGG-3'
Phosphoglycerate kinase 1	PGK-1	Sense: 5' -CGGTAGTCCTTATGAGCC-3'
		Anti-sense: 5'-CATGAAAGCGGAGGTTCT-3'
Phosphoglycerate mutase 1	PGAM-1	Sense: 5'-CCTGGAGAACCGCTTC-3'
		Anti-sense: 5'-CATGGGCTGCAATCAGTACAC-3'
Enolase	Enolase	Sense: 5'-CTGATGCTGGAGTTGGATGG-3'
		Anti-sense: 5'-CCATTGATCACGTTGAAGGC-3'
M1 isoform of pyruvate kinase	PKM1	Sense: 5'-CTATCCTCTGGAGGCTGTGC-3'
		Anti-sense: 5'-CCATGAGGTCTGTGGAGTGA-3'
M2 isoform of pyruvate kinase	PKM2	Sense: 5'-GGGTTCGGAGGTTTGATG-3'
		Anti-sense: 5'-ACGGCGGTGGCTTCTGT-3'
Lactate dehydrogenase B	LDHB	Sense: 5'-CCTAGAGCTCACTAGTCACAG-3'
		Anti-sense: 5'-CTCCTGTGCAAAATGGCAAC-3'
Lactate dehydrogenase A	LDHA	Sense: 5'-CAGCTTGGAGTTTGCAGTTAC-3'
		Anti-sense: 5'-TGATGGATCTCCAACATGG-3'
Glyceraldehyde-3-phosphate dehydrogenase	GAPDH	Sense: 5'-TGACGCTGGGGCTGGCATTG-3'
		Anti-sense: 5'-GCTCTTGCTGGGGCTGGTGG-3'

LDH activity, lactate production, glucose utilization assay and the intracellular ATP level

NPC cells were transfected transiently with plasmids and siRNAs, with/without treatment of oxamate (20 mmol/L). 1×10^6 cells were used to test LDH activity. Lactate production was detected by Lactate Dehydrogenase Activity Assay Kit and Lactate Assay Kit (Sigma, St. Louis, MO, USA). For glucose utilization assay, NPC cells were transiently transfected. After 24 h, phenol-red free RPMI supplemented with 1% FBS or with 1% FBS and 20 mmol/L oxamate replaced the previous media, and cultured for 72 h. A colorimetric glucose assay kit (BioVision, Milpitas, CA, USA) was supplied to measure the glucose concentrations [19]. Intracellular ATP levels were detected using a firefly luciferase-based ATP assay kit (Beyotime Institute of Biotechnology, Haimen, China). The protein concentration was also tested using a BCA protein assay kit (Beyotime Institute of Biotechnology, Haimen, China). The relative ATP level is expressed as the ATP concentration/protein concentration.

Chromatin Immunoprecipitation (ChIP) assay

ChIP assays were performed using cell lines DNA by ChIP kit purchased from CST. Briefly, about 5×10^6 cells were treated with 1% formaldehyde aimed for cross-linking procedure, and the reaction was then stopped by the adding 0.125 M glycine. The NPC cells were scraped and collected after centrifugation at the speed of 800 g for 5 min at 4 °C. Next, the cross-linked segments were resuspended using SDS lysis buffer which contained protease inhibitor cocktail II, and the soluble chromatin was pieced to fragment the DNA using nuclear lysis buffer. The fragmented chromatin were aliquoted, each as genomic input DNA or immunoprecipitated with JMJD2A or IgG antibodies. The mixed solutios were incubated at 4 °C with rotation overnight. The complexes were collected with a magnetic separator, followed by washing and eluting with ChIP elution buffer. The spin columns were used to purify DNA. The ChIP products and genomic input DNA were analyzed by Reverse transcription quantitative real-time PCR

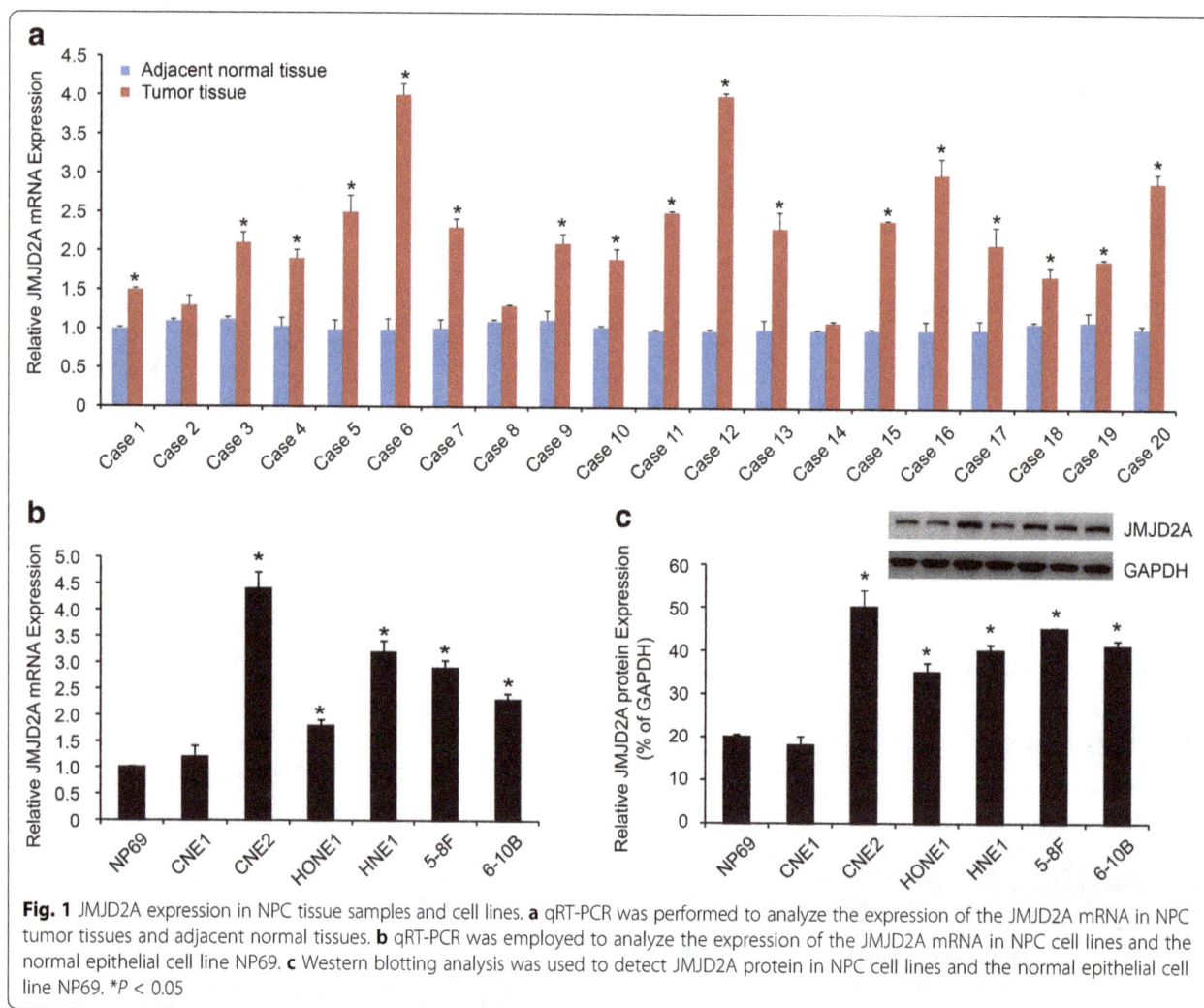

Fig. 1 JMJD2A expression in NPC tissue samples and cell lines. **a** qRT-PCR was performed to analyze the expression of the JMJD2A mRNA in NPC tumor tissues and adjacent normal tissues. **b** qRT-PCR was employed to analyze the expression of the JMJD2A mRNA in NPC cell lines and the normal epithelial cell line NP69. **c** Western blotting analysis was used to detect JMJD2A protein in NPC cell lines and the normal epithelial cell line NP69. *$P < 0.05$

analysis. The three pairs of LDHA primers used for ChIP assays were the following:

sense, 5′-caagccactgacagttcttg-3′
antisense, 5′-ACCTAAGTCGAGTGACCTCC-3′
sense, 5′-GTGCTATTTTGGAGCTGAGGTT-3′
antisense, 5′-AGCCCTTGAGTATGCCAAAAT-3′
sense, 5′-TATCTCAAAGCTGCACTGGGC-3′,
antisense, 5′-TGCTGATTCCATTGCCTAGC-3′

MTT assay

A MTT assay was performed to evaluate cell proliferation ability. About 5000 cells were seeded into each wells and transfected with plasmid and followed by the treatment with or without oxamate sodium (20 mmol/L) with 24, 48 and 72 h, relatively. Next, 5 mg/L of the MTT solution was added to each wells, and incubated at 37 °C for 4 h.

Discarding the supernatant and adding 150 μL DMSO for disolving. At last, the absorbances were measured by a microplate reader (Bio-Tek Instruments, Inc., Winooski, VT, USA) at the wave length of 570 nm.

NPC cell migration and invasion assays

NPC cells were transfected with control, siJMJD2A or pJMJD2A. 1×10^5 cells in 600 μL of serum-free medium were placed in the upper chamber with or without a Matrigel-coated membrane (Millipore, Billerica, MA, USA). RPMI-1640 supplemented with 10% FBS or with 10% FBS and 20 mmol/L oxamate place in the lower chamber was used as a chemoattractant.

Promoter reporter construction and dual luciferase assay

A fragment containing the sequences from −1330 to +150 bp of the LDHA gene relative to the transcription

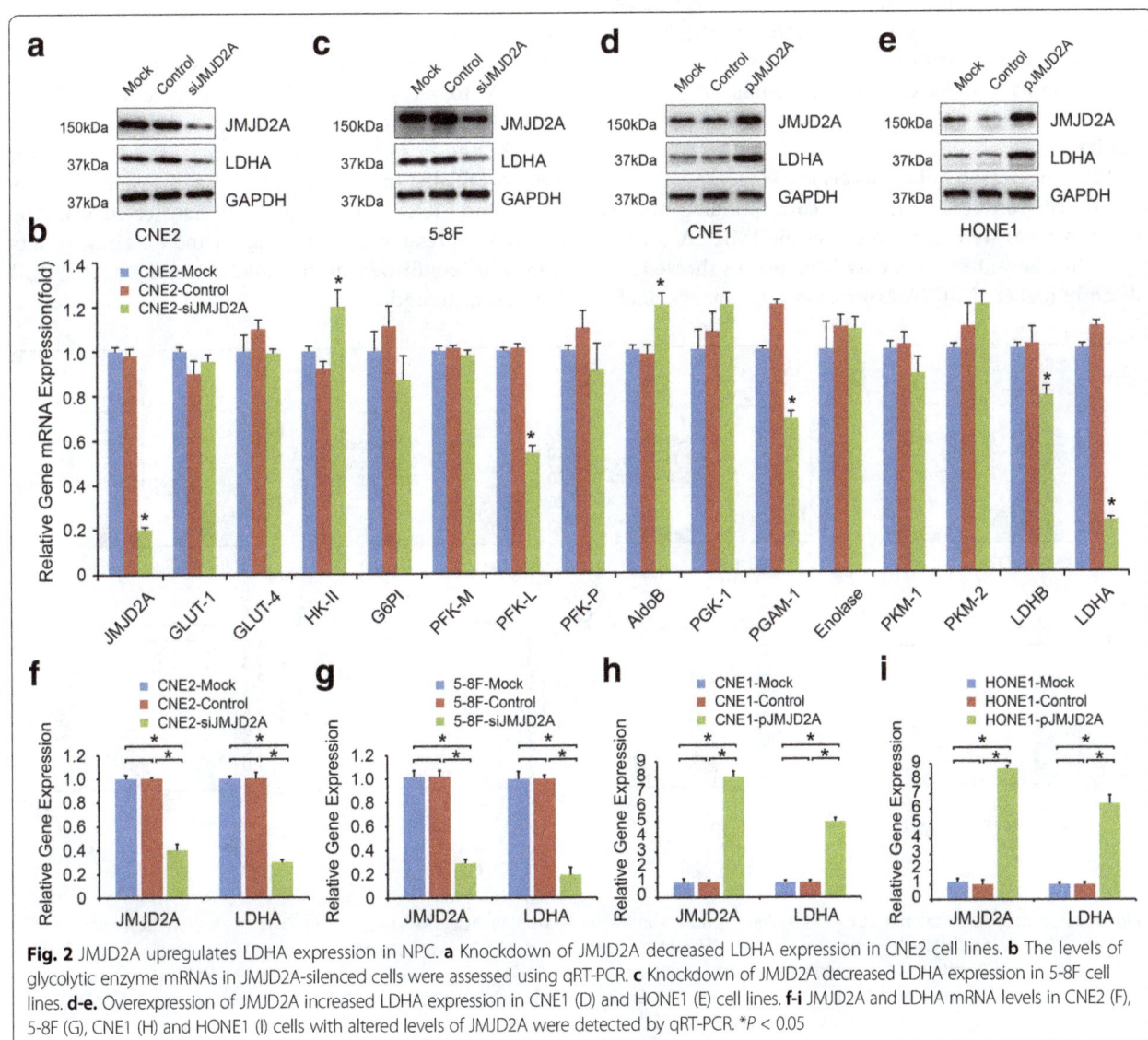

Fig. 2 JMJD2A upregulates LDHA expression in NPC. **a** Knockdown of JMJD2A decreased LDHA expression in CNE2 cell lines. **b** The levels of glycolytic enzyme mRNAs in JMJD2A-silenced cells were assessed using qRT-PCR. **c** Knockdown of JMJD2A decreased LDHA expression in 5-8F cell lines. **d-e.** Overexpression of JMJD2A increased LDHA expression in CNE1 (D) and HONE1 (E) cell lines. **f-i** JMJD2A and LDHA mRNA levels in CNE2 (F), 5-8F (G), CNE1 (H) and HONE1 (I) cells with altered levels of JMJD2A were detected by qRT-PCR. *P < 0.05

initiation site was subcloned into the pGL3-basic vector [20] (the vector was constructed and verified by Obio Bioengineering Co., Ltd.). The NPC cells were transfected by the constructed LDHA promoter reporter, siJMJD2A, or overexpression plasmid. Co-transfecting a β-actin/Renilla luciferase reporter, which includes a full-length Renilla luciferase gene, was used as normalizing the LDHA promoter activity. A dual luciferase assay kit (Promega, Madison, WI, USA) was employed to detect the luciferase activity in 24 h after transfection.

Statistical analysis

All data are measured and presented as means ± standard deviations. Two groups were compared using Student's t-test, whereas three or more groups were compared using one-way analysis of variance with SPSS 13.0 (SPSS, Inc., Chicago, IL, USA). The analysis of the correlations between the clinicopathological characteristics and JMJD2A and LDHA expression was using χ^2 test. A Univariate and Cox regression analysis was also performed. The Kaplan-Meier method was used to assess overall survival. A value of $P < 0.05$ was considered statistically significant.

Results

JMJD2A is expressed at high levels in NPC

Twenty pairs of NPC tissues and corresponding normal tissues samples were used to detect the JMJD2A mRNA expression. Seventeen of twenty NPC tissues showed significantly higher JMJD2A expression (Fig. 1a; $P < 0.05$).

We also used cell lines to confirm this result. Compared with NP69, the other NPC cell lines showed higher expression of both the JMJD2A mRNA and protein (Fig. 1b and c; $P < 0.05$).

JMJD2A upregulates LDHA expression in NPC

Aerobic glycolysis is the major feature for cancer metabolism; thus, we paid attention to the regulatory effects of JMJD2A on glycolysis in NPC cells. We assessed the effects of JMJD2A on the glycolytic enzymes expression. We first used RNAi to knockdown JMJD2A expression and confirmed the knockdown efficacy (Fig. 2a; $P < 0.05$). Next, we used CNE2-siJMJD2A cells to detect the levels of glycolytic enzyme mRNAs by qRT-PCR. JMJD2A silencing did not alter the most of the enzymes, with the exception of the downregulation the expression of PFK-L, PGAM-1, LDHB and LDHA (Fig. 2b; $P < 0.05$). Among the enzymes listed above, LDHA exhibited the greatest decrease in expression. We then confirm the effects of JMJD2A expression on the LDHA protein. We used CNE2 and 5-8F cells, which express higher levels of JMJD2A, to verify the siJMJD2A results and found that JMJD2A silencing downregulated LDHA expression (Fig. 2a and c; $P < 0.05$). Meanwhile, LDHA expression was upregulated in the low-JMJD2A expressing cell lines CNE1 and HONE1 that had been transfected with the JMJD2A expression plasmid (Fig. 2d and e). These results were also confirmed at the mRNA level by qRT-PCR (Fig. 2f, g, h, and i; $P < 0.05$).

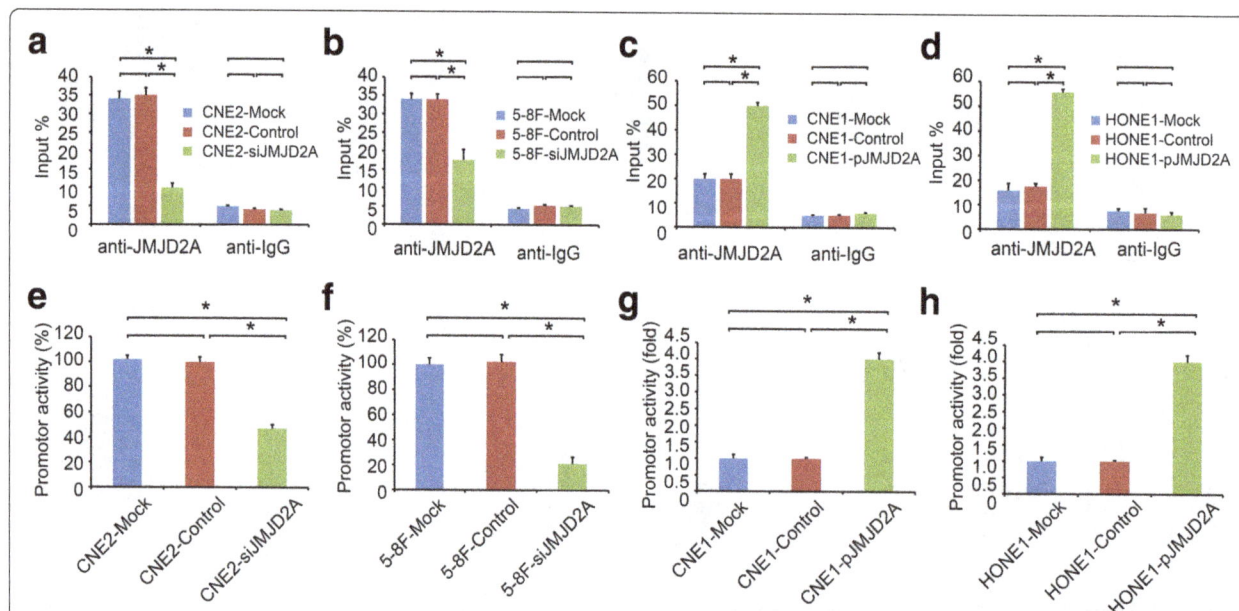

Fig. 3 Transcriptional activation of LDHA expression by JMJD2A in NPC cells. **a-b** Chip assays revealed that JMJD2A knockdown decreased the binding of JMJD2A to the LDHA promoter in CNE2 (A) and 5-8F (B) cell lines. **c-d** JMJD2A overexpression increased JMJD2A binding to the LDHA promoter in CNE1 (C) and HONE1 (D) cells. **e-h** Luciferase reporter assay were performed to detect the effect of JMJD2A on LDHA transcription. Silencing of JMJD2A decreased LDHA promoter activity in CNE2 (E) and 5-8F (F) cell lines, whereas JMJD2A overexpression elevated the LDHA promoter activity in CNE1 (G) and HONE1 (H) cell lines. *$P < 0.05$

JMJD2A activates LDHA expression at transcriptional level by in NPC cells

Our data revealed a direct correlation between JMJD2A and LDHA expression. ChIP assay were conducted to further explore the mechanisms by which JMJD2A regulated LDHA expression. We designed three pairs of primers

targeting the LDHA promoter region (Additional file 1: Figure S1A). JMJD2A bound to the LDHA promoter, and among the primers, primer b showed the largest difference (Additional file 1: Figure S1B; $P < 0.05$). Thus, the subsequent investigations were only performed using primer b. We used both the overexpression and RNAi systems to

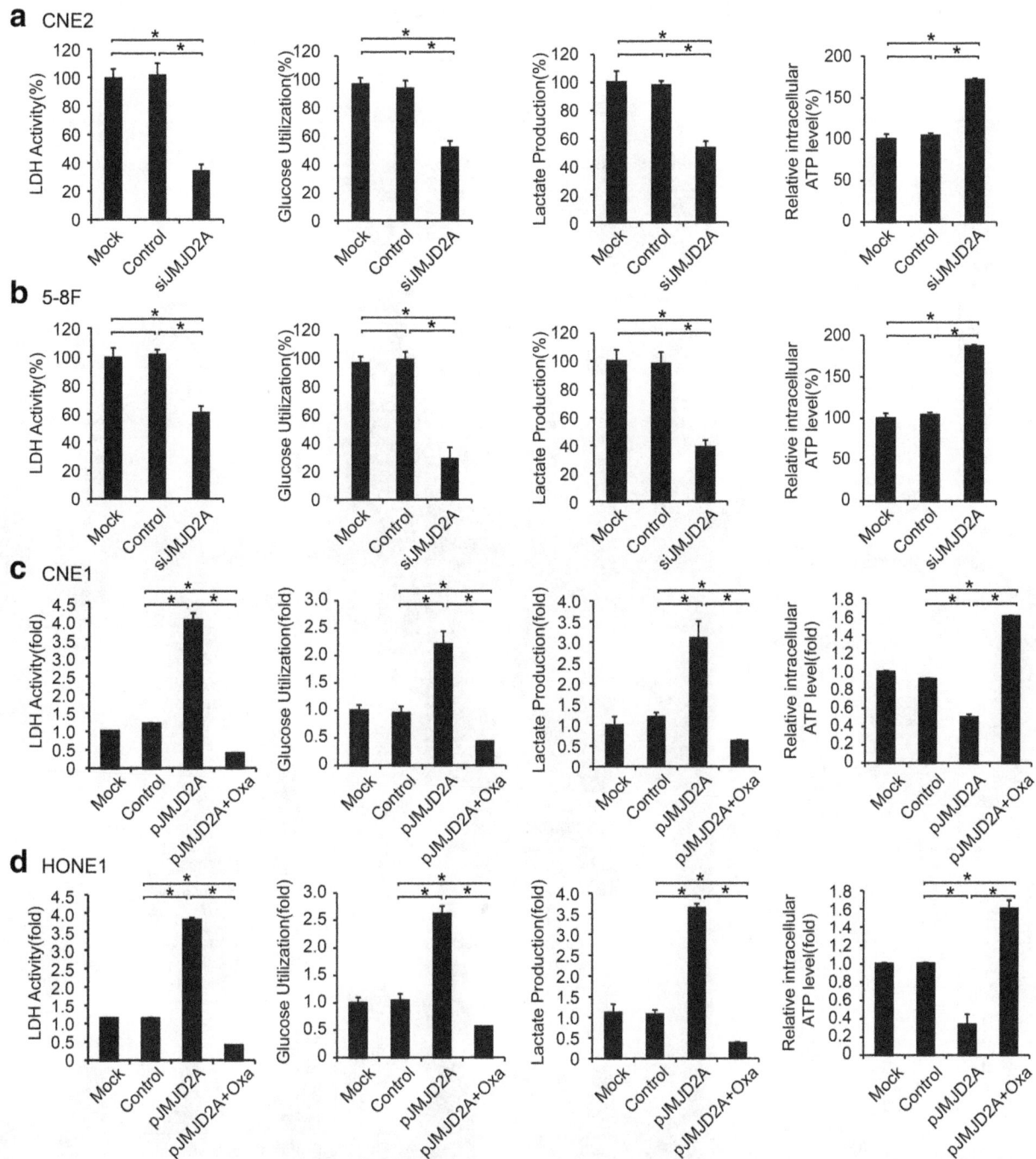

Fig. 4 JMJD2A promoted the Warburg effect in NPC cells. **a-b** LDHA activity, glucose utilization, lactate production, and increase in intracellular ATP levels were assessed in CNE2 (A) and 5-8F (B) cell lines transfected with siJMJD2A. **c-d** LDHA activity, glucose utilization, lactate production, and increase in intracellular ATP levels were assessed in CNE1 (C) and HONE1 (D) cell lines transfected with pJMJD2A and treated with or without 20 mmol/L oxamate sodium. *$P < 0.05$

confirm the results and found that JMJD2A knockdown decreased the binding of JMJD2A to the LDHA promoter in the CNE2 and 5-8F cell lines, leading to the downregulation of LDHA expression (Fig. 3a and b; $P < 0.05$). Meanwhile, JMJD2A overexpression increased JMJD2A binding to the LDHA promoter in the CNE1 and HONE1 cell lines, leading to the upregulation of LDHA expression (Fig. 3c and d; $P < 0.05$). Then, a luciferase reporter assay was to detect the effects of JMJD2A on

LDHA transcription. Silencing of JMJD2A decreased LDHA promoter activity (Fig. 3e and f; $P < 0.05$), whereas JMJD2A overexpression elevated the LDHA promoter activity (Fig. 3g and h; $P < 0.05$). Based on these data, JMJD2A bound to the LDHA promoter and activated LDHA expression transcriptionally. Further study will be emphasized on looking for possible transcriptional factors that bind to JMJD2A and directly interact with the LDHA promoter.

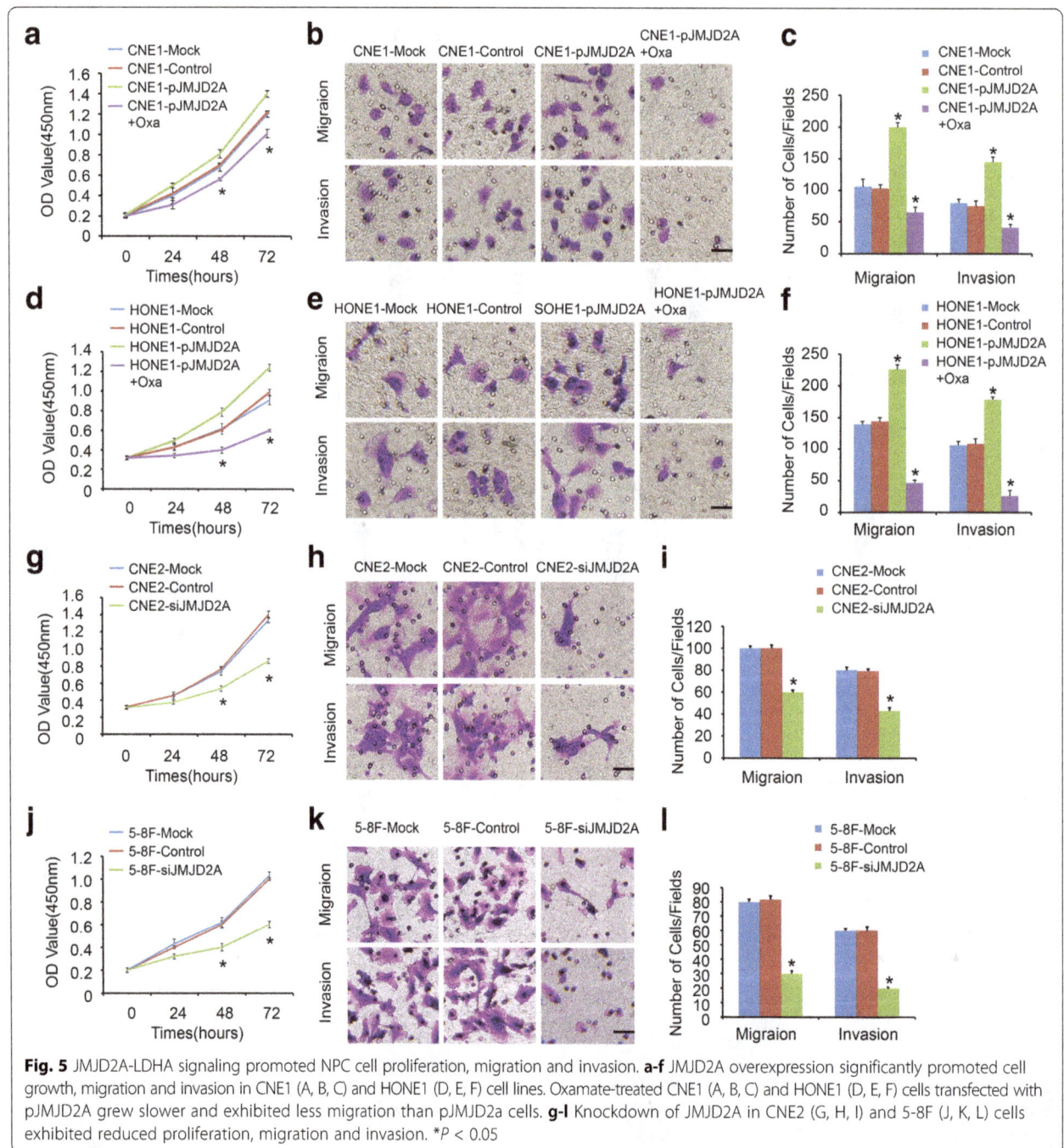

Fig. 5 JMJD2A-LDHA signaling promoted NPC cell proliferation, migration and invasion. **a-f** JMJD2A overexpression significantly promoted cell growth, migration and invasion in CNE1 (A, B, C) and HONE1 (D, E, F) cell lines. Oxamate-treated CNE1 (A, B, C) and HONE1 (D, E, F) cells transfected with pJMJD2A grew slower and exhibited less migration than pJMJD2a cells. **g-l** Knockdown of JMJD2A in CNE2 (G, H, I) and 5-8F (J, K, L) cells exhibited reduced proliferation, migration and invasion. *$P < 0.05$

JMJD2A promotes the Warburg effect in NPC cells

Because we have observed that JMJD2A is associated with LDHA expression, we further explored the impact of JMJD2A on the Warburg effect, including LDH activity, glucose utilization, lactate production, and the intracellular ATP level. After knocking down JMJD2A, we observed significant decreases in LDH activity, glucose utilization, and lactate production, as well as an increase in the intracellular ATP level (Fig. 4a and b; $P < 0.05$). In comparison, JMJD2A upregulation markedly increased LDH activity, lactate production, glucose utilization, and also decreased the intracellular ATP level in cells (Fig. 4c and d; $P < 0.05$). LDHA activity inhibition by oxamate sodium attenuated the JMJD2A-induced increase in glucose utilization, lactate production, and LDH activity (Fig. 4c and d; $P < 0.05$). Thus, JMJD2A may regulate lactate production and glucose utilization by regulating LDHA activity.

JMJD2A-LDHA signaling promotes NPC cell proliferation, migration and invasion

We overexpressed JMJD2A in CNE1 cells treated with or without oxamate to detect the effects of JMJD2A-LDHA signaling on the biological features of NPC.

JMJD2A overexpression significantly promoted cell growth (Fig. 5a; $P < 0.05$), migration and invasion (Fig. 5b and c; $P < 0.05$). Oxamate-treated CNE1 cells transfected with pJMJD2A grew slower and exhibited less migration than pJMJD2a cells (Fig. 5a, b, and c; $P < 0.05$). These results were confirmed in the HONE1 cell line (Fig. 5d, e, and f; $P < 0.05$). Consistently, two siJMJD2A cell lines, CNE2 (Fig. 5g, h, and i; $P < 0.05$) and 5-8F (Fig. 5j, k, and l; $P < 0.05$), exhibited reduced proliferation, migration and invasion.

Direct correlations between JMJD2A and LDHA expression with the pathologic features of NPC

We provided evidences that JMJD2A transcriptionally regulated LDHA gene expression and NPC glycolysis. We investigated JMJD2A and LDHA expression in NPC tumor specimens using IHC. The expression of both JMJD2A and LDHA was positively correlated with the T, M classification and clinical stage (Table 2; $P < 0.05$). As shown in representative figures, JMJD2A and LDHA expression were positively associated with advanced tumor stages (Fig. 6a, b, c, and d; $P < 0.05$). Additionally, the level of JMJD2A was positively correlated with LDHA expression in NPC tissues (Table 3, $r = 0.642$, $P < 0.05$).

Table 2 Associations between JMJD2A, LDHA protein expression and clinicopathological characteristics in NPC

Variable	Cases	JMJD2A expression		P-value	LDHA expression		P-value
		Low ($n = 24$)	High ($n = 26$)		Low ($n = 21$)	High ($n = 29$)	
Gender							
Male	22	10	12	0.749	9	13	0.890
Female	28	14	14		12	16	
Age(years)							
< 50	21	9	12	0.536	7	14	0.291
≥ 50	29	15	14		14	15	
Histological type							
DNKC	25	11	14	0.571	10	15	0.774
UDC	25	13	12		11	14	
T classification							
T1-T2	31	20	11	0.003*	18	13	0.003*
T3-T4	19	4	15		3	16	
N classification							
N0-N1	32	14	18	0.423	13	19	0.793
N2-N3	18	10	8		8	10	
M classification							
M0	37	21	16	0.037*	19	18	0.024*
M1	13	3	10		2	11	
Clinical stage							
I-II	24	17	7	0.002*	16	8	0.001*
III-IV	26	7	19		5	21	

DNKC differentiated non-keratinizing carcinoma, UDC undifferentiated carcinoma, T tumor size, N lymph node metastasis, M distant metastasis

*$P < 0.05$ indicates a significant association among the variables (2-tailed)

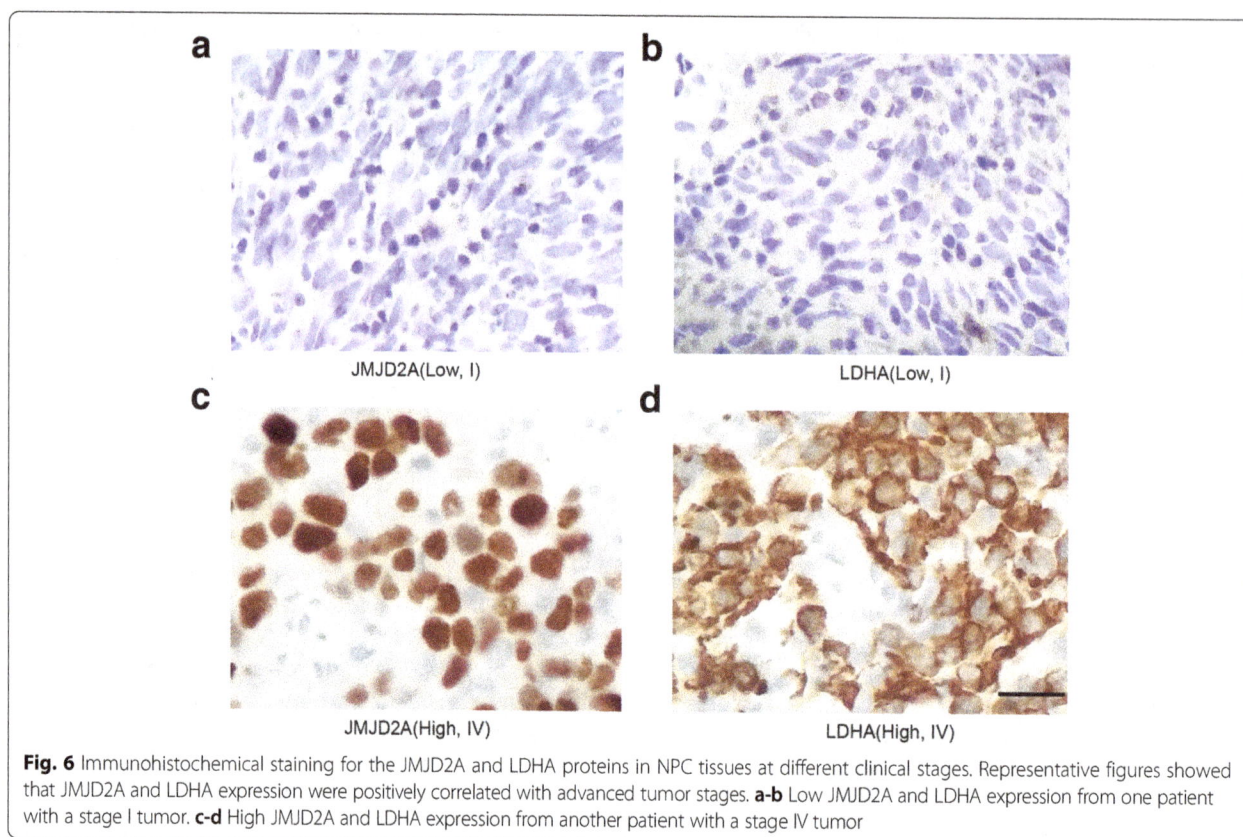

Fig. 6 Immunohistochemical staining for the JMJD2A and LDHA proteins in NPC tissues at different clinical stages. Representative figures showed that JMJD2A and LDHA expression were positively correlated with advanced tumor stages. **a-b** Low JMJD2A and LDHA expression from one patient with a stage I tumor. **c-d** High JMJD2A and LDHA expression from another patient with a stage IV tumor

Further, we performed a Kaplan-Meier analysis and found that higher JMJD2A or LDHA expression predicted a worse prognosis (Fig. 7a and b; $P < 0.05$). Patients with higher expression of both JMJD2A and LDHA had the worst prognosis (Fig. 7c; $P < 0.05$). According to the Cox analysis, both JMJD2A and LDHA may be predictive markers for patients with NPC (Table 4; $P < 0.05$). Based on these data, JMJD2A-LDHA signaling regulates NPC development and progression.

Discussion

In our research, we have investigated the role of JMJD2A in NPC metabolism and JMJD2A-LDHA signaling in NPC tumorigenesis. We provided evidences supporting a critical role for JMJD2A in the glycolysis regulation via the transcriptional activation of LDHA gene expression. First, JMJD2A was upregulated in NPC tumor tissues and cell lines. Second, JMJD2A silencing decreased the

LDHA expression at mRNA and protein level and increased LDH activity, glucose utilization, lactate production, and the ATP level, and JMJD2A overexpression had the opposite effects. Third, JMJD2A directly bound the LDHA promoter region and transcriptionally regulated LDHA gene expression. Fourth, activated JMJD2A-LDHA signaling pathway promoted NPC cell proliferation, migration and invasion. Additionally, both JMJD2A and LDHA expression were positively correlated with the TNM classification and clinical stage. Moreover, JMJD2A expression was positively correlated with LDHA expression in NPC tissues, and higher JMJD2A and LDHA expression predicted a worse prognosis. Thus, JMJD2A regulates glycolysis in NPC by modulating LDHA expression. This novel JMJD2A-LDHA signaling pathway could contribute to the Warburg effect in NPC cells and tumorigenesis and progression.

JMJD2A, as a histone demethylase, plays vital role in various cancer types. Its function as an oncogene or suppressor gene remains unclear. In bladder cancer, JMJD2A is expressed at significantly lower levels in cancer samples than in normal tissues [21]. Lower JMJD2A expression is correlated with a poorer prognosis [21]. However, JMJD2A is upregulated at malignant gastric cancer tissues in comparison with that of normal control. JMJD2A regulates gastric cancer cell growth and serves as an independent prognostic factor [18]. Furthermore, JMJD2A

Table 3 Correlation analysis between JMJD2A and LDHA protein expression in NPC

Tissue sample	LDHA expression		r	P-value
	Low	High		
JMJD2A Low	18	6	0.642	<0.001*
JMJD2A High	3	23		

*$P < 0.05$ indicates that correlation is significant at the 0.05 level (2-tailed)

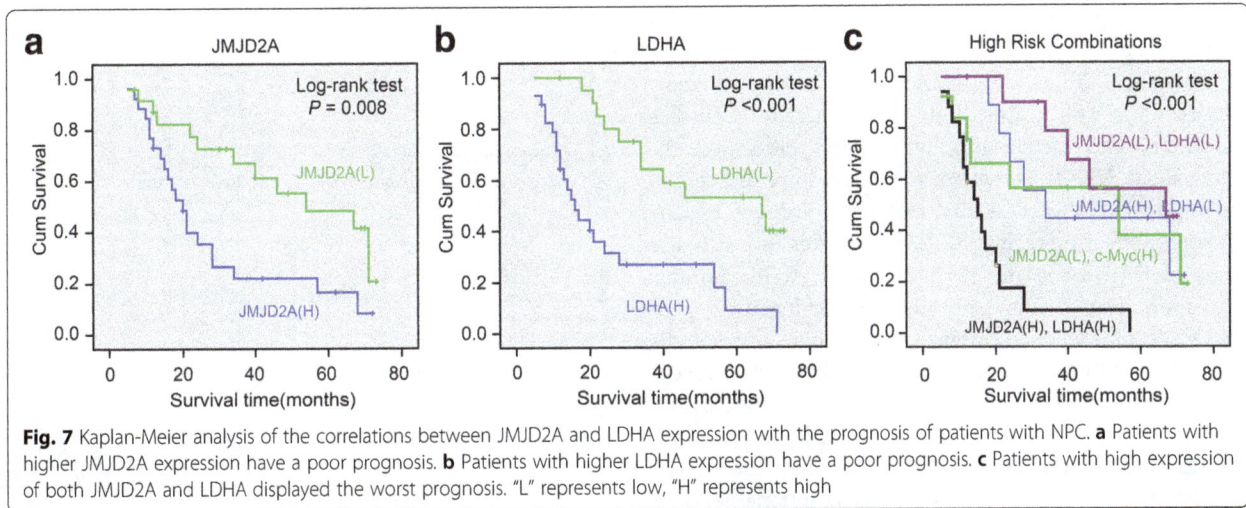

Fig. 7 Kaplan-Meier analysis of the correlations between JMJD2A and LDHA expression with the prognosis of patients with NPC. **a** Patients with higher JMJD2A expression have a poor prognosis. **b** Patients with higher LDHA expression have a poor prognosis. **c** Patients with high expression of both JMJD2A and LDHA displayed the worst prognosis. "L" represents low, "H" represents high

participates in carcinogenesis by regulating the G1/S transition in lung cancers and bladder cancers [19]. Additionally, JMJD2A is overexpressed in breast cancer [9, 10, 22], lung cancer [11, 19], prostate cancer [23], colorectal cancer [24], and head and neck squamous cell carcinoma [25]. In our study, we first observed JMJD2A overexpression in human NPC and showed that it was correlated with the TNM classification and clinical stage, promoting NPC progression.

We have revealed a critical role for JMJD2A in NPC progression, but the previous studies provide little evidence of revealing JMJD2A function in the cancer metabolism. The Warburg effect is considered a hallmark of cancer [12]. The Warburg effect means that tumor cells predominantly produce energy through glycolysis and followed by the lactic acid fermentation [26], rather than through a comparatively low level of glycolysis rate, followed by the oxidation of pyruvate in mitochondria, as occurs in most normal cells [27–29]. Upregulated enzymes and glucose transporters of glycolytic pathway as the results of oncogene activation are main reasons for the Warburg effects [30]. In our study, JMJD2A silencing did not alter the most glycolytic enzymes expression, with the exception of PFK-L, PGAM-1, LDHB and LDHA. Because LDHA exhibited the greatest decrease in expression and mainly converts pyruvate to lactate, we mainly explored the function of JMJD2A in glycolysis through activating LDHA expression in this study.

LDHA, which catalyzes the last step of anaerobic glycolysis, is a major subunit of LDH. Abnormal LDHA expression is universal in many human cancers, such as pancreatic cancer [31], hepatocellular carcinoma [32], and breast cancer [33], suggesting that the overexpression of this gene promotes cancer development and progression. LDHA is reported to be an adverse independent prognostic factor for NPC [34]. In our present study, the LDHA level was elevated, and correlated with the TNM and clinical stage in NPC tissue samples. Based on these results, the level of LDHA expression was associated with NPC development and progression. Moreover, LDHA was positively correlated with JMJD2A expression in tumor specimens. Next, we evaluated whether altering JMJD2A

Table 4 Summary of univariate and multivariate Cox regression analysis of overall survival duration in all NPC patients (n = 50)

Clinicopathological parameters	Univariate analysis			Multivariate analysis		
	HR	95% CI	P-value	HR	95% CI	P-value
JMJD2A(High/Low)	2.539	1.233–5.228	0.011*	2.652	1.245–5.650	0.011*
LDHA(High/Low)	3.652	1.721–7.749	0.001*	3.433	1.560–7.556	0.002*
Gender (Female/Male)	2.324	0.954–5.662	0.063			
Age(years)(≥50/<50)	0.681	0.341–1.357	0.681			
Histological type(UDC/DNKC)	0.614	0.308–1.224	0.166			
T classification(T3 + T4/T1 + T2)	1.351	0.679–2.687	0.391			
N classification (N2 + N3/N0 + N1)	2.941	1.160–7.455	0.023*			
M classification (M1/M0)	2.349	1.107–4.984	0.026*			
Clinical stage (III + IV/I + II)	2.291	1.096–4.788	0.028*			

HR hazard ratio, 95% CI 95% confidence interval, *indicates P < 0.05

expression could exert effects on LDHA expression, LDH activity, glucose utilization, lactate production, and the intracellular ATP level. JMJD2A overexpression markedly increased LDHA expression, LDH activity, glucose utilization, and lactate production, and decreased the intracellular ATP level, whereas JMJD2A knockdown had the opposite effects. Thus, JMJD2A influences the Warburg effect by regulating LDHA expression. A major focus of JMJD2A studies was its role in transcriptional regulation, where it may either activate or inactivate genetic transcription. The latter function may involve the correlation with histone deacetylases or the nuclear receptor co-repressor complex [35, 36] or direct binding to a transcription factor, as observed for the p53 gene [37]. We further studied whether JMJD2A could regulate LDHA expression by modulating through transcriptional level. In the present study, JMJD2A directly bound to LDHA promoter region and activated LDHA expression transcriptionally. However, the detailed molecular mechanisms by which JMJD2A regulates LDHA expression require further exploration. Next, we analyzed the effects of JMJD2A-LDHA signaling alterations on NPC cell growth and invasion in vitro. Elevated JMJD2A-LDHA signaling promotes cell proliferation and invasion, whereas decreased JMJD2A-LDHA signaling had the opposite effects. Taken together, our results have implied that JMJD2A regulates the Warburg effect in NPC by transcriptionally regulating LDHA expression.

Conclusions

In summary, our study is the first to share some critical insights into the role of JMJD2A in NPC glycolysis metabolism and identified a role of a novel JMJD2A-LDHA signaling in NPC tumorigenesis. We identified and demonstrated a novel JMJD2A-LDHA signaling pathway alteration, which could be promising molecular target for new therapeutic exploration to control NPC.

Abbreviations

ChIP: Chromatin immunoprecipitation; JMJD2A: Jumonji C domain 2A; MTT: 3-(4,5-dimethylthiazol-2-yl)-2,5-diphenyl-tetrazolium bromide; NPC: Nasopharyngeal carcinoma

Acknowledgments

We sincerely appreciate the patients who participated in this study.

Funding

The authors did not receive funding from any source for this study.

Authors' contributions

YS and QHY performed the cellular and histological studies, the statistical analyses, and drafted the manuscript. XYW and LPY collected tumor tissues and followed the patients. ZFW and YCC helped perform the cellular and histological studies. JDL participated in designing the study. All authors read and approved the final manuscript.

Competing interests

The authors declare that they have no competing interests.

Author details

[1]Department of E.N.T., Dongying People's Hospital, Shandong 257091, China. [2]Department of E.N.T., Kenli People's Hospital, Shandong, China.

References

1. Ferlay J, Soerjomataram I, Ervik M, et al. GLOBOCAN 2012 v1.0, Cancer incidence and mortality worldwide: IARC CancerBase No. 11. http://globocan.iarc.fr/Default.aspx. Accessed 25 Aug 2015.
2. Wei WI, Sham JS. Nasopharyngeal carcinoma. Lancet. 2005;365(9476):2041–54.
3. Jiang W, Liu N, Chen XZ, Sun Y, Li B, Ren XY, Qin WF, Jiang N, Xu YF, Li YQ, et al. Genome-wide identification of a methylation gene panel as a prognostic biomarker in nasopharyngeal carcinoma. Mol Cancer Ther. 2015;14(12):2864–73.
4. Sun Q, Liu H, Li L, Zhang S, Liu K, Liu Y, Yang C. Long noncoding RNA-LET, which is repressed by EZH2, inhibits cell proliferation and induces apoptosis of nasopharyngeal carcinoma cell. Med Oncol. 2015;32(9):226.
5. Kooistra SM, Helin K. Molecular mechanisms and potential functions of histone demethylases. Nat Rev Mol Cell Biol. 2012;13(5):297–311.
6. Whetstine JR, Nottke A, Lan F, Huarte M, Smolikov S, Chen Z, Spooner E, Li E, Zhang G, Colaiacovo M, et al. Reversal of histone lysine trimethylation by the JMJD2 family of histone demethylases. Cell. 2006;125(3):467–81.
7. Cloos PA, Christensen J, Agger K, Maiolica A, Rappsilber J, Antal T, Hansen KH, Helin K. The putative oncogene GASC1 demethylates tri- and dimethylated lysine 9 on histone H3. Nature. 2006;442(7100):307–11.
8. Berry WL, Shin S, Lightfoot SA, Janknecht R. Oncogenic features of the JMJD2A histone demethylase in breast cancer. Int J Oncol. 2012;41(5):1701–6.
9. Li BX, Zhang MC, Luo CL, Yang P, Li H, Xu HM, Xu HF, Shen YW, Xue AM, Zhao ZQ. Effects of RNA interference-mediated gene silencing of JMJD2A on human breast cancer cell line MDA-MB-231 in vitro. J Exp Clin Cancer Res. 2011;30:90.
10. Li BX, Luo CL, Li H, Yang P, Zhang MC, Xu HM, Xu HF, Shen YW, Xue AM, Zhao ZQ. Effects of siRNA-mediated knockdown of jumonji domain containing 2A on proliferation, migration and invasion of the human breast cancer cell line MCF-7. Exp Ther Med. 2012;4(4):755–61.
11. Mallette FA, Richard S. JMJD2A promotes cellular transformation by blocking cellular senescence through transcriptional repression of the tumor suppressor CHD5. Cell Rep. 2012;2(5):1233–43.
12. Hanahan D, Weinberg RA. Hallmarks of cancer: the next generation. Cell. 2011;144(5):646–74.
13. Xie P, Yue JB, Fu Z, Feng R, Yu JM. Prognostic value of 18F-FDG PET/CT before and after radiotherapy for locally advanced nasopharyngeal carcinoma. Ann Oncol. 2010;21(5):1078–82.
14. Chan SC, Chang JT, Wang HM, Lin CY, Ng SH, Fan KH, Chin SC, Liao CT, Yen TC. Prediction for distant failure in patients with stage M0 nasopharyngeal carcinoma: the role of standardized uptake value. Oral Oncol. 2009;45(1):52–8.
15. Shen YA, Wang CY, Hsieh YT, Chen YJ, Wei YH. Metabolic reprogramming orchestrates cancer stem cell properties in nasopharyngeal carcinoma. Cell Cycle. 2015;14(1):86–98.
16. Luo W, Fang W, Li S, Yao K. Aberrant expression of nuclear vimentin and related epithelial-mesenchymal transition markers in nasopharyngeal carcinoma. Int J Cancer. 2012;131(8):1863–73.
17. Han T, Jiao F, Hu H, Yuan C, Wang L, Jin ZL, Song WF, Wang LW. EZH2 promotes cell migration and invasion but not alters cell proliferation by suppressing E-cadherin, partly through association with MALAT-1 in pancreatic cancer. Oncotarget. 2016;7(10):11194–207.
18. Hu CE, Liu YC, Zhang HD, Huang GJ. JMJD2A predicts prognosis and regulates cell growth in human gastric cancer. Biochem Biophys Res Commun. 2014;449(1):1–7.

19. Kogure M, Takawa M, Cho HS, Toyokawa G, Hayashi K, Tsunoda T, Kobayashi T, Daigo Y, Sugiyama M, Atomi Y, et al. Deregulation of the histone demethylase JMJD2A is involved in human carcinogenesis through regulation of the G(1)/S transition. Cancer Lett. 2013;336(1):76–84.

20. Cui J, Shi M, Xie D, Wei D, Jia Z, Zheng S, Gao Y, Huang S, Xie K. FOXM1 promotes the warburg effect and pancreatic cancer progression via transactivation of LDHA expression. Clin Cancer Res. 2014;20(10):2595–606.

21. Kauffman EC, Robinson BD, Downes MJ, Powell LG, Lee MM, Scherr DS, Gudas LJ, Mongan NP. Role of androgen receptor and associated lysine-demethylase coregulators, LSD1 and JMJD2A, in localized and advanced human bladder cancer. Mol Carcinog. 2011;50(12):931–44.

22. Cicatiello L, Addeo R, Sasso A, Altucci L, Petrizzi VB, Borgo R, Cancemi M, Caporali S, Caristi S, Scafoglio C, et al. Estrogens and progesterone promote persistent CCND1 gene activation during G1 by inducing transcriptional derepression via c-Jun/c-Fos/estrogen receptor (progesterone receptor) complex assembly to a distal regulatory element and recruitment of cyclin D1 to its own gene promoter. Mol Cell Biol. 2004;24(16):7260–74.

23. Shin S, Janknecht R. Activation of androgen receptor by histone demethylases JMJD2A and JMJD2D. Biochem Biophys Res Commun. 2007; 359(3):742–6.

24. Roque L, Rodrigues R, Martins C, Ribeiro C, Ribeiro MJ, Martins AG, Oliveira P, Fonseca I. Comparative genomic hybridization analysis of a pleuropulmonary blastoma. Cancer Genet Cytogenet. 2004;149(1):58–62.

25. Ding X, Pan H, Li J, Zhong Q, Chen X, Dry SM, Wang CY. Epigenetic activation of AP1 promotes squamous cell carcinoma metastasis. Sci Signal. 2013;6(273):ra28 21–13. S20-15

26. Alfarouk KO, Verduzco D, Rauch C, Muddathir AK, Adil HH, Elhassan GO, Ibrahim ME, David Polo Orozco J, Cardone RA, Reshkin SJ, et al. Glycolysis, tumor metabolism, cancer growth and dissemination. A new pH-based etiopathogenic perspective and therapeutic approach to an old cancer question. Oncoscience. 2014;1(12):777–802.

27. Alfarouk KO, Muddathir AK, Shayoub ME. Tumor acidity as evolutionary spite. Cancers (Basel). 2011;3(1):408–14.

28. Gatenby RA, Gillies RJ. Why do cancers have high aerobic glycolysis? Nat Rev Cancer. 2004;4(11):891–9.

29. Kim JW, Dang CV. Cancer's molecular sweet tooth and the Warburg effect. Cancer Res. 2006;66(18):8927–30.

30. Chen JQ, Russo J. Dysregulation of glucose transport, glycolysis, TCA cycle and glutaminolysis by oncogenes and tumor suppressors in cancer cells. Biochim Biophys Acta. 2012;1826(2):370–84.

31. Shi M, Cui J, Du J, Wei D, Jia Z, Zhang J, Zhu Z, Gao Y, Xie K. A novel KLF4/ LDHA signaling pathway regulates aerobic glycolysis in and progression of pancreatic cancer. Clin Cancer Res. 2014;20(16):4370–80.

32. Sheng SL, Liu JJ, Dai YH, Sun XG, Xiong XP, Huang G. Knockdown of lactate dehydrogenase A suppresses tumor growth and metastasis of human hepatocellular carcinoma. FEBS J. 2012;279(20):3898–910.

33. Zhao YH, Zhou M, Liu H, Ding Y, Khong HT, Yu D, Fodstad O, Tan M. Upregulation of lactate dehydrogenase A by ErbB2 through heat shock factor 1 promotes breast cancer cell glycolysis and growth. Oncogene. 2009;28(42):3689–701.

34. Li AC, Xiao WW, Wang L, Shen GZ, Xu AA, Cao YQ, Huang SM, Lin CG, Han F, Deng XW, et al. Risk factors and prediction-score model for distant metastasis in nasopharyngeal carcinoma treated with intensity-modulated radiotherapy. Tumour Biol. 2015;36(11):8349–57.

35. Zhang D, Yoon HG, Wong J. JMJD2A is a novel N-CoR-interacting protein and is involved in repression of the human transcription factor achaete scute-like homologue 2 (ASCL2/Hash2). Mol Cell Biol. 2005;25(15):6404–14.

36. Gray SG, Iglesias AH, Lizcano F, Villanueva R, Camelo S, Jingu H, Teh BT, Koibuchi N, Chin WW, Kokkotou E, et al. Functional characterization of JMJD2A, a histone deacetylase- and retinoblastoma-binding protein. J Biol Chem. 2005;280(31):28507–18.

37. Kim TD, Shin S, Berry WL, Oh S, Janknecht R. The JMJD2A demethylase regulates apoptosis and proliferation in colon cancer cells. J Cell Biochem. 2012;113(4):1368–76.

PD-L1 expression in malignant salivary gland tumors

Koji Harada*, Tarannum Ferdous and Yoshiya Ueyama

Abstract

Background: Programmed death-1 ligand-1 (PD-L1) an important cancer biomarker that can suppress the immune system and its high expression is often reported to be related with increased tumor aggressiveness in some cancers. Here, we examined and evaluated PD-L1 expression in patients with malignant salivary gland tumor. Moreover, the relationship between PD-L1 immunolocalization and clinical pathological features, as well as the prognosis of malignant salivary gland tumors was investigated.

Methods: We examined PD-L1expression in 47 patients with malignant salivary gland tumor by immunohistochemical staining. PD-L1 positivity was defined as ≥5% in tumor cell membrane and evaluated according to three categories (0% = 0, < 5% = 1, ≥5% = 2) in tumor-infiltrating mononuclear cells (TIMCs). Fisher's exact test was used to compare between PD-L1 expression and clinico-pathological features, and Kaplan–Meier method was used to estimate the distribution of OS by PD-L1 positivity.

Results: PD-L1 expression was detected in 51.1% of malignant salivary gland tumor tissues. No association was observed between PD-L1 immunolocalization in tumor and patient gender, or age. However, PD-L1 immunodetection of tumor cell membranes was significantly associated to stage, recurrence or metastasis after surgery, and patient outcome. On the other hand, PD-L1 immunodetection of tumor-infiltrating mononuclear cells (TIMCs) was significantly associated to recurrence or metastasis after surgery, and patient outcome. PD-L1 positivity in both tumor cell membrane and TIMCs was associated with shorter overall survival (OS) ($p = 0.002$ and $p = 0.016$, respectively).

Conclusion: These findings suggested that patients with PD-L1 positive tumors or TIMCs appear to have poor clinical outcomes in malignant salivary gland tumors.

Keywords: PD-L1, Malignant salivary gland tumor, Prognosis, Immunohistochemistry

Background

The incidence of malignant salivary gland tumors is relatively low compared to other head and neck cancers. They account for more than 0.5% of all malignancies and approximately 3–6.5% of all head and neck cancers [1, 2]. These tumors show varied histological features, and are largely present in the parotid and submandibular glands. The standard treatment for salivary gland cancers is surgical operation because they show resistance to chemotherapy and radiotherapy generally; however, its treatment often requires complex multidisciplinary approach [3, 4]. We often select post-operative radiotherapy when the tumor could not be removed

completely by surgery [5]. Unfortunately, these are the only treatment options currently available for malignant salivary gland tumors. As these tumors are often slow growing and are detected at an advanced, non-surgical stage; sometimes they are difficult to treat. Conventional chemotherapies often shows poor efficacy in managing locally advanced or metastatic tumors [3, 4, 6]. Molecular targeted therapies might be useful for the treatment of these patients, although no significant guidelines or tools for selecting candidate patients are available [7]. Thus, novel therapeutic strategies need to be developed and established for the treatment of malignant salivary gland tumors.

It is well known that development and prognosis of malignant tumors are closely associated with host immune functions. Anti-tumor immune responses are

* Correspondence: harako@yamaguchi-u.ac.jp
Department of Oral and Maxillofacial Surgery, Yamaguchi University Graduate School of Medicine, 1-1-1 Minamikogushi, Ube 755-8505, Japan

induced when the host immune system efficiently identifies the tumor antigen and various T cells are activated. Co-stimulatory molecules and regulative networks play an important role in this progression. There are two groups of co-stimulatory molecules: the tumor necrosis factor TNF receptor (TNFr) superfamily and the immunoglobulin (Ig) superfamily [8]. Programmed death-1 (PD-1) is a co-stimulatory molecule that functions as an immune checkpoint. It is expressed on T cells and pro-B cells, and negatively regulates T cell activation and responses [9]. Two binding ligands have been identified for PD-1, Programmed death-1 ligand-1 (PD-L1, also known as B7-H1) and PD-L2, and both belong to the B7 family [10, 11]. PD-L1 is expressed in resting T cells, B cells, dendritic cells (DCs) and in various tumor cells; and the formation of PD-1 and PD-L1 receptor-ligand complex leads to the inhibition of the cytotoxic T cells and induces special apoptosis of T cells, which results in tumor immune escape [12–14]. Moreover, it has been reported that overexpression of PD-L1 is closely associated with the poor prognosis of renal cell carcinoma, esophageal cancer, gastric cancer, urothelial cancer, pancreatic cancer, and malignant melanoma [12, 15–19]. However, the levels and clinical significance of PD-L1 expression in malignant salivary gland tumor is still unknown.

The purpose of our study was to characterize the PD-L1 expression in patients with malignant salivary gland tumor, and to investigate the relationship between PD-L1 expression levels with clinico-pathological features as well as disease outcomes of the patients.

Methods

Patients and samples

Institutional review board (IRB) of the ethical committee of the Yamaguchi University Hospital approved this study (Ref H26–179). Our study was a retrospective one; therefore, informed consent was waived by the IRB.

Forty-seven patients ($n = 47$) with salivary gland cancers (Adenoid cystic carcinoma, Mucoepidermoid carcinoma, Adenocarcinoma and Mucinous adenocarcinoma) treated surgically at Yamaguchi University Hospital from April 1990 to March 2011 were included in this study. Clinico-pathological characteristics such as gender, age, stage and follow-up data (recurrence, metastasis and outcome) were retrospectively collected from patients' medical records.

Immunohistochemistry

Tissue samples obtained from biopsy or operation specimens were used to prepare Formalin-Fixed Paraffin-Embedded (FFPE) blocks. Four-micron-thick tumor sections were prepared from these blocks were used for the immunohistochemical analysis. These paraffin-embedded tissue sections were deparaffinized in 100% xylene (Wako

Pure Chemical Industries, Ltd.) for 10 min at room temperature, followed by rehydration using graded (100–70% v/v, 5 min/each concentration) ethyl alcohol (Muto Pure Chemicals Co., Ltd., Tokyo, Japan). Then, the sections were washed with phosphate-buffered saline (PBS), and heated in a microwave in a Tris-EDTA buffer solution (pH 9.0). The slides were then allowed to cool down, and inserted into a 0.3% hydrogen peroxide/methanol mixture for 20 min at room temperature. After PBS wash, the tissue sections were incubated with Dako REAL™ Peroxidase-Blocking solution (Agilent Technologies, Inc., Santa Clara, CA, USA) for 30 min at room temperature; then incubated overnight at 4 °C with a rabbit polyclonal anti-PD-L1 antibody (Abcam, Cambridge, UK). After PBS wash, Dako REAL™ EnVision™ Detection system (Agilent Technologies) was used according to the manufacturer's protocol to detect the immunostaining. Tissues were then lightly counterstained with hematoxylin (Muto Pure Chemicals Co., Tokyo, Japan), and were subsequently dehydrated in graded (70–100% v/v) ethyl alcohol (Muto Pure Chemicals Co., Ltd.), inserted in xylene (Wako Pure Chemical Industries Ltd.) and mounted with glass coverslips using DPX mounting medium (Sigma-Aldrich; Merck KGaA). In case of negative controls, primary antibody was omitted.

Quantification of PD-L1 expression in tumor cell membrane

Immunoreactivity for PD-L1 expression was evaluated in tumor cell membrane by three authors (KH, TF, and YU), who had no knowledge of the patient's clinical status. Briefly, five randomly selected areas were examined. The proportion of tumor cells showing high and low immunolabeling in each selected field was determined by counting individual tumor cells at high magnification (× 400). At least 200 tumor cells were counted. PD-L1 tumor positivity was defined as ≥5% tumor cell membrane staining. PD-L1-positive immunolabeling was predominantly located in the cytoplasm and with some nuclear membrane localization (Fig. 1).

Quantification of PD-L1 expression in tumor-infiltrating mononuclear cells

The extent of tumor-infiltrating mononuclear cells (TIMCs) (i.e. lymphocytes and macrophages) was assessed in hematoxylin and eosin-stained slides and evaluated as absent (0), focal (1), mild (2), moderate (3) and marked (4) by three authors (KH, TF, and YU), who had no knowledge of the patient's clinical status. The percentage of PD-L1-positive TIMCs was also evaluated independently. Immunoreactivity for PD-L1 expression was evaluated according to three categories (0% = 0, < 5% = 1, ≥5% = 2). An adjusted score representing PD-L1 expression was calculated multiplying the percentage of TIMCs that stained

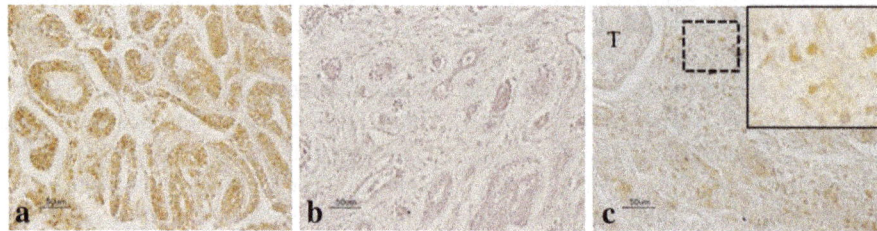

Fig. 1 PD-L1 expression in FFPE samples stained with anti-PD-L1 antibody. **a** Positive staining is present in tumor cells membrane. **b** Negative staining is present in tumor cells membrane. **c** Tumor cells are negative (T) and TIMCs are positive for PD-L1, magnified view of TIMCs was shown in the upper right corner

positive for PD-L1 and the extent of mononuclear cell infiltration.

Statistical analysis

In the present study, we investigated PD-L1 expression and its association with clinical outcome in patients with malignant salivary gland tumor. Overall survival (OS) defined as time from diagnosis to death was analyzed as an end point. In the absence of an event, the end point was censored at last follow-up time. Patient and tumor characteristics were summarized descriptively. PD-L1 positivity was defined as 5% or greater of tumor cell membrane staining. For PD-L1 expression in TIMCs, any score greater than five was considered high. Comparisons between PD-L1 expression and clinico-pathological features were evaluated using Fisher's exact test for categorical variables. Kaplan–Meier method estimated the distribution of OS by the PD-L1 positivity. All statistical computations were carried out using the StatView software (version 5.0 J, SAS Institute Inc. Cary, NC, USA) and a p value (two-sided) < 0.055 was considered statistically significant.

Results

Patients and tumor characteristics

Characteristics of 47 patients with malignant salivary gland tumor included in this study are summarized in Table 1. The histological subtypes included adenoid cystic carcinoma ($n = 25$), mucoepidermoid carcinoma ($n = 9$), adenocarcinoma ($n = 11$) and mucinous adenocarcinoma ($n = 2$). The median follow-up time was 7.4 years [interquartile range (IQR): 1.8–12.8], and the median age was 62 years (range 24–80 years). For malignant salivary gland tumor, clinical stages I, II, III and IV at diagnosis was identified in 9, 18, 5 and 15 patients, respectively.

PD-L1 expression in tumor cells and clinico-pathological features

Table 2 shows the association between PDL-1 expression in tumor cell membrane and clinico-pathological

features of patients. Among 47 patients with malignant salivary gland tumor, 23 patients (48.9%) showed negative PD-L1 expression in tumor cell membrane; whereas 24 patients (51.1%) showed positive expression. Specifically, PD-L1 positivity in tumor cell membrane was detected in 11 of 25 (44.0%) adenoid cystic carcinoma patients, 7 of 11 (63.6%) mucoepidermoid carcinoma patients, 5 of 9 (55.6%) adenocarcinoma patients, and 1 of 2 (50.0%) mucinous

Table 1 Patient characteristics

Characteristic	Total ($n = 47$) No. of patients	%
Gender		
Male	26	55.3
Female	21	44.7
Stage		
I	9	19.1
II	18	38.3
III	5	10.6
IV	15	31.9
Histology		
adenoid cystic carcinoma	25	40.4
mucoepidermoid carcinoma	9	17.0
adenocarcinoma	11	23.4
mucinous adenocarcinoma	2	6.4
Recurrence or metastasis after surgery		
No	31	66.0
Yes	16	34.0
PD-L1 expression in tumor cells membrane		
< 5% (negative)	23	48.9
≥ 5% (positive)	24	51.1
PD-L1 expression in tumor-infiltrating mononuclear cells (TIMC)		
Score < 4 (negative)	27	57.4
Score ≥ 4 (positive)	20	42.6
	Median	Min-max
Age (years)	62.0	24–80

Table 2 Association between PD-L1 expression in malignant salivary gland tumor membrane and clinico-pathological factors[a]

Characteristic	% Positive tumor cell membrane			p-value
	< 5% (negative) (n = 23, 48.9%), n	5% or more (positive) (n = 24, 51.1%), n	Total (n = 47), n	
Gender				> 0.999
Male	13	13	26	
Female	10	21	21	
Age				> 0.999
65≥	13	12	25	
65<	10	12	22	
Stage				0.047
I + II	17	10	27	
III + IV	6	14	20	
Recurrence or metastasis after surgery				0.028
No	19	12	31	
Yes	4	12	16	
Outcome				0.002
Alive	22	13	35	
Death	1	11	12	

[a]Fisher's exact test

Table 3 Association between PD-L1 expression in tumor-infiltrating mononuclear cells (TIMCs) and clinico-pathological factors[a]

Characteristic	% Positive tumor- infiltrating mononuclear cells			p-value
	Score < 5 (low) (n = 27, 57.4%), n	Score ≥ 5 (high) (n = 20, 42.6%), n	Total (n = 47), n	
Gender				> 0.999
Male	15	11	26	
Female	12	9	21	
Age				0.769
65≥	14	11	25	
65<	13	9	22	
Stage				0.073
I + II	19	8	27	
III + IV	8	12	20	
Recurrence or metastasis after surgery				0.011
No	19	12	31	
Yes	8	8	16	
Outcome				0.049
Alive	23	12	35	
Death	4	8	12	

[a]Fisher's exact test

adenocarcinoma patients. PD-L1 positivity in tumor cell membrane was significantly associated with higher stage ($p = 0.047$), recurrence or metastasis after surgery ($p = 0.028$), and fatal outcome ($p = 0.002$). On the other hand, PD-L1 positivity was not associated with gender, age at diagnosis.

PD-L1 expression in TIMCs and clinico-pathological features

Association between PDL-1 expression in TIMC and clinico-pathological factors are presented in Table 3. Overall, the extent of TIMCs infiltration was: absent in 0 patients, focal in 23 patients, mild in 17 patients, moderate in 6 patients and marked in 1 patient. PD-L1 expression in TIMCs was low (score < 5) in 27 patients (57.4%). Twenty patients (42.6%) were considered as PD-L1 high (score ≥ 5) in the TIMCs. Among the cases with PD-L1 high TIMCs, all patients showed positive expression in more than 5% of immune cells. There was a significant association between PD-L1 expression levels in TIMCs and recurrence or metastasis after surgery ($p = 0.011$), as well as PD-L1 expression levels and outcome of patients ($p = 0.049$). PD-L1 positivity in TIMCs was not significantly associated with gender ($p > 0.999$), age ($p = 0.769$), stage ($p = 0.073$).

PD-L1 expression in malignant salivary gland tumors and survival time

The overall median follow-up of the cohort was 7.4 years, 12 patients died and 16 patients had recurrence or metastasis after surgery. PD-L1 positivity on tumor cell membrane and TIMCs both were associated with OS ($p = 0.002$ and $p = 0.016$, respectively) (Fig. 2).

Discussion

This study demonstrated significant association between PD-L1 positivity in tumor cells and higher stage, recurrence or metastasis after surgery, fatal outcome or survival time in patients with malignant salivary gland tumors. In addition, significant association was also observed between PD-L1 expression levels in TIMCs and recurrence or metastasis after surgery or patient outcome. Therefore, we can assume that patients with PD-L1 positive malignant salivary gland tumors or TIMCs cannot be expected to show favorable prognosis, especially when conventional therapy or surgical operation is used as the treatment method. Hence, novel and advanced therapeutic approaches against locally advanced or metastatic malignant salivary gland tumors are needed to ensure favorable treatment outcome of patients. It was reported that, blocking the interactions between PD-1 and PD-L1 can inhibit antitumor

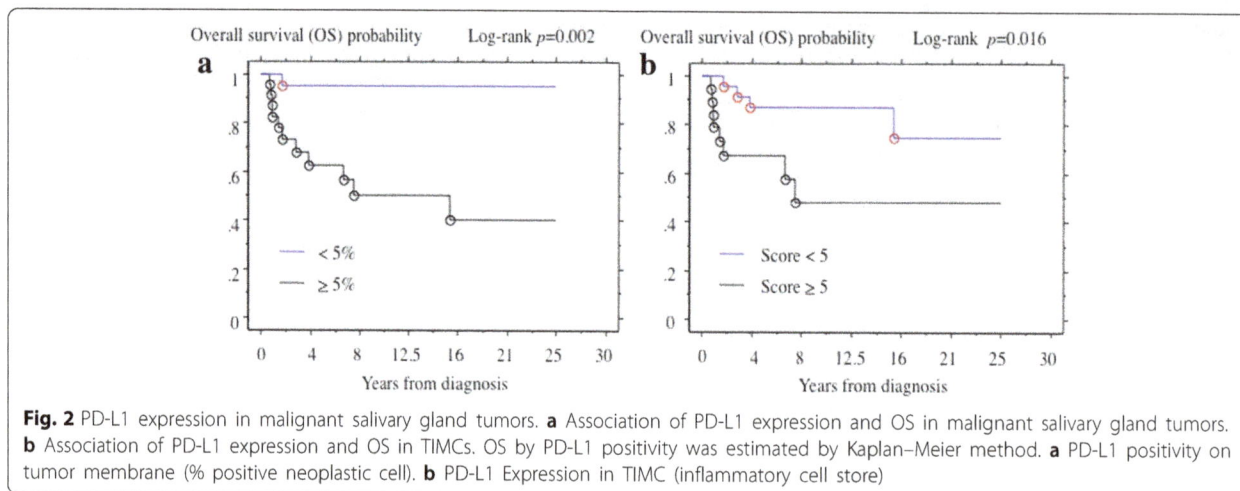

Fig. 2 PD-L1 expression in malignant salivary gland tumors. **a** Association of PD-L1 expression and OS in malignant salivary gland tumors. **b** Association of PD-L1 expression and OS in TIMCs. OS by PD-L1 positivity was estimated by Kaplan–Meier method. **a** PD-L1 positivity on tumor membrane (% positive neoplastic cell). **b** PD-L1 Expression in TIMC (inflammatory cell store)

immunity, enhance T-cell-mediated immune function and promote antitumor activity of therapeutic agents in preclinical models and in vitro [20]. Brahmer et al. showed the efficacy of anti-PD-L1 antibody (BMS-93655) in his multicenter phase 1 trial study with patients with advanced cancer, including non-small-cell lung cancer, melanoma and renal-cell cancer [20]. Recently, anti-PD-1 monoclonal antibody (nivolumab) is considered as a new therapeutic option for the treatment of unresectable malignant melanoma [21]. Moreover, some clinical studies that evaluated the safety and efficacy of nivolumab in patients with advanced cancer showed encouraging results [21–24]. However, higher PD-L1 expression in tumor cells is not always associated with unfavorable outcome [25, 26].

Until now, there were no available reports that indicated any relationship between PD-L1 expression and clinical outcomes in malignant salivary gland tumor patients. To our knowledge, this is the first study that demonstrated the association between PD-L1 expression in tumor cells or TIMCs with recurrence or metastasis after surgery, fatal outcome and shorter OS in patients with malignant salivary gland tumors treated by surgical operation. We could detect PD-L1 expression both in tumor cells and TIMCs. The detail mechanisms of PD-L1 expression in tumor cells or TIMCs are still unknown. It is reported that, Natural killer cells as well as T-cells expresses cytokines such as interferon-γ (IFN-γ), tumor necrosis factor-α (TNF-α) and interleukin-2 (IL-2) which in turn can induce PD-L1 expression on surrounding immune and tumor cells when T-cells recognize antigen and become activated [27]. TIMCs also have an important role in induction of PD-L1 expressions, and various cytokines derived from TIMCs promotes tumor growth as well as impairs antitumor immune responses. The expression mechanisms of PD-L1 must be complicated with different circumstances

involved; however, the extent of TIMCs could be an important predictive factor for anti-PD-1 monoclonal antibody therapy including nivolumab [21]. In this study, we found high extent of TIMCs, as well as high PD-L1 expression in both tumor cells and TIMCs. Nivolumab has just got marketing approval as a drug for the treatment of unresectable malignant melanoma, and it might also be effective for locally advanced or metastatic malignant salivary gland tumors [21]. Further in vitro, in vivo and clinical studies with anti-PDL-1 antibody (BMS-93655) against salivary gland tumors might also generate favorable results.

Our study is a retrospective analysis of PD-L1 expression and we have only analyzed 47 cases of malignant salivary gland tumors. Further prospective studies are needed to understand the role of PD-L1 expression more precisely in immune cells as a predictive and prognostic biomarker in malignant salivary gland tumors.

Conclusion

This is the first study that demonstrated the association between PD-L1 positive expression and clinical stage, recurrence or metastasis after surgery and survival time of patients with malignant salivary gland tumors. Our data also showed significant association between PD-L1 expression levels in TIMCs and recurrence or metastasis after surgery or patient outcome.

Abbreviations
DC: dendritic cells; FFPE: Formalin-Fixed Paraffin-Embedded; IFN-γ: Interferon-γ; Ig: Immunoglobulin; IL-2: Interleukin-2; OS: Overall survival; PBS: Phosphate-buffered saline; PD-1: Programmed death-1; PDL1: Programmed death ligand 1; TIMC: Tumor-infiltrating mononuclear cell; TNFr: TNF receptor; TNF-α: Tumor necrosis factor-α

Acknowledgements
Not applicable

Funding
This study was supported in part by a Grant-in-Aid from the Japanese Ministry of Education, Science and Culture (Grant no. 24593034). Funding body had no contribution in designing the study, data collection, interpretation or analysis of data, or writing the manuscript.

Authors' contributions
KH was involved in the study design, data analysis, and writing of the manuscript. TF carried out the immunohistochemical studies, data collection and evaluation, and assisted in manuscript writing. YU revised and edited the manuscript. All the authors read and approved the final version of the manuscript.

Authors' information
KH is assistant professor, TF is academic researcher and UY is professor in Department of Oral and Maxillofacial Surgery, Yamaguchi University Graduate School of Medicine, Ube, Japan.

Competing interests
The authors declare that they have no competing interests.

References
1. Speight PM, Barrett AW. Salivary gland tumours. Oral Dis. 2002;8:229–40.
2. Carvalho AL, Nishimoto IN, Califano JA, Kowalski LP. Trends in incidence and prognosis for head and neck cancer in the United States: a site-specific analysis of the SEER database. Int J Cancer. 2005;114:806–16.
3. Kaplan MJ, Johns ME, Cantrell RW. Chemotherapy for salivary gland cancer. Otolaryngol Head Neck Surg. 1986;95:165–70.
4. Belani CP. Preliminary experience with chemotherapy in advanced salivary glands neoplasms. Med Pediat Oncol. 1988;16:197–202.
5. Noh JM, Ahn YC, Nam H, Park W, Baek CH, Son YI, Jeong HS. Treatment results of major salivary gland cancer by surgery with or without postoperative radiation therapy. Clin Exp Otorhinolaryngol. 2010;3:96–101.
6. Licitra L, Cavina R, Grandi C, Palma SD, Guzzo M, Demicheli R, Molinari R. Cisplatin, doxorubicin and cyclophosphamide in advanced salivary gland carcinoma: a phase II trial of 22 patients. Ann Oncol. 1996;7:640–2.
7. Caballero M, E Sosa A, Tagliapietra A, Grau JJ: Metastatic adenoid cystic carcinoma of the salivary gland responding to cetuximab plus weekly paclitaxel after no response to weekly paclitaxel alone. Head Neck 2013, 35: 52–54.
8. Chambers CA, Allison JP. Costimulatory regulation of T cell function. Curr Opin Cell Biol. 1999;11:203–10.
9. Pardoll DM. Spinning molecular immunology into successful immunotherapy. Nat Rev Immunol. 2002;2:227–38.
10. Dong H, Zhu G, Tamada K, Chen L. B7-H1, a third member of the B7 family, co-stimulates T-cell proliferation and interleukin-10 secretion. Nat Med. 1999;5:1365–9.
11. Tseng SY, Otsuji M, Gorski K, Huang X, Slansky JE, Pai SI, Shin T, Pardoll DM, Tsuchiya H. B7-DC, a new dendritic cell molecule with potent costimulatory properties for T cells. J Exp Med. 2001;193:839–46.
12. Ohigashi Y, Sho M, Yamada Y, Tsurui Y, Hamada K, Ikeda N, Mizuno T, Yoriki R, Kashizuka H, Yane K, Tsushima F, Otsuki N, Yagita H, Azuma M, Nakajima Y. Clinical significance of programmed death-1 ligand-1 and programmed death-1 ligand-2 expression in human esophageal cancer. Clin Cancer Res. 2005;11:2947–53.
13. Yamazaki T, Akiba H, Iwai H, Matsuda H, Aoki M, Tanno Y, Shin T, Tsuchiya H, Pardoll DM, Okumura K, Azuma M, Yagita H. Expression of programmed death 1 ligands by murine T cells and APC. J Immunol. 2002;169:5538–45.
14. Yuan Y, He Y, Wang X, Zhang H, Li D, Feng Z, Zhang G. Investigation on the effects of soluble programmed death-1 (sPD-1) enhancing anti-tumor immune response. J Huazhong Univ Sci Technolog Med Sci. 2004;24:531–4.
15. Thompson RH, Gillett MD, Cheville JC, Lohse CM, Dong H, Webster WS, Krejci KG, Lobo JR, Sengupta S, Chen L, Zincke H, Blute ML, Strome SE, Leibovich BC, Kwon ED. Costimulatory B7-H1 in renal cell carcinoma patients: Indicator of tumor aggressiveness and potential therapeutic target. Proc Natl Acad Sc. 2004;101:17174–9.
16. Wu C, Zhu Y, Jiang J, Zhao J, Zhang XG, Xu N. Immunohistochemical localization of programmed death-1 ligand-1 (PD-L1) in gastric carcinoma and its clinical significance. Acta Histochem. 2006;108:19–24.
17. Nakanishi J, Wada Y, Matsumoto K, Azuma M, Kikuchi K, Ueda S. Overexpression of B7-H1 (PD-L1) significantly associates with tumor grade and postoperative prognosis in human urothelial cancers. Cancer Immunol Immunother. 2007;56:1173–82.
18. Nomi T, Sho M, Akahori T, Hamada K, Kubo A, Kanehiro H, Nakamura S, Enomoto K, Yagita H, Azuma M, Nakajima Y. Clinical significance and therapeutic potential of the programmed death-1 ligand/programmed death-1 pathway in human pancreatic cancer. Clin Cancer Res. 2007;13:2151–7.
19. Hino R, Kabashima K, Kato Y, Yagi H, Nakamura M, Honjo T, Okazaki T, Tokura Y. Tumor cell expression of programmed cell death-1 ligand 1 is a prognostic factor for malignant melanoma. Cancer. 2010;116:1757–66.
20. Brahmer JR, Tykodi SS, Chow LQ, Hwu WJ, Topalian SL, Hwu P, Drake CG, Camacho LH, Kauh J, Odunsi K, Pitot HC, Hamid O, Bhatia S, Martins R, Eaton K, Chen S, Salay TM, Alaparthy S, Grosso JF, Korman AJ, Parker SM, Agrawal S, Goldberg SM, Pardoll DM, Gupta A, Wigginton JM. Safety and activity of anti-PD-L1 antibody in patients with advanced cancer. N Engl J Med. 2012;366:2455–65.
21. Brahmer JR, Drake CG, Wollner I, Powderly JD, Picus J, Sharfman WH, Stankevich E, Pons A, Salay TM, McMiller TL, Gilson MM, Wang C, Selby M, Taube JM, Anders R, Chen L, Korman AJ, Pardoll DM, Lowy I, Topalian SL. Phase I study of single-agent anti-programmed death-1 (MDX-1106) in refractory solid tumors: safety, clinical activity, pharmacodynamics, and immunologic correlates. J Clin Oncol. 2010;28:3167–75.
22. Topalian SL, Hodi FS, Brahmer JR, Gettinger SN, Smith DC, McDermott DF, Powderly JD, Carvajal RD, Sosman JA, Atkins MB, Leming PD, Spigel DR, Antonia SJ, Horn L, Drake CG, Pardoll DM, Chen L, Sharfman WH, Anders RA, Taube JM, McMiller TL, Xu H, Korman AJ, Jure-Kunkel M, Agrawal S, McDonald D, Kollia GD, Gupta A, Wigginton JM, Sznol M. Safety, activity, and immune correlates of anti-PD-1 antibody in cancer. N Engl J Med. 2012;366:2443–54.
23. Motzer RJ, Rini BI, McDermott DF, Redman BG, Kuzel TM, Harrison MR, Vaishampayan UN, Drabkin HA, George S, Logan TF, Margolin KA, Plimack ER, Lambert AM, Waxman IM, Hammers HJ. Nivolumab for Metastatic Renal Cell Carcinoma: Results of a Randomized Phase II Trial. J Clin Oncol. 2015;33:1430–7.
24. Rizvi NA, Mazières J, Planchard D, Stinchcombe TE, Dy GK, Antonia SJ, Horn L, Lena H, Minenza E, Mennecier B, Otterson GA, Campos LT, Gandara DR, Levy BP, Nair SG, Zalcman G, Wolf J, Souquet PJ, Baldini E, Cappuzzo F, Chouaid C, Dowlati A, Sanborn R, Lopez-Chavez A, Grohe C, Huber RM, Harbison CT, Baudelet C, Lestini BJ, Ramalingam SS. Activity and safety of nivolumab, an anti-PD-1 immune checkpoint inhibitor, for patients with advanced, refractory squamous non-small-cell lung cancer (CheckMate 063): a phase 2, single-arm trial. Lancet Oncol. 2015;16:257–65.
25. Bellmunt J, Mullane SA, Werner L, Fay AP, Callea M, Leow JJ, Taplin ME, Choueiri TK, Hodi FS, Freeman GJ, Signoretti S. Association of PD-L1 expression on tumor-infiltrating mononuclear cells and overall survival in patients with urothelial carcinoma. Ann Oncol. 2015;26:812–7.
26. Schalper KA, Velcheti V, Carvajal D, Wimberly H, Brown J, Pusztai L, Rimm DL. In situ tumor PD-L1 mRNA expression is associated with increased TILs and better outcome in breast carcinomas. Clin Cancer Res. 2014;20:2773–82.
27. Ritprajak P, Azuma M. Intrinsic and extrinsic control of expression of the immunoregulatory molecule PD-L1 in epithelial cells and squamous cell carcinoma. Oral Oncol. 2015;51:221–8.

18

Cathepsin K associates with lymph node metastasis and poor prognosis in oral squamous cell carcinoma

Frank K. Leusink[1*], Eleftherios Koudounarakis[1†], Michael H. Frank[2†], Ronald Koole[2], Paul J. van Diest[3] and Stefan M. Willems[3]

Abstract

Background: Lymph node metastasis (LNM) is a major determinant of prognosis and treatment planning of oral squamous cell carcinoma (OSCC). Cysteine cathepsins constitute a family of proteolytic enzymes with known role in the degradation of the extracellular matrix. Involvement in pathological processes, such as inflammation and cancer progression, has been proved. The aim of the study was to discover the clinicopathological and prognostic implications of cathepsin K (CTSK) expression in oral squamous cell carcinoma.

Methods: Eighty-three patients with primary OSCC, treated surgically between 1996 and 2000, were included. Gene expression data were acquired from a previously reported study. Human papilloma virus (HPV) status was previously determined by an algorithm for HPV-16. CTSK Protein expression was semi-quantitatively determined by immunohistochemistry in tumor and stromal cells. Expression data were correlated with various clinicopathological variables.

Results: Elevated gene and protein expression of CTSK were strongly associated to LNM and perineural invasion ($p < 0.01$). Logistic regression analysis highlighted increased CTSK protein expression in tumor cells as the most significant independent factor of lymphatic metastasis (OR = 7.65, CI:2.31–23.31, $p = 0.001$). Survival analysis demonstrated CTSK protein expression in both stromal and tumor cells as significant indicators of poor 5-year disease specific survival (HR = 2.40, CI:1.05–5.50, $p = 0.038$ for stromal cells; HR = 2.79, CI:1.02–7.64, $p = 0.045$ for tumor cells).

Conclusion: Upregulation of CTSK seems to be associated with high incidence of lymphatic spread and poor survival in OSCC. CTSK could therefore serve as a predictive biomarker for OSCC.

Keywords: Oral squamous cell carcinoma, Cathepsin K, Lymph node metastasis, Prognosis

Background

Oral squamous cell carcinoma (OSCC) constitutes the most common malignancy of the head and neck region [1]. Lymph node metastasis (LNM) has been shown to be the most significant, independent prognostic factor and is related to a decrease of the 5-year survival rate by 50% [2]. Thus, revealing the presence of occult metastasis is of the utmost importance for early and proper

management of the neck. Variable imaging studies have been used for this purpose, including ultrasound combined with fine needle aspiration cytology, computed tomography, magnetic resonance imaging and, more recently, positron emission tomography, with variable results [3]. Moreover, the sentinel node procedure has been currently adopted by some oncological centers and embodied in the staging algorithm of early OSCC. However, its greater disadvantage is that the patient undergoes an interventional procedure. In the context of molecular biology, a significant amount of research has been focused during the last decades on biomarkers that may have additional diagnostic value. Roepman et al. showed that gene expression

* Correspondence: frankleusink@hotmail.com
†Equal contributors
[1]Department of Head and Neck Oncology and Surgery, Netherlands Cancer Institute – Antoni van Leeuwenhoek, Plesmanlaan 121, 1066, CX, Amsterdam, The Netherlands
Full list of author information is available at the end of the article

profiling revealed a strong signature predicting LNM in OSCC [4]. Reanalysis and multicenter validation ($n = 222$) of the entire data set identified more genes with predictive power [5, 6]. Cathepsin K (CTSK) was one of the significantly upregulated genes.

Cathepsin K (also known as cathepsin O2), encoded by the CTSK gene on chromosome 1q21, is one of the 11 lysosomal protein degradation enzymes called cysteine cathepsins, which participate in a considerable number of physiological processes, including MHC-II-mediated antigen presentation, bone remodeling, keratinocyte differentiation and prohormone activation [7]. It is a unique collagenolytic cysteine peptidase and it is highly expressed in osteoclasts and in many other cell types, i.e. macrophages, dendritic cells, adipocytes, fibroblasts and most epithelial cells [8, 9]. Cathepsin K is the sole matrix-degrading enzyme for which a fundamental role in bone resorption has been unequivocally documented in mice and humans [7]. However, increased expression of this lysosomal enzyme is also observed in various pathological conditions, such as neurological disorders, inflammatory diseases and cancer. The role of cathepsins in cancer progression and invasion, mainly through degradation of and remodeling in the tumor microenvironment, is supported by several experimental studies and clinical reports in various types of tumors [10]. In OSCC, both cathepsins B (CTSB) and cathepsin D (CTSD) are correlated with invasion and progression [11, 12] and more specifically CTSD with LNM [12]. Furthermore, CTSB was reported as the promotor of motility and invasiveness [13]. More recently, CTSB was found correlated with survival and LNM, with stronger correlations for the subsite buccal mucosa [14]. Regarding CTSK in OSCC, silencing of CTSK was reported to reduce invasion of aggressive tongue HSC-3 cells in 3D models [15] which could be caused by decreased cell migration and adhesion [16]. To date, there is little data about the relation of CTSK expression in OSCC with clinical and pathological parameters. In the present study, gene and protein expression data of CTKS in OSCC was acquired and the correlation with clinicopathological variables, particularly LNM, was examined.

Methods

Patients and tissue samples

The study work-flow is presented in Fig. 1. The study included 83 consecutive patients with OSCC who were diagnosed and surgically treated at the University Medical Center in Utrecht, The expressioNetherlands, between 1996 and 2000, described in an earlier reported study [17]. Detailed patient characteristics are shown in Table 1. Tissues were used in line with the code 'Proper Secondary Use of Human Tissue' as installed by the Dutch Federation of Biomedical Scientific Societies. Table 2

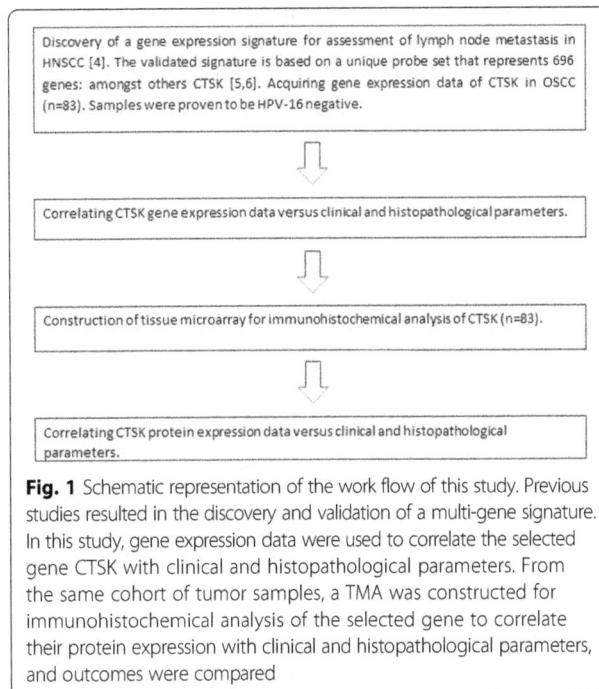

Fig. 1 Schematic representation of the work flow of this study. Previous studies resulted in the discovery and validation of a multi-gene signature. In this study, gene expression data were used to correlate the selected gene CTSK with clinical and histopathological parameters. From the same cohort of tumor samples, a TMA was constructed for immunohistochemical analysis of the selected gene to correlate their protein expression with clinical and histopathological parameters, and outcomes were compared

demonstrates the pathological features of the study population. All oral carcinomas included in the current study tested negative for HPV-16 [17], which is in line with other data [18] reporting the incidence of HPV in OSCC to be less than 4%. A previously constructed [17] tissue microarray (TMA) was used for immunohistochemical analysis of CTSK.

CTSK gene expression analysis

Genome-wide gene expression was measured using dual-channel microarrays with a pool of tumor samples, as described in an earlier study [4]. CTSK was represented by a sole, unique feature on this array.

Immunohistochemistry

Five μm thick sections of FFPE tonsil control tissue and the TMA were cut and mounted on silane-coated glass slides. After deparaffinization the endogenous peroxidase activity was blocked for 30 min in a 0.3% H_2O_2 phosphate-citrate buffer solution of pH 5.8 with sodium azide. Then, tissue sections were subjected to antigen retrieval by boiling in sodium citrate solution (pH 6) for 15 min at 37 °C. Subsequently, the tissue slides were washed with PBS, 0.05% (v/v) Tween-20 and incubated with a dilution of the primary mouse monoclonal antibody against CTSK (clone CK4, Novocastra, Newcastle, UK) for 1 h at RT. Slides were washed and incubated with the following species-specific secondary antibodies: 1:250 diluted rabbit anti-mouse (RAMPO, Dako, Glostrup, Denmark) followed by Powervision anti-rabbit/HRP conjugated (Klinipath, Duiven, The Netherlands). All antibodies were

Table 1 Clinical characteristics of the included OSCC patients

	No.	(%)
All cases	83	(100)
Gender		
Female	36	(43)
Male	47	(57)
Age at diagnosis		
0–60	53	(44)
≥ 61	30	(56)
Median (range)	62	(37–87)
Smoking history		
Current smoker or ceased < 1 year	58	(70)
Ex-smoker, ceased > 1 year	9	(11)
Never smoker	15	(18)
Alcohol consumption		
≥ 5 U/day	19	(23)
1–4 U/day	28	(34)
Occasionally	17	(20)
Never	19	(23)
Clinical T-stage		
cT1	13	(16)
cT2	31	(37)
cT3	8	(10)
cT4	31	(37)
Clinical N-Stage		
cN0	53	(64)
cN1–3	30	(36)
Sub-site		
Tongue	30	(36)
Floor of mouth	35	(42)
Buccal cavity	10	(12)
Gum	8	(10)
Mean follow-up (months)	45	

Table 2 Pathological characteristics of the included OSCC patients

	No.	(%)
All cases	83	(100)
Pathological T-Stage		
pT1	17	(20)
pT2	27	(33)
pT3	10	(12)
pT4	29	(35)
Pathological N-Stage		
pN0	38	(46)
pN1–3	45	(54)
Stage grouping		
I	14	(17)
II	9	(11)
III	22	(26)
IVA-IVB	38	(46)
Infiltration depth		
≥ 4.0 mm	72	(87)
< 4.0 mm	11	(13)
Differentiation grade		
Good / Moderate	67	(81)
Poor / Undifferentiated	16	(19)
Keratinization		
Present	60	(72)
Absent	20	(24)
Missing	3	(4)
Vaso-invasion		
Present	18	(22)
Absent	62	(75)
Missing	3	(3)
Bone-invasion		
Present	25	(30)
Absent	58	(70)
Perineural growth		
Present	34	(41)
Absent	39	(47)
Missing	10	(12)
Spidery growth		
Present	65	(78)
Absent	18	(22)
High risk HPV status		
positive	0	(0)
negative	83	(100)

diluted in PBS/1%BSA. After washing with PBS, the bound antibodies were visualized using 3,3′-diamino-benzidine (0.6 mg/ml). Slides were counterstained with hematoxylin.

Evaluation of protein expression

Intensity and percentages of positive tumor cells were semi-quantitatively and independently evaluated by 3 observers (SMW, PJvD and FKL) who were blinded to patient outcome. Stromal positive cells were evaluated separately in a likewise fashion. In case of disagreement, the observers reanalyzed the staining results until they reached consensus. To determine the score for each TMA-core, appropriate controls of normal squamous epithelium were used. Protein expression was scored for both its intensity in tumor cells relative to normal epithelium (strong expression = 2, normal expression = 1, no expression = 0) and the percentage of tumor cells in the tissue section with such a specific intensity. Multiplying of these two scoring variables resulted in a scoring range of 0 up to 200, in which a score of 0 represents a complete loss or no expression of protein in all tumor cells and a score of 200 represents a high expression throughout the tumor (Fig. 2a-d). Cores were considered lost if less than 10% of cells contained tumor ('sampling error') or when less than 10% of tissue was present ('absent core'). Cases were excluded if more than 2 cores were lost per case. When the scores between the cores of a particular case differed, the most frequent score determined the overall score. In case of 4 different scores in one case, the average score was calculated.

Statistical analysis

The non-parametric Mann-Whitney U test was used to determine differences in CTSK expression between various clinicopathologically defined groups. Logistic regression techniques were used to assess correlations between CTSK expression and the incidence of neck LNM. Overall survival (OS) was defined as the length of the time from surgery to death from any cause. Disease-specific survival (DSS) was defined as the time from surgery to death due to disease. Receiver operating characteristic (ROC) curves were designed to determine optimal cut-off values. The association between CTSK and the primary and secondary outcomes was analysed with crosstabs, chi-square test (or Fisher's Exact Test when appropriate), logistic

regression, Kaplan Meier/logrank survival analyses, and Cox-regression.

All p values were based on two-tailed statistical analysis and $p < 0.05$ was considered significant. Statistical analysis was performed using the SPSS 25.0 statistical package (IBM Corp. IBM SPSS Statistics for OSx, Version 25.0. Armonk, NY: IBM Corp).

Results

Gene expression and clinicopathological variables

A statistically significant association of high CTSK mRNA levels to lymphatic metastasis ($p < 0.01$) was observed, as wells as to vaso- and perineural invasion ($p < 0.01$ in both cases; Table 3). In contrast, no significant correlation was found to other pathological characteristics, such as pT status, depth of invasion and tumor grade.

Among the various clinical parameters, a strong correlation of increased gene expression was found only to alcohol consumption ($p < 0.01$). No significant relationship was found to smoking history, age, tumor subsite and clinical T or N stage.

CTSK gene expression and survival

A Cox regression analysis was performed in order to determine the prognostic significance of the CTSK gene expression. Dichotomization was based on the cut-off value of -0.26, determined by ROC analysis. Patients with high CTSK gene expression demonstrated a significantly worse 5-year DSS (HR = 2.29, CI: 1.01–5.21, $p = 0.047$; Table 4). The pathological N status was shown to have the strongest impact for DSS

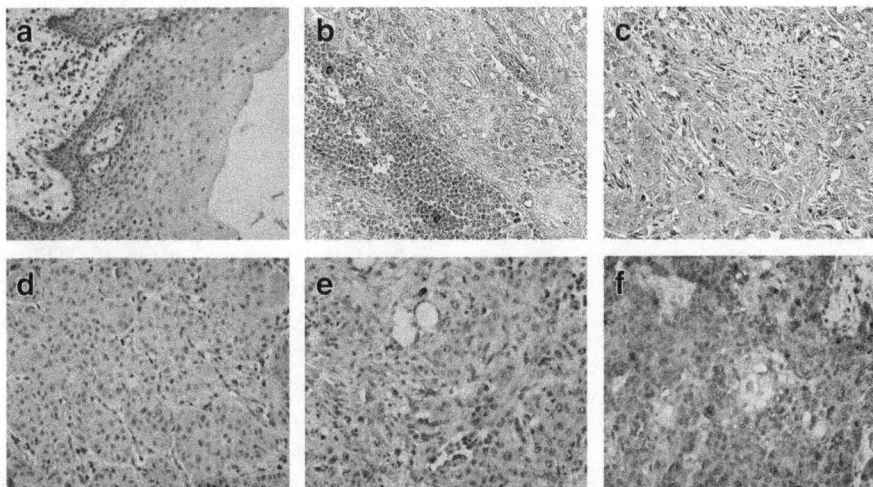

Fig. 2 CTSK expression in OSCC and normal mucosa. Representative stainings of the TMA, consisting of 83 OSCC cases, are presented. CTSK is diffusely expressed, is stained both in tumor as in stromal cells and varies in expression from non to strong expression. Staining scores were calculated by the product of intensity (normal = 1, strong = 2) and the proportion of stained tumor or stromal cells (%). Panels **a-f** represent examples of CTSK staining; **a**) normal mucosa, **b**) OSCC negative for CTSK in stromal cells, **c**) OSCC with normal staining in tumor cells and in stromal cells, **d**) OSCC negative for CTSK, **e**) OSCC with a normal intensity (score = 1 × 50% = 50), **f**) OSCC with a strong intensity (score = 2 × 75% = 150)

Table 3 Correlations between gene (mRNA) and protein (IHC) expression of CTSK and clinical and pathological parameters of the included OSCC cohort (n = 83)

		CTSK	
	mRNA	IHC tumor	IHC stroma
Clinical characteristic			
Smoking history	NS	NS	NS
Alcohol consumption	p < 0.01	NS	NS
Age	NS	NS	NS
cT status	NS	NS	NS
cN status	NS	NS	NS
Subsite	NS	NS	NS
Pathological characteristic			
pN-status	p < 0.01	p < 0.01	p < 0.01
pT-status	NS	NS	NS
Infiltration depth	NS	NS	NS
Differentiation grade	NS	NS	NS
Vaso-invasion	p < 0.01	NS	NS
Bone-invasion	NS	NS	NS
Peri-neural invasion	p < 0.01	p < 0.01	NS
Spidery growth	NS	NS	NS

Cases were stratified according to clinical and pathological characteristics. Smoking history was dichotomized to current smoker or ceased < 1 year versus ex-smoker (ceased > 1 year) and never smoker. Alcohol consumption was dichotomized to 1–4 or ≥ 5 U/day versus occasionally or never. Clinical and pathological nodal status (cN and pN) were dichotomized to cN0 versus cN+ and to pN0 versus pN+. Infiltration was dichotomized to < 4 mm versus ≥4 mm. Differentiation was dichotomized to well and moderate versus poor and undifferentiated. P-values represent the Mann-Whitney U test of these comparisons. IHC: immunohistochemistry; mRNA: messenger ribonucleic acid; NS: non-significant

Table 4 Univariate and multivariate DSS Cox regression model for gene and protein CTSK expression

	Univariate		
	HR	95% CI	p-value
Age[a]	1.01	0.48–2.12	0.978
Tumor stage[b]	4.01	1.21–13.29	0.023
pN[c]	4.10	1.66–10.15	0.002
CTSK protein expression (stroma)	2.40	1.05–5.50	0.038
CSTK protein expression (tumor)	2.79	1.02–7.64	0.045
CTSK gene expression	2.29	1.01–5.21	0.047
	Multivariate		
pN status	3.61	1.12–11.57	0.030
corrected for CTSK protein expression (tumor)			

Dichotomization was made according to the cut-off values into high and low expression. The most important prognostic parameters (age, stage and pN) were added in the regression model
[a] < 60 vs. ≥60 years; [b] I, II vs. III, IV; c pN0 vs. pN+

(HR = 4.10, CI:1.66–10.15, p = 0.002). The prognostic significance of CTSK gene expression did not hold for overall survival (OS) (p = 0.2). The Kaplan-Meier survival plot is shown in Fig. 3a (p = 0.040).

CTSK protein expression and clinicopathological variables
A total of 213 (64%) cores with tumor and 246 (74%) cores with stroma stained with the CTSK antibody were available for analysis. Due to our inclusion criteria (≥2 tumor cores available per case), 19 cases were missing. The majority of the OSCCs in this cohort showed a weak expression for CTSK (42% in tumor cells and 54% in stromal cells), whereas only 5% demonstrated no expression in tumor cells. All stromal samples showed some expression (Additional file 1: Table S1).

A cut-off value of 25 was determined by ROC analysis, in order to divide patients into low and high protein expression groups. No statistically significant correlation to clinical variables was found (Table 3). In contrast, there was a significant association with histopathologically proven LNM (p < 0.01) and increased CTSK expression in both tumor and stromal cells. A similar strong relationship to peri-neural invasion was also demonstrated (p = 0.01) for CTSK tumor cell expression. No association to other pathological variables was evident.

In logistic regression analysis, factors with known impact to nodal disease were incorporated into the model, including T stage, perineural and vaso-invasion, depth of infiltration and spidery growth pattern, along with CTSK protein expression in tumor and in stroma cells (Table 5). In univariate analysis, high CTSK expression (tumor and stroma) appeared to be an important independent predictive factor of lymph node involvement (tumor: OR = 7.65, CI: 2.51–23.32; p < 0.001 and stroma: OR = 4.04, CI: 1.57–10.36; p = 0.004). In multivariate analysis, CTSK protein expression (tumor), corrected for pathological T stage, remained a strong prognostic factor for regional disease, demonstrating an odds ratio of 9 (CI: 2.83–31.65; p < 0.01).

Next, the predictive value of CTSK as a biomarker of occult metastasis in early stage (cT1-T2 N0) OSCC was examined. A total of 24 patients had early T stage without clinically detectable nodal disease. Out of the ten patients with yet occult metastases in the neck dissection specimen, nine had a high protein CTSK expression, whereas only one patient showed a value lower than the cut-off (Table 6). The sensitivity of high protein expression in detecting occult metastasis in early stage OSCC was, thus, calculated at 90%, whereas the specificity was 57%. Additionally, the positive predictive value was found at 60%, with a negative predictive value of 89%.

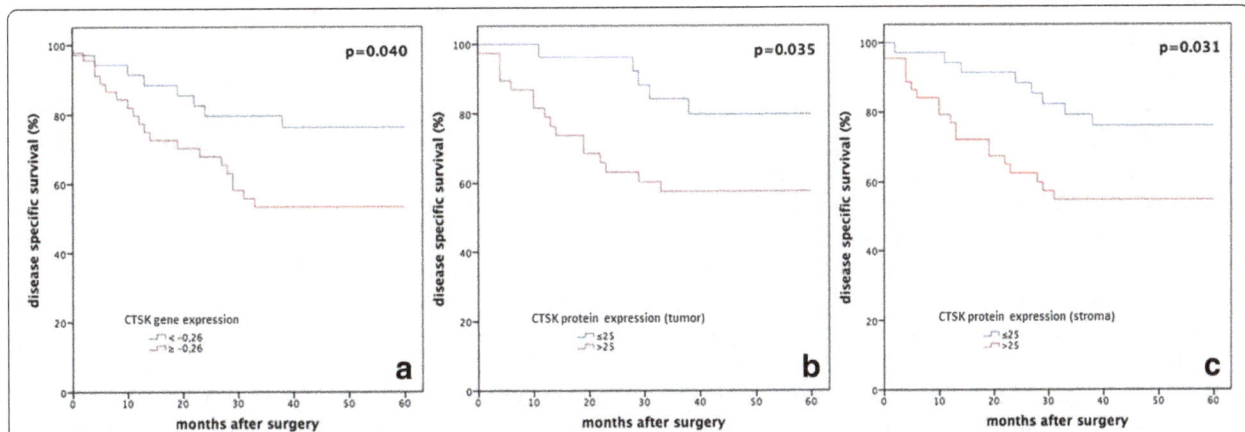

Fig. 3 Kaplan Meier disease specific survival (DSS) plots for all patients with OSCC (n = 83). Cases were stratified according to differential expression of CTSK, and were dichotomized into low and high expression according to the determined cut-off point in panel **a** for gene expression (− 0.26) and in panel **b** and **c** for protein expression (25). P-values in **a-c** represent the Log-rank test of this group comparison and therefore differ from the significance levels of the Cox-regression analysis in Table 4. In all three analyses, high CTSK expression was strongly associated with a worse 5-year DSS

CTSK protein expression and survival

In Cox regression, CTSK protein expression of tumor and stromal cells was dichotomized into low versus high based on the previously reported cut-off value, demonstrating a significantly worse DSS in OSCC subjects with increased CTSK protein expression (tumor: HR = 2.79, CI 1.02–7.64, $p = 0.045$ and stroma: HR = 2.40, CI 1.05–5.50, $p = 0.038$; Table 4). No prognostic impact on overall survival was found. The Kaplan-Meier survival plot is shown in Fig. 3b ($p = 0.035$, tumor) and in Fig. 3c ($p = 0.031$, stroma).

In multivariate analysis, pN status was corrected for CTSK protein expression (tumor), and pathological N

status showed once more a strong correlation (HR = 3.61, CI:1.12–11.57, p = 0.03), with a change though of the beta coefficient greater than 10%, confirming the role of CTSK as a significant confounder for DSS.

Discussion

Cancer metastasis is a complex process that includes a number of different events, referred as the invasion-metastasis cascade. The first critical step of the process is the invasion of the malignant cells into the surrounding extracellular matrix (ECM) and stromal cell layers [19]. The biological role of CTSK in promoting tumor invasion and migration has been proved ex vivo in cell-based systems [15, 16]. Apart from their well-known function of ECM degradation and remodeling, cathepsins are also suggested to participate in the activation cascade of pro-urokinase-type plasminogen activator and other proteases, enhancing thus their effect in the dissolution of the tumor matrix and basic membrane [20]. In addition to their extracellular function, there is evidence that intracellular cathepsins promote tumor progression by affecting processes acting both as pro-tumorigenic and anti-tumorigenic [21]. Intracellular

Table 5 Univariate and multivariate logistic regression model for CTSK protein expression and LNM

	Univariate		
	OR	95% CI	p-value
pT[a]	1.49	1.01 - 2.20	0.044
Peri-neural invasion[a]	5.20	1.87–14.45	0.002
Vaso-invasion[a]	9.71	2.06–45.89	0.004
Depth of invasion	1.51	0.85–2.69	0.165
Spidery growth	4.44	1.41–14.00	0.011
CTSK protein expression (stroma)	4.04	1.57–10.36	0.004
CTSK protein expression (tumor)	7.65	2.51–23.32	< 0.001
	Multivariate		
CTSK protein expression (tumor) corrected for pT-status	9.46	2.83–31.65	< 0.01

Dichotomization was made into low expression (score 0–25) versus high expression (score 26–200). The most important predictive parameters (pT, peri-neural invasion, vaso-invasion, depth of invasion, spidery growth) were added in the model

LNM = lymph node metastasis, OR = odds ratio, HR = hazard ratio, 95% CI = 95% confidence interval, p-value of the Cox regression model

[a]age: < 60 vs ≥ 60 years, tumor stage I, II vs III, IV, pN status pN0 vs pN+

Table 6 Allocation of cT1-T2 N0 patients based on their pathological N-status and CTSK protein expression

		pN status		Total
		pN0	pN+	
CTSK	≤25	8	1	9
	> 25	6	9	15
Total		14	10	24

The value of CTSK protein expression in predicting occult metastasis (≤25 predicts pN0, > 25 predicts pN+) in cT1-T2 N0 patients is calculated as follows: sensitivity (9/9 + 1) × 100% = 90%; specificity (8 + 6) × 100% =57%; positive predictive value (9/6 + 9) × 100% = 60%; negative predictive value (8/8 + 1) × 100% = 89%

collagen degradation is an example of the potential intracellular pro-tumorigenic activity of cathepsins.

The pathophysiological role of the cathepsins in cancer metastasis has attracted the interest of studying its value as a biomarker of metastasis and prognosis in various types of malignancy. Increased protein expression of cathepsins V, B and D has been associated with distant metastasis and worse DSS in breast cancer [22]. Similar results have been found for cathepsin A in malignant melanoma and cathepsin B in non-small cell lung carcinoma [23, 24] and in OSCC [11–14]. Overexpression of CTSK has been observed in invasive ductal carcinoma of the breast, lung and prostate adenocarcinoma [25–27]. In all these studies, increased protein expression was related to high metastatic potential. Interestingly, high expression of CTSK was found in the desmoplastic reactive stroma of the lung adenocarcinoma, indicating that stromal production of CTSK can favor or modulate the invasion of tumor cells [28]. In oral and oropharyngeal SCC, downregulation of the cognate inhibitor of CTSK [29], SERPINB13, was reported to be associated with LNM and poor prognosis [30]. However, only one study exists in the literature regarding the prognostic value of CTSK in tongue SCC [15]. In that study, Bitu et al. reported that CTSK was expressed in both stromal and tumor cells by immunohistochemistry. The only significant finding was that CTSK expression in stromal cells exhibited a potential protective role, since a poorer prognosis in early stage tumors was correlated to weak CTSK expression in the tumor microenvironment front. However, the same study found decreased invasion of HSC-3 tumor cells when cathepsin K silencing was applied. It was, thus, concluded that different prognosis could be exhibited, depending on whether CTSK is expressed more in tumor or stromal cells.

The present study is the first conducted to explore the predictive and prognostic value of CTSK in patients with OSCC. Combined evaluation of both gene and protein expression was used to augment the validity of clinicopathological correlations. Although some discrepancies were found in the associations with the clinicopathological parameters between gene and protein expression, the results are likewise. Some variation may be expected since mRNA levels are not directly proportional to the protein concentration due to post-translational mechanisms, that control protein turnover and abundance, and different translational rates, which are determined by constants that are not completely known [31]. Another factor could also be that gene expression data were acquired using biopsies taken at the border of the primary tumor and samples were included if they consisted of at least 50% tumor cells. The other part of the sample consisted of stromal cells and epithelial cells adjacent to the tumor. Consequently, gene expression was measured using tumor, stromal and epithelial cells, whereas protein expression was scored semi-quantitatively by immunoreactivity in tumor cells and in stromal cells separately. Finally, the semi-quantitative nature of immunoreactivity could cause a potential difficulty in accurate measurement of CTKS levels in paraffin tissue compared to the mRNA CTSK levels determined in fresh frozen biopsies. This could be another reason for the discrepancy between mRNA and protein data.

There are various explanations for the disagreement with the results reported by Bitu et al. Our findings show that CTSK expressed in either tumor cells or stroma cells correlates with a higher risk for lymph node metastases and a worse DSS. This corresponds with other reports on CTSK expression in different tumor entities [28] but is discrepant with Bitu et al. suggesting that stromal CTSK seems to have a protective role in the complex progression of tongue cancer. After scoring CTSK staining of both tumor cells and of the tumor micro environment (TME), Bitu determined staining gradients (TME: tumor) into higher, lower or no gradient. 'No gradient' can only be achieved if there is complete lack of TME staining. Next, they combined in the survival analyses 'no gradient' samples with 'higher gradient' samples to be compared with the 'lower gradient' samples which is biologically inappropriate, but explains their suggestion and the discrepancy. Although not reported, there were probably more 'no gradient' samples than 'higher gradient' samples combined and compared in the survival analyses with 'lower gradient' samples. Furthermore, the different scoring system as well as the different antibody clone used to detect cathepsin K could play a role. In the previous study, there is also insufficient information about the diagnostic approach to the lymph node status and incomplete pathological data, such as infiltration depth and perineural invasion, of the studied cohort. Lack of these data could underestimate the clinicopathological correlations. Third, the findings of the previous study were solely based on immunohistochemistry and were, partly, contradictory with the observation, reported by the same authors, of the diminished invasion potential of the HSC-3 tumor cells, when cathepsin K was silenced or inhibited.

The results of the current study suggest that CTSK may be used as a predictive biomarker in patients with OSCC. Its high sensitivity (90%) combined to the high negative predictive value (89%) makes it particularly valuable in excluding occult metastasis in early T1-2 N0 OSCC, allowing to perhaps rely on a "wait and see" policy for the management of the neck. Moreover, it is shown that tumors with up-regulation of CTSK harbored a high potential for perineural invasion. This can be interpreted by the proteolytic action on the nerves' epineurium and perineurium, facilitating tumor cell migration into the nerve fasciculus. Hence, CTSK can be a molecular determinant of perineural invasion, apart from the various neurotrophins and chemokines that are involved in this process [32]. The strong relationship of CTSK with both lymphatic spread and perineural invasion is also reflected by its significant impact on DSS.

The current study was based on a relatively limited cohort of 83 patients with OSCC. The results should be further validated by studies using different CTSK antibodies and including higher number of patients with emphasis on predicting occult metastasis in cases of N0 stage. Furthermore, serum levels of CTSK can be also evaluated at different stages of the disease and correlate them to clinicopathological variables. Important prognostic implications of elevated serum levels of cathepsins have been observed in other types of malignancies, such as in prostate cancer [33]. Finally, the emergence of new CTSK inhibitors, like odanacatib [16], can provide in the future a new tool for the suppression of tumor progression in patients with inoperable disease.

Conclusion

In conclusion, our findings provide evidence that increased CTSK expression is associated with lymphatic spread and poor prognosis of OSCC. Due to the high negative predictive value (89%) of CTSK protein expression, this biomarker can be a simple and useful tool in the diagnostic work-up of cT1-T2 N0 OSCC, however it should be validated first in a larger prospective cohort study.

Abbreviations
CI: Confidence interval; CTSK: Cathepsin K; DSS: Disease-specific survival; FFPE: Formalin-fixed, paraffin-embedded; HE: Hematoxylin and eosin; HPV: Human papilloma virus; HR: Hazard ratio; IHC: Immunohistochemistry; LNM: Lymph node metastasis; OR: Odds ratio; OS: Overall survival; OSCC: Oral squamous cell carcinoma; PCR: Polymerase chain reaction; ROC: Receiver operating characteristic; TMA: Tissue microarray

Acknowledgements
A special thanks to the technicians of the laboratory of pathology for their valuable help.

Funding
No funding was received for this study.

Authors' contributions
FKL and SMW planned and designed the study. FKL is the principal investigator and performed data analysis. MHF conducted the statistical analyses. FKL and EK wrote the manuscript. PJvD and RK critically reviewed the article. All authors read and approved the final manuscript.

Competing interests
The authors declare that they have no competing interests.

Author details
[1]Department of Head and Neck Oncology and Surgery, Netherlands Cancer Institute – Antoni van Leeuwenhoek, Plesmanlaan 121, 1066, CX, Amsterdam, The Netherlands. [2]Department of Oral and Maxillofacial Surgery, University Medical Centre Utrecht, Heidelberglaan 100, 3584, CX, Utrecht, The Netherlands. [3]Department of Pathology, University Medical Centre Utrecht, Heidelberglaan 100, 3584, CX, Utrecht, The Netherlands.

References
1. Jemal A, Bray F, Center MM, Ferlay J, Ward E, Forman D. Global cancer statistics. CA Cancer J Clin. 2011;61(2):69–90.
2. Sanderson RJ, Ironside JAD. Squamous cell carcinomas of the head and neck. BMJ. 2002;325(7368):822–7.
3. Leusink FK, van Es RJ, de Bree R, Baatenburg de Jong RJ, van Hooff SR, Holstege FC, et al. Novel diagnostic modalities for assessment of the clinically node-negative neck in oral squamous-cell carcinoma. Lancet Oncol. 2012;13(12):e554–61.
4. Roepman P, Wessels LF, Kettelarij N, Kemmeren P, Miles AJ, Lijnzaad P, et al. An expression profile for diagnosis of lymph node metastases from primary head and neck squamous cell carcinomas. Nat Genet. 2005;37(2):182–6.
5. Roepman P, Kemmeren P, Wessels LF, Slootweg PJ, Holstege FC. Multiple robust signatures for detecting lymph node metastasis in head and neck cancer. Cancer Res. 2006;66:2361–6.
6. van Hooff SR, Leusink FK, Roepman P, Baatenburg de Jong RJ, Speel EJ, van den Brekel MW, et al. Validation of a gene expression signature for assessment of lymph node metastasis in oral squamous cell carcinoma. J Clin Oncol. 2012;30(33):4104–10.
7. Turk V, Turk B, Turk D. Lysosomal cysteine proteases: facts and opportunities. EMBO J. 2001;20(17):4629–33.
8. Wen X, Yi LZ, Liu F, Wei JH, Xue Y. The role of cathepsin K in oral and maxillofacial disorders. Oral Dis. 2016;22:109–15.
9. Siponen M, Bitu CC, Al-Samadi A, Nieminen P, Salo T. Cathepsin K expression is increased in oral lichen planus. J Oral Pathol Med. 2016;45:758–65.
10. Turk V, Stoka V, Vasiljeva O, Renko M, Sun T, Turk B, et al. Cysteine cathepsins: from structure, function and regulation to new frontiers. Biochim Biophys Acta. 2012;1824(1):68–88.
11. Kawasaki G, Kato Y, Mizuno A. Cathepsin expression in oral squamous cell carcinoma: relationship with clinicopathological factors. Oral Surg Oral Med Oral Pathol Oral Radiol Endod. 2002;93:446–54.
12. Vigneswaran N, Zhao W, Dassanayake A, Muller S, Miller DM, Zacharias W. Variable expression of cathepsin B and D correlates with highly invasive and metastatic phenotype of oral cancer. Human Pathol. 2000;31:931–7.
13. Wickramasinghe NS, Nagaraj NS, Vigneswaran N, Zacharias W. Cathepsin B promotes both motility and invasiveness oral carcinoma cells. Arch Biochem Biophys. 2005;436:187–95.
14. Yang W-E, Ho C-C, Yang S-F, Lin S-H, Yeh K-T, Lin C-W, et al. Cathepsin B expression and the correlation with clinical aspects of oral squamous cell carcinoma. PLoS One. 2016;11(3):e0152165.
15. Bitu CC, Kauppila JH, Bufalino A, Nurmenniemi S, Teppo S, Keinänen M, et al. Cathepsin K is present in invasive oral tongue squamous cell carcinoma in vivo and in vitro. PLoS One. 2013;8(8):e70925.
16. Yamashita K, Iwatake M, Okamoto K, Yamada S-i, Umeda M, Tsukuba T. Cathepsin K modulates invasion, migration and adhesion of oral squamous cell carcinomas in vitro. Oral Dis. 2017;23:518–25.
17. Leusink FK, van Diest PJ, Frank MH, Broekhuizen R, Braunius W, van Hooff SR, et al. The Co-Expression of Kallikrein 5 and Kallikrein 7 Associates with Poor Survival in Non-HPV Oral Squamous-Cell Carcinoma. Pathobiology. 2015;82(2):58–67.
18. Psyrri A, Gouveris P, Vermorken JB. Human papillomavirus-related head and neck tumors: clinical and research implication. Curr Opin Oncol. 2009;21:201–5.
19. Valastyan S, Weinberg RA. Tumor metastasis: molecular insights and evolving paradigms. Cell. 2011;147(2):275–92.
20. Guo M, Mathieu PA, Linebaugh B, Sloane BF, Reiners JJ Jr. Phorbol ester activation of a proteolytic cascade capable of activating latent transforming growth factor-betaL a process initiated by the exocytosis of cathepsin B. J Biol Chem. 2002;277(17):14829–37.

21. Vasiljeva O, Turk B. Dual contrasting roles of cysteine cathepsins in cancer progression: apoptosis versus tumor invasion. Biochimie. 2008;90(2):380–6.
22. Sun T, Jiang D, Zhang L, Su Q, Mao W, Jiang C. Expression profile of cathepsins indicates the potential of cathepsins B and D as prognostic factors in breast cancer patients. Oncol Lett. 2016;11(1):575–83.
23. Kozlowski L, Wojtukiewicz MZ, Ostrowska H. Cathepsin a activity in primary and metastatic human melanocytic tumors. Arch Dermatol Res. 2000;292(2–3):68–71.
24. Chen Q, Fei J, Wu L, Jiang Z, Wu Y, Zheng Y, et al. Detection of cathepsin B, cathepsin L, cystatin C, urokinase plasminogen activator and urokinase plasminogen activator receptor in the sera of lung cancer patients. Oncol Lett. 2011;2(4):693–9.
25. Brubaker KD, Vessella RL, True LD, Thomas R, Corey E. Cathepsin K mRNA and protein expression in prostate cancer progression. J Bone Miner Res. 2003;18(2):222–30.
26. Littlewood-Evans AJ, Bilbe G, Bowler WB, Farley D, Wlodarski B, Kokubo T, et al. The osteoclast-associated protease cathepsin K is expressed in human breast carcinoma. Cancer Res. 1997;57(23):5386–90.
27. Cordes C, Bartling B, Simm A, Afar D, Lautenschläger C, Hansen G, et al. Simultaneous expression of Cathepsins B and K in pulmonary adenocarcinomas and squamous cell carcinomas predicts poor recurrence-free and overall survival. Lung Cancer. 2009;64(1):79–85.
28. Rapa I, Volante M, Cappia S, Rosas R, Scagliotti GV, Papotti M. Cathepsin K is selectively expressed in the stroma of lung adenocarcinoma but not in bronchioloalveolar carcinoma. A useful marker of invasive growth. Am J Clin Pathol. 2006;125(6):847–54.
29. Jayakumar A, Kang Y, Frederick MJ, Pak SC, Henderson Y, Holton PR, Mitsudo K, Silverman GA, EL-Naggar AK, Bromme D, Clayman GL. Inhibition of the cysteine proteinases cathepsins K and L by the serpin headpin (SERPINB13): a kinetic analysis. Arch Biochem Biophys. 2003;409:367–74.
30. de Koning PJ, Bovenschen N, Leusink FK, Broekhuizen R, Quadir R, van Gemert JT, et al. Downregulation of SERPINB13 expression in head and neck squamous cell carcinomas associates with poor clinical outcome. Int J Cancer. 2009;125(7):1542–50.
31. Schwanhäusser B, Busse D, Li N, Dittmar G, Schuchhardt J, Wolf J, et al. Global quantification of mammalian gene expression control. Nature. 2011;473(7347):337–42.
32. Marchesi F, Piemonti L, Mantovani A, Allavena P. Molecular mechanisms of perineural invasion, a forgotten pathway of dissemination and metastasis. Cytokine Growth Factor Rev. 2010;21(1):77–82.
33. Miyake H, Hara I, Eto H. Serum level of cathepsin B and its density in men with prostate cancer as novel markers of disease progression. Anticancer Res. 2004;24(4):2573–7.

19

Identification of novel enriched recurrent chimeric *COL7A1-UCN2* in human laryngeal cancer samples using deep sequencing

Ye Tao[1†], Neil Gross[2], Xiaojiao Fan[3†], Jianming Yang[4†], Maikun Teng[3], Xu Li[3], Guojun Li[2], Yang Zhang[1*] and Zhigang Huang[1*]

Abstract

Background: As hybrid RNAs, transcription-induced chimeras (TICs) may have tumor-promoting properties, and some specific chimeras have become important diagnostic markers and therapeutic targets for cancer.

Methods: We examined 23 paired laryngeal cancer (LC) tissues and adjacent normal mucous membrane tissue samples (ANMMTs). Three of these pairs were used for comparative transcriptomic analysis using high-throughput sequencing. Furthermore, we used real-time polymerase chain reaction (RT-PCR) for further validation in 20 samples. The Kaplan-Meier method and Cox regression model were used for the survival analysis.

Results: We identified 87 tumor-related TICs and found that *COL7A1-UCN2* had the highest frequency in LC tissues (13/23; 56.5%), whereas none of the ANMMTs were positive (0/23; $p < 0.0001$). *COL7A1-UCN2*, generated via alternative splicing in LC tissue cancer cells, had disrupted coding regions, but it down-regulated the mRNA expression of *COL7A1* and *UCN2*. Both *COL7A1* and *UCN2* were down-expressed in LC tissues as compared to their paired ANMMTs. The *COL7A1*:β-actin ratio in *COL7A1-UCN2*-positive LC samples was significantly lower than that in *COL7A1-UCN2*-negative samples ($p = 0.019$). Likewise, the *UCN2*:β-actin ratio was also decreased ($p = 0.21$). Furthermore, *COL7A1-UCN2* positivity was significantly associated with the overall survival of LC patients ($p = 0.032$; HR, 13.2 [95%CI, 1.2–149.5]).

Conclusion: LC cells were enriched in the recurrent chimera *COL7A1-UCN2*, which potentially affected cancer stem cell transition, promoted epithelial-mesenchymal transition in LC, and resulted in poorer prognoses.

Keywords: Laryngeal cancer, Transcription-induced chimera, Gene fusion, COL7A1, UCN2

Background

There were an estimated 26,400 new cases of and 3620 deaths from laryngeal cancer in China in 2015 [1]. Like other carcinomas of the respiratory system, carcinogen exposure via tobacco smoke causes DNA damage, and the accumulation of this DNA damage can alter genetic and epigenetic regulatory functions and thereby transform normal cells into cancer cells [2, 3]. This cell transformation usually takes multiple steps to complete, and it is affected by the sensitivity of the individual and the degree of damage [4]. This process is called tumorigenesis [5].

Tumorigenesis often presents with chromosomal and DNA abnormalities, and one common chromosomal rearrangement is gene fusion [6]. Some specific gene fusions have become important diagnostic markers of and therapeutic targets in cancer over the past several decades [7]. These chimeric products are often associated with neoplastic behavior [7, 8]. Typically, the *BCR-ABL1* fusion gene is rearranged via the t(8;14)(q24;q32) translocation in Burkitt lymphoma cells. This rearrangement is caused by this gene's juxtaposition with regulatory elements of the immunoglobulin heavy chain gene at 14q32, where the *MYC* gene is constitutively activated due to its expression, which is driven by immunoglobulin enhancers [7, 9]. Other fusion genes, including *PRCC-TFE3* in papillary renal cell carcinoma [10], *PAX8-PPARG* in follicular thyroid carcinoma [11], *FUS-CREB3L2* in soft

* Correspondence: zhangyangent@163.com; huangzhigang1963@sohu.com
†Equal contributors
1Department of Otolaryngology-Head and Neck Surgery, Key Laboratory of Otolaryngology Head and Neck Surgery, Beijing Tongren Hospital, Capital Medical University, Beijing 100730, China
Full list of author information is available at the end of the article

tissue sarcoma [12], and *TMPRSS2-ETS* in prostate cancer [13], have gradually been identified with various potential gene regulation mechanisms.

As in the fusion of two DNA genes, the two adjacent RNA genes, which are in the same orientation and are usually transcribed independently, are occasionally transcribed into a single fused RNA sequence. The various splicing mechanisms involved in such a transcription include RNA editing, alternative splicing (AS), *trans*-splicing, alternative transcription start sites, and alternative polyadenylation transcription termination sites [14–17]. This single fused RNA sequence is called a transcription-induced chimera (TIC) [14]. Unlike a single transcript that can be translated into various proteins in prokaryotes, TICs usually do not produce chimeric proteins or independent transcripts. Instead, they have tumor-promoting properties as hybrid RNAs [14]. For example, the expression of the chimeric transcript *HBx-LINE1* was associated with hepatocellular carcinoma development and correlated with poor survival [18]. Also, the chimeric transcript *SLC45A3-ELK4*, generated by *cis*-splicing between the adjacent *SLC45A3* and *ELK4* genes, did not involve DNA rearrangements or *trans*-splicing and could augment prostate cancer cell proliferation [19].

In comprehensively analyzing novel TICs in transcriptomes in LC cells using a paired-end strategy for RNA deep sequencing, we found that *COL7A1*-urocortin 2 (*UCN2*) is a novel TIC. We could not elucidate the intrinsic genetic and epigenetic mechanism responsible for *COL7A1-UCN2* generation; however, both the *COL7A1* and *UCN2* genes had explicit suppressor roles in tumor regulation, specifically the regulation of the epithelial-mesenchymal transition (EMT) [20–22]. Therefore, we hypothesized that *COL7A1-UCN2* may down-regulate the mRNA expression of both *COL7A1* and *UCN2* in LC tissues and that such down-regulation may promote tumor invasion via EMT regulation. Furthermore, we also speculate that *COL7A1-UCN2* generation can reflect the degree of DNA damages and that this TIC positivity may be associated with LC prognosis.

Methods

Patients and tissue samples

The Institutional Review Board approval for this laryngeal cancer research project (No. TRECKY 2009–33; Date: Jan, 2009) was obtained from the Beijing Tongren Hospital of Capital Medical University. A total of 23 patients who underwent surgery for pathologically confirmed LC from 2009 to 2016 were enrolled in this study. All patients received and signed a written informed consent. These patients had archived tumor specimens and data available, with a minimum of 36 months of cancer-free or censored-death follow-up after surgery. The follow up was completed through monitoring of their medical records or conducting

telephone interviews. To confirm the diagnosis, the tumors' histological classifications and differentiation were defined based on the 1999 World Health Organization's histological classification standards for LC. Tumor staging was carried out using the 2009 TNM staging criteria of the Union for International Cancer Control. Clinicopathological data were available for all 23 patients (Table 1).

All tumor samples contained more than 50% tumor cells and were stored at − 80 °C until use. Paired LC and adjacent normal mucous membrane tissue samples (ANMMTs) were obtained from the 23 patients. Paired samples from three male patients with T4N2aM0 disease and various degrees of differentiation (well, moderately, and poorly differentiated) who were 61–63 years old, smokers, and alcohol drinkers and had undergone total laryngectomy with selective bilateral neck dissection and

Table 1 Correlation of *COL7A1-UCN2* expression with LC clinical characteristics

Characteristics	Cases (%)	COL7A1-UCN2 mRNA expression		*p*
		mRNA positive (+) N, %	mRNA negative (−) N, %	
Age (years)				0.685
≥ 60	15 (65.2)	9 (39.1)	6 (26.1)	
< 60	8 (34.8)	4 (17.4)	4 (17.4)	
Gender				1.000
Male	20 (87.0)	11 (47.8)	9 (39.1)	
Female	3 (13.0)	2 (8.7)	1 (4.3)	
Tumor stage				0.221
I—II	8 (34.8)	3 (13.0)	5 (21.7)	
III—IV	15 (65.2)	10 (43.5)	5 (21.7)	
Differentiation				1.000
Well	4 (17.4)	2 (8.7)	2 (8.7)	
Moderate	16 (69.6)	9 (39.1)	7 (30.4)	
Poor	3 (13.0)	2 (8.7)	1 (4.3)	
LNM				0.685
N0	10 (43.5)	5 (15.6)	5 (15.6)	
N+	13 (56.5)	8 (34.8)	5 (15.6)	
Treatment				0.685
S only	8 (34.8)	4 (17.4)	4 (17.4)	
S + C/X	15 (65.2)	9 (39.1)	6 (26.1)	
Smoking				0.435
Ever	22 (95.7)	13 (56.5)	9 (39.1)	
Never	1 (4.3)	0 (0.00)	1 (4.3)	
Alcohol				1.000
Ever	21 (91.3)	12 (37.5)	9 (39.1)	
Never	2 (8.7)	1 (4.3)	1 (4.3)	

LNM lymph node metastasis, + positive, *C* chemotherapy, *X* radiation, *S* surgery without preoperative chemotherapy or radiotherapy were prepared for transcriptomic analysis. The paired samples from the remaining 20 patients were used to validate the TIC using real-time polymerase chain reaction (RT-PCR). Adjacent normal tissue samples were obtained at least 5 mm from the tumor margins [23].

Pathological review

Slides with hematoxylin and eosin staining were used to contain the paired frozen tumor and normal tissue sections. These slides were subjected to pathological examination twice to ensure that tumor tissues carrying high-density cancer foci (> 75%) were used and that the normal tissue samples had no tumor components. All samples were examined and reviewed by two pathologists independently, and disagreements between them were resolved via negotiation.

Preparation and sequencing of cDNA library

The total RNA was isolated from the fresh tissues using TRIzol reagent (Sigma-Aldrich, Missouri, St. Louis, US) according to the manufacturer's instructions. Poly(A) mRNA was isolated from the total RNA using beads containing oligo(dT). A fragmentation buffer was used to fragment the purified mRNA. Using these short mRNA fragments as templates, random hexamer primers were applied to synthesize first-strand cDNA. The fragmentation buffer, RNase H, and DNA polymerase I were used to synthesize the second-strand cDNA. Short double-stranded cDNA fragments were purified using a QIA quick PCR extraction kit (Qiagen, Hilden, Germany) and eluted with EB buffer for end repair and the addition of an "A" base. The short fragments were then ligated to Illumina sequencing adaptors (San Diego, CA, U.S.A.). DNA fragments of a selected size were gel--purified and amplified using PCR. The amplified library of fragments was sequenced using an Illumina HiSeq 4000 sequencing machine.

Raw read filtering

The images of the nucleotides generated by the Illumina HiSeq 4000 sequencing machine were converted into nucleotide sequences using a base-calling pipeline. The raw reads of the nucleotide sequences were saved in FASTQ format. The dirty raw reads were removed before the data analysis. Three removal criteria were used in filtering out dirty raw reads: 1) reads with sequence adapters, 2) reads with more than 2% "N" bases, and 3) low-quality reads. This ensured that clean reads were used for the subsequent mapping to the human genome and transcriptome.

Reads mapped to the human genome and transcriptome

The Burrows-Wheeler Aligner software program was used to map clean reads to a reference genome, and the Bowtie software program was used to map them to a reference gene. The expression level of each gene was measured via the number of specific fragment reads mapped per kilobase exon model per million reads (RPKM). The formula used for mapping is as follows: $RPKM = \frac{10^9 C}{NL}$. In this formula, C stands for the number of fragments specifically mapped to a given gene, N stands for the number of fragments specifically mapped to all genes, and L stands for the overall length of exons for the given gene. For genes with more than one alternative transcript, the longest transcript was chosen for the calculation of the RPKM. The RPKM calculation avoids the effect of differing gene lengths and sequencing discrepancies. Thus, the differences in the gene's expressions between samples were directly compared using the RPKM.

Differentially expressed gene analysis

Differentially expressed genes were identified in the tumor and matched normal tissue samples according to two criteria — a false-discovery rate no greater than 0.001 and a log2 ratio of at least 1. This approach was chosen based on the significance of digital gene expression profiles.

Fusion of human gene detection

During the read alignment of the short RNA and the reference genome, when the reads were divided into two fragments, only some of them could be aligned. Two-segment alignments could be read to the reference genome using the gene fusion-detection doctrines of the SOAPfuse software program, which can detect gene fusions using span and junction reads [24]. This basic method includes 1) comparing the reads to the reference genome alignment and the transcripts to the notes; 2) using the local genome library, which contains an exhaustive algorithm, to construct the fusion site sequence; and 3) retaining highly credible fusion transcripts using a series of filtering means. The requirements for the alignment detection of the divided reads were as follows: a length of at least 8 bp for the shorter read segment and an intron boundary within one of the three canonical bounds (GT-AG, GC-AG, and AT-AC). Regardless of where the intron was derived, the boundaries always should be the same. For the DNA positive strand, for both read segment alignments, a maximum of one mismatch and an unmapped alignment was required. Based on the information on the alignments of the two segments, gene fusion sites identified from the mapping of the human genome and transcriptome were retrieved using a Perl script. A fused gene certainly existed if the fusion site was located at the known exon boundaries of the two genes, with at least one paired-end read support-ing it [25–27].

Detection of alternative splicing (AS)

AS is a fundamental mechanism of the generation of transcript diversity. The base-calling pipeline used in this study to detect AS events in the transcriptome cDNA library consisted of two major steps. 1) SOAPsplice (Version 1.1) was used to map the reads to the human reference sequence and report the splice junctions according to the junction reads of the alignments [24]. With SOAPsplice, the default parameters were used as much as possible; three mismatches were set for intact alignments, and no more than one mismatch was set for splicing alignments. 2) Abased on AS mechanisms, both the junctions of splicing [e.g., known splice junctions ob-tained from the National Center for Biotechnology Information RefSeq database (Bethesda, MD, US)] and the results derived from the mapping were applied for the detection of the four basic AS events: the skipping of exons, sites of alternative 5′ splicing, sites of alternative 3′ splicing, and the retention of introns.

By detecting the four types of AS events, those that occurred in the tumors, rather than in the matched nor-mal tissue, were detected as specifically tumor-related AS events. The AS events that were detected in both LC and ANMMT samples were then filtered. Finally, for each sample, a list of highly reliable tumor-specific AS events was generated.

Validation of transcriptome cDNA library using RT-PCR

To determine the frequency of *COL7A1-UCN2* and *COL7A1* and *UCN2* mRNA expression, the other 20 paired LC and ANMMT samples were subjected to RT-PCR analysis. The primer sequences used for this RT-PCR are listed in Table 2.

For the cDNA of *COL7A1-UCN2* and *COL7A1*, the PCR conditions were 10 min at 95 °C, 30 cycles of 30 s at 95 °C, 30 s at 62 °C, 90 s at 72 °C, and 10 min at 72 ° C. For *UCN2* cDNA, the PCR conditions were 10 min at 95 °C, 30 cycles of 30 s at 95 °C, 30 s at 70 °C, 30 s at

Table 2 Primer sequences used for RT-PCR in the study

Primers	Sequences
COL7A1-UCN2	F: 5′-CGCCAAGAGATGAGTCAGCAC-3′
	R: 5′-GCACTCAGATCTGATATGACCTGC-3′
COL7A1	F:5′-CGCCAAGAGATGAGTCAGCAC-3′
	R:5′-CTCTGCAGGTAGGGCAGGGT-3′
UCN2	F:5′-ATGACCAGGTGTGCTCTGCTGTTGC-3′
	R: 5′-TCAGCAGTGGCCGACACG-3′
β-actin	F:5′-TTGCCGACAGGATGCAGAA-3′
	R:5′-GCCGATCCACACGGAGTACTT-3′

72 °C, and 10 min at 72 °C. β-actin was used as a loading control. The RT-PCR products were analyzed using gel electrophoresis.

Quantitative analysis of PCR products was carried out using a Rotor-Gene 3000 (Corbett Research, Sydney, Australia) and a commercially available SYBR Premix Ex Taq Perfect Real-Time Kit (Takara Biotechnology, Dalian, China), which were used according to the manu-facturer's instructions. The primer sequences used were those described above. The PCR conditions were 30 s at 95 °C, 40 cycles of 5 s at 95 °C, and 30 s at 60 °C. The data were analyzed using the $\Delta\Delta Ct$ method, and values were expressed as the fold difference from the house-keeping gene, β-actin.

Statistical analysis

Data were expressed as means ± standard deviation. Differences between the two groups were examined using Fisher's exact test (two-sided, $n < 40$) or a paired or unpaired Mann-Whitney U-test. The Kaplan-Meier method and Cox regression model were used to perform the overall survival analysis of the 23 patients, who were grouped according to their positivity or negativity for *COL7A1-UCN2*. *P*-values less than 0.05 were considered statistically significant. The data were analyzed using the SPSS 20.0 statistical software program (IBM Corporation, Armonk, NY, USA).

Results

Transcriptome sequences in human LC and ANMMT samples

We compared the transcriptome sequences in LC and paired normal tissue samples and identified a series of gene fusions and differentially expressed genes. The RNA sequencing data for the three pairs of LC and ANMMT samples subjected to transcriptomic analysis are listed in Table 3.

Landscapes of the TIC genome in LC tissues

In the comparative transcriptome analysis of the three paired LC and ANMMT samples with distinct patterns of tumor differentiation, we identified 87 TICs. We detected the novel chimeric transcript fusion *COL7A1-UCN2* in two of the three LC samples but not in their paired ANMMT samples. Also, we did find a coding frameshift in this TIC (Fig. 1 and Additional file 1: Figure S1; Table 4).

Both the *COL7A1* and *UCN2* genes are located at 3p21.3. In *COL7A1-UCN2*, *COL7A1* is located at exons 113–117 (from Chr. 3: 48602216 to Chr. 3: 48603724) and is 587 nt long. *UCN2* is located at exon 2 (from Chr. 3: 48600032 to Chr. 3:48600569) and is 538 nt long. In *COL7A1-UCN2*, the exon 2 sequence of *UCN2* was

Table 3 RNA sequencing data for three pairs of LC and ANMMT samples for transcriptomic analysis

Sample		Clean reads	Expressed genes	Expressed Transcripts		Chimeric Transcripts		Alternative splicing	SNP
ID	Tissue			Number	Novel- Transcripts	Number	COL7A1-UCN2 TIC	Number	
1	Tumor a	51,217,028	17,083	24,932	665	55	+	110,548	112,177
	Normal b	51,478,578	17,010	24,521	624	33	−	85,635	112,710
2	Tumor c	51,098,090	17,278	25,427	789	42	−	108,219	120,160
	Normal d	51,157,672	16,901	24,108	540	34	−	85,393	100,871
3	Tumor e	50,846,034	18,089	26,379	1194	32	+	105,866	134,840
	Normal f	51,363,004	17,590	25,339	1005	26	−	103,312	164,495

frameshifted during the transcript fusion process (Fig. 2).

COL7A1-UCN2 cDNA validation

In the 20 other tissue sample pairs, RT-PCR analysis revealed *COL7A1-UCN2* cDNA expression in eleven of the LC samples but no TIC transcripts in the ANMMT samples (Fig. 3a). Thus, in this study of 23 LC patients, we detected *COL7A1-UCN2* in 13 patients (57%), and a comparison of the positive TIC distribution in the LC and ANMMT samples demonstrated that positive LC samples were statistically significantly more common than positive ANMMT samples ($p < 0.0001$) (Fig. 3b).

Expression of COL7A1 and UCN2 mRNA

Among all 23 LC patients, the *COL7A1*:β-actin ratio in the ANMMT samples (12.61 ± 15.52) was significantly higher than that in the LC samples (5.99 ± 11.68; $p = 0.028$)

(Fig. 4a). Likewise, the *UCN2*:β-actin ratio in the ANMMT samples (17.02 ± 21.69) was significantly higher than that in the LC samples (7.34 ± 14.90; $p = 0.021$) (Fig. 4b). Furthermore, among all 23 LC tissues, the *COL7A1*:β-actin ratio in the *COL7A1-UCN2* TIC-positive samples (3.89 ± 8.56) was significantly lower than that in the *COL7A1-UCN2* TIC-negative samples (8.71 ± 14.87; $p = 0.019$) (Fig. 4c); likewise, the *UCN2*:β-actin ratio in *COL7A1-UCN2* TIC-positive samples (3.17 ± 2.62) was also lower than that in the *COL7A1-UCN2* TIC-negative samples (12.84 ± 21.85; $p = 0.21$) (Fig. 4d).

Disrupted coding regions of both COL7A1 and UCN2 in COL7A1-UCN2

We compared the DNA sequences in the recurrent hybrid *COL7A1* (rh*COL7A1*, the sequence of *COL7A1* in *COL7A1-UCN2*) and *COL7A1*. The rh*COL7A1* is located from exon 113 to exon 117 in a normal *COL7A1* gene

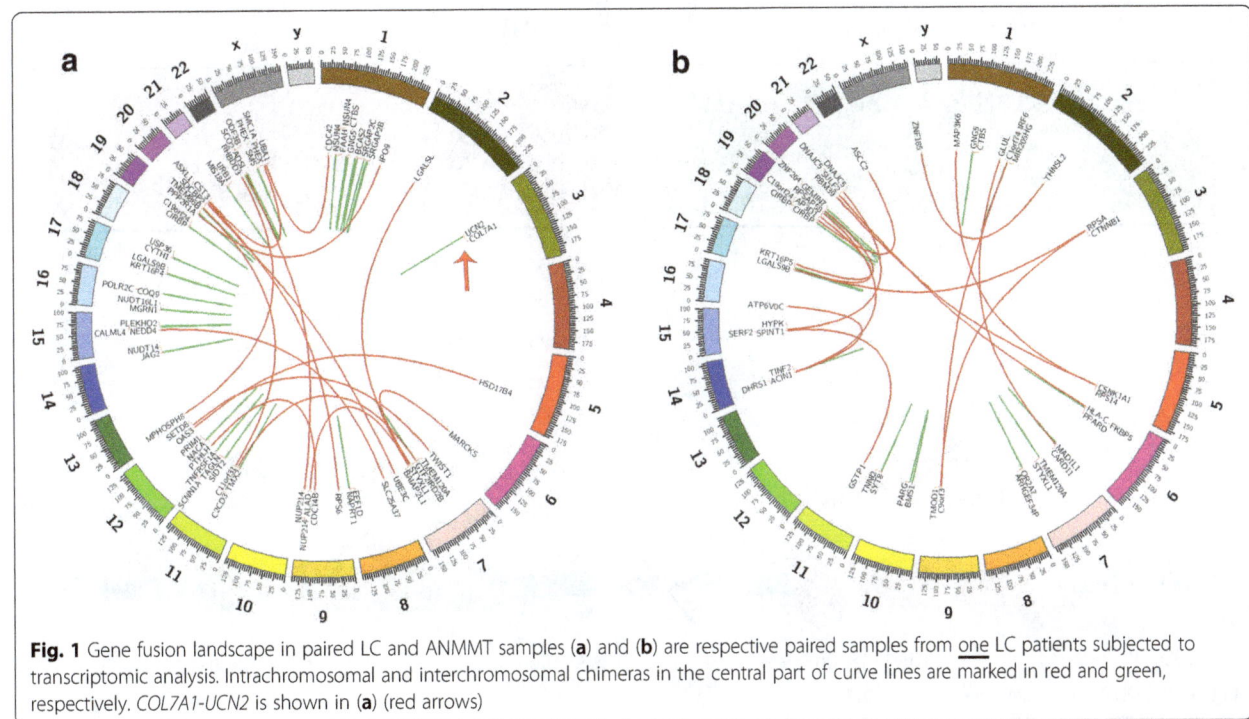

Fig. 1 Gene fusion landscape in paired LC and ANMMT samples (**a**) and (**b**) are respective paired samples from one LC patients subjected to transcriptomic analysis. Intrachromosomal and interchromosomal chimeras in the central part of curve lines are marked in red and green, respectively. *COL7A1-UCN2* is shown in (**a**) (red arrows)

Table 4 Selected chimeras (10 out of 87 total) identified in three LC samples subjected to transcriptomic analysis

Category	Up-stream Gene	Up-genome position	Down-stream Gene	Down-genome position	Frameshift
Interchromosomal	ALAD	chr9: 116149551	LAMTOR4	chr7: 99751605	NA
Interchromosomal	ARHGAP8	chr22: 45221411	NUP214	chr9: 134103680	frame-shift
Interchromosomal	ASXL1	chr20: 31024580	RPS6	chr9: 19378798	frame-shift
Interchromosomal	BAIAP2L1	chr7: 97984354	MARCKS	chr6: 114180859	frame-shift
Interchromosomal	C2CD3	chr11: 73840431	SMOX	chr20: 4101628	NA
Interchromosomal	CDC14B	chr9: 99284788	PTHLH	chr12: 28116703	frame-shift
Interchromosomal	PPP2R1A	chr19: 52714563	IPO9	chr1: 201827608	frame-shift
Interchromosomal	CST3	chr20: 23618257	UBE3C	chr7: 157060279	frame-shift
Interchromosomal	HSD17B4	chr5: 118809616	OAS3	chr12: 113410220	NA
Interchromosomal	KMT2E	chr7: 104654982	LGALSL	chr2: 64685419	frame-shift
Intrachromosomal	COL7A1	chr3: 48602216	UCN2	chr3: 48600569	frame-shift
Intrachromosomal	COQ9	chr16: 57494016	POLR2C	chr16: 57496472	frame-shift
Intrachromosomal	DENND2C	chr1: 115128157	BCAS2	chr1: 115124012	NA
intrachromosomal	EEF1D	chr8: 144661949	NAPRT1	chr8: 144660113	NA
Intrachromosomal	GBP3	chr1:89474630	CCBL2	chr1: 89435150	frame-shift
Intrachromosomal	HDGF	chr1: 156713444	MRPL24	chr1: 156711380	frame-shift
Intrachromosomal	KRT16P4	chr17: 18354079	LGALS9C	chr17:18387189	NA
Intrachromosomal	MAP2K5	chr15: 68065090	SKOR1	chr15: 68118274	frame-shift
Intrachromosomal	MGRN1	chr16: 4733933	NUDT16L1	chr16: 4744959	frame-shift
Intrachromosomal	NSUN4	chr1: 46826500	FAAH	chr1: 46867763	frame-shift
Intrachromosomal	NUDT14	chr14: 105642871	JAG2	chr14: 105624100	frame-shift
Intrachromosomal	ODF3B	chr22: 50968332	SCO2	chr22: 50962852	NA

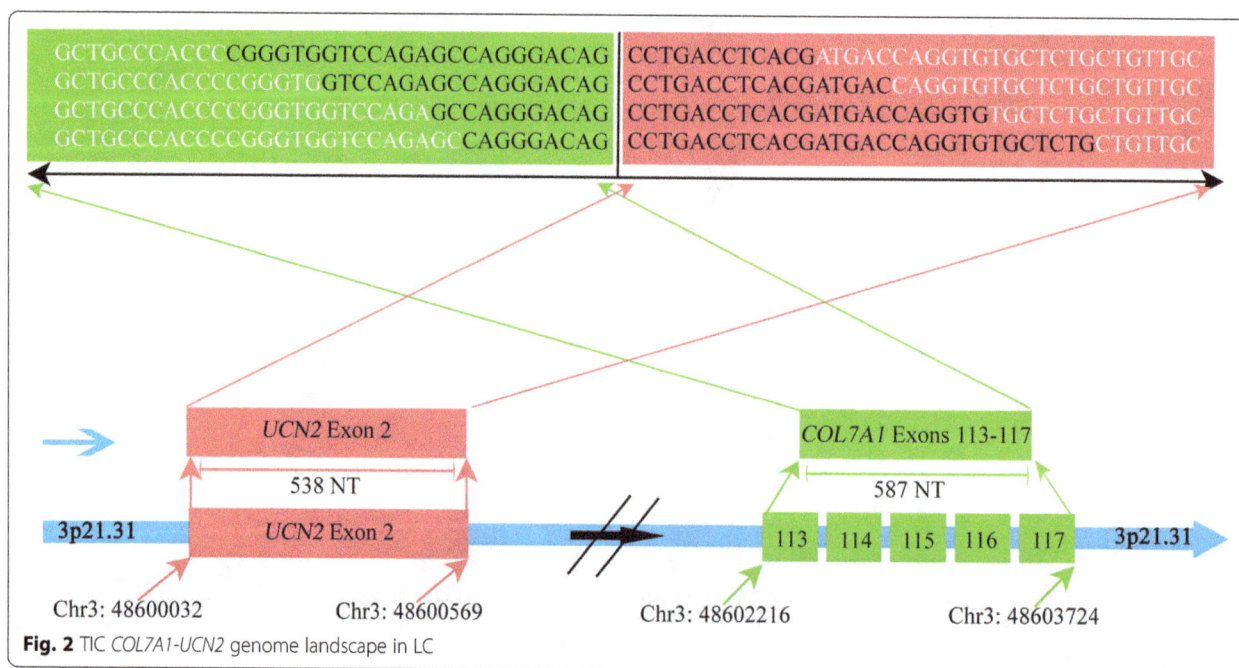

Fig. 2 TIC *COL7A1-UCN2* genome landscape in LC

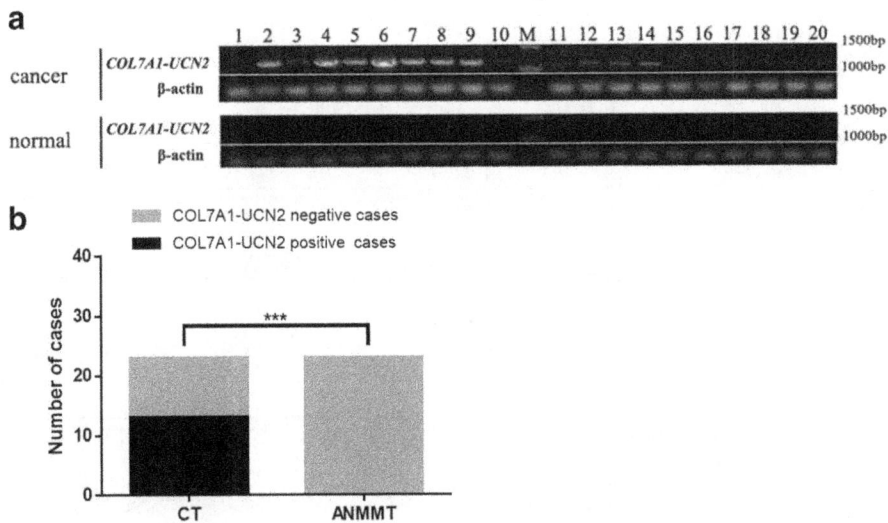

Fig. 3 RT-PCR validation of expression of TIC *COL7A1-UCN2* cDNA in LC and ANMMT samples

(Fig. 5a). <u>Besides,</u> the DNA sequences in recurrent hybrid *UCN2* (rh*UCN2*; the sequence of *UCN2* in *COL7A1-UCN2*) and *UCN2* were also compared. The rh*UCN2* was composed of reversed nucleotides 1–540 of exon 2 in a normal *UCN2* gene (Fig. 5b).

From the above, we found the *COL7A1-UCN2* cDNA sequence and its predicted amino acid sequence, in which AG (highlighted in yellow) represents the last two nucleotides of *COL7A1*, which may translate into S (a serine amino acid, also highlighted in yellow), the first nucleotide of *UCN2* (Fig. 6). Based on the above prediction, both the COL7A1 and UCN2 coding regions of *COL7A1-UCN2* were disrupted.

Effect of COL7A1-UCN2 expression on overall survival in patients with LC

A Kaplan-Meier analysis revealed that LC patients who were positive for *COL7A1-UCN2* had a significantly

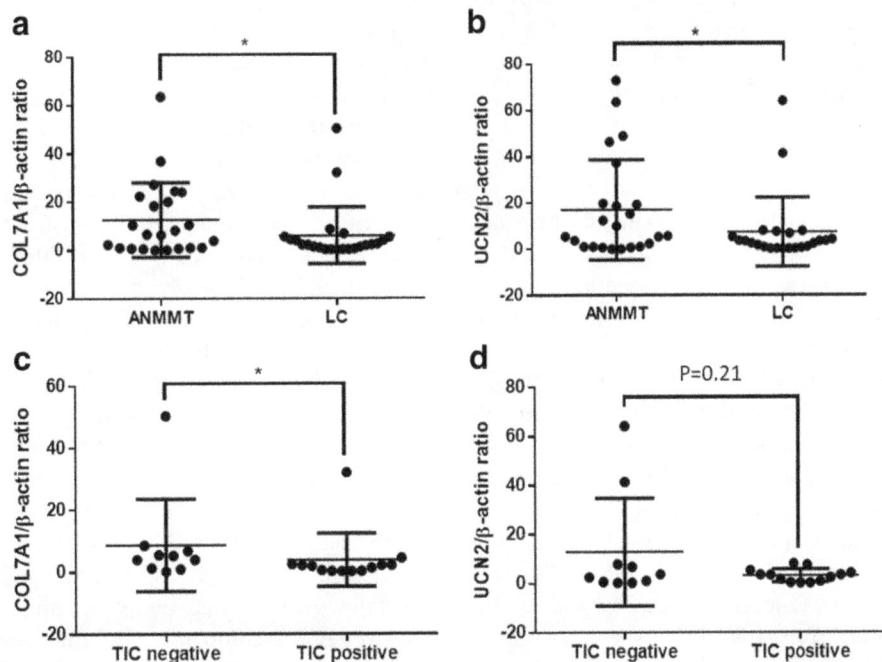

Fig. 4 Comparison of *COL7A1* and *UCN2* mRNA expression. LC, laryngeal cancer tissue; ANMMT, adjacent normal membrane mucous Tissue. (**a**) and (**b**) are comparison between LC and ANMMT samples; (**c**) and (**d**) are comparison between TIC *COL7A1-UCN2* negativity and positivity LC samples. *$p < 0.05$

a

rhCOL7A1 / COL7A1 (ex113-117)

b

rhUCN2 / UCN2 (ex2)

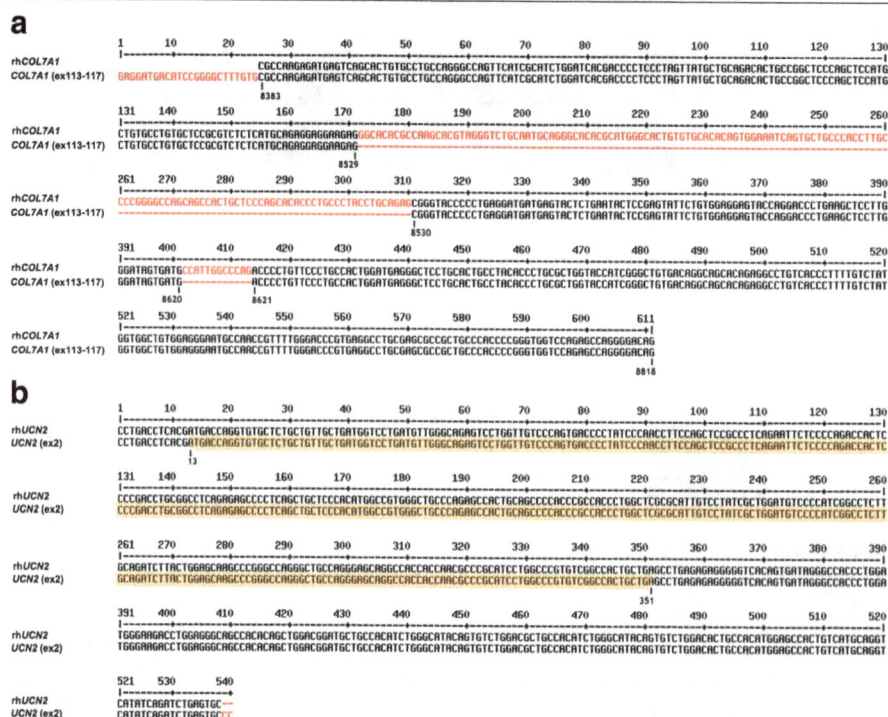

Fig. 5 Comparison of DNA sequences between recurrent-hybrid genes and normal genes. **a** Comparison of DNA sequences in recurrent-hybrid *COL7A1* (rh*COL7A1*; the sequence of *COL7A1* in *COL7A1-UCN2*) and *COL7A1* (from exon 113 to exon 117 in a normal *COL7A1* gene). 8383, 8529, 8530, 8620, 8621, and 8818 are the gene sequence numbers in the encoding protein sequence. **b** Comparison of DNA sequences in recurrent-hybrid *UCN2* (rh*UCN2*; the sequence of *UCN2* in *COL7A1-UCN2*) and *UCN2* (nucleotides 1–540 of exon 2 in a normal *UCN2* gene). The gene sequences encoding for the final protein sequences are highlighted in orange. The consensus and inconsistent sequences are shown in black and red, respectively

worse overall survival time than those patients who were negative did (*p* = 0.032 [log-rank test]) (Fig. 7). Multivariable analysis demonstrated a significant association between *COL7A1-UCN2* expression and overall survival (hazard ratio, 13.2 [95% confidence interval, 1.2–149.5]).

Discussion

High-throughput transcriptome sequencing provides sufficient information with which to identify candidate oncogenic mRNA chimeras. These chimeric isoforms are usually generated by AS, which is a fundamental mechanism of transcript diversity generation [26–31]. AS generated the TIC *COL7A1-UCN2* between neighboring genes, which is referred to as a read-through event [32]. In the present study, we found *COL7A1-UCN2* positivity in 13 of 23 LC samples, whereas all 23 paired ANMMT samples were negative. This TIC was generated via alternative splicing in the cells of LC tissues. Furthermore, those LC tissues with *COL7A1-UCN2* positivity had lower levels of *COL7A1* and *UCN2* mRNAs as compared to negative LC tissues. Therefore, this TIC potentially down-regulated the expression of the *COL7A1* and *UCN2* genes during and after chimera fusion; and it is thereby associated with poor clinical

prognosis because both *COL7A1* and *UCN2* possessed explicit suppressor roles in tumor EMT regulation.

In a previous study, low or nonexistent *COL7A1* expression was associated with the loss of the membrane basement, a specific extracellular matrix (ECM) component, and the promotion of the EMT process in cutaneous squamous cells (CSCCs) [33]. *COL7A1*-produced type VII collagen (ColVII) is the primary component of anchoring fibril protein, which constructs the membrane basement that separates the epithelium from the stroma in epithelial and mucous cells. Invasive epithelial-mucous tumors can be distinguished from benign and pre-invasive lesions by the consistent loss of the surrounding linear basement membrane in a wide variety tissues [33–39]. The breakdown of the basement membrane is a critical early step in EMT, in which oncogenic derivatives of epithelial stem cells are thought to act as intrinsic cancer stem cells that disrupt the basement membrane via the secretion of matrix metalloproteinases (MMPs) [33]. In CSCCs, tumor cells with *COL7A1* knockdown manifested increased migration and higher invasiveness, accompanied by the alteration of EMT marker expression (the decreased expression of E-cadherin and the increased expression of MMP2 and vimentin). Furthermore, ColVII knockdown can decrease

The cDNA sequence of *COL7A1-UCN2* chimera

CGCCAAGAGATGAGTCAGCACTGTGCCTGCCAGGGCCAGTTCATCGCATCTGGATCACGACCCCTCCCTAGT
TATGCTGCAGACACTGCCGGCTCCCAGCTCCATGCTGTGCCTGTGCTCCGCGTCTCTCATGCAGAGGAGGAA
GAGGGCACACGCCAAGCACGTAGGGTCTGCAATGCAGGGCACACGCATGGGCACTGTGTGCACACAGTG
GAAATCAGTGCTGCCCACCTTGCCCCGGGGCCAGCAGCCACTGCTCCCAGCACACCCTGCCCTACCTGCAG
AGCGGGTACCCCCTGAGGATGATGAGTACTCTGAATACTCCGAGTATTCTGTGGAGGAGTACCAGGACCCTG
AAGCTCCTTGGGATAGTGATGCCATTGGCCCAGACCCCTGTTCCCTGCCACTGGATGAGGGCTCCTGCACTG
CCTACACCCTGCGCTGGTACCATCGGGCTGTGACAGGCAGCACAGAGGCCTGTCACCCTTTTGTCTATGGTG
GCTGTGGAGGGAATGCCAACCGTTTTGGGACCCGTGAGGCCTGCGAGCGCCGCTGCCCACCCCGGGTGGT
CCAGAGCCAGGGGAC==AG==

CCTGACCTCACGATGACCAGGTGTGCTCTGCTGTTGCTGATGGTCCTGATGTTGGGCAGAGTCCTGGTTGTC
CCAGTGACCCCTATCCCAACCTTCCAGCTCCGCCCTCAGAATTCTCCCCAGACCACTCCCCGACCTGCGGCCT
CAGAGAGCCCCTCAGCTGCTCCCACATGGCCGTGGGCTGCCCAGAGCCACTGCAGCCCCCACCCGCCACCCT
GGCTCGCGCATTGTCCTATCGCTGGATGTCCCCATCGGCCTCTTGCAGATCTTACTGGAGCAAGCCCGGGCC
AGGGCTGCCAGGGAGCAGGCCACCACCAACGCCCGCATCCTGGCCCGTGTCGGCCACTGCTGAGCCTGAG
AGAGGGGGTCACAGTGATAGGGCCACCCTGGATGGGAAGACCTGGAGGGCAGCCACACAGCTGGACGGA
TGCTGCCACATCTGGGCATACAGTGTCTGGACGCTGCCACATCTGGGCATACAGTGTCTGGACACTGCCACA
TGGAGCCACTGTCATGCAGGTCATATCAGATCTGAGTGC   (1125 nts)

Predicted amino acid sequence

RQEMSQHCACQGQFIASGSRPLPSYAADTAGSQLHAVPVLRVSHAEEEEGTRQARRVCNAGHTHGHCVHTV
EISAAHLAPGPAATAPSTPCPTCRAGTP-G--VL-ILRVFCGGVPGP-SSLG--CHWPRPLFPATG-GLLHCLHPALVP
SGCDRQHRGLSPFCLWWLWRECQPFWDP-GLRAPLPTPGGPEPGD==S==LTSR-PGVLCCC-WS-CWAESWLSQ-
PLSQPSSSALRILPRPLPDLRPQRAPQLLPHGRGLPRATAAPPATLARALSYRWMSPSASCRSYWSKPGPGLPGS
RPPPTPASWPVSATAEPERGGHSDRATLDGKTWRAATQLDGCCHIWAYSVWTLPHLGIQCLDTATWSHCHAG
HIRSEC

Fig. 6 The *COL7A1-UCN2* cDNA sequence and its predicted amino acid sequence. AG (highlighted in yellow) represents the last two nucleotides of *COL7A1*, which may translate into S (Serine, also highlighted in yellow) with the first nucleotide of *UCN2*

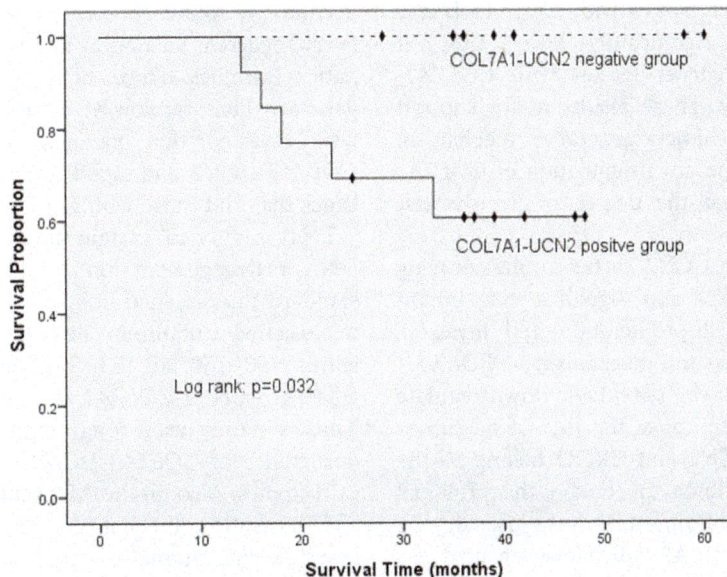

Fig. 7 Effect of *COL7A1-UCN2* expression on overall survival in patients positive and negative for this TIC

epithelial cancer cell differentiation and increase the expression of the chemokine ligand receptors CXCL10-CXCR3 and PLC-β4, which can further facilitate EMT and increase tumor invasion through an autocrine forward loop [22].

In our present study, COL7A1 mRNA levels were down-regulated in cancer tissues, and the COL7A1-UCN2 chimera generation mechanism circumvented TGF-β1's tumor-suppressive effects and thereby promoted tumor invasion and proliferation. TGF-β1 maintained normal tissue homeostasis and could both suppress and promote tumor proliferation in a time- and concentration-dependent manner [20, 40, 41]. Within this homeostasis, TGF-β1 broadly controlled the ECM, providing transcription regulation for the following genes: COL1A1, COL1A2, COL3A1, COL5A2, COL6A1, COL6A3, COL7A1, etc. The ECM is a dense latticework of collagen and elastin that serves as a selective macromolecular filter, it plays a role in mitogenesis and differentiation [42, 43]. Therefore, abnormal ECM homeostasis is a hallmark of cancer. It may be associated with the dysregulation of various collagens and increased tumor invasion because COL7A1-produced collagen VII is an essential component of various collagens [20, 43]. TGF-β1 can up-regulate collagen VII in tissues given normal homeostasis, a high concentration, and long-term exposure to TGF-β1 [42]. Collagen VII was found to be down-regulated in cancer tissues, and homeostasis was lost through epigenetic transcription regulation [44], canonical pathway inactivation in TGF-β1 (i.e., TGFR mutation) in cancer cells [45], or ECM alteration in the tumor microenvironment [46]. In our study, we found that cancer tissues had significantly decreased COL7A1 mRNA levels as compared to paired normal tissues, and we also found that cancer tissues with COL7A1-UCN2 chimera positivity had significantly lower COL7A1 mRNA levels than the cancer tissues with COL7A1-UCN2 chimera negativity. These results might support that the COL7A1-UCN2 chimera generation mechanism may be associated with the down-regulation of COL7A1 mRNA, which is reflected the degree of invasiveness found in tumor cells.

The activation of the UCN2/corticotropin-releasing factor receptor 2 (CRFR2) axis signaling can inhibit tumor vascularization, cell proliferation and invasion, and EMT [21, 47], whereas the mechanism of COL7A1-UCN2 chimera generation can potentially down-regulate UCN2 mRNA and thereby cause the loss of its tumor suppressor role. Both UCN2 and CRFR2 belong to the CRH family, which is known to contain the principal neuroendocrine regulators of stress response in the central nervous system [21, 47, 48]. However, previous studies found that the dysregulation of UCN2/CRFR2 signaling was associated with prostate cancer [49], non-

small cell lung carcinoma [50], colorectal cancer (CRC) [21], Lewis lung carcinoma (LLC) [47], and human adrenal and ovarian tumors [51]. Specifically, in vivo and in vitro studies found that UCN2/CRFR2 activation inhibited tumor vascularization and cell proliferation and invasion [21, 47]. Furthermore, in CRC cell lines, the blockage of the UCN2/CRFR2 axis promoted EMT (the altered expression of EMT marker, decreased vimentin, and increased E-cadherin and glycogen synthase kinase 3β expression) via persistent interleukin-6/Stat3 signaling (colonic inflammation regulation) [21].

The coding regions of both COL7A1 and UCN2 were disrupted or destroyed in COL7A1-UCN2, and this TIC did not encode a fusion protein. COL7A1 protein includes a Kunitz domain, the deactivation of which induces tumorigenesis [52]. In the rhCOL7A1 coding region, the Kunitz domain is the first 49 residues in the predicted amino acid sequence of COL7A1-UCN2, whereas the remaining 96 residues of the Kunitz domain may be disrupted by UCN2 sequence insertion. In the rhUCN2 coding region, UCN2 was frame-shifted, and a discontinuous sequence in the coding region may also disrupt normal UCN2 expression, although COL7A1-UCN2 includes the complete nucleotides for encoding UCN2 (13–351 nt; 112 amino acids) (Figs. 5 and 6). Therefore, in line with the results of a previous study [14], COL7A1-UCN2 produced no fusion proteins or independent transcripts.

The presence of COL7A1-UCN2 in LCs was not the result of stochastic processes. Instead, it was a reflection of DNA damage to a severe degree, and thus it may be associated with poor prognosis. First, we found COL7A1-UCN2 positivity in 13 of 23 LC samples, whereas all 23 paired ANMMT samples were negative. Second, we found consistent, precise RNA junctions in every recurrent validation in all COL7A1-UCN2-positive patient samples. Third, highly expressed genes did not generate TICs randomly. Fourth, a Kaplan-Meier analysis revealed that patients who were positive for COL7A1-UCN2 had significantly worse overall survival times than did those who were negative.

This study had certain limitations. To validate the DNA rearrangements in chromosomes, the use of a standard fluorescence in situ hybridization (FISH) assay necessitated a minimum distance between the two fused genes (100–150 kb) [53], but the distance between the adjacent ends of COL7A1 and UCN2 is less than 20 kb. Thus, we only used long-range RT-PCR to detect the occurrence of COL7A1-UCN2 cDNA expression in the LC samples. Also, in the AS events, whether the intrinsic TIC-generation mechanism occurs via cis-splicing or trans-splicing remains unknown [29]. Determining whether TICs function as noncoding RNAs or regulatory RNAs in cancer cell lines without protein participation requires further in vitro evidence. Finally, although our patient sample size was small and potential selection bias could exist, our findings on *COL7A1-UCN2* TIC may provide some novel information to help generate new hypothesis for our future study.

Conclusion

Our results indicated that the TIC *COL7A1-UCN2* is highly common and enriched in LC samples and that its expression may be associated with LC-cell transition, EMT promotion, and poor LC prognosis. Although its intrinsic generation mechanisms remain largely unknown, *COL7A1-UCN2* may serve as a diagnostic biomarker for early the detection of LC, as well as LC prognosis.

Abbreviations

ANMMT: Adjacent normal mucous membrane tissue; AS: Alternative splicing; ColVII: Type VII collagen; CRC: Colorectal cancer; CRFR2: Corticotropin-releasing factor receptor 2; ECM: Extracellular matrix; EMT: Epithelial-mesenchymal transition; FISH: Fluorescence in situ hybridization; LC: Laryngeal cancer; LLC: Lewis lung carcinoma; MMPs: Matrix metalloproteinases; RPKM: Reads per kilobase exon model per million reads; RT-PCR: Real-time polymerase chain reaction; TIC: Transcription-induced chimera; UCN2: Urocortin 2

Acknowledgments
None.

Funding
This work was supported by China National Science Foundation (Grant N0.81670946), which supported the design of the study and collection, analysis, and interpretation of data and in writing the manuscript. The funding body had no role in the design of the study and collection, analysis, and interpretation of data and in writing the manuscript.

Authors' contributions
YT, XF, JY, YZ and ZH carried out the majority of the experiment, data analysis, and wrote the manuscript. YT, XF, NG, JY, MT, XL, GL, YZ, and ZH made substantial contributions to conception and design, or acquisition of data, or analysis and interpretation of data. All authors reviewed and approved the final manuscript.

Competing interests
The authors declare that they have no competing interests.

Author details
[1]Department of Otolaryngology-Head and Neck Surgery, Key Laboratory of Otolaryngology Head and Neck Surgery, Beijing Tongren Hospital, Capital Medical University, Beijing 100730, China. [2]Department of Head and Neck Surgery, The University of Texas MD Anderson Cancer Center, Houston, TX 77030, USA. [3]Hefei National Laboratory for Physical Sciences at Microscale, Innovation Centre for Cell Signaling Network, School of Life Science, University of Science and Technology of China, Hefei, Anhui 230026, People's Republic of China. [4]Department of Otolaryngology-Head and Neck Surgery, the Second Affiliated Hospital of Anhui Medical University, Hefei 230601, China.

References

1. Chen W, Zheng R, Baade PD, Zhang S, Zeng H, Bray F, Jemal A, Yu XQ, He J. Cancer statistics in China, 2015. CA Cancer J Clin. 2016;66(2):115–32.
2. Teyssier JR. The chromosomal analysis of human solid tumors a triple challenge. Cancer Genet Cytogenet. 1989;37(1):103–25.
3. Brugere J, Guenel P, Leclerc A, Rodriguez J. Differential effects of tobacco and alcohol in cancer of the larynx, pharynx, and mouth. Cancer. 1986;57(2):391–5.
4. Incze J, Vaughan CW, Lui P, Strong MS, Kulapaditharom B. Premalignant changes in normal appearing epithelium in patients with squamous cell carcinoma of the upper aerodigestive tract. Am J Surg. 1982;144(4):401–5.
5. Shin DM, Kim J, Ro JY, Hittelman J, Roth JA, Hong WK, Hittelman WN. Activation of p53 gene expression in premalignant lesions during head and neck tumorigenesis. Cancer Res. 1994;54(2):321–6.
6. Soda M, Choi YL, Enomoto M, Takada S, Yamashita Y, Ishikawa S, Fujiwara S-I, Watanabe H, Kurashina K, Hatanaka H. Identification of the transforming EML4–ALK fusion gene in non-small-cell lung cancer. Nature. 2007; 448(7153):561–6.
7. Mitelman F, Johansson B, Mertens F. The impact of translocations and gene fusions on cancer causation. Nat Rev Cancer. 2007;7(4):233–45.
8. Mertens F, Antonescu CR, Mitelman F. Gene fusions in soft tissue tumors: recurrent and overlapping pathogenetic themes. Genes Chromosomes Cancer. 2016;55(4):291–310.
9. Dave SS, Fu K, Wright GW, Lam LT, Kluin P, Boerma E-J, Greiner TC, Weisenburger DD, Rosenwald A, Ott G. Molecular diagnosis of Burkitt's lymphoma. N Engl J Med. 2006;354(23):2431–42.
10. Sidhar SK, Clark J, Gill S, Hamoudi R, Crew AJ, Gwilliam R, Ross M, Linehan WM, Birdsall S, Shipley J. The t (X; 1)(p11. 2; q21. 2) translocation in papillary renal cell carcinoma fuses a novel gene PRCC to the TFE3 transcription factor gene. Hum Mol Genet. 1996;5(9):1333–8.
11. Kroll TG, Sarraf P, Pecciarini L, Chen C-J, Mueller E, Spiegelman BM, Fletcher JA. PAX8-PPARγ1 fusion in oncogene human thyroid carcinoma. Science. 2000;289(5483):1357–60.
12. Panagopoulos I, Tiziana Storlazzi C, Fletcher CD, Fletcher JA, Nascimento A, Domanski HA, Wejde J, Brosjö O, Rydholm A, Isaksson M. The chimeric FUS/CREB3l2 gene is specific for low-grade fibromyxoid sarcoma. Genes Chromosom Cancer. 2004;40(3):218–28.
13. Tomlins SA, Rhodes DR, Perner S, Dhanasekaran SM, Mehra R, Sun X-W, Varambally S, Cao X, Tchinda J, Kuefer R. Recurrent fusion of TMPRSS2 and ETS transcription factor genes in prostate cancer. Science. 2005; 310(5748):644–8.
14. Parra G, Reymond A, Dabbouseh N, Dermitzakis ET, Castelo R, Thomson TM, Antonarakis SE, Guigo R. Tandem chimerism as a means to increase protein complexity in the human genome. Genome Res. 2006;16(1):37–44.
15. Li H, Wang J, Mor G, Sklar J. A neoplastic gene fusion mimics trans-splicing of RNAs in normal human cells. Science. 2008;321(5894):1357–61.
16. Iyer MK, Chinnaiyan AM, Maher CA. ChimeraScan: a tool for identifying chimeric transcription in sequencing data. Bioinformatics. 2011;27(20):2903–4.
17. McPherson A, Hormozdiari F, Zayed A, Giuliany R, Ha G, Sun MG, Griffith M, Heravi Moussavi A, Senz J, Melnyk N, et al. deFuse: an algorithm for gene fusion discovery in tumor RNA-Seq data. PLoS Comput Biol. 2011;7(5):e1001138.
18. Lau C-C, Sun T, Ching AK, He M, Li J-W, Wong AM, Co NN, Chan AW, Li P-S, Lung RW. Viral-human chimeric transcript predisposes risk to liver cancer development and progression. Cancer Cell. 2014;25(3):335–49.
19. Zhang Y, Gong M, Yuan H, Park HG, Frierson HF, Li H. Chimeric transcript generated by cis-splicing of adjacent genes regulates prostate cancer cell proliferation. Cancer Discov. 2012;2(7):598–607.
20. Martins VL, Caley MP, Moore K, Szentpetery Z, Marsh ST, Murrell DF, Kim MH, Avari M, McGrath JA, Cerio R, et al. Suppression of TGF beta and Angiogenesis by type VII collagen in cutaneous SCC. J Natl Cancer Inst. 2016;108(1)
21. Rodriguez JA, Huerta-Yepez S, Law IK, Baay-Guzman GJ, Tirado-Rodriguez B, Hoffman JM, Iliopoulos D, Hommes DW, Verspaget HW, Chang L, et al. Diminished expression of CRHR2 in human colon cancer promotes tumor growth and EMT via persistent IL-6/Stat3 signaling. Cell Mol Gastroenterol Hepatol. 2015;1(6):610–30.
22. Martins VL, Vyas JJ, Chen M, Purdie K, Mein CA, South AP, Storey A, McGrath JA, O'Toole EA. Increased invasive behaviour in cutaneous squamous cell carcinoma with loss of basement-membrane type VII collagen. J Cell Sci. 2009;122(11):1788–99.

23. Furusaka T, Matuda H, Saito T, Katsura Y, Ikeda M. Long-term observations and salvage operations on patients with T2N0M0 squamous cell carcinoma of the glottic larynx treated with radiation therapy alone. Acta Otolaryngol. 2012;132(5):546–51.

24. Jia W, Qiu K, He M, Song P, Zhou Q, Zhou F, Yu Y, Zhu D, Nickerson ML, Wan S. SOAPfuse: an algorithm for identifying fusion transcripts from paired-end RNA-Seq data. Genome Biol. 2013;14(2):R12.

25. Ge H, Liu K, Juan T, Fang F, Newman M, Hoeck W. FusionMap: detecting fusion genes from next-generation sequencing data at base-pair resolution. Bioinformatics. 2011;27(14):1922–8.

26. Edgren H, Murumagi A, Kangaspeska S, Nicorici D, Hongisto V, Kleivi K, Rye IH, Nyberg S, Wolf M, Borresen-Dale AL, et al. Identification of fusion genes in breast cancer by paired-end RNA-sequencing. Genome Biol. 2011;12(1):R6.

27. Sbone A: FusionSeq: a modular framework for finding gene fusions by analyzing paired-end 2010.

28. Wang K, Singh D, Zeng Z, Coleman SJ, Huang Y, Savich GL, He X, Mieczkowski P, Grimm SA, Perou CM, et al. MapSplice: accurate mapping of RNA-seq reads for splice junction discovery. Nucleic Acids Res. 2010;38(18):e178.

29. Kannan K, Wang L, Wang J, Ittmann MM, Li W, Yen L. Recurrent chimeric RNAs enriched in human prostate cancer identified by deep sequencing. Proc Natl Acad Sci U S A. 2011;108(22):9172–7.

30. Zhao Q, Caballero OL, Levy S, Stevenson BJ, Iseli C, de Souza SJ, Galante PA, Busam D, Leversha MA, Chadalavada K, et al. Transcriptome-guided characterization of genomic rearrangements in a breast cancer cell line. Proc Natl Acad Sci U S A. 2009;106(6):1886–91.

31. Gingeras TR. Implications of chimaeric non-co-linear transcripts. Nature. 2009;461(7261):206–11.

32. Maher CA, Kumar-Sinha C, Cao X, Kalyana-Sundaram S, Han B, Jing X, Sam L, Barrette T, Palanisamy N, Chinnaiyan AM. Transcriptome sequencing to detect gene fusions in cancer. Nature. 2009;458(7234):97–101.

33. Horejs CM. Basement membrane fragments in the context of the epithelial-to-mesenchymal transition. Eur J Cell Biol. 2016;95:427–40.

34. Barsky SH, Rao NC, Restrepo C, Liotta LA. Immunocytochemical enhancement of basement membrane antigens by pepsin: applications in diagnostic pathology. Am J Clin Pathol. 1984;82(2):191–4.

35. Birembaut P, Caron Y, Adnet JJ, Foidart JM. Usefulness of basement membrane markers in tumoural pathology. J Pathol. 1985;145(4):283–96.

36. Gelse K. Collagens—structure, function, and biosynthesis. Adv Drug Deliv Rev. 2003;55(12):1531–46.

37. Pozzi A, Yurchenco PD, Iozzo RV. The nature and biology of basement membranes. Matrix Biol. 2017;57-58:1–11.

38. Uitto J, Christiano AM. Molecular genetics of the cutaneous basement membrane zone. Perspectives on epidermolysis bullosa and other blistering skin diseases. J Clin Invest. 1992;90(3):687–92.

39. Uitto J, Pulkkinen L. Molecular complexity of the cutaneous basement membrane zone. Mol Biol Rep. 1996;23(1):35–46.

40. Fuxe J, Vincent T, Garcia de Herreros A. Transcriptional crosstalk between TGF-beta and stem cell pathways in tumor cell invasion: role of EMT promoting Smad complexes. Cell Cycle. 2010;9(12):2363–74.

41. Knaup J, Gruber C, Krammer B, Ziegler V, Bauer J, Verwanger T. TGF beta-signaling in squamous cell carcinoma occurring in recessive dystrophic epidermolysis bullosa. Anal Cell Pathol. 2011;34(6):339–53.

42. Vindevoghel L, Kon A, Lechleider RJ, Uitto J, Roberts AB, Mauviel A. Smad-dependent transcriptional activation of human type VII collagen gene (COL7A1) promoter by transforming growth factor-beta. J Biol Chem. 1998;273(21):13053–7.

43. Verrecchia F, Chu M-L, Mauviel A. Identification of novel TGF-β/Smad gene targets in dermal fibroblasts using a combined cDNA microarray/promoter transactivation approach. J Biol Chem. 2001;276(20):17058–62.

44. Chernov AV, Strongin AY. Epigenetic regulation of matrix metalloproteinases and their collagen substrates in cancer. Biomol Concepts. 2011;2(3):135–47.

45. Massagué J. TGFβ in cancer. Cell. 2008;134(2):215–30.

46. Kessenbrock K, Plaks V, Werb Z. Matrix metalloproteinases: regulators of the tumor microenvironment. Cell. 2010;141(1):52–67.

47. Hao Z, Huang Y, Cleman J, Jovin IS, Vale WW, Bale TL, Giordano FJ. Urocortin2 inhibits tumor growth via effects on vascularization and cell proliferation. Proc Natl Acad Sci U S A. 2008;105(10):3939–44.

48. Reubi JC, Waser B, Vale W, Rivier J. Expression of CRF1 and CRF2 receptors in human cancers. J Clin Endocrinol Metab. 2003;88(7):3312–20.

49. Tezval H, Jurk S, Atschekzei F, Serth J, Kuczyk MA, Merseburger AS. The involvement of altered corticotropin releasing factor receptor 2 expression in prostate cancer due to alteration of anti-angiogenic signaling pathways. Prostate. 2009;69(4):443–8.

50. Wang J, Jin L, Chen J, Li S. Activation of corticotropin-releasing factor receptor 2 inhibits the growth of human small cell lung carcinoma cells. Cancer Investig. 2009;28(2):146–55.

51. Suda T, Tomori N, Yajima F, Odagiri E, Demura H, Shizume K. Characterization of immunoreactive corticotropin and corticotropin-releasing factor in human adrenal and ovarian tumours. Acta Endocrinol. 1986;111(4):546–52.

52. Ranasinghe S, McManus DP. Structure and function of invertebrate Kunitz serine protease inhibitors. Dev Comp Immunol. 2013;39(3):219–27.

53. Rickman DS, Pflueger D, Moss B, VanDoren VE, Chen CX, de la Taille A, Kuefer R, Tewari AK, Setlur SR, Demichelis F. SLC45A3-ELK4 is a novel and frequent erythroblast transformation–specific fusion transcript in prostate cancer. Cancer Res. 2009;69(7):2734–8.

20

Pretreatment neutrophil to lymphocyte ratio in determining the prognosis of head and neck cancer

Yalian Yu[1], Hongbo Wang[2], Aihui Yan[1], Hailong Wang[3], Xinyao Li[1], Jiangtao Liu[4] and Wei Li[1*]

Abstract

Background: Recent studies have reported a relationship between prognosis and neutrophil-to-lymphocyte ratio (NLR) in patients with head and neck cancer (HNC). As the results are still controversial, we conducted a meta-analysis of pretreatment NLR in peripheral blood and prognosis in HNC patients.

Methods: We retrieved articles from PubMed, Medline, Cochrane Library, Embase and Web of Science. A comparative analysis was conducted for the effect of pretreatment NLR in peripheral blood on overall survival (OS), progression-free survival, disease-free survival (DFS), disease-specific survival, metastasis-free survival, and recurrence-free survival of HNC patients. The analysis applied the criteria for systematic reviews described in the Cochrane Handbook and was conducted using hazard ratios (HRs) to estimate effect size, and calculated by Stata/SE version 13.0.

Results: The meta-analysis included eligible cohort studies (5475 cases). The OS data indicated increased mortality risk in HNC patients with a high NLR (HR = 1.84, 95% confidence interval (CI): 1.53–2.23; $P < 0.001$; heterogeneity, $I^2 = 37.2\%$, $P = 0.074$). Analysis of subgroups stratified by NLR cutoff values revealed increased mortality risk and significantly shorter DFS in patients with high NLR compared to those with low NLR (HR = 2.18, 95% CI: 1.46–3.24; $P < 0.001$). Patients with high NLR had a higher probability of tumor recurrence after treatment than those with low NLR (HR = 1.63, 95% CI: 1.09–2.45; $P = 0.017$; heterogeneity, $I^2 = 68.7\%$; $P = 0.022$). The probability of distant metastasis following treatment was greater in patients with high compared with low NLR (HR = 1.92, 95% CI: 1.36–2.72; $P < 0.001$; heterogeneity, $I^2 = 0.0\%$; $P = 0.614$). Funnel plots of the meta-analysis results were stable, as shown by sensitivity analysis. No publication bias was detected by the Egger test ($P = 0.135$).

Conclusions: HNC patients with elevated pretreatment NLR in peripheral blood have poor prognosis and are prone to local invasion and distant metastasis. NLR values are easily obtained from routinely collected blood samples and could assist clinicians to determine prognosis of HNC patients.

Keywords: Head and neck cancer, Neutrophil-to-lymphocyte ratio, Prognosis, Meta-analysis

Background

Head and neck cancer (HNC) is currently the fifth most common malignancy worldwide, with > 600,000 new cases and > 300,000 deaths annually [1, 2]. Despite effective surgical interventions and adjuvant therapy, the 5-year HNC survival rate of nearly 50% is still lower than that of most other cancers [3]. HNC originates in the mucosal epithelium of the oropharynx, nasopharynx, nasal and paranasal sinuses, larynx and hypopharynx. Many patients are diagnosed with HNC at an advanced stage. Data from the United States show that more than two-thirds of HNC patients present with lymph node invasion or distant metastasis at the time of diagnosis. More than half the patients need more surgery or radiotherapy because of recurrence within 2 years of initial surgery [4]. Therefore, simple, effective and economically feasible laboratory indices that can predict increased risk of recurrence, metastasis or death in HNC patients are essential for early diagnosis and improved survival in clinical practice.

* Correspondence: wli@mail.cmu.edu.cn
[1]Department of Otorhinolaryngology, the First Affiliated Hospital of China Medical University, Shenyang, Liaoning Province, People's Republic of China
Full list of author information is available at the end of the article

Awareness of the presence of inflammation in the tumor microenvironment has spurred research on the relationship between inflammation and malignancy [5–10]. The progression of cancer requires interactions between tumor cells and their microenvironment, including inflammatory, immune and metabolic responses to stimuli from the surrounding tissue. The systemic inflammatory response plays a key role in tumor cell invasion by promoting microvascular regeneration, tumor metastasis, and tumor cell proliferation [8, 9, 11]. Moreover, the systemic inflammatory response facilitates the differentiation of tumor cells and suppresses activity of host immune cells [6, 12–14]. Neutrophil-to-lymphocyte ratio (NLR) is an accurate and reliable index of systemic inflammation. NLR is closely associated with prognosis of solid tumors, such as colorectal, non-small cell lung, stomach and prostate cancer [15–19]. However, the association of NLR and prognosis of HNC remains controversial. For that reason, we conducted this meta-analysis of the prognostic value of NLR in HNC.

Methods
Literature search strategy
A systematic research was performed according to the Preferred Reporting Items for Systematic Reviews and Meta-Analysis (PRISMA) guidelines [20]. The research of PubMed, Embase, Cochrane Library and Web of Science identified relevant studies published in English or Chinese up to June 2016. The search strings included "head and neck cancer", "head and neck carcinoma", "head and neck neoplasms", "neutrophil-to-lymphocyte ratio", "neutrophils", "lymphocytes", and "NLR". Manual searches of reference lists in articles retrieved online were conducted to identify additional relevant studies.

Literature inclusion and exclusion criteria
Articles were included following independent searches by two of the authors (YY and XL). Disagreements were resolved by discussion or intervention by a third researcher (HW). To be included, a study had to report findings on the association between prognosis in head and neck tumors and NLR in peripheral blood before therapeutic intervention. The interventions included surgical resection, radiotherapy, chemotherapy, or combined therapy. Prognosis-related survival data included hazard ratio (HR) with 95% confidence intervals (CIs), or curves of overall survival (OS), progression-free survival (PFS), disease-free survival (DFS), disease-specific survival (DSS), metastasis-free survival (MFS), or recurrence-free survival (RFS). Studies were excluded using the criteria of the Cochrane Nonrandomized Studies Methods Group [21]. Duplicate reports and duplicate cases (with multiple reports of the same study, the most recent publication was selected), and case reports were excluded. We also excluded articles without available full text; articles with incomplete survival data that could

not be obtained following communication with the authors; literature reviews; and conference abstracts that lacked sufficient data for meta-analysis quality assessment.

Data extraction
We extracted data indicating country or region, author, title, year of publication, journal name, postal or e-mail address, type of research, sample size, age, gender, intervention measure, tumor type, AJCC or UICC cancer stage, lesion site, duration of or lost to follow-up, HR and 95% CI, and NLR cutoff value used to define OS, PFS and DFS. For studies that lacked complete data, the results of multivariate analysis were preferable to those of univariate analysis, but in the absence of multivariate analysis, univariate analysis was accepted. If HRs were not presented, they were calculated from the survival curve data as described by Tierney et al. [22].

Assessment of included studies
There are no criteria for evaluation of treatment described in prognostic cohort studies included in systematic reviews. Consequently, each study was assessed by two researchers (YY and XL) following the Newcastle–Ottawa Scale (NOS) for assessing the quality of cohort studies [23]. The maximum NOS score is 9 points, and studies with scores > 5 points were classified as high quality. Disagreements were resolved by discussion with a third researcher (HW).

Statistical analysis
Data analysis and processing were carried out using Stata/SE version 13.0 (StataCorp LP, College Station, TX, USA) provided by the Cochrane Collaboration. Disagreements were resolved through discussion. OS, PFS and DFS were evaluated using HR and 95% CI to describe the size of the treatment effect. χ^2 tests were conducted at $\alpha = 0.05$, with $P < 0.1$ as significant. The measure of heterogeneity was I^2, and < 25% indicated low heterogeneity, 25–50% indicated moderate heterogeneity, and > 50% indicated high heterogeneity. A fixed effects model was used for studies without heterogeneity, and a random effects model was used for studies with heterogeneity. Meanwhile, subgroup analysis and meta-regression methods were used for heterogeneity analysis. Publication bias was assessed by the Egger test using Stata/SE version 13.0, and the results are shown in funnel plots. Sensitivity analysis was conducted by the meta-trim method.

Results
Included studies and quality assessment
A total of 122 relevant studies were retrieved; 98 of which were excluded at the initial assessment of titles and abstracts, and the full-text of the remaining 24 was further screened. Nineteen eligible nonrandomized studies

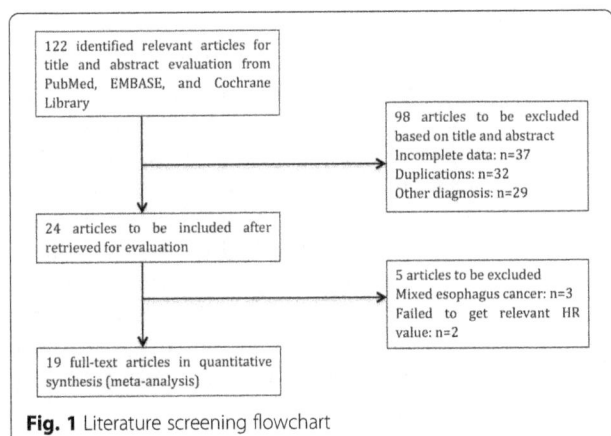

Fig. 1 Literature screening flowchart

[24–42], all of which were cohort studies and included a total of 5475 patients, were included in the analysis. A flowchart of the inclusion and exclusion criteria of each study is shown in Fig. 1. Two researchers agreed on the 19 studies that were finally selected. All studies included patients with pretreatment NLR and survival data, and the study data and quality assessment results of each study are summarized in Table 1. The Cox regression hazard

model used to adjust for potential confounding bias included the majority but not all of the included studies. If multivariate analysis of survival data was unavailable, univariate analysis was adopted for assessment of the survival data. The HNC tumor sites included the mouth, nasal and paranasal sinuses, nasopharynx, larynx and hypopharynx.

OS of HNC patients and subgroup analysis by NLR cutoff value

Fourteen studies were included in the meta-analysis of OS. The mortality risk of patients with high NLR was 1.84 times that of patients with low NLR. The difference was significant (HR = 1.84, 95% CI: 1.53–2.23; $P < 0.001$; heterogeneity, $I^2 = 37.2\%$, $P = 0.074$; Fig. 2a). Subgroup analysis by NLR cutoff value revealed a higher mortality risk in patients with high NLR compared to those with low NLR. The difference reached significance (2.1 < cutoff < 3, HR = 1.71, 95% CI: 1.34–2.17, $P < 0.001$; heterogeneity, $I^2 = 47.6\%$, $P = 0.064$; 3 ≤ cutoff < 4, HR = 1.94, 95% CI: 1.235–3.064, $P = 0.005$; heterogeneity, $I^2 = 18.3\%$, $P = 0.294$; cutoff ≥4, HR = 2.414, 95% CI: 1.696–3.436, $P < 0.001$, heterogeneity: $I^2 = 0.0\%$, $P = 0.675$; Fig. 2b). In the subgroup-

Table 1 Characteristics and quality assessment results for each included publications

Study	Country	Ethnicity	Tumors	Patients(female/male)	Age(range)	Result	Follow-up (month)	Uni\Multi	Cutoff value	NOS Score
Sun et al, 2016 [24]	China	Asian	NC	251 (71\180)	46 (15-76)	OS PFS	50 (5-84)	Multi	2.6	8
Wong et al, 2015 [25]	UK	Caucasian	LSCC	140 (19\121)	66 (36-92)	OS DFS	41 (2-103)	Multi	3.1	8
Fu et al, 2016 [26]	China	Asian	LSCC	420 (7\413)	60 (33-84)	OS CSS	ungiven	Multi	2.59	7
An et al, 2011 [27]	China	Asian	NC	363 (89\274)	47 (12-76)	DSS MFS	62 (2-92)	Multi	3.73	7
Li et al, 2015 [28]	China	Asian	NC	363 (89\274)	47 (12-76)	DSS	14.7 (3.22-92.9)	Multi	2.81	8
He et al, 2012 [29]	China	Asian	NC	1410 (383\1027)	46.1 (13-79)	OS PFS	41 (2-60)	Multi	2.74	7
Fang et al, 2013 [30]	China	Asian	OCSCC	226 (19\207)	52.47 (27.0-84.0)	OS DFS	ungiven	Uni	2.44	6
Nakahira et al, 2016 [31]	Japan	Asian	NS	100 (14\86)	65.2 (37-85)	CSS	37.85 (4-92)	Multi	3	8
Perisanidis et al, 2013 [32]	Austria	Caucasian	OCSCC	97 (30\67)	ungiven	DSS	> 5 years or until death	Multi	1.9	7
Charles et al, 2016 [33]	Australia	Caucasian	HNSCC	145 (30\115)	63 (23-86)	OS RFS	29 (1.5-84)	Multi	5	8
Tu et al, 2015 [34]	China	Asian	LSCC	141 (4\137)	59 (36-87)	OS DFS	51 (5-102)	Multi	2.17	7
Moon et al, 2016 [35]	Korea	Asian	HNSCC	153 (24\129)	57 (16-78)	OS PFS CSS	39.5 (4.7-62.6)	Multi	3.3	8
Rachidi et al, 2016 [36]	America	Caucasian	HNSCC	543 (123\420)	58.8	OS	64.4 (2-156)	Multi	4.39	8
Song et al, 2015 [37]	China	Asian	HSCC	146 (10\136)	57.5 (34-89)	OS	33.2 (2-128)	Uni	2.3	7
Salim et al, 2015 [38]	Turkey	Caucasian	HNSCC	79 (8\71)	59 (28-85)	OS	ungiven	Uni	2.93	6
Haddad et al, 2015 [39]	Australia	Caucasian	HNC	46 (8\38)	59 (43-81)	OS MFS RFS	34 (13-47)	Uni	5	5
Rassouli et al, 2015 [40]	Canada	Caucasian	HNSCC	273 (75\198)	64 + _12	DFS	45 (42-48)	Uni	4.27	6
Selzer et al, 2015 [41]	Austria	Caucasian	HNC	318 (121\247)	ungiven	OS	ungiven	Uni	1.58	7
Kim et al, 2016 [42]	Korea	Asian	HNC	104 (9\95)	58 (20-82)	OS PFS	39 (4.8-82.5)	Multi	3	8

NC nasopharyngeal carcinoma, *LSCC* laryngeal squamous cell carcinoma, *OCSCC* Oral Cavity Squamous Cell Carcinoma, *HNSCC* Head and neck squamous cell carcinoma, *HSCC* hypopharyngeal squamous cell carcinoma, *HNC* head and neck cancer, *Uni* univariate analysis, *MFS* metastasis-free survival, *Multi* multivariate analysis, *NOS score* Newcastle-Ottawa Scale score, > 5 meant relative good quality

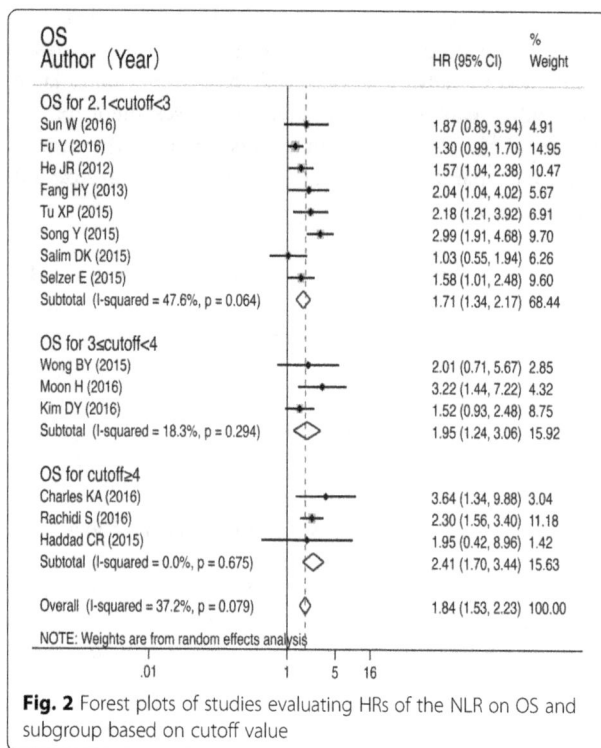

Fig. 2 Forest plots of studies evaluating HRs of the NLR on OS and subgroup based on cutoff value

analysis of ethnicity, either Asian [24, 26, 29, 30, 34, 35, 37, 42] or Caucasian [25, 33, 36, 38, 39, 41] patients with an evaluated indicated NLR a poor predictor of overall survival. All the results above are shown in Table 2.

PFS and DFS for HNC patients

The meta-analysis of PFS showed that malignancy was more likely to progress in patients with high NLR than in those with low NLR. The difference was significant (HR = 2.17, 95% CI: 1.20–3.92; $P < 0.001$; Fig. 3a). Patients with high NLR had shorter DFS than those with low NLR. The difference reached significance (HR = 2.18, 95% CI: 1.46–3.24; $P < 0.001$; Fig. 3b).

RFS and MFS for HNC patients

The meta-analysis of RFS showed that the probability of tumor recurrence after treatment was greater in patients with high NLR than in those with low NLR. The difference was significant (HR = 1.63, 95% CI: 1.09–2.45; $P = 0.017$; heterogeneity, $I^2 = 68.7\%$, $P = 0.022$; Fig. 4a). There were three studies [27, 28, 39] that analyzed the correlation between the MFS and NLR. Patients with an elevated NLR had a higher probability of distant metastasis after treatment compared with those with a low NLR, the HR was 1.92 (95% CI: 1.36–2.72; $P < 0.001$; Fig. 4b). There was no statistically significant heterogeneity ($I^2 = 0.0\%$; $P = 0.614$).

Publication bias and sensitivity analysis

In the sensitivity analysis, the trim and fill method was used to combine six sets of data. The corrected data were consistent with the original results (HR = 1.459, 95% CI: 1.174–1.813; $P = 0.001$), indicating stable funnel plots of the meta-analysis (Fig. 5a). Publication bias was tested by the Egger test ($P = 0.135$), which indicated the absence of publication bias for OS (Fig. 5b).

Discussion

This study was the first to evaluate the association of NLR in peripheral blood and prognosis in HNC patients. We found that patients with elevated pretreatment NLRs had predictable decreases in OS, DSS and PFS. Also, with increasing NLR cutoff value, mortality risk had a corresponding increasing trend, and patients were increasingly prone to local recurrence and distant metastasis. Our meta-analysis was consistent with previous studies of other malignant tumors. Other meta-analyses revealed better prognosis in patients with colorectal, non-small cell lung, stomach and prostate cancer who had low pretreatment NLR compared to those who had high pretreatment NLR [15–19]. Pretreatment NLR reflects the status of systemic inflammation and the immune system.

Table 2 Summary of meta-analysis results

Outcomes	Variable	N	References	Fixed-effect model		Random-reffect model		Heterogeneity	
				HR(95%CI)	p	HR(95%CI)	p	I2	p
OS	Ethnicity								
	Asian	8	[24, 26, 29, 30, 34, 35, 37, 42]	1.72 (1.46,2.03)	< 0.001	1.87 (1.46,2.40)	< 0.001	49%	0.056
	Caucasian	6	[25, 33, 36, 38, 39, 41]	1.85 (1.44,2.37)	< 0.001	1.83 (1.34,2.51)	< 0.001	26%	0.239
	cutoff value								
	2.1 < cutoff< 3	8	[24, 26, 29, 30, 34, 37, 38, 41]	1.63 (1.39,1.91)	< 0.001	1.71 (1.43,2.17)	< 0.001	47.60%	0.064
	3 < =cutoff< 4	3	[25, 35, 42]	1.88 (1.28,2.77)	0.001	1.95 (1.24,3.06)	0.04	18.30%	0.249
	cutoff> = 4	3	[33, 36, 39]	2.41 (1.70,3.44)	< 0.001	2.41 (1.70,3.44)	< 0.001	0	0.675
DFS		4	[25, 30, 34, 40]	1.99 (1.46,2.71)	< 0.001	1.99 (1.46,2.71)	< 0.001	0	0.457
MFS		3	[27, 28, 39]	1.92 (1.36,2.72)	< 0.001	1.92 (1.36,2.72)	< 0.001	0	0.614
PFS		5	[24, 29, 35, 38, 42]	1.60 (1.37,1.87)	< 0.001	2.17 (1.20,3.92)	0.01	91.30%	0

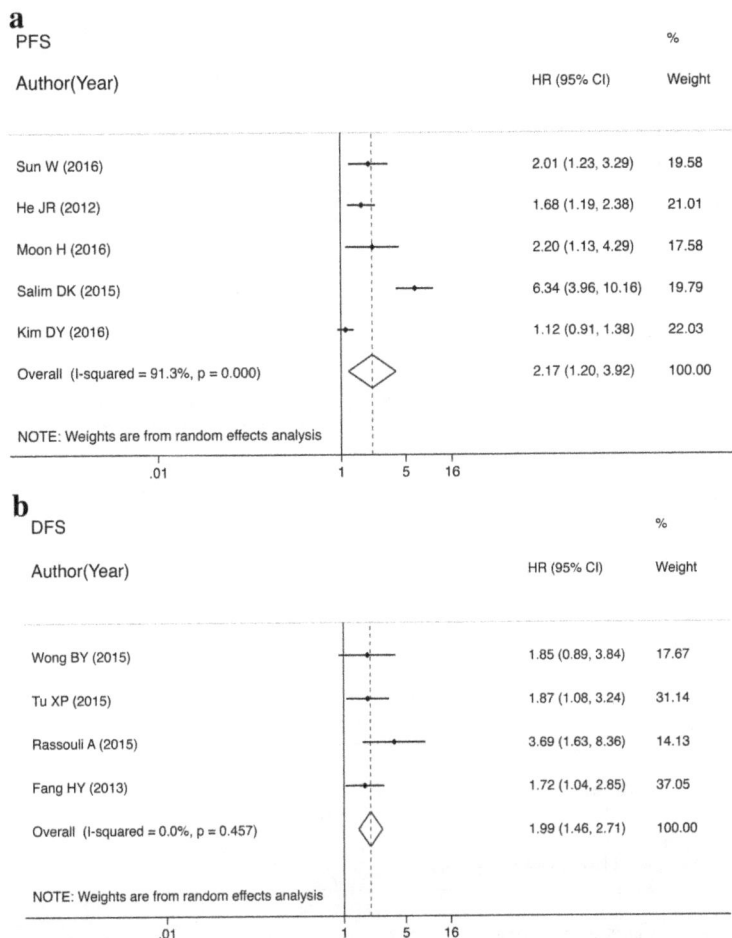

Fig. 3 a Forest plots of studies evaluating HRs of the NLR on PFS for head and neck cancer. **b** Forest plots of studies evaluating HRs of the NLR on DFS for head and neck cancer

However, the cause of poor prognosis in HNC patients with elevated NLR requires further investigation.

Elevation of neutrophils reflects systemic as well as local inflammatory responses. Neutrophils provide a microenvironment conducive to the growth of tumor cells, and they promote tumor progression and invasion of malignant tumor cells [43]. Neutrophils produce and secrete tumor-promoting growth factors, such as epidermal growth factor, vascular endothelial growth factor, interleukin (IL)-6 and IL-8, that can promote tumor cell activation and facilitate tumor development, invasion and metastasis [8, 9]. In addition to producing cytokines, neutrophils secrete proteases, such as specific matrix metalloproteinases [44, 45], cysteine cathepsins [46, 47] and serine proteases [48]. These proteases can disrupt the connections between cells and degrade extracellular matrix and basement membrane proteins, thereby facilitating the migration of tumor cells [46–49]. They also promote epithelial cell proliferation, activate dormant tumor cells, and trigger revascularization [50], forming a link between inflammation and cancer. An increase in the number of neutrophils surrounding cancerous tissue can suppress antitumor immune responses while activating T lymphocytes and natural killer (NK) cells [51]. Thus, elevation of neutrophils and release of associated cytokines play a role in tumor metastasis and indicate poor prognosis in patients with malignant tumors.

In contrast, a reduction in the number of lymphocytes reflects decreased activity of lymphokine-activated killer cells [52], with inhibition of the monitoring of the host immune response [53]. The reduction of lymphocytes includes cells of the innate immune system, such as B lymphocytes, NK cells, CD4$^+$ helper T lymphocytes and CD8$^+$ cytotoxic T lymphocytes, leading to suppression of the immune response [7, 54]. Additionally, reduction of the number of lymphocytes results in decreased release of cytokines, such as interferon and tumor necrosis factor-α by tumor macrophages. These cytokines promote apoptosis of tumor cells, which is a key host defense against tumor cell invasion. The collective effect of these changes is attenuation of the antitumor-specific immune system [55, 56]. There is also a link

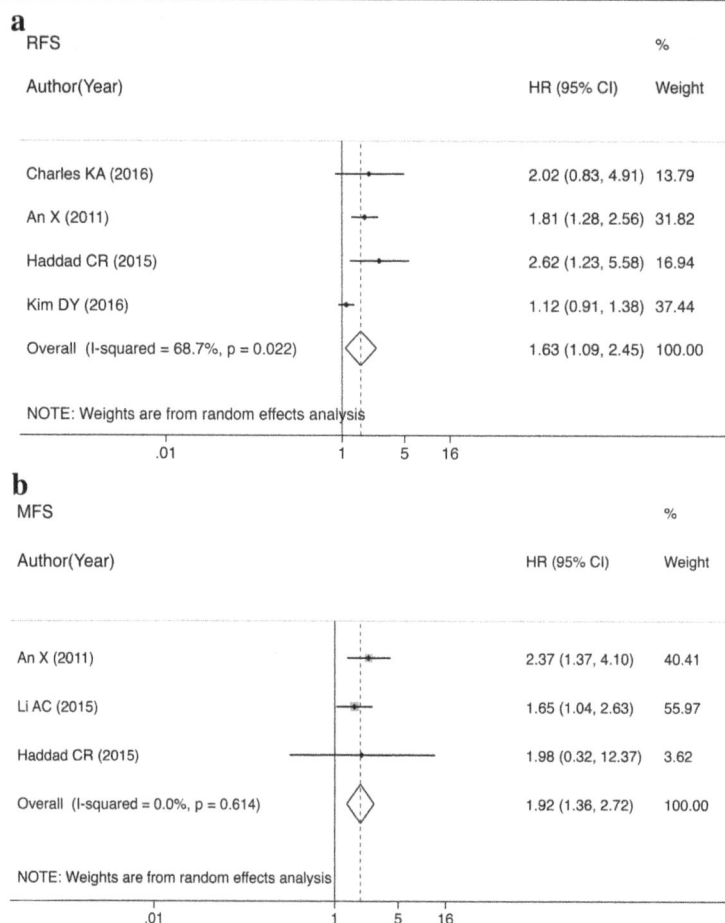

Fig. 4 **a** Forest plots of studies evaluating HRs of the NLR on RFS for head and neck cancer. **b** Forest plots of studies evaluating HRs of NLR on MFS for head and neck cancer

between the immune system and systemic inflammation. Wong et al. [25] proposed that chronic inflammation is associated with increased myeloid-derived suppressor cells (MDSCs), which suppress the immune response. They also found that MDSC-mediated immune suppression resulted in dysfunction of the acquired (T cells) and innate (NK cells) immune systems; both of which play a major role in scavenging pathogens and mutant cells under normal conditions.

This study demonstrated that pretreatment NLR can be used to evaluate prognosis in HNC patients, but the optimum NLR cutoff value remains unclear. In the studies we analyzed, the NLR cutoff values ranged from 2.1 to 4.39 and were selected from the means of all patients in each study, or on the basis of previous research. Different studies used different cutoff values, making it difficult to perform the meta-analysis using a single, defined cutoff value. In order to obtain the optimal range of cutoff values, we divided the range into three equal groups for subgroup analysis using NLR cutoff values of 3.0 and 4.0, and a performed a meta-analysis of each subgroup. It is

noteworthy that the increase in NLR resulted in similar mortality risks in subgroups 1 and 2, whereas the risk was significantly greater in subgroup 3 than in the other two subgroups. We infer that the prognostic value of NLR in HNC patients is influenced by a range of cutoff values. Optimally, we recommend using a continuous range of NLR values, rather than point values when selecting and comparing NLR cutoff values in future studies.

This meta-analysis had several limitations. First, all included studies were retrospective observational studies, and although multivariate analysis can control for confounding factors to a certain degree, selection bias was inevitable. Second, the NLR values could easily have been affected by infectious diseases, chronic infections, and use of glucocorticoid hormones that might have been present in the same period. Inflammation and NLR elevation are also believed to be associated with coronary heart diseases including acute coronary syndrome [57]. Interference of the NLR values by potential confounding factors associated with other diseases was thus inevitable. Third, NLR is closely associated with other variables

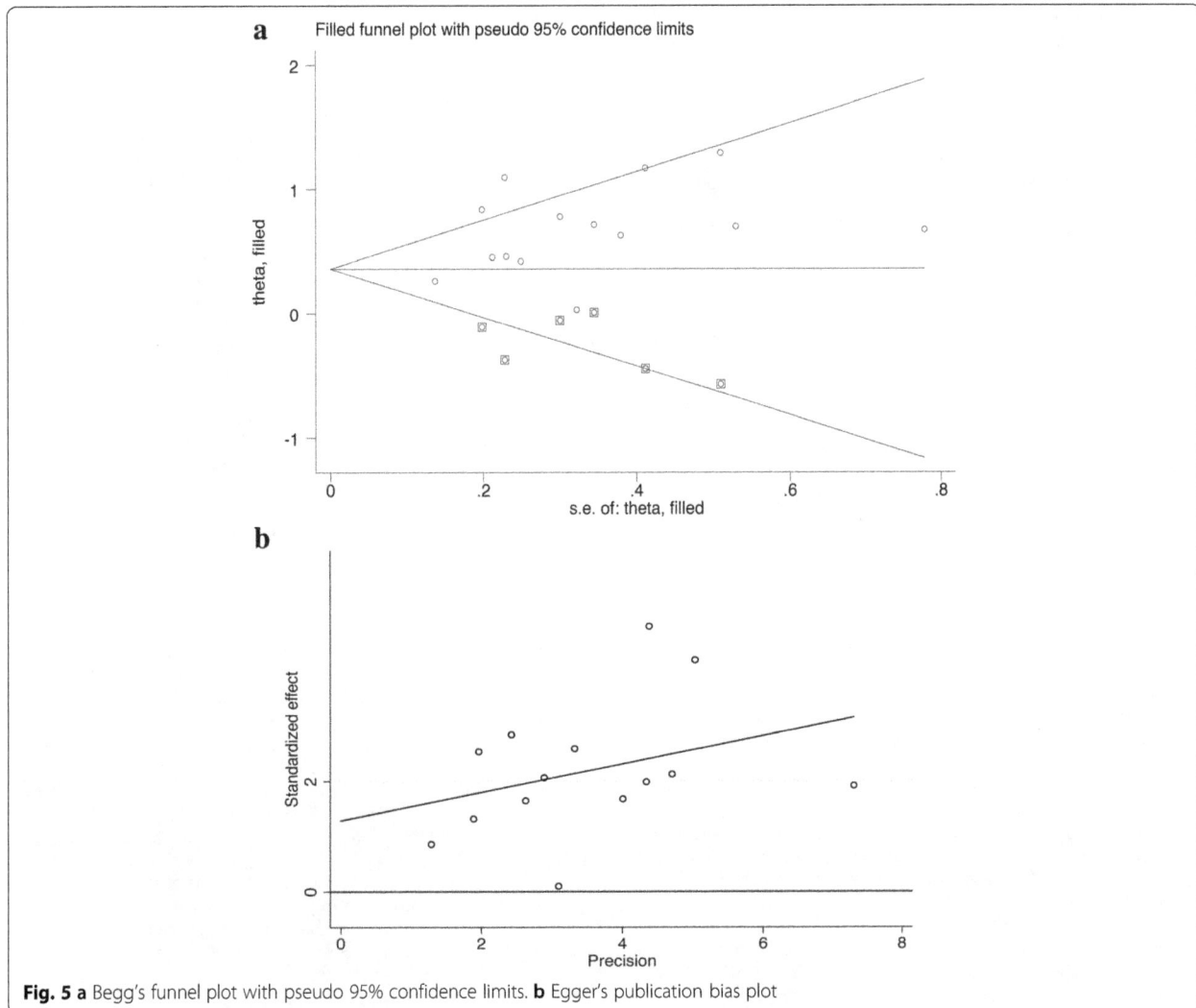

Fig. 5 a Begg's funnel plot with pseudo 95% confidence limits. **b** Egger's publication bias plot

associated with systemic inflammation, such as C-reactive protein and platelet-to-lymphocyte ratio. Interactions among these factors might have resulted in high collinearity in multivariate analysis by the Cox regression model, thereby influencing the evaluation of prognosis by NLR alone. Finally, there was a risk of reporting bias related to the method of retrieving full-text studies. Some studies did not report clinically significant results, and thus did not contribute to the calculated HR values, and some studies only included positive results in the data analysis.

Conclusion

This meta-analysis showed that HNC patients with elevated pretreatment NLR had poor prognosis and were prone to local invasion and distant metastasis. NLR, which is easily obtained from peripheral blood samples, can help clinicians to determine the prognosis of HNC patients. Preoperative and postoperative interventions to regulate inflammatory and immune responses have a place in the long-term treatment of HNC, but future studies are required to validate the clinical use of NLR.

Abbreviations

CIs: Confidence intervals; DFS: Disease-free survival; DSS: Disease-specific survival; HR: Hazard ratio; IL: Interleukin; MFS: Metastasis-free survival; Multi: Multivariate analysis; NLR: Neutrophil-to-lymphocyte ratio; NOS: Newcastle–Ottawa Scale; OS: Overall survival; PFS: Progression-free survival; RFS: Recurrence-free survival

Acknowledgments

The authors thank the study participants in each of the individual studies for their involvement.

Funding

National Science Foundation of China No. 81102057 supported this work. The funding body had no role in the design of the study and collection, analysis, and interpretation of data and in writing the manuscript.

Authors' contributions

WL, JTL and AHY were responsible for conception and design of the study. YLY and XYL did the studies selection, data extraction, statistical analyses and the writing of paper. HLW and AHY participated in studies selection and data extraction and provided statistical expertise. YLY, XYL and HBW contributed to the literature search, studies selection, and figures. JTL and WL reviewed and edited the manuscript extensively. All of the authors were involved in interpretation of results, read and approved the final manuscript.

Competing interests

The authors declare that they have no competing interests.

Author details

[1]Department of Otorhinolaryngology, the First Affiliated Hospital of China Medical University, Shenyang, Liaoning Province, People's Republic of China. [2]Department of Radiology, Shengjing Hospital of China Medical University, Shenyang, Liaoning Province, People's Republic of China. [3]Department of Clinical Epidemiology and Center of Evidence Based Medicine, the First Affiliated Hospital of China Medical University, Shenyang, Liaoning Province, People's Republic of China. [4]Department of Cardiovascular Surgery & Electro-chemotherapy, China-Japan Friendship Hospital, Beijing, People's Republic of China.

Reference

1. Torre LA, Bray F, Siegel RL, Ferlay J, Lortet-Tieulent J, Jemal A. Global cancer statistics, 2012. CA Cancer J Clin. 2015;65(2):87–108.
2. Siegel RL, Miller KD, Jemal A. Cancer statistics, 2016. CA Cancer J Clin. 2016; 66(1):7–30.
3. Dasgupta S, Koch R, Westra WH, Califano JA, Ha PK, Sidransky D, Koch WM. Mitochondrial DNA mutation in normal margins and tumors of recurrent head and neck squamous cell carcinoma patients. Cancer Prev Res (Phila). 2010;3(9):1205–11.
4. Argiris A, Karamouzis MV, Raben D, Ferris RL. Head and neck cancer. Lancet. 2008;371(9625):1695–709.
5. Balkwill F, Charles KA, Mantovani A. Smoldering and polarized inflammation in the initiation and promotion of malignant disease. Cancer Cell. 2005;7(3):211–7.
6. Baniyash M, Sade-Feldman M, Kanterman J. Chronic inflammation and cancer: suppressing the suppressors. Cancer Immunol Immunother. 2014; 63(1):11–20.
7. Hanahan D, Coussens LM. Accessories to the crime: functions of cells recruited to the tumor microenvironment. Cancer Cell. 2012;21(3):309–22.
8. Hanahan D, Weinberg RA. Hallmarks of cancer: the next generation. Cell. 2011;144(5):646–74.
9. Hanahan D, Weinberg RA. The hallmarks of cancer. Cell. 2000;100(1):57–70.
10. Hainaut P, Plymoth A. Targeting the hallmarks of cancer: towards a rational approach to next-generation cancer therapy. Curr Opin Oncol. 2013;25(1):50–1.
11. Kim S, Miller BJ, Stefanek ME, Miller AH. Inflammation-induced activation of the indoleamine 2,3-dioxygenase pathway: relevance to cancer-related fatigue. Cancer. 2015;121(13):2129–36.
12. Baniyash M. Myeloid-derived suppressor cells as intruders and targets: clinical implications in cancer therapy. Cancer Immunol Immunother. 2016; 65(7):857–67.
13. OuYang LY, Wu XJ, Ye SB, Zhang RX, Li ZL, Liao W, Pan ZZ, Zheng LM, Zhang XS, Wang Z, et al. Tumor-induced myeloid-derived suppressor cells promote tumor progression through oxidative metabolism in human colorectal cancer. J Transl Med. 2015;13:47.
14. de Raaf PJ, Sleijfer S, Lamers CH, Jager A, Gratama JW, van der Rijt CC. Inflammation and fatigue dimensions in advanced cancer patients and cancer survivors: an explorative study. Cancer. 2012;118(23):6005–11.
15. Malietzis G, Giacometti M, Kennedy RH, Athanasiou T, Aziz O, Jenkins JT. The emerging role of neutrophil to lymphocyte ratio in determining colorectal cancer treatment outcomes: a systematic review and meta-analysis. Ann Surg Oncol. 2014;21(12):3938–46.
16. Yin Y, Wang J, Wang X, Gu L, Pei H, Kuai S, Zhang Y, Shang Z. Prognostic value of the neutrophil to lymphocyte ratio in lung cancer: a meta-analysis. Clinics (Sao Paulo). 2015;70(7):524–30.
17. Sun J, Chen X, Gao P, Song Y, Huang X, Yang Y, Zhao J, Ma B, Gao X, Wang Z. Can the neutrophil to lymphocyte ratio be used to determine gastric Cancer treatment outcomes? A systematic review and Meta-analysis. Dis Markers. 2016;2016:7862469.
18. Kacan T, Babacan NA, Seker M, Yucel B, Bahceci A, Eren AA, Eren MF, Kilickap S. Could the neutrophil to lymphocyte ratio be a poor prognostic factor for non small cell lung cancers? Asian Pac J Cancer Prev. 2014;15(5):2089–94.
19. Templeton AJ, Pezaro C, Omlin A, McNamara MG, Leibowitz-Amit R, Vera-Badillo FE, Attard G, de Bono JS, Tannock IF, Amir E. Simple prognostic score for metastatic castration-resistant prostate cancer with incorporation of neutrophil-to-lymphocyte ratio. Cancer. 2014;120(21):3346–52.
20. Moher D, Liberati A, Tetzlaff J, Altman DG, Group P. Preferred reporting items for systematic reviews and meta-analyses: the PRISMA statement. BMJ. 2009;339:b2535.
21. Higgins JP, Green S Cochrane Handbook for Systematic Reviews of Interventions. Available at http://handbook.cochrane.org/. Accessed 05 Jan 2013.
22. Tierney JF, Stewart LA, Ghersi D, Burdett S, Sydes MR. Practical methods for incorporating summary time-to-event data into meta-analysis. Trials. 2007;8:16.
23. Wells GA, Shea B, O'Connell D, et al. The Newcastle-Ottawa scale (NOS) for assessing the quality of nonrandomised studies in meta- analyses. 2008. http://www.ohri.ca/programs/clinical_epidemiology/oxford.asp
24. Sun W, Zhang L, Luo M, Hu G, Mei Q, Liu D, Long G, Hu G. Pretreatment hematologic markers as prognostic factors in patients with nasopharyngeal carcinoma: neutrophil-lymphocyte ratio and platelet-lymphocyte ratio. Head Neck. 2016;38(Suppl 1):E1332–40.
25. Wong BY, Stafford ND, Green VL, Greenman J. Prognostic value of the neutrophil-to-lymphocyte ratio in patients with laryngeal squamous cell carcinoma. Head Neck. 2016;38(Suppl 1):E1903–8.
26. Fu Y, Liu W, OuYang D, Yang A, Zhang Q. Preoperative neutrophil-to-lymphocyte ratio predicts long-term survival in patients undergoing Total laryngectomy with advanced laryngeal squamous cell carcinoma: a single-center retrospective study. Medicine (Baltimore). 2016;95(6):e2689.
27. An X, Ding PR, Wang FH, Jiang WQ, Li YH. Elevated neutrophil to lymphocyte ratio predicts poor prognosis in nasopharyngeal carcinoma. Tumour Biol. 2011;32(2):317–24.
28. Li AC, Xiao WW, Wang L, Shen GZ, Xu AA, Cao YQ, Huang SM, Lin CG, Han F, Deng XW, et al. Risk factors and prediction-score model for distant metastasis in nasopharyngeal carcinoma treated with intensity-modulated radiotherapy. Tumour Biol. 2015;36(11):8349–57.
29. He JR, Shen GP, Ren ZF, Qin H, Cui C, Zhang Y, Zeng YX, Jia WH. Pretreatment levels of peripheral neutrophils and lymphocytes as independent prognostic factors in patients with nasopharyngeal carcinoma. Head Neck. 2012;34(12):1769–76.
30. Fang HY, Huang XY, Chien HT, Chang JT, Liao CT, Huang JJ, Wei FC, Wang HM, Chen IH, Kang CJ, et al. Refining the role of preoperative C-reactive protein by neutrophil/lymphocyte ratio in oral cavity squamous cell carcinoma. Laryngoscope. 2013;123(11):2690–9.
31. Nakahira M, Sugasawa M, Matsumura S, Kuba K, Ohba S, Hayashi T, Minami K, Ebihara Y, Kogashiwa Y. Prognostic role of the combination of platelet count and neutrophil-lymphocyte ratio in patients with hypopharyngeal squamous cell carcinoma. Eur Arch Otorh inolaryngol. 2016;273(11):3863–7.
32. Perisanidis C, Kornek G, Poschl PW, Holzinger D, Pirklbauer K, Schopper C, Ewers R. High neutrophil-to-lymphocyte ratio is an independent marker of poor disease-specific survival in patients with oral cancer. Med Oncol. 2013; 30(1):334.
33. Charles KA, Harris BD, Haddad CR, Clarke SJ, Guminski A, Stevens M, Dodds T, Gill AJ, Back M, Veivers D, et al. Systemic inflammation is an independent predictive marker of clinical outcomes in mucosal squamous cell carcinoma of the head and neck in oropharyngeal and non-oropharyngeal patients. BMC Cancer. 2016;16(1):124.
34. Tu XP, Qiu QH, Chen LS, Luo XN, Lu ZM, Zhang SY, Chen SH. Preoperative neutrophil-to-lymphocyte ratio is an independent prognostic marker in patients with laryngeal squamous cell carcinoma. BMC Cancer. 2015;15:743.
35. Moon H, Roh JL, Lee SW, Kim SB, Choi SH, Nam SY, Kim SY. Prognostic value of nutritional and hematologic markers in head and neck squamous cell carcinoma treated by chemoradiotherapy. Radiother Oncol. 2016;118(2):330–4.
36. Rachidi S, Wallace K, Wrangle JM, Day TA, Alberg AJ, Li Z. Neutrophil-to-lymphocyte ratio and overall survival in all sites of head and neck squamous cell carcinoma. Head Neck. 2016;38(Suppl 1):E1068–74.
37. Song Y, Liu H, Gao L, Liu X, Ma L, Lu M, Gao Z. Preoperative neutrophil-to-lymphocyte ratio as prognostic predictor for hypopharyngeal squamous cell carcinoma after radical resections. J Craniofac Surg. 2015;26(2):e137–40.
38. Salim DK, Mutlu H, Eryilmaz MK, Salim O, Musri FY, Tural D, Gunduz S,

Coskun HS. Neutrophil to lymphocyte ratio is an independent prognostic factor in patients with recurrent or metastatic head and neck squamous cell cancer. Mol Clin Oncol. 2015;3(4):839–42.

39. Haddad CR, Guo L, Clarke S, Guminski A, Back M, Eade T. Neutrophil-to-lymphocyte ratio in head and neck cancer. J Med Imaging Radiat Oncol. 2015;59(4):514–9.

40. Rassouli A, Saliba J, Castano R, Hier M, Zeitouni AG. Systemic inflammatory markers as independent prognosticators of head and neck squamous cell carcinoma. Head Neck. 2015;37(1):103–10.

41. Selzer E, Grah A, Heiduschka G, Kornek G, Thurnher D. Primary radiotherapy or postoperative radiotherapy in patients with head and neck cancer: comparative analysis of inflammation-based prognostic scoring systems. Strahlenther Onkol. 2015;191(6):486–94.

42. Kim DY, Kim IS, Park SG, Kim H, Choi YJ, Seol YM. Prognostic value of posttreatment neutrophil-lymphocyte ratio in head and neck squamous cell carcinoma treated by chemoradiotherapy . Auris Nasus Larynx. 2017;44(2):199–204

43. Grivennikov SI, Greten FR, Karin M. Immunity, inflammation, and cancer. Cell. 2010;140(6):883–99.

44. Egeblad M, Werb Z. New functions for the matrix metalloproteinases in cancer progression. Nat Rev Cancer. 2002;2(3):161–74.

45. Lynch CC, Matrisian LM. Matrix metalloproteinases in tumor-host cell communication. Differentiation. 2002;70(9-10):561–73.

46. Gocheva V, Joyce JA. Cysteine cathepsins and the cutting edge of cancer invasion. Cell Cycle. 2007;6(1):60–4.

47. Mohamed MM, Sloane BF. Cysteine cathepsins: multifunctional enzymes in cancer. Nat Rev Cancer. 2006;6(10):764–75.

48. Laufs S, Schumacher J, Allgayer H. Urokinase-receptor (u-PAR): an essential player in multiple games of cancer: a review on its role in tumor progression, invasion, metastasis, proliferation/dormancy, clinical outcome and minimal residual disease. Cell Cycle. 2006;5(16):1760–71.

49. Joyce JA, Pollard JW. Microenvironmental regulation of metastasis. Nat Rev Cancer. 2009;9(4):239–52.

50. Schwartsburd PM. Age-promoted creation of a pro-cancer microenvironment by inflammation: pathogenesis of dyscoordinated feedback control. Mech Ageing Dev. 2004;125(9):581–90.

51. Petrie HT, Klassen LW, Kay HD. Inhibition of human cytotoxic T lymphocyte activity invitro by autologous peripheral blood granulocytes. J Immunol. 1985;134(1):230–4.

52. Teramukai S, Kitano T, Kishida Y, Kawahara M, Kubota K, Komuta K, Minato K, Mio T, Fujita Y, Yonei T, et al. Pretreatment neutrophil count as an independent prognostic factor in advanced non-small-cell lung cancer: an analysis of Japan multinational trial organisation LC00-03. Eur J Cancer. 2009;45(11):1950–8.

53. Schreiber RD, Old LJ, Smyth MJ. Cancer immunoediting: integrating immunity's roles in cancer suppression and promotion. Science. 2011;331(6024):1565–70.

54. Ishigami S, Natsugoe S, Tokuda K, Nakajo A, Che X, Iwashige H, Aridome K, Hokita S, Aikou T. Prognostic value of intratumoral natural killer cells in gastric carcinoma. Cancer. 2000;88(3):577–83.

55. Avci N, Deligonul A, Tolunay S, Cubukcu E, Fatih Olmez O, Altmisdortoglu O, Tanriverdi O, Aksoy A, Kurt E, Evrensel T. Prognostic impact of tumor lymphocytic infiltrates in patients with breast cancer undergoing neoadjuvant chemotherapy. J BUON. 2015;20(4):994–1000.

56. Song MK, Chung JS, Seol YM, Kim SG, Shin HJ, Choi YJ, Cho GJ, Shin DH. Influence of low absolute lymphocyte count of patients with nongerminal center type diffuse large B-cell lymphoma with R-CHOP therapy. Ann Oncol. 2010;21(1):140–4.

57. Bhat T, Teli S, Rijal J, Bhat H, Raza M, Khoueiry G, Meghani M, Akhtar M, Costantino T. Neutrophil to lymphocyte ratio and cardiovascular diseases: a review. Expert Rev Cardiovasc Ther. 2013;11(1):55–9.

21

Compared characteristics of current vs. past smokers at the time of diagnosis of a first-time lung or head and neck cancer

Corinne Vannimenus[1]*, Hélène Bricout[2], Olivier Le Rouzic[1], François Mouawad[3], Dominique Chevalier[3], Eric Dansin[4], Laurence Rotsaert[4], Gautier Lefebvre[4], Olivier Cottencin[5], Henri Porte[6], Arnaud Scherpereel[1], Asmaa El Fahsi[2], Florence Richard[7], Benjamin Rolland[8] and The ALTAK Study Group

Abstract

Background: Active smoking at the time of diagnosis of a first head & neck (H&N) or lung cancer is associated with a worse cancer outcome and increased mortality. However, the compared characteristics of active vs. former smokers at cancer diagnosis are poorly known.

Methods: In 371 subjects with a first H&N or lung cancer, we assessed: 1) socio-demographic features; 2) lifelong types of smoking; 3) alcohol use disorder identification test (AUDIT); 4) cannabis abuse screening test (CAST); and 5) Mini International Neuropsychiatric Interview (MINI). Using a multivariable regression model, we compared the profile of current smokers and past smokers.

Results: Current smokers more frequently exhibited H&N cancer (OR 3.91; 95% CI [2.00–6.51]; $p < 0.0001$) and ever smoking of hand-rolled cigarettes (OR 2.2; 95% CI [1.25–3.88]; $p = 0.007$). Among subjects with lung cancer ($n = 177$), current smoking was primarily associated with ever smoking of hand-rolled cigarettes (OR 2.88; 95% CI [1.32–6.30]; $p = 0.008$) and negatively associated with age (OR 0.92; 95% CI [0.89–0.96]; $p < 0.001$). Among subjects with H&N cancer ($n = 163$), current smokers exhibited a significantly greater AUDIT score (OR = 1.08; 95% CI [1.01–1.16]; $p = 0.03$).

Conclusion: At the time of diagnosis of the first lung or H&N cancer, current smoking is highly associated with previous type of smoking and alcohol drinking patterns.

Keywords: Tobacco use, Lung neoplasms, Head & Neck Neoplasms, Alcohol-related disorders

Background

Tobacco smoking is the most important risk factor for lung cancer [1], while tobacco and alcohol conjointly account for the occurrence of 67–84% of the head and neck (H&N) cancers [2]. Continuing to smoke after the diagnosis of cancer is associated with higher risks of complications, secondary cancers, and death [3]. Moreover, in patients with a lung or H&N cancer, persistent smoking is associated with decreased quality of life, general health, and emotional and social functioning [4–6]. Intensive smoking cessation programs are thus warranted in current smokers with a first tobacco-related cancer [7].

In recent years, the implementation of tobacco control policies has enhanced the level of information on tobacco-related harm, which has promoted tobacco cessation [8], and subsequently reduced the incidence of tobacco-related cancers [9]. Despite the impact of such policies, some individuals continue to smoke tobacco until they experience a first-time tobacco-related health problem, including a first-time tobacco-related cancer. In contrast, some other individuals who experience a tobacco-related cancer had already stopped tobacco use

* Correspondence: corinne.vannimenus@chru-lille.fr
[1]Service de Tabacologie, Clinique de Pneumologie, Hôpital Calmette, CHRU de Lille CS70001, 59037 Lille cedex, France
Full list of author information is available at the end of the article

long before the cancer diagnosis. Thus, the profile of patients with a first-time tobacco-related cancer can be divided into three categories at cancer diagnosis: 1) current smokers (CSs); 2) former smokers (FSs); and 3) never smokers.

Many previous studies have compared the profile of current vs. former smokers at the time of cancer diagnosis. A comprehensive review has recently listed these studies [10]. However, these studies essentially consisted of un-adjusted analyses on the smoking status at cancer diagnosis, and, in most cases, they did not explore the contribution of the psychiatric history and other substance use patterns. Consequently, little is known about whether the smoking status at the time of diagnosis of a first-time lung or H&N cancer is related to specific social or psychiatric features, lifelong smoking patterns, or history of other substance uses. In the non-cancer population, it was found that the overall outcome of tobacco dependence is associated with the age of first cigarette, lifelong smoking patterns, and poorer psychosocial conditions [11]. Moreover, concurrent psychiatric and other substance use disorders are also associated with a poorer outcome [12, 13]. In patients with a first lung or H&N cancer, the role of these risk factors was never investigated. Enhancing the knowledge of the psychosocial determinants of the CS status among subjects with a first lung or H&N cancer could strengthen the impact of smoking cessation programs proposed to these patients.

In a multicenter one-year cohort study among 371 subjects with a first-time lung or H&N cancer (i.e., the ALTAK study), we conducted a cross-sectional study using the baseline assessment to investigate the differences in social factors, psychiatric condition, and other substance use patterns between current and past-smokers at the time of the cancer diagnosis. The presentation of the study is provided according to the 'strengthening the reporting of observational studies in epidemiology' (STROBE) statement [14].

Methods

Study design and centers

Data used in this study originated from the baseline screening of the ALTAK cohort study, conducted among 372 subjects with a first lung or H&N cancer. Participants were recruited by otorhinolaryngologists, clinical oncologists, or pulmonologists of the participating centers, at the end of the consultation of cancer announcement. Physicians explained the study and received written consent for participation. The study took place between September 2012 and December 2014 in three different centers: 1) the *Centre Oscar Lambret*, i.e., the Regional Comprehensive Cancer Center of Lille; 2) the Department of Respiratory Diseases of the University Hospital of Lille; and 3) the Department of Otolaryngology-Head and Neck Surgery of the University Hospital of Lille.

The main objectives of the ALTAK cohort study were: 1) to measure the proportion of subjects that maintain tobacco smoking or alcohol abuse despite the occurrence of cancer; and 2) to identify the social and psychiatric features and addictive comorbidities that could constitute vulnerability factors for not stopping tobacco or alcohol after cancer diagnosis. More information on the study protocol can be found at https://clinicaltrials.gov/ct2/show/NCT01647425. Here, we have used the baseline data of the cohort to explore the determinants of the smoking status at time of cancer diagnosis.

Participants and measures

Inclusion criteria were: 1) age of 18 or more; 2) first lung or H&N cancer excluding mesothelioma and esophagus cancer; and 3) no history of any other cancer over the last five years. The type of cancer (lung or H&N), and the TNM classification grade [15] were noted by the clinician who received the initial consent.

Participants were assessed by an addiction specialist in the week following the announcement of the cancer diagnosis. The information collected at baseline and used in the present study was: 1) socioeconomic conditions: age, gender, familial status, employment, and educational level; 2) cancer status: localization, TNM grade, Eastern Cooperative Oncology Group / World Health Organization (ECOG/WHO) score; 3) smoking status and smoking habits: CS, i.e., at last one smoking episode in previous month; FS, i.e., no smoking episode over the previous month; and lifelong non-smoker; 4) alcohol use patterns: use of alcohol during the last 12 months (yes/no); misuse of alcohol during the last 12 months (yes/no), defined by an average alcohol use exceeding the recommended national thresholds, i.e., ≥210 g of alcohol per week for a man and 140 g for a woman, and ≥ 50 g per occasion for a man and 40 g for a woman [16], Alcohol Use Disorder Identification Test (AUDIT) [17]; 5) Severity of use of cannabis using the Cannabis Abuse Screening Test (CAST) [18], i.e., at least one positive item; and 6) Psychiatric assessment using the Mini International Neuropsychiatric Interview (MINI) [19], which is a validated structured interview for diagnosing mental health disorders.

Statistical analyses

Descriptive statistics of each variable are reported in Table 1. Quantitative values are presented as the mean (standard deviation [sd]) when normally distributed or as the median (interquartile range) when there is skewed distribution. Qualitative data are presented as n (percent). To compare smoker and ex-smoker groups, Student's t-test or the Kruskal-Wallis test were used for quantitative data, and the Chi-squared test or Fisher's exact test were used for categorical data. Logistic regression models were used

Table 1 Descriptive statistics and univariate comparisons between current and past smokers at the time of the cancer onset

	Past Smokers	Current Smokers	p-value
Number of subjects (n; %)	177 (52.1%)	163 (47.9%)	
Gender (n females; %)	27 (15.3%)	35 (21.5%)	0.14
Age (m ± SD)	61.9 ± 9.7	56.0 ± 8.0	< 0.0001
Educational level			0.45
Elementary / primary school	75 (42.4%)	68 (41.7%)	
Secondary / high school	75 (42.4%)	77 (47.2%)	
Undergraduate and more/ college or university	27 (15.2%)	18 (11.1%)	
Workers (n; %)	58 (32.8%)	98 (60.1%)	< 0.0001
Married (n; %)	124 (70.1%)	97 (59.5%)	0.04
Living alone (n; %)	35 (19.8%)	45 (27.6%)	0.09
Cancer			
Localization			< 0.0001
1 = lung	119 (67.2%)	58 (35.6%)	
2 = head & neck	58 (32.8%)	105 (64.4%)	
"0" score at the ECOG performance status (n; %)	77 (43.5%)	47 (28.8%)	0.005
TNM Grade 4 (N = 299) (n; %)	97 (59.2%)	73 (54.1%)	0.38
Presence of metastases (N = 296) (n; %)	72 (44.7%)	40 (29.6%)	0.008
Tobacco			
Age of first cigarette (years; m ± SD)	15.6 ± 3.8	15.6 ± 4.1	0.95
Lifelong reported types of smoking, (N = 339) (n; %)			
Manufactured cigarettes	172 (97.2%)	154 (95.1%)	0.31
Roll-up cigarettes	64 (36.2%)	91 (56.2%)	0.0002
Cigarillos	82 (46.3%)	58 (35.8%)	0.05
Cigars	55 (31.1%)	40 (24.7%)	0.19
Pipe	50 (28.3%)	26 (16.1%)	0.007
Alcohol			
12-month use (n; %)	140 (79.1%)	122 (74.8%)	0.35
12-month misuse (n; %)	51 (28.8%)	70 (42.9%)	0.007
AUDIT, (N = 322) (median [IQ])	4 [2–6]	6 [2–11]	0.002[a]
AUDIT-C, (N = 322) (median [IQ])	4 [1–5]	5 [1–7]	0.01[a]
CAST (m ± SD)	0.10 ± 0.43	0.22 ± 0.59	0.019[a]
MINI 5.0 (N = 337)			
TOTAL (n; %)	61 (34.9%)	72 (44.4%)	0.07
Current MDD (n; %)	23 (13.1%)	29 (17.9%)	0.22
Dysthymia (n; %)	2 (1.1%)	3 (1.9%)	0.67[b]
Suicide risk (n; %)	39 (22.3%)	43 (26.5%)	0.36
Lifelong mania/hypomania (n; %)	2 (1.1%)	7 (4.3%)	0.09[b]
Schizophrenia (n; %)	10 (5.7%)	14 (8.6%)	0.30
Panic disorder/ agoraphobia (n; %)	16 (9.1%)	27 (16.7%)	0.04
Eating Disorder (n; %)	0 (0.0%)	0 (0.0%)	NA
Generalized anxiety (n; %)	7 (4.0%)	3 (1.9%)	0.34[b]
Antisocial personality disorder (n; %)	0 (0.0%)	3 (1.9%)	0.12[b]

Table 1 Descriptive statistics and univariate comparisons between current and past smokers at the time of the cancer onset (Continued)

	Past Smokers	Current Smokers	p-value
Obsessive-compulsive disorder (n; %)	1 (0.6%)	2 (1.2%)	0.61[b]
PTSD (n; %)	1 (0.6%)	4 (2.5%)	0.20[b]
Other SUD (n; %)	0 (0.0%)	1 (0.6%)	0.48[b]

Abbreviations: *AUDIT*: Alcohol Use Disorder Identification Test, AUDIT-C: AUDIT "consumptions" i.e., the 3 first questions of the AUDIT, which pertain to the drinking levels, *CAST*: Cannabis Abuse Screening Test, *ECOG*: Eastern Cooperative Oncology Group, *MINI*: Mini International Neuropsychiatric Interview, version 5.0, *TNM*: Tumor/Nodules/Metastases, *PTSD*: Post-Traumatic Stress Disorder, *SUD*: Substance Use Disorder

*a "0" score at the ECOG performance status means "Fully active, able to carry on all predisease activities without restriction"

[a]Mann Whitney test

[b]Fischer's exact test

to estimate OR with 95% confidence interval (95%CI). A backward stepwise regression method was used to select variables (with $p < 0.20$) associated with smoking status in a multiple logistic regression model, adjusted for age and sex. Significance levels were set at $p < 0.05$. The final multiple logistic regression model was also stratified by localization. Analyses were performed using the SAS software release 9.02 (SAS Institute INC, Cary, NC, USA).

Ethics approval

The protocol of the ALTAK study (NCT01647425) was declared to and approved by the Comité de Protection des Personnes Nord-Ouest (#CPP12/09) and the Agence Nationale des Médicaments et produits de santé (#B111675–10).

Results

In total, 389 subjects were proposed to participate in the ALTAK study, of whom 371 accepted (response rate: 95. 4%). Among them, 163 (43.9%) were CSs at the time of cancer diagnosis, and 177 (47.7%) were PSs. The characteristics of these participants are summarized in Table 1, according to their smoking status. Bivariable comparisons between the CS and FS groups are also provided in Table 1.

Bivariable comparisons found that belonging to the CS group was significantly associated with younger age ($p < 0.0001$), being professionally active (p < 0.0001), and being unmarried ($p = 0.04$). Moreover, the CS status was significantly associated with a H&N localization of the cancer, with no alteration in daily life activities at the time of diagnosis ($p = 0.005$), and with the absence of metastases ($p = 0.008$). With respect to recent substance use patterns, being CS was associated with smoking roll-up cigarettes ($p < 0.0002$), with reporting alcohol misuse in the past 12 months ($p = 0.007$) as well as with the AUDIT ($p = 0.002$) and AUDIT-C ($p = 0.01$) scores. Finally, the CS status was significantly associated with the CAST score for cannabis use ($p = 0.019$). By contrast, the CS status was not found associated with sex ($p = 0.14$), educational level ($p = 0.45$), or living alone ($p = 0.09$). Furthermore, being CS was not related to the age of first

cigarette ($p = 0.95$) and the presence of any psychiatric disorder according to the MINI ($p = 0.07$).

A separate multivariable analysis of the CS status was conducted among patients with lung and H&N cancer (see Table 2). In subjects with a lung cancer, the CS status was positively associated with ever use of hand-rolled cigarettes and negatively associated with age and ever use of cigarillos. There were trends for positive statistical associations between the CS status and positive MINI, never use of a pipe, and being single. In subjects with H&N cancer, the CS status was positively associated with the AUDIT score. Trends for positive statistical associations were found between the CS status and younger age, ever use of hand-rolled cigarettes, and never use of a pipe.

Discussion

The main objective of the study was to compare the sociodemographic features, psychiatric history, and substance use patterns, of CSs and FSs at the time of initial diagnosis of a first lung or H&N cancer. The main results of the multivariable regression models were that the CS status was associated with younger age and ever use of hand-roll cigarettes in subjects with a first lung cancer, and increased AUDIT score in subjects with a first H&N cancer. Overall, we found a prevalence of 43. 9% CSs, i.e., smokers over the preceding month. This figure is relatively consistent with the estimation provided by a recent literature review, which estimated approximately 50% the rate of CSs over the year preceding the diagnosis of a lung or H&N cancer [10]. Though most of the studies have used a one-year period prior to cancer to define the CS status [10], we chose to follow the recommendations of the National Cancer Institute that deem a one-month period to be more precise [20].

Regarding the sociodemographic features of CSs, we have found in bivariable comparisons that being CS was significantly associated with younger age, being inactive, and being unmarried. Previous studies that explored the smoking status among subjects with a first lung or H&N cancer found relatively similar results. For example, Schnoll et al. found that only a single marital status was

Table 2 Association between patient characteristics and current smoking status. Logistic regression model adjusted for age and sex and stratified by localization

	Lung cancer			Head & neck cancer		
	OR	95% CI	p-value	OR	95% CI	p-value
Age	0.92	0.89–0.96	< 0.001	0.97	0.92–1.01	0.15
Marital status						
Married or in couple	1			1		
Single or widowed	0.49	0.23–1.07	0.07	0.70	0.30–1.61	0.40
Hand-rolled cigarettes						
Never use	1			1		
Ever use	2.88	1.32–6.30	0.008	1.98	0.93–4.25	0.08
Cigarillos						
Never use	1			1		
Ever use	0.43	0.19–0.97	0.04	1.09	0.46–2.58	0.85
Pipe						
Never use	1			1		
Ever use	0.46	0.16–1.37	0.16	0.37	0.14–1.00	0.05
AUDIT	1.01	0.92–1.10	0.87	1.08	1.01–1.16	0.03
Psychiatric disorder						
No	1			1		
Yes	1.89	0.86–4.13	0.11	1.36	0.60–3.11	0.46

AUDIT = Alcohol use disorders identification test

significantly associated with increased CS status [21]. In subjects with H&N cancer only, Duffy et al. found that smoking at cancer diagnosis was associated with younger age, single status, and lower education level [22]. Another study by the same team of authors also found that active smoking at the time of diagnosis of an H&N cancer was associated with a single status, but not with age or education level [23].

Though younger age was not consistently found as a substantial contributor of the CS status in previous studies among subjects with lung or H&N cancer, it is a well-known factor in the general population, both in the US and in Europe [24, 25]. In this respective, our result could thus be reflective of this general finding. Moreover, the CS status was significantly more important among subjects with a H&N cancer, compared to those with a lung cancer.

Another important result was that the CS rate was much higher in the subjects with a first H&N cancer than in those with a first lung cancer. To our knowledge, our study was the first to directly compare these two types of populations. The risk of experiencing a lung cancer, especially adenocarcinoma, is still significantly increased compared with never smokers more than 30 years after smoking cessation [26]. In contrast, quitting tobacco smoking fosters a more rapid decrease in the relative risk of H&N cancer [27]. The gap observed

in the CS rates between lung and H&N cancer populations may thus be attributable to this difference in longitudinal risk reduction among FSs.

More importantly, it was recently noted that almost no previous studies have addressed the relative rates of the types of tobacco ever used among CSs and FSs with a lung or H&N cancer and that it was a significant issue to explore [10]. In this regard, our study is also the first to provide important findings on this subject. We have notably found that reporting ever smoking of roll-up cigarettes was highly associated with being a CS at the time of cancer diagnosis of a first lung cancer. In the French population, it has been previously found that 24.3% of smokers were used handrolling tobacco, while 7.5% of smokers use only this type of tobacco [28]. These figures are difficult to compare to other countries, as the prevalence of roll-you-own smokers is very variable depending on countries and their specific regulations on tobacco [29]. Regardless, in France, compared to smokers of manufactured cigarettes, handrolling smokers reported much lower average personal incomes and higher rates of unemployment [28]. This finding is consistent with other data out of France [30]. In the general population, it was previously shown that quitting smoking is inversely associated with impaired social conditions (10). Our findings in patients with cancer could thus be explained by unexplored social factors, even if our analyses were adjusted for the level of education.

Moreover, as early alterations in daily life activities and the presence of metastases at the time of cancer diagnosis were significantly associated with the FS status in bivariable comparisons, it could be suggested that the FS status is actually partially explained by symptom burden, in particular the fact that some people have become too sick to smoke before cancer was diagnosed. However, these two variables were involved in the step-by-step regression model, but they were not retained as relevant explanatory parameters by the modeling.

Finally, we identified that concurrent alcohol misuse, reflected by the AUDIT score, was significantly associated with the CS status only in patients with a H&N cancer (see Table 2), which could be underlain by the fact that alcohol and tobacco are combined risk factors for this type of cancer.

Several limitations should be acknowledged with regard to the present study. First, the study was multicenter, but the recruitment was regional. Some findings could thus be skewed by local features. Moreover, patients with esophageal cancers were not included in the study, and thus, the findings cannot be applied to all types of H&N cancers. Finally, we did not assess the use of non-smoking types of tobacco, notably chewing or snuff tobacco. However, this type of tobacco use is very rare in Europe [25]. The main objective of our study was to assess the lifelong types of tobacco used by the patients. This retrospective assessment could be found to be rather imprecise. However, a detailed and quantitative assessment of the specific periods of time during which each type of tobacco was used over the entire lifetime period would have been very difficult to carry out and would have suffered from memory bias and imprecision.

Conclusions

The study highlights important risk factors associated with a CS status at the time of diagnosis of a first lung or H&N cancer. Some risk factors are specific to H&N cancer (i.e., concurrent alcohol misuse), whereas some others are associated with both types of cancer, i.e., young age, ever use of hand-rolled cigarettes, and possibly some psychiatric comorbidities. These findings should warrant a specific screening of these risk factors in subjects with a first lung or H&N cancer, with the aim to treat comorbid conditions and to act on impaired social situations, together with treating cancer and offering tobacco cessation programs to the patients.

Abbreviations
AUDIT: Alcohol Use Disorders Identification Test; CAST: Cannabis Abuse Screening Test; CSs: Current Smokers; ECOG: Eastern Cooperative Oncology Group; FSs: Former Smokers; H&N: Head and Neck; MINI: Mini International Neuropsychiatric Interview; STROBE: 'Strengthening The Reporting of OBservational studies in Epidemiology'; WHO: World Health Organization

Acknowledgements
The authors wish to thank Françoise WEINGERTNER, Stéphanie CLISANT, and Yvette VENDEL for their significant organizational help. The ALTAK Study Group is composed of the following members: Corinne VANNIMENUS, Françoise WEINGERTNER, Hélène BRICOUT, Olivier LE ROUZIC, François MOUAWAD, Dominique CHEVALIER, Eric DANSIN, Stéphanie CLISANT, Laurence ROTSAERT, Gautier LEFEBVRE, Olivier COTTENCIN, Henri PORTE, Arnaud SCHERPEREEL, Asmaa EL FAHSI, Dienabou SYLLA, Florence RICHARD, and Benjamin ROLLAND.

Funding
ALTAK was funded by the Institut National du Cancer (INCa): Grant #RECF1764. The study design and the conduct of the study are independent and remain the full responsibility of the investigators.

Authors' contributions
BR, HB, FR, and CV designed the study and obtained the grant. CV was the grant holder. CV, AEF, OC, OLR, FM, DC, ED, GL, HP, AS, and LR collected the data. BR, HB, and FR performed the statistical analyses. BR wrote the first draft of the manuscript. CV, HB, FR, OLR, FM, DC, ED, LR, GL, OC, HP, AS, AEF were involved in revising the manuscript critically. All authors have read and approved the final version of the manuscript, and have agreed to be accountable for all aspects of the work in ensuring that questions related to the accuracy or integrity of any part of the work are appropriately investigated and resolved.

Competing interests
The authors declare that they have no competing interests.

Author details
[1]Service de Tabacologie, Clinique de Pneumologie, Hôpital Calmette, CHRU de Lille CS70001, 59037 Lille cedex, France. [2]Centre de Référence Régionale en Cancérologie, Lille, France. [3]Service d'Oto-rhino-laryngologie, CHRU de Lille, Lille, France. [4]Département de Cancérologie Cervico-Faciale, Centre de Lutte Contre le Cancer Oscar Lambret, Lille, France. [5]Service d'Addictologie, CHRU de Lille, Lille, France. [6]Clinique de Chirurgie Thoracique, CHRU de Lille, Lille, France. [7]Santé Publique et Epidémiologie, Institut Pasteur, Université de Lille, INSERM UMR744, Lille, France. [8]Univ Lyon; UCBL; INSERM U1028 ; CNRS UMR5292 ; Service Universitaire d'Addictologie de Lyon, CH le Vinatier, Lyon, France.

References
1. Alberg AJ, Samet JM. Epidemiology of lung cancer. Chest. 2003;123(1 Suppl):21S–49S.
2. Anantharaman D, Marron M, Lagiou P, Samoli E, Ahrens W, Pohlabeln H, et al. Population attributable risk of tobacco and alcohol for upper aerodigestive tract cancer. Oral Oncol. 2011;47(8):725–31.
3. Toll BA, Brandon TH, Gritz ER, Warren GW, Herbst RS. AACR Subcommittee on tobacco and Cancer. Assessing tobacco use by cancer patients and facilitating cessation: an American Association for Cancer Research policy statement. Clin Cancer Res. 2013;19(8):1941–8.
4. Gritz ER, Carmack CL, de Moor C, Coscarelli A, Schacherer CW, Meyers EG, et al. First year after head and neck cancer: quality of life. J Clin Oncol. 1999; 17(1):352–60.
5. Duffy SA, Terrell JE, Valenstein M, Ronis DL, Copeland LA, Connors M. Effect of smoking, alcohol, and depression on the quality of life of head and neck cancer patients. Gen Hosp Psychiatry. 2002;24(3):140–7.

6.   Garces YI, Schroeder DR, Nirelli LM, Croghan GA, Croghan IT, Foote RL, et al. Tobacco use outcomes among patients with head and neck carcinoma treated for nicotine dependence: a matched-pair analysis. Cancer. 2004; 101(1):116–24.

7.   Karam-Hage M, Cinciripini PM, Gritz ER. Tobacco use and cessation for cancer survivors: an overview for clinicians. CA Cancer J Clin. 2014;64(4): 272–90.

8.   Farrelly MC, Pechacek TF, Thomas KY, Nelson D. The impact of tobacco control programs on adult smoking. Am J Public Health. 2008;98(2):304–9.

9.   Jemal A, Cokkinides VE, Shafey O, Thun MJ. Lung cancer trends in young adults: an early indicator of progress in tobacco control (United States). Cancer Causes Control. 2003;14(6):579–85.

10. Burris JL, Studts JL, DeRosa AP, Ostroff JS. Systematic review of tobacco use after lung or head/neck Cancer diagnosis: results and recommendations for future research. Cancer Epidemiol Biomark Prev. 2015;24(10):1450–61.

11. Vangeli E, Stapleton J, Smit ES, Borland R, West R. Predictors of attempts to stop smoking and their success in adult general population samples: a systematic review. Addiction. 2011;106(12):2110–21.

12. Goodwin RD, Pagura J, Spiwak R, Lemeshow AR, Sareen J. Predictors of persistent nicotine dependence among adults in the United States. Drug Alcohol Depend. 2011;118(2–3):127–33.

13. Goodwin RD, Kim JH, Weinberger AH, Taha F, Galea S, Martins SS. Symptoms of alcohol dependence and smoking initiation and persistence: a longitudinal study among US adults. Drug Alcohol Depend. 2013;133(2): 718–23.

14. von Elm E, Altman DG, Egger M, Pocock SJ, Gøtzsche PC, Vandenbroucke JP, et al. The strengthening the reporting of observational studies in epidemiology (STROBE) statement: guidelines for reporting observational studies. Lancet. 2007;370(9596):1453–7.

15. Travis WD, Giroux DJ, Chansky K, Crowley J, Asamura H, Brambilla E, et al. The IASLC lung Cancer staging project: proposals for the inclusion of broncho-pulmonary carcinoid tumors in the forthcoming (seventh) edition of the TNM classification for lung Cancer. J Thorac Oncol. 2008;3(11):1213–23.

16. French Alcohol Society. Good Practice Recommendations. Alcohol misuse: screening, diagnosis and treatment. 2015. http://www.sfalcoologie.asso.fr/ download/SFA-GPR-AlcoholMisuse.pdf?PHPSESSID=4e400010332fdc95b 8572ae6e0e7d9d7 (Accessed 10 Jul 2017).

17. Saunders JB, Aasland OG, Babor TF, de la Fuente JR, Grant M. Development of the alcohol use disorders identification test (AUDIT): WHO collaborative project on early detection of persons with harmful alcohol consumption–II. Addiction. 1993;88(6):791–804.

18. Legleye S, Karila L, Beck F, Reynaud M. Validation of the CAST, a general population Cannabis abuse screening test. J Subst Use. 2007;12(4):233–42.

19. Sheehan DV, Lecrubier Y, Sheehan KH, Amorim P, Janavs J, Weiller E, et al. The Mini-International Neuropsychiatric Interview (M.I.N.I.): the development and validation of a structured diagnostic psychiatric interview for DSM-IV and ICD-10. J Clin Psychiatry. 1998;59(Suppl 20):22–33. quiz 34–57

20. National Cancer Institute, American Association for Cancer Research. NCI-AACR cancer patient tobacco use questionnaire. https://www.gem-measures.org/ Public/DownloadMeasure.aspx?mid=2003 (Accessed 20 July 2017).

21. Schnoll RA, James C, Malstrom M, Rothman RL, Wang H, Babb J, Miller SM, Ridge JA, Movsas B, Langer C, Unger M, Goldberg M. Longitudinal predictors of continued tobacco use among patients diagnosed with cancer. Ann Behav Med. 2003;25(3):214–22.

22. Duffy SA, Ronis DL, Valenstein M, Fowler KE, Lambert MT, Bishop C, Terrell JE. Depressive symptoms, smoking, drinking, and quality of life among head and neck cancer patients. Psychosomatics. 2007;48(2):142–8.

23. Duffy SA, Khan MJ, Ronis DL, Fowler KE, Gruber SB, Wolf GT, Terrell JE. Health behaviors of head and neck cancer patients the first year after diagnosis. Head Neck. 2008;30(1):93–102.

24. American Lung Association. Trends in Tobacco Use. 2011. http://www.lung.org/ assets/documents/research/tobacco-trend-report.pdf (Accessed 20 July 2017).

25. European Commission. Special Eurobarometer 385: « Attitudes of European towards tobacco ». 2012. http://ec.europa.eu/health/tobacco/docs/ eurobaro_attitudes_towards_tobacco_2012_en.pdf. (Accessed 20 July 2017).

26. Ebbert JO, Yang P, Vachon CM, Vierkant RA, Cerhan JR, Folsom AR, et al. Lung cancer risk reduction after smoking cessation: observations from a prospective cohort of women. J Clin Oncol. 2003;21(5):921–6.

27. Marron M, Boffetta P, Zhang Z-F, Zaridze D, Wünsch-Filho V, Winn DM, et al. Cessation of alcohol drinking, tobacco smoking and the reversal of head and neck cancer risk. Int J Epidemiol. 2010;39(1):182–96.

28. Guignard R, Beck F, Richard JB, Peretti-Watel P. Le tabagisme en France: analyse de l'enquête Baromètre santé 2010 [Tobacco use in France: results of the 2010 "Health Barometer"].. Saint-Denis, Inpes, coll. Baromètres santé, 2013: 56 p. http://inpes.santepubliquefrance.fr/CFESBases/catalogue/pdf/ 1513.pdf (Accessed 24 Dec 17).

29. Young D, Borland R, Hammond D, Cummings KM, Devlin E, Yong HH, O'Connnor RJ, ITC Collaboration. Prevalence and attributes of roll-your-own smokers in the international tobacco control (ITC) four country survey. Tob Control. 2006;15(Suppl 3):iii76–82.

30. Curti D, Shang C, Ridgeway W, Chaloupka FJ, Fong GT. The use of legal, illegal and roll-your-own cigarettes to increasing tobacco excise taxes and comprehensive tobacco control policies: findings from the ITC Uruguay survey. Tob Control. 2015;24(Suppl 3):iii17–24.

22

Effect of surgery and radiotherapy on complete blood count, lymphocyte subsets and inflammatory response in patients with advanced oral cancer

Tadej Dovšak[1,2*], Alojz Ihan[3], Vojko Didanovič[1,2], Andrej Kansky[1,2], Miha Verdenik[1,2] and Nataša Ihan Hren[1,2]

Abstract

Background: The immune system has a known role in the aetiology, progression and final treatment outcome of oral squamous cell cancers. The aim of this study was to evaluate the influence of radical surgery and radiotherapy on advanced oral squamous cell carcinoma blood counts, lymphocyte subsets and levels of acute inflammatory response markers.

Methods: Blood samples were obtained from 56 patients 5 days before and 10 days after surgery, 30 days and 1 year after radiotherapy. The whole blood count, lymphocyte subsets and inflammatory response markers (C-reactive protein, erythrocyte sedimentation rate, leukocyte count, expression of index CD64 and index CD163 on neutrophils and monocytes) were measured, statistically analysed and correlated with clinical treatment outcomes.

Results: The post-operative period was characterised by the onset of anaemia, thrombocytosis, lymphopenia with reduced B lymphocyte, T helper cell and NK cell counts, and a rise in acute phase reactants. Immediately after radiotherapy, the anaemia improved, the lymphopenia worsened, and thrombocyte levels returned to pre-treatment values. There was a drop in counts across the T and B cell lines, including a reduction in B lymphocytes, naïve and memory T cells with reduced CD4+ and CD8+ counts and a decreased CD4/CD8 ratio. One year after radiotherapy all the lymphocyte subsets remained depressed, the only exception being NK cells, whose levels returned to pre-treatment values.

Conclusions: We concluded that surgery resulted in a stronger acute phase response than radiotherapy, while radiotherapy caused a long-lasting reduction in lymphocyte counts. There was no correlation between any of the pre-treatment parameters and the clinical outcome.

Keywords: Oral cancer, Surgery, Radiotherapy, Lymphopenia, Treatment outcome

Background

Oral and pharyngeal cancer is the 7th most common cancer and the 9th most lethal in the European Union [1]. The treatment for early-stage oral squamous cell cancers (OSCC) is generally single modality, either surgery or radiotherapy. Treatment of early-stage oral squamous cell cancers (OSCC) is generally unimodal

using either surgery or radiotherapy (RT). The treatment for locoregionally advanced OSCC is multimodal, with either surgery followed by adjuvant radiation or chemoradiation (as indicated by pathologic features), or definitive chemoradiation. Survival of patients with oral cancer mainly depends on the stage of disease. More than 50% of patients with oral cancer have advanced disease at the time of diagnosis [2]. By introducing new cytotoxic therapies to patients' treatment regimens, the survival rates have improved in the last decade [3].

Lymphocytes are involved in most human immune system mechanisms aimed at identifying and removing

* Correspondence: tadej.dovsak@gmail.com
[1]Clinical Department of Maxillofacial and Oral Surgery, |University Medical Center, Ljubljana, Slovenia
[2]Department of Maxillofacial and Oral Surgery, Faculty of Medicine, University of Ljubljana, Vrazov trg 2, 1104 Ljubljana, Slovenia
Full list of author information is available at the end of the article

cancer cells [4]. Patients with cancer are known to have abnormalities in T-cell and B-cell counts [5].

The microenvironment of head and neck squamous cell carcinomas (HNSCC), which include OSCC amongst them, is characterized by an imbalanced cytokine profile, favouring immunosuppressive over stimulatory cytokines [6]. It is also known that immunodeficiency increases HNSCC risk [7]. Infiltration of regulatory T cells into the tumour microenvironment was shown to promote tumour-induced immune modulation and subsequent tumour progression [8].

Patients with HNSCC have reduced levels of CD3+, CD4+, and CD8+ T cells in peripheral blood and CD4+ levels show correlation with the stage of disease [9].

Injury from surgical trauma follows dynamic pattern and results in haemodynamic, metabolic and immune changes in patients in the postoperative period. The initial systemic inflammatory response is mediated primarily by the cells of the innate immune system. Once healing of the injured site has begun, an anti-inflammatory response becomes prominent. This anti-inflammatory or immuno-suppressive phenotype is mediated primarily by the cells of the adaptive immune system. After major surgery, the functions of innate and of cell- mediated immunity are dramatically paralyzed [10].

Radiotherapy is one of three treatment modalities in oral cancer patients. Depending on the site and dose of radiation majority of patients will experience signs of acute toxicity that are self-limited in duration [11]. Lymphocytes are sensitive to radiation and radiation of areas rich in lymphatics and large vessels produces significant and long lasting immune alterations [12].

The aim of our prospective non-randomized study was to evaluate the effect of major surgical procedures and RT on the complete blood count, lymphocyte subpopulations and acute inflammatory response markers in the peripheral blood of patients with advanced oral squamous cell carcinoma (AOSCC). Partial preliminary results have already been published [13].

Methods

Patients were selected from the prospective non-randomized study, running from 2008 to 2013 on the Clinical Department for Oral and Maxillofacial Surgery, University Clinical Center in Ljubljana, according to the following inclusion criteria:

- Histologically verified squamous cell carcinoma of the oral cavity Stage III and IV according to the American Joint Committee on Cancer 2010 staging.
- Surgery and radiotherapy as the only treatment modalities.
- Patients' first malignant tumour.
- No prior radiotherapy.

- Completed blood sampling prior to surgery, after surgery, after radiotherapy, 1 year after the radiotherapy.

The study protocol was approved by the Republic of Slovenia National Medical Ethics Committee (No. 79/06/07; 19 April 2007), and an adequate written consent was obtained from each patient. Protocol of the study did not affect the standard treatment protocol of the patients in any way. The primary treatment modality of oral cancer is generally determined by the stage of the disease, with surgical treatment remaining the mainstay of multimodal treatment. In treatment selection our multidisciplinary board follows the national guidelines, which were adopted from the National Comprehensive Cancer Network (NCCN).

Seventy two patients were enrolled in the study in line with the inclusion criteria. At the end of the study 10 patients, who had been clinically assigned to advanced cancer, were down staged based on the histopathological report, 4 patients did not have complete blood samples and 2 patients no longer wanted to participate in the study. Of the remaining 56 patients, there were 44 men and 12 women with median age of 68 years (range, 47-89 years). Additional examinations required for the purpose of our study were blood sampling 5 days before surgery (T1), 10 days after surgery (T2), 30 days after radiotherapy (T3) and 1 year after radiotherapy (T4). The treatment outcome was evaluated 2 years after the radiotherapy. Main characteristics of patients are presented in Table 1.

Flow cytometry: The samples (100 μl of blood) were incubated with 10 μl of the appropriate MoAb. Antibodies against the following cell surface structures were applied: CD3, CD4, CD8, CD19, HLA-DR, CD56, CD45RA+, CD45RO, CD95 (Exalpha Biologicals, Boston, MA, USA. Non-specific isotype mouse MoAb were used as negative controls. Cells were analyzed on FACSCantoII™ Flow Cytometer (BDBiosciences), equipped with blue (488-nm solid-state) and red (633-nm helium-neon) laser. Digital data was acquired with FACSDiva software (BDBiosciences) and analyzed using FlowJo software (Tree Star Inc.).

Neutrophil CD64 expression was measured with a diagnostic kit Leuko64™ following the manufacturer's instructions. Additionally, we used the Leuko64™ QuantiCALC automated software (Trillium Diagnostic) that reports neutrophil expression of CD64 as an index using fluorescein-labelled calibration beads. An internal negative control of the assay was provided by the automated measurement of the lymphocyte CD64 index, which had to be less than 1.0, and an internal positive control of the assay was provided by automated measurement of the monocyte CD64 index, which had to be more than 3.0. Isotype-control antibodies were routinely used in each experiment to detect a non-specific staining.

Table 1 The main patient characteristics together with AOC stages, localizations of tumours, type of neck dissection, reconstruction type and blood sampling times

Number of patients	56		
Gender	♂ 44		♀ 12
Age (mean (range))		62 (42-84)	
Cancer Stage AJCC2010		III (12)	
		IVA (44)	
Tumour location	Tongue	22	
	Floor of mouth	17	
	Retromolar trigonum	6	
	Gum Maxilla	5	
	Gum Mandible	6	
Neck dissection	Unilateral	25	
	Bilateral	31	
Reconstruction	None		5
	Local flap	Tongue	2
	Distal flap	Temporalis	2
		PMMF	6
	Free flap	RFF	22
		ALT	8
		Iliac crest	3
		Fibula	6
		LMF	2
Blood samples	T1- 5 days before surgery		
	T2- 10 days after surgery		
	T3- 30 days after radiotherapy		
	T4- 1 year after radiotherapy		

PMMF Pectoralis Major Muscular Flap, *RFF* Radial Forearm Flap, *LMF* Latissimus Myocutaneous Flap, *ALT* Anterior Lateral Thigh, *T1* blood sample before surgery, *T2* blood sample after surgery, *T3* blood sample before radiotherapy, *T4* blood sample 1 year after radiotherapy

Data were presented as the average and 95% confidence interval for the average. Comparison between groups at different time intervals was performed using the Student's t- test.

One year after last blood sampling (T4), patients were divided into two groups: the first one with no evidence of disease or with death of other cause, and the second with local, locoregional or distal failure and death of the disease. We checked for possible prognostic factors in the immune state of the patients, prior to the performance of a Student's t-test between these two groups.

The differences were considered to be statistically significant at the level of $p < 0.05$. Statistical analysis was performed using Statistical Package for the Social Sciences for Windows, version 12.0 (SPSS Inc., Chicago, USA).

Results

Of 56 patients that matched the inclusion criteria, 37 were free of disease at final check-up (1 year after last blood sampling - T4). Of the remaining 19, 4 patients died of other causes during the time of our study, 9 patients died of disease-related complications, 4 patients developed local progression of the disease, 1 patient developed distant metastases, and 1 patient developed a secondary tumour. Thirty seven patients that were free of disease and 4 patients that died of other causes constituted the "success" group, while the remaining 15 patients constituted the "failure" group.

Blood samples prior to surgery (T1) were collected between 5 to 13 days before surgery (mean 8 ± 2). All patients were surgically treated with en-bloc excision of tumour and modified neck dissection (31 of them bilateral), and a subsequent reconstruction (41 with free flaps and 10 with pedicled flaps). In only 5 cases it was possible to close the defect primarily. The average blood loss during surgery was 470 ml (range 250 - 1200 ml) as assessed by the anaesthesiologist and the surgeon. All except one patient were tracheotomised at the time of surgery, with 3 patients subsequently remaining tube dependent, and the remainder having the tracheostomy tube removed between 2 to 22 days after the surgical procedure (mean 8 ± 5).

Blood samples prior to radiotherapy (T2) were taken between 8 and 11 days after surgery (mean 8 ± 2). Patients were irradiated with an external beam by a 6 MV linear accelerator. They received a dose between 60 and 66 Gy (mean 62 ± 2), divided over 2 Gy daily fractions, five times a week. No patient received hyperfractionated RT or chemotherapy. RT was performed within 28 to 54 days after surgery (mean 34 ± 7). The lower border of the irradiation field was always two centimetres above the clavicle, to avoid irradiation of the thymus.

The period of time between the last dose of RT and the next blood sample collection (T3) ranged from 24 to 44 days (mean 36 ± 6). The last blood sample (T4) was collected between 206 and 517 days after radiotherapy (mean 398 ± 57).

The mean values of measured parameters at all blood sampling times are presented in Table 2 together with their standard deviations and normal reference values for peripheral blood of our hospital laboratory.

Surgery resulted in anaemia, leucocytosis, lymphopenia, thrombocytosis, rise in neutrophils, CRP, erythrocyte sedimentation rate (ESR) and a reduction in albumin levels. In lymphocyte subpopulations the reductions in B lymphocyte, T helper cell, NK cell and naïve helper T lymphocyte counts were statistically significant. Out of the measured indexes, the only statistically significant increase was in the level of index CD64 on monocytes.

Radiotherapy caused a marked reduction in total lymphocyte counts, the levels of T, B lymphocytes, T

Table 2 Mean values and standard deviations of all measured parameters in blood samples in observed times (T1, T2, T3, T4) together with normal values

	T1 (mean ± SD)	T2 (mean ± SD)	T3 (mean ± SD)	T4 (mean ± SD)	Normal values
Erci (10*12/L)	4.32 ± 0.52	3.75 ± 0.48	4.45 ± 0.62	4.33 ± 0.44	4.20- 6.30
Hb (g/L)	139.2 ± 12.6	114.6 ± 17.9	134.9 ± 16.7	135.3 ± 12.2	120-180
Leu. (10*9/L)	8.53 ± 2.81	9.34 ± 3.06	6.9 ± 2.37	7.78 ± 5.39	4.0- 10.0
Lym (10*9/L)	1.9 ± 0.62	1.7 ± 0.62	1.1 ± 0.49	1.24 ± 0.64	1.4- 3.3
Pt (10*9/L)	278.7 ± 83.5	511.6 ± 202.2	270.7 ± 76.3	278.2 ± 92.1	140- 340
Neutr (10/9/l)	5.50 ± 2.26	6.56 ± 2.79	4.99 ± 2.12	5.54 ± 3.99	1.6- 7.5
CRP (mg/L)	9.1 ± 12.2	33.8 ± 37.4	13.3 ± 28.6	11.9 ± 23.8	< 5
ESR (mm/h)	32.1 ± 20.9	59.8 ± 21.2	39.8 ± 25.3	28.2 ± 19.6	< 15
Albumin (g/L)	42.7 ± 3.9	39.1 ± 4.2	43.9 ± 3.9	45.0 ± 3.3	32- 55
iCD64 mono.	7.5 ± 2.5	9.1 ± 3.9	11.0 ± 20.6	8.0 ± 2.9	4.34–8.70
iCD64 nevt.	0.73 ± 0.22	1.09 ± 1.46	0.93 ± 0.58	0.75 ± 0.32	0.45–2.16
iCD163 mono.	8586 ± 4129	8538 ± 4885	8667 ± 5288	8372 ± 6002	1061- 2740
iCD163 nevt.	223.4 ± 109.6	238.5 ± 153.8	252.9 ± 173.3	253.7 ± 172.9	301-435
HLA/DR3 (10*9/L)	0.26 ± 0.19	0.27 ± 0.25	0.28 ± 0.25	0.21 ± 0.21	0.06-0.30
CD3+ (10*9/L)	1.44 ± 0.52	1.32 ± 0.55	0.79 ± 0.41	0.81 ± 0.56	1.00-2.20
CD19+ (10*9/L)	0.17 ± 0.10	0.13 ± 0.07	0.06 ± 0.04	0.10 ± 0.06	0.11-0.57
CD4+ (10*9/L)	0.92 ± 0.32	0.82 ± 0.32	0.37 ± 0.17	0.38 ± 0.22	0.53-1.30
CD8+ (10*9/L)	0.53 ± 0.28	0.50 ± 0.32	0.41 ± 0.29	0.43 ± 0.38	0.33-0.92
CD4/CD8	2.10 ± 1.14	2.12 ± 1.27	1.11 ± 0.64	1.11 ± 0.59	1.0- 2.0
NK (10*9/L)	0.30 ± 0.16	0.24 ± 0.12	0.26 ± 0.14	0.34 ± 0.18	0.07-0.48
CD45RA + CD4+	0.27 ± 0.18	0.22 ± 0.13	0.06 ± 0.04	0.07 ± 0.05	0.23-0.77
CD45RO + CD4+	0.65 ± 0.25	0.59 ± 0.26	0.31 ± 0.15	0.31 ± 0.20	0.24 – 0.70

Legend: *Leu* leukocytes, *Lym* lymphocytes, *CD3+* T lymphocytes, *CD19+* B lymphocytes, *CD4+* T helper cells, *CD8+* cytotoxic T cells, *HLA/DR3* activated T lymphocytes, *NK* natural killer cells, *iCD64 mono* index of CD64 expression on monocytes, *iCD64 neutr* index of CD64 expression on neutrophils, *iCD163 mono* index of CD163 expression on monocytes, *iCD163 neutr* index of CD163 expression on neutrophils, *CD45 + RA + CD4+* naïve helper T lymphocytes, *CD45 + RO + CD4+* memory helper T lymphocytes, *CD95 + CD4+* apoptosis destined T helper cells, *Erci* erythrocytes, *Hb* haemoglobin, *Pt* platelets, *Neutr* neutrophils, *ESR* erythrocyte sedimentation rate; *CRP* C-reactive protein

helper lymphocytes, and cytotoxic T lymphocytes. CD4+ lymphocytes levels changed more than CD8+ levels, thereby also decreasing the CD4/CD8 ratio. Neither the CD64 index nor CD163 index showed any statistically significant changes during the observational period. The levels of NK cells did not change after radiotherapy and after 1 year rose to levels that were just above the pre-treatment values. CD45RA + CD4+ (naïve) T lymphocytes levels were diminished to 20% of the starting value and their value remained unchanged even after 1 year. CD45RO + CD4+ (memory) T lymphocyte levels were halved and did not recover after 1 year. After 1 year, there was still a statistically significant reduction, compared to pre-treatment values, in the levels of haemoglobin, lymphocytes, activated T lymphocytes, T lymphocytes, B lymphocytes, CD8+ and CD4+ lymphocytes, while the CD4/CD8 ratio was essentially half of that measured at T1.

The results of T-test comparing values of observed parameters at different blood sampling types are presented in Table 3.

One year after last blood sampling, at final check-up, we statistically correlated the measured parameters between the "success" group (no evidence of disease and death of other cause) and the "failure" group (locoregional, distant failure, secondary tumour and death of disease) at T1 for possible prognostic markers. Table 4 summarizes statistical analysis of selected parameters between both groups.

Levels of measured lymphocyte subpopulations indexed on T1 levels are shown in Fig. 1.

Figure 2 shows the levels of acute phase proteins (ESR, Albumin, CRP), neutrophyls and marker of activated T helpers (HLA/DR3) at blood sampling times indexed to T1 values.

Discussion

Radical surgical removal of the tumour is commonly the first and most important step toward the elimination of the disease. Nonetheless, during the perioperative period in oncological surgery, there might be some shedding of malignant cells, increased proliferation of tumour cells,

Table 3 Comparison of the observed parameters between T1/T2, T2/T3, T1/T3, T3/T4, T1/T4, T2/T4 blood samples as p values of the t- test between compared parameters at stated blood sampling times. Statistical significant differences according to the compared value ($p \leq 0.05$) are marked by * and ($p \leq 0.005$) with **

	T1/T2	T2/T3	T1/T3	T3/T4	T1/T4	T2/T4
Erci (10*12/L)	0.000**	0.000**	0.064	0.043*	0.719	0.000**
Hb (g/L)	0.000**	0.000**	0.042*	0.967	0.028*	0.000**
Leu. (10*9/L)	0.128	0.000**	0.001**	0.313	0.442	0.086
Lym (10*9/L)	0.011*	0.000**	0.000**	0.040*	0.000**	0.000**
Pt (10*9/L)	0.000**	0.000**	0.501	0.683	0.784	0.000**
Neutr (10/9/l)	0.024*	0.000**	0.192	0.443	0.887	0.131
CRP (mg/L)	0.000**	0.004**	0.223	0.707	0.466	0.001**
ESR (mm/h)	0.000**	0.000**	0.008*	0.000**	0.273	0.000**
Albumin (g/L)	0.000**	0.000**	0.049*	0.050	0.000**	0.000**
iCD64 mono.	0.011*	0.496	0.241	0.286	0.185	0.121
iCD64 nevt.	0.090	0.385	0.021*	0.008*	0.500	0.111
iCD163 mono.	0.915	0.861	0.979	0.931	0.555	0.585
iCD163 nevt.	0.378	0.618	0.164	0.725	0.297	0.683
HLA/DR3 (10*9/L)	0.989	0.534	0.436	0.002**	0.04*	0.122
CD3+ (10*9/L)	0.060	0.000**	0.000**	0.605	0.000**	0.000**
CD19+ (10*9/L)	0.006*	0.000**	0.000**	0.000**	0.000**	0.008*
CD4+ (10*9/L)	0.023*	0.000**	0.000**	0.347	0.000**	0.000**
CD8+ (10*9/L)	0.189	0.045*	0.002**	0.762	0.061	0.225
CD4/CD8	0.576	0.000**	0.000**	0.140	0.000**	0.000**
NK (10*9/L)	0.008*	0.592	0.050	0.001**	0.125	0.000**
CD45RA + CD4+	0.003**	0.000**	0.000**	0.005*	0.000**	0.000**
CD45RO + CD4+	0.045	0.000**	0.000**	0.646	0.000**	0.000**

Legend: *Leu* leukocytes, *Lym* lymphocytes, *CD3+* T lymphocytes, *CD19+* B lymphocytes; *CD4+* T helper cells, *CD8+* cytotoxic T cells, *HLA/DR3* activated T lymphocytes, *NK* natural killer cells, *iCD64 mono* index of CD64 expression on monocytesm, *iCD64 neutr* index of CD64 expression on neutrophils, *iCD163 mono* index of CD163 expression on monocytes, *iCD163 neutr* index of CD163 expression on neutrophils, *CD45 + RA + CD4+* naïve helper T lymphocytes, *CD45 + RO + CD4+* memory helper T lymphocytes, *CD95 + CD4+* apoptosis destined T helper cells, *Erci* erythrocytes, *Hb* haemoglobin, *Pt* platelets, *Neutr* neutrophils, *ESR* erythrocyte sedimentation rate, *CRP* C-reactive protein

excess release of pro-angiogenic and/or pro-invasive factors, abundant release of growth factors, psychological distress, and suppression of cell mediated immunity, which may act in synergy to render the patient temporarily vulnerable to metastases, which could otherwise have been controlled [14].

Free tissue transfer represents one of the most popular and reliable techniques for reconstruction after large primary tumours resection [15]. In only 5 of our patients it was possible to close the defect primarily or with a local flap, all others needed distal or free flap reconstruction. During such major surgery substantial blood loss may occur, varying between 500 and 1500 ml [16]. Anaemia is expected after major surgery of the head and neck, however, moderate anaemia also developed in our patients despite the loss of small volumes of blood. Hypoxia because of anaemia can decrease radiation efficacy [17]. The level of haemoglobin in our study was just below the proposed level of Hb before RT, which is 120 g/l, although in our study blood samples were taken within 8 and 12 days after surgery, thus the expected spontaneous rise prior to radiotherapy probably did occur. Microvascular reconstruction leads to prolonged operative times, and major, prolonged, surgical procedures are known to cause immunosuppression [18].

Inflammatory proteins (ESR, CRP) are non-specific markers related to infection, injury and neoplasia. They have been also correlated to cancer progression and prognosis in different malignancies [19], which was not the case in our study. In our patients, the ESR was elevated above normal before commencement of any treatment, and doubled after surgery (T2). At the T3 blood sampling the ESR remained above the initial value but with a gradual reduction towards pre-treatment values. It is of interest that ESR at T4 fell below the starting values, although the reduction failed to reach statistical significance. C-reactive protein (CRP) is an acute phase protein synthesized in the hepatocytes. CRP levels rise approximately 4 to 12 h after surgery, and peak at 24 to

Table 4 is showing p values of the t- test at T1 between the "success" ($N = 41$) and the "failure" ($N = 15$) group of patients. Statistical significant differences according to the compared value ($p \leq 0.05$) are marked by * and ($p \leq 0.005$) with **

Marker	Success group	Failure Group	Significany	Normal values
CRP (mg/L)	8.5	11.0	0,496	< 5
Neutr/Lym	2.9	3.3	0,414	
Pt (10*9/L)	277	282	0,844	140-340
CD3+ (10*9/L)	1.50	1.25	0,111	1.00-2.20
CD19+ (10*9/L)	0.17	0.16	0,717	0.11-0.57
CD45RA + CD4+	0.29	0.22	0,263	
CD45RO + CD4+	0.66	0.60	0,391	
Pt/Lym	153	173	0.363	

Legend: *CRP* C-reactive protein, *Neutr* neutrophils, *Lym* lymphocytes, *CD3+* T lymphocytes, *CD19+* B lymphocytes, *CD45 + RA + CD4+* naïve helper T lymphocytes, *CD45 + RO + CD4+* memory helper T lymphocytes, *Pt* platelets

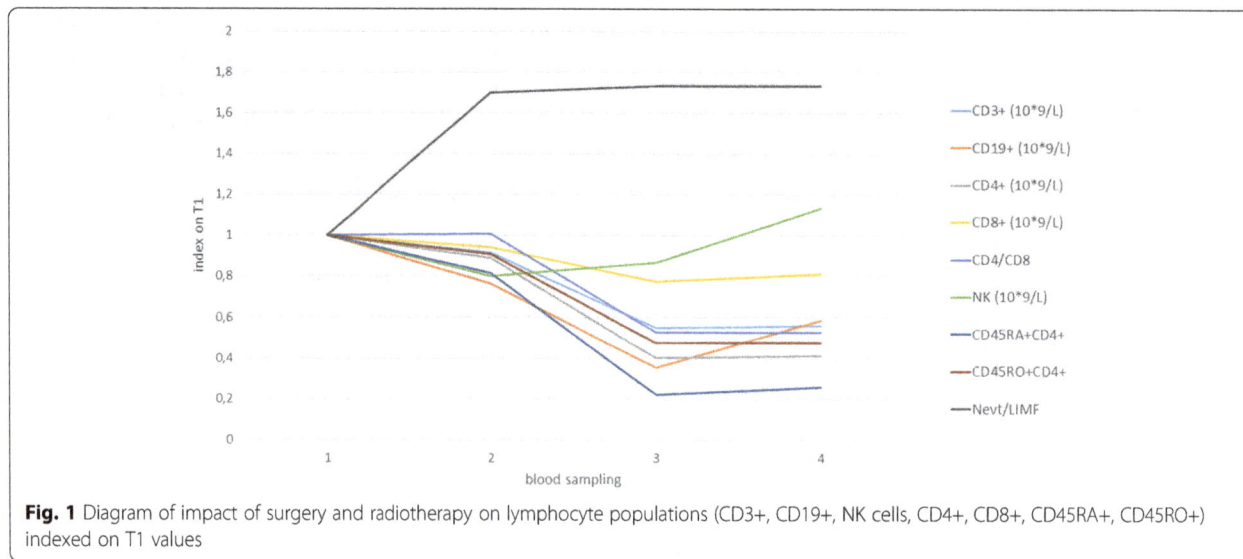

Fig. 1 Diagram of impact of surgery and radiotherapy on lymphocyte populations (CD3+, CD19+, NK cells, CD4+, CD8+, CD45RA+, CD45RO+) indexed on T1 values

72 h [20]. Once the tissue injury is resolved, CRP levels fall rapidly due to a short half-life of 6 h. Khandavilli et al. reported that increased preoperative CRP was associated with worse overall survival in patients with oral cancer [21], but a study by Krusse et al. failed to prove any correlation between preoperative CRP levels and disease progression in head and neck cancer [22]. Our results failed to show any correlation between the preoperative levels of the CRP and disease outcome. Surgery caused a 4-fold increase in CRP levels, while at T3 the levels of CRP showed a trend of returning to the pre-treatment values, although still at more than double the normal values. This is in accordance with the study by Mohammed et al. and Cheethana et al., who used ESR and CRP as biomarkers of radiation induced mucositis [23, 24]. After 1 year the CRP levels were practically identical to the preoperative values, but still above normal, which could indicate an ever-present subtle inflammation in the radiation-damaged mucosa.

There are several reports regarding the potential utility of CD64 (Fc receptor on monocytes, neutrophils, macrophages and eosinophils) on neutrophils for the diagnostic assessment of infection and systemic inflammatory response syndrome (SIRS) in adults [25].

CD163 is a monocyte/macrophage-associated antigen, which possesses anti-inflammatory properties and has an immunoregulatory role [26]. Since both indexes are only increased for short periods of a few days [27], this might explain why we failed to find any differences in the index values at various sampling times.

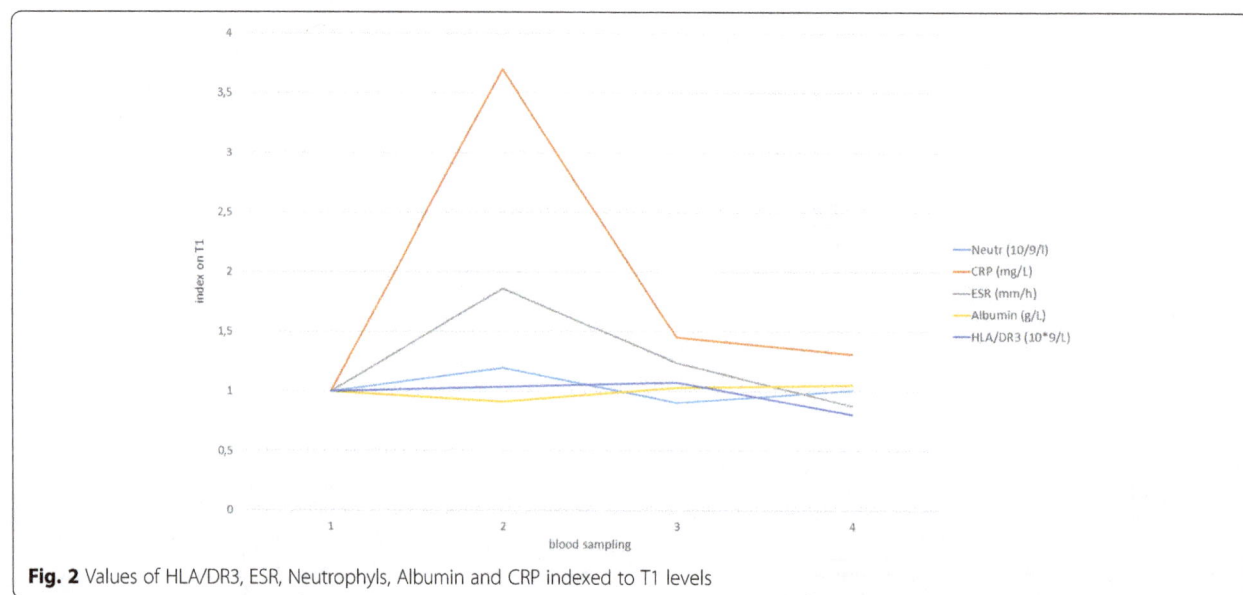

Fig. 2 Values of HLA/DR3, ESR, Neutrophyls, Albumin and CRP indexed to T1 levels

Various early studies have shown that cancer patients have depressed cell-mediated immune functions [28, 29]. Although we did not use a control group to match the T1 levels with healthy volunteers, it is worth noting that the average values of our measured parameters did not fall outside of reference values used by our hospital laboratory.

Leaver et al. and Ogawa et al. reported a fall in NK cells and T lymphocytes after surgery, and the levels were reduced up to 14 days after surgery [18, 30]. Additionally, the study conducted by Kuss et al. showed a persistent reduction in CD4+ cell counts in patients with a history head and neck cancer which was discovered long after surgery [29]. In our study the levels of NK cells and CD4+ cells also fell, but in contrast with the abovementioned studies, we observed a reduction in B lymphocyte levels. There was a trend towards reduced levels of T lymphocytes, but no other measured immunological parameter reached statistical significance. Although our T2 blood samples were taken within 8 and 12 days of surgery (mean 8 ± 2), one of the reasons for this discrepancy might be the small sample group.

In our group of patients radiotherapy was delivered between 28 to 54 days after surgery (mean 34 ± 7), and it only exceeded the prescribed 6 weeks' time in 8 patients (15%), providing the appropriate treatment regimen to most of the patients in the recommended time [31].

In our study we observed that even after more than a year, post-radiotherapy levels of lymphocytes, B lymphocytes, T lymphocytes, CD4+ and CD8+ lymphocytes remained significantly diminished compared to their pre-treatment levels. A study by Verastegui et al. [12] showed that CD4+ lymphocytes have a tendency to recover better than CD8+ cells, however, we did not see the expected trend in our study. In contrast, the levels of NK cells after a year were higher (although the increase was not statistically significant) than pre-treatment levels, indicating a probable compensatory increase. The levels of B lymphocytes in the study of Verastegui et al. [12] returned to normal after 1 year, which was not the case in our study, where they remained significantly reduced even more than a year after radiotherapy.

The large amount of accumulated evidence indicates that CD4+ T cells have a pivotal role in generating and maintaining anti-tumour immune responses through their interactions with cytotoxic T lymphocytes, B lymphocytes, macrophages and NK cells [32]. The levels of CD4+ lymphocytes more than halved after radiotherapy, and they remained at the same extremely low level even a year after radiotherapy. On the other hand, radiotherapy reduced the levels of CD8+ to 80% of pre-treatment values, and there was a trend towards the normalisation of their values a year after treatment completion, due to a faster effective doubling time of CD8+ cells, confirmed

also in the study by Kuss et al. [29]. As a consequence, the CD4/CD8 index halved after radiotherapy and remained at the value of 1.1 1 year after radiotherapy. The ineffectiveness of the immune cell response mechanisms against tumour antigens may be in part due to the reduction in the number and activity of CD4+ T lymphocytes, also confirmed in our study, which impacts the function and activity of CD8+ T cells. CD4+ T cells play a key role in initiating and sustaining the CD8+ T lymphocyte-led immune responses directed against tumour cells. CD4+ T cells are important in preventing cytotoxic lymphocyte anergy, and are involved in the formation of the memory CD8+ subpopulation. They also stimulate macrophages and eosinophils present in the tumour stroma [33, 34].

Most striking was the effect of radiotherapy on naïve T lymphocytes (CD45 + RA+), whose levels plummeted to 20% of pre-treatment values in contrast to memory T lymphocytes (CD45 + RO+), whose levels merely halved after radiotherapy. Both values remained unchanged afterwards. Although the thymus was spared from radiation, probably due to partial thymus involution in elderly patients [35] and higher radiosensitivity of naïve cells [36], the reconstitution of T lymphocytes was significantly depressed. As noted before, even in the setting of exposing a small percentage of body surface to radiation therapy, when the irradiated area is rich in large blood vessels, this will cause prolonged immune alterations [12].

The immune defects of OSCC patients as well as other cancer patients are most likely due to a multitude of mechanisms, making the reversal of immune inhibition more difficult. Radiotherapy even worsens these defects, which could have a negative influence on the efficacy of RT itself and it might just be that reduced immunity induced by radiotherapy in selected group of patients within OSCC group makes them more susceptible to tumour recurrence and worse survival [12, 37].

Using biomarkers to stratify oral cancer patients' risk of neck metastasis [38] is a rapidly developing field. We planned to search for possible markers to predict disease progression. We therefore divided patients into a treatment success and treatment failure group 2 years after radiotherapy, since recurrence most often appears within 2 years of treatment [39]. Although many authors have linked survival in head and neck cancer to many variables, such as CRP [21], lymphocyte/neutrophil ratio [40], monocytes [41] and thrombocytes [42] we did not find any correlation between pre-treatment values and disease progression or survival. The small sample size, which is the major limitation of our study, is probably the reason for this.

It should also be emphasized that the results of most of the cited publications regarding the head and neck region have dealt with a heterogeneous group of cancers, which are characterized by vastly different biological properties. Our study focused only on the immune changes in advanced squamous cell carcinoma of the oral cavity. Larger prospective studies are needed not only to confirm these findings, but also to address the possible underlying mechanisms that might link treatment-related lymphopenia to disease recurrence and survival.

Conclusions

Our study has shown that surgery causes a profound inflammatory reaction and a fall in the levels of B lymphocytes as well as NK cells, while radiotherapy produces long lasting immune depression with levels of T, B lymphocytes, CD4+ T lymphocytes and CD4/CD8 index almost halved after 1 year. Even more striking was the influence on the naïve T lymphocytes that did not recover to levels above 20% of the starting values. None of the measured parameters allowed us to predict the clinical outcome before the commencement of treatment.

Abbrevations

AOSCC: Advanced oral squamous cell carcinoma; CRP: C-reactive protein; ESR: Erythrocyte sedimentation rate; HNSCC: Head and neck squamous cell carcinoma; OSCC: Oral squamous cell cancers; RT: Radiotherapy

Acknowledgements
Thanks to Didanovic Gorenc Nina for her proofreading and Ivan Verdenik for support regarding statistics.

Funding
This research did not receive any specific grant from funding agencies in the public, commercial, or not-for-profit sectors.

Authors' contributions
All authors contributed to the study design, read and approved the final manuscript. TD and VD treated patients. NIH and TD contributed to the writing of the manuscript. AI analyzed immunological status, while AK, MV, NIH and TD analysed results.

Competing interests
None declared

Author details
[1]Clinical Department of Maxillofacial and Oral Surgery, |University Medical Center, Ljubljana, Slovenia. [2]Department of Maxillofacial and Oral Surgery, Faculty of Medicine, University of Ljubljana, Vrazov trg 2, 1104 Ljubljana, Slovenia. [3]Institute of Microbiology and Immunology, Faculty of Medicine, University of Ljubljana, Ljubljana, Slovenia.

References

1. Boyle P, Ferlay J. Cancer incidence and mortality in Europe, 2004. Ann Oncol. 2005;16(3):481–8.
2. Warnakulasuriya S. Global epidemiology of oral and oropharyngeal cancer. Oral Oncol. 2009;45(4-5):309–16.
3. Amit M, Yen TC, Liao CT, Chaturvedi P, Agarwal JP, Kowalski LP, Ebrahimi A, Clark JR, Kreppel M, Zoller J, et al. Improvement in survival of patients with oral cavity squamous cell carcinoma: an international collaborative study. Cancer. 2013;119(24):4242–8.
4. Mellman I, Coukos G, Dranoff G. Cancer immunotherapy comes of age. Nature. 2011;480(7378):480–9.
5. Lee JJ, Lin CL, Chen THH, Kok SH, Chang MC, Jeng JH. Changes in peripheral blood lymphocyte phenotypes distribution in patients with oral cancer/oral leukoplakia in Taiwan. Int J Oral Maxillofac Surg. 2010; 39(8):806–14.
6. Gildener-Leapman N, Ferris RL, Bauman JE. Promising systemic immunotherapies in head and neck squamous cell carcinoma. Oral Oncol. 2013;49(12):1089–96.
7. Badoual C, Sandoval F, Pere H, Hans S, Gey A, Merillon N, Van Ryswick C, Quintin-Colonna F, Bruneval P, Brasnu D, et al. Better understanding tumor-host interaction in head and neck cancer to improve the design and development of immunotherapeutic strategies. Head Neck. 2010; 32(7):946–58.
8. Liu H, Wang SH, Chen SC, Chen CY, Lo JL, Lin TM. Immune modulation of CD4+CD25+ regulatory T cells by zoledronic acid. BMC Immunol. 2016;17(1):45.
9. Kuss I, Hathaway B, Ferris RL, Gooding W, Whiteside TL. Imbalance in absolute counts of T lymphocyte subsets in patients with head and neck cancer and its relation to disease. Adv Otorhinolaryngol. 2005;62:161–72.
10. Greenfeld K, Avraham R, Benish M, Goldfarb Y, Rosenne E, Shapira Y, Rudich T, Ben-Eliyahu S. Immune suppression while awaiting surgery and following it: dissociations between plasma cytokine levels, their induced production, and NK cell cytotoxicity. Brain Behav Immun. 2007;21(4):503–13.
11. Purdy J, Klein E. External photon beam dosimetry and treatment planning. Princ Pract Radiat Ther. 1997;3:308–12.
12. Verastegui EL, Morales RB, Barrera-Franco JL, Poitevin AC, Hadden J. Long-term immune dysfunction after radiotherapy to the head and neck area. Int Immunopharmacol. 2003;3(8):1093–104.
13. Dovšak T, Ihan A, Didanovič V, Kansky A, Hren N. Influence of surgical treatment and radiotherapy of the advanced intraoral cancers on complete blood count, body mass index, liver enzymes and leukocyte CD64 expression. Radiol Oncol. 2009;43(4):282–92.
14. Neeman E, Ben-Eliyahu S. Surgery and stress promote cancer metastasis: new outlooks on perioperative mediating mechanisms and immune involvement. Brain Behav Immun. 2013;30(Suppl):S32–40.
15. Omura K. Current status of oral cancer treatment strategies: surgical treatments for oral squamous cell carcinoma. Int J Clin Oncol. 2014;19(3): 423–30.
16. Scott SN, Boeve TJ, McCulloch TM, Fitzpatrick KA, Karnell LH. The effects of Epoetin alfa on transfusion requirements in head and neck cancer patients: a prospective, randomized, placebo-controlled study. Laryngoscope. 2002; 112(7):1221–9.
17. Grau C, Overgaard J. Significance of hemoglobin concentration for treatment outcome. In: Molls M. Vaupel P, editors. Blood perfusion and microenviroment of human tumors. Berlin: Springer; 1998. p. 101–112.
18. Leaver HA, Craig SR, Yap PL, Walker WS. Lymphocyte responses following open and minimally invasive thoracic surgery. Eur J Clin Investig. 2000;30(3):230–8.
19. Brigden ML. Clinical utility of the erythrocyte sedimentation rate. Am Fam Physician. 1999;60(5):1443–50.
20. Giannoudis PV, Smith MR, Evans RT, Bellamy MC, Guillou PJ. Serum CRP and IL-6 levels after trauma: not predictive of septic complications in 31 patients. Acta Orthop Scand. 1998;69(2):184–8.
21. Khandavilli SD, Ceallaigh PO, Lloyd CJ, Whitaker R. Serum C-reactive protein as a prognostic indicator in patients with oral squamous cell carcinoma. Oral Oncol. 2009;45(10):912–4.
22. Kruse AL, Luebbers HT, Gratz KW. C-reactive protein levels: a prognostic marker for patients with head and neck cancer? Head Neck Oncol. 2010;2:21.
23. Mohammed FF, Poon I, Zhang L, Elliott L, Hodson ID, Sagar SM, Wright J. Acute-phase response reactants as objective biomarkers of radiation-induced mucositis in head and neck cancer. Head Neck. 2012;34(7):985–93.

24. Chethana RPS, Madathil LP, Rao S, Shetty P, Patidar M. Quantitative analysis of acute phase proteins in post chemo-radiation mucositis. J Clin Diagn Res. 2015;9(10):Zc28–31.

25. Qureshi S, Lewis S, Gant V, Treacher D, Davis B, Brown K. Increased distribution and expression of CD64 on blood polymorphonuclear cells from patients with the systemic inflammatory response syndrome (SIRS). Clin Exp Immunol. 2001;125(2):258–65.

26. Zuwała-Jagiełło J. Haemoglobin scavenger receptor: function in relation to disease. Acta Biochim Pol. 2005;53(2):257–68.

27. Fjaertoft G, Douhan Håkansson L, Pauksens K, Sisask G, Venge P. Neutrophil CD64 (FcγRI) expression is a specific marker of bacterial infection: a study on the kinetics and the impact of major surgery. Scand J Infect Dis. 2007;39(6-7):525–35.

28. Olkowski ZL, Wilkins SA Jr. T-lymphocyte levels in the peripheral blood of patients with cancer of the head and neck. Am J Surg. 1975;130(4):440–4.

29. Kuss I, Hathaway B, Ferris RL, Gooding W, Whiteside TL. Decreased absolute counts of T lymphocyte subsets and their relation to disease in squamous cell carcinoma of the head and neck. Clin Cancer Res. 2004;10(11):3755–62.

30. Ogawa K, Hirai M, Katsube T, Murayama M, Hamaguchi K, Shimakawa T, Naritake Y, Hosokawa T, Kajiwara T. Suppression of cellular immunity by surgical stress. Surgery. 2000;127(3):329–36.

31. Graboyes EM, Garrett-Mayer E, Sharma AK, Lentsch EJ, Day TA. Adherence to National Comprehensive Cancer Network guidelines for time to initiation of postoperative radiation therapy for patients with head and neck cancer. Cancer. 2017;123(14):2651–60.

32. Toes RE, Ossendorp F, Offringa R, Melief CJ. CD4 T cells and their role in antitumor immune responses. J Exp Med. 1999;189(5):753–6.

33. Kuss I, Donnenberg AD, Gooding W, Whiteside TL. Effector CD8+CD45RO-CD27-T cells have signalling defects in patients with squamous cell carcinoma of the head and neck. Br J Cancer. 2003;88(2):223–30.

34. Caserta S, Kleczkowska J, Mondino A, Zamoyska R. Reduced functional avidity promotes central and effector memory CD4 T cell responses to tumor-associated antigens. J Immunol. 2010;185(11):6545–54.

35. Weinberg K, Parkman R. Age, the thymus, and T lymphocytes. N Engl J Med. 1995;332(3):182–3.

36. Tabi Z, Spary LK, Coleman S, Clayton A, Mason MD, Staffurth J. Resistance of CD45RA- T cells to apoptosis and functional impairment, and activation of tumor-antigen specific T cells during radiation therapy of prostate cancer. J Immunol. 2010;185(2):1330–9.

37. Brown JS, Blackburn TK, Woolgar JA, Lowe D, Errington RD, Vaughan ED, Rogers SN. A comparison of outcomes for patients with oral squamous cell carcinoma at intermediate risk of recurrence treated by surgery alone or with post-operative radiotherapy. Oral Oncol. 2007;43(8):764–73.

38. Uchida K, Veeramachaneni R, Huey B, Bhattacharya A, Schmidt BL, Albertson DG. Investigation of HOXA9 promoter methylation as a biomarker to distinguish oral cancer patients at low risk of neck metastasis. BMC Cancer. 2014;14:353.

39. Kissun D, Magennis P, Lowe D, Brown JS, Vaughan ED, Rogers SN. Timing and presentation of recurrent oral and oropharyngeal squamous cell carcinoma and awareness in the outpatient clinic. Br J Oral Maxillofac Surg. 2006;44(5):371–6.

40. Fang HY, Huang XY, Chien HT, Chang JT, Liao CT, Huang JJ, Wei FC, Wang HM, Chen IH, Kang CJ, et al. Refining the role of preoperative C-reactive protein by neutrophil/lymphocyte ratio in oral cavity squamous cell carcinoma. Laryngoscope. 2013;123(11):2690–9.

41. Bobdey S, Ganesh B, Mishra P, Jain A. Role of monocyte count and neutrophil-to-lymphocyte ratio in survival of oral cancer patients. Int Arch Otorhinolaryngol. 2017;21(1):21–7.

42. Lu CC, Chang KW, Chou FC, Cheng CY, Liu CJ. Association of pretreatment thrombocytosis with disease progression and survival in oral squamous cell carcinoma. Oral Oncol. 2007;43(3):283–8.

23

Occupational exposure to petroleum-based and oxygenated solvents and hypopharyngeal and laryngeal cancer in France: the ICARE study

Christine Barul[1,2], Matthieu Carton[3], Loredana Radoï[4,5], Gwenn Menvielle[6], Corinne Pilorget[7,8], Simona Bara[9], Isabelle Stücker[4], Danièle Luce[1*] (iD) ICARE study group

Abstract

Background: To examine associations between occupational exposure to petroleum-based and oxygenated solvents and the risk of hypopharyngeal and laryngeal cancer.

Methods: ICARE is a large, frequency-matched population-based case-control study conducted in France. Lifetime occupational history, tobacco smoking and alcohol consumption were collected. Analyses were restricted to men and included 383 cases of hypopharyngeal cancer, 454 cases of laryngeal cancer, and 2780 controls. Job–exposure matrices were used to assess exposure to five petroleum-based solvents (benzene; gasoline; white spirits; diesel, fuels and kerosene; special petroleum products) and to five oxygenated solvents (alcohols; ketones and esters; ethylene glycol; diethyl ether; tetrahydrofuran). Odds ratios (ORs) adjusted for smoking, alcohol drinking and other potential confounders and 95% confidence intervals (CI) were estimated with unconditional logistic models.

Results: No significant association was found between hypopharyngeal or laryngeal cancer risk and exposure to the solvents under study. Non-significantly elevated risks of hypopharyngeal cancer were found in men exposed to high cumulative levels of white spirits (OR = 1.46; 95% CI: 0.88–2.43) and tetrahydrofuran (OR = 2.63; 95CI%: 0.55–12.65), with some indication of a dose-response relationship (p for trend: 0.09 and 0.07 respectively).

Conclusion: This study provides weak evidence for an association between hypopharyngeal cancer and exposure to white spirits and tetrahydrofuran, and overall does not suggest a substantial role of exposure to petroleum-based or oxygenated solvents in hypopharyngeal or laryngeal cancer risk.

Keywords: Solvents, Occupational exposure, Cancer, Larynx, Hypopharynx

Background

Despite a decrease in the last decades, incidence of hypopharyngeal cancer and laryngeal cancer in France among men remains among the highest in Europe, with annual incidence rates of about 5/100,000 and 7/100,000 respectively [1]. Tobacco smoking and alcohol consumption are the major risk factors [2], their joint effect being at least multiplicative [3].

Several occupational exposures are also known or suspected to be associated with these cancers. Exposure to strong acid mists [4] and to asbestos [5] are recognized risk factors for laryngeal cancer, and there is also some evidence that exposure to asbestos increases the risk of hypopharyngeal cancer [5]. Other possible occupational risk factors include exposure to polycyclic aromatic hydrocarbons, engine exhausts, and solvents [6]. Exposure to solvents in general was found to be associated with an increased risk of laryngeal or hypopharyngeal cancer in several studies [7–9], but the role of specific solvents was rarely investigated.

* Correspondence: daniele.luce@inserm.fr
[1]Univ Rennes, Inserm, EHESP, Irset (Institut de recherche en santé, environnement et travail)-UMR_S 1085, Pointe-à-Pitre F-97110, France
Full list of author information is available at the end of the article

We previously examined the role of chlorinated solvents in head and neck cancer risk, and found an association between exposure to perchloroethylene and laryngeal cancer [10]. In our study population, increased risks of laryngeal and/or hypopharyngeal cancer were also observed among building caretakers, cleaners, farm workers, toolmakers, rubber and plastic workers, who may be exposed to other types of solvents [11]. Therefore, our objective in this study was to examine the associations between exposure to petroleum-based and oxygenated solvents and the risk of hypopharyngeal and laryngeal cancers.

Methods

Study design and population

The present study is based on data from the ICARE study, a French multicenter population-based case-control study, conducted between 2001 and 2007 in ten geographical areas covered by a cancer registry. Eligible cases were patients aged between 18 and 75 years, with histologically confirmed tumor of the oral cavity, pharynx, sinonasal cavities and larynx first diagnosed during the study period.

Population controls were selected in the same geographical areas using incidence density sampling, with frequency-matching by gender and age (< 40, 40–54, 55–64, ≥65 years old). A further stratification was performed to make controls comparable to the general population on socioeconomic status. The participation rates were 82.5% among cases and 80.6% among controls. Details about the study design have been described elsewhere [12]. The present study was restricted to squamous cell carcinomas of the larynx (International Classification of Diseases for Oncology 3rd revision codes: C32) and hypopharynx (C12-C13). Analyses were restricted to men and women were analyzed separately [13]. Overall, 383 cases of hypopharyngeal cancer and 454 cases of laryngeal cancer, and 2780 controls were included.

Data collection

Standardized questionnaires were used by trained interviewers during face-to-face interviews to collect data. Those included sociodemographic characteristics, smoking and alcohol consumption histories, and a detailed lifetime occupational history, with a description of each job held for at least one month.

Trained coders blinded to case-control status coded occupations and industries, according to the International Standard Classification of Occupations (ISCO) [14] and the French Nomenclature of Activities (NAF) [15].

Exposure assessment

Exposures to five petroleum-based solvents (benzene; gasoline; white spirits and other light aromatic mixtures; diesel, fuels and kerosene; special petroleum products) and five oxygenated solvents (alcohols; ketones and esters; ethylene glycol; diethyl ether; tetrahydrofuran) were assessed by job-exposures matrices (JEMs) developed for the French population in the context of the Matgéné program [16]. The JEMs assessed both inhalation and dermal exposures, with no distinction in exposure rating by route of exposure. Inhalation is, however, the main route of exposure for the solvents under study.

For each combination of ISCO and NAF codes, three indices of exposure were provided by the JEMs: (i) probability of exposure expressed as the percentage of exposed workers; (ii) intensity of exposure; and (iii) frequency of exposure as a percentage of working time. For these three indices, different categories were used according to the solvent (See Additional file 1). Exposure indices were provided for different calendar periods to take into account variations due to changes in exposure over time. Specific JEMs were also used to assess exposure to asbestos [17] and perchloroethylene [10]. Exposure to strong inorganic acids was obtained for each job from specific questions in the questionnaire.

Two variables were computed by linking lifetime occupational history with these indices: 'ever/never' exposed ('ever' defined as having worked in at least one job with probability of exposure greater than zero), and the Cumulative Exposure Index (CEI). CEIs were the results of summation over the entire work history of the product of exposure probability, frequency, intensity and duration of each job period, using the central value of the classes. CEIs were categorized in four categories: 'never exposed', and three categories according to the percentiles of the distribution among exposed controls (low: < 50th; medium: 50th–90th; high: > 90th). We estimated lifetime exposure prevalence to the various solvents as the mean of the maximum probability of exposure of each subject over his working life, using the central values of the classes.

Other variables

Analyses were adjusted for age at interview in categories (< 40, 40–49, 50–59; 60–69, ≥70 years), residence area, alcohol consumption in categories (≤0.03, 0.04–2.00, 2.01–4.99, 5.00–7.99, 8.00–11.99, ≥12 glasses/day), smoking status (never; former: time since stopping smoking > 2 years at the interview; current), daily amount of tobacco in categories (1–10, 11–20, 20–25, > 25 g/day), duration of tobacco smoking in categories (1–20, 21–30, 31–40, > 40 years), and cumulative asbestos exposure in 4 categories (never exposed, and tertiles of the distribution among exposed controls).

Statistical analysis

Adjusted odds ratios (ORs) and corresponding 95% confidence intervals (95% CI) were obtained by use of multivariable unconditional logistic regression models. Main analyses were performed separately for each solvent. Tests for linear trends were performed by modelling the median of each category as a continuous variable. We also examined the risks associated with joint exposure to several solvents by families of solvents (i) petroleum-based, (ii) oxygenated solvents. These analyses were restricted to combinations of solvents with at least 10 exposed cases.

In additional analyses we also adjusted for socioeconomic status, assessed by occupational class of the longest job held. As we previously found that exposure to perchloroethylene [10] was associated with laryngeal cancer, adjustment for this exposure was also performed but did not modify ORs estimates. Similarly, adjustment for self-reported exposure to strong inorganic acids did not change the ORs. Therefore, strong inorganic acids and perchloroethylene were not included in the models presented here.

Results

Table 1 shows the main characteristics of cases and controls, as well as lifetime prevalence of exposure to the various solvents. Cases of hypopharyngeal and laryngeal cancers were generally older, more often blue collar workers, daily drank more alcohol and were more often smokers than controls. Exposure to petroleum-based solvents was relatively frequent, and exposure prevalences were higher in cases than in controls. Exposure prevalences were lower for oxygenated solvents, and were roughly similar in cases and in controls.

The solvents studied are used as cleaners, degreasers and reagents in varied industrial processes, and are used in a number of formulations such as paints, adhesives, inks and dyes, dry cleaning solutions, pesticides, fuels, cosmetics and pharmaceuticals.

In our study population, men exposed to petroleum solvents were mainly employed as machinery fitters, and to a lesser extent as transport drivers (diesel/fuels/kerosene, gasoline) and construction workers (white spirits). Machinery fitters was the most frequent occupation among men exposed to ketones, esters, and ethylene glycol. Men exposed to ether and alcohols were mostly employed as medical workers. Exposure to tetrahydrofuran occurred primarily among plumbers and welders, due to the use of PVC pipe glues (data not shown).

Exposures to the solvents under study were correlated. The stronger correlations were found between exposures to benzene and white spirits ($r = 0.62$), gasoline and diesel/fuels/kerosene ($r = 0.69$) and ketones/esters and alcohols ($r = 0.64$) (see Additional file 2).

Table 1 Main characteristics of cases and controls

	Hypopharyngeal cancer $n = 383$		Laryngeal cancer $n = 454$		Controls $n = 2780$	
	n	%	n	%	n	%
Age						
< 40	0	0.0	5	1.10	76	2.7
40–49	51	13.3	56	12.3	555	20.0
50–59	164	42.8	175	38.6	825	29.7
60–69	118	30.8	147	32.4	939	33.8
≥ 70	50	13.1	71	15.6	385	13.9
Socioeconomic status						
Farmers	8	2.1	18	4.0	168	6.0
Self-employed workers	25	6.6	34	7.5	152	5.5
Managers	21	5.5	34	7.5	544	19.6
Intermediate occupations	32	8.4	55	12.2	564	20.3
Employees	40	10.4	45	10.0	297	10.7
Blue collar workers	252	65.8	265	58.8	1053	37.9
Alcohol consumption, glasses/day						
≤ 0.03	11	2.9	19	4.2	206	7.5
0.04–2.00	34	8.9	70	15.4	1190	42.8
2.01–4.99	89	23.2	110	24.2	849	30.5
5.00–7.99	78	20.4	108	23.8	305	10.9
8.00–11.99	82	21.4	74	16.3	134	4.8
≥ 12	70	18.3	54	11.9	73	2.6
Smoking status						
Never	3	0.8	13	2.9	753	27.1
Former	121	31.6	122	26.9	1271	45.7
Current	256	66.9	317	69.8	751	27.0
Lifetime exposure prevalence						
Petroleum-based solvents						
Benzene		16.9		15.6		11.7
Gasoline		11.6		11.1		8.7
Special petroleum-based products		3.6		2.6		2.5
Diesel, fuels and kerosene		20.0		18.4		14.4
White spirits		21.3		18.7		14.4
Oxygenated solvents						
Ketones and esters		13.5		11.8		9.5
Alcohols		12.2		11.5		12.9
Diethyl ether		0.4		0.6		1.4
Ethylene glycol		6.5		7.0		6.1
Tetrahydrofuran		1.6		1.0		0.7

Table 2 reports the associations between occupational exposure to petroleum-based solvents and hypopharyngeal and laryngeal cancer risk. Overall, no significant association was found. For hypopharyngeal cancer, the

Table 2 Association between hypopharyngeal and laryngeal cancers and occupational exposure to petroleum-based solvents

Petroleum based solvents	Controls n	Hypopharynx n	OR[a]	[95% CI]	Larynx n	OR[a]	[95% CI]
Benzene							
Never	2120	237	–		314	–	
Ever	552	102	1.07	[0.80–1.45]	109	0.94	[0.71–1.24]
CEI							
Low	279	51	1.15	[0.78–1.69]	46	0.81	[0.55–1.18]
Medium	220	39	1.02	[0.67–1.57]	56	1.27	[0.87–1.84]
High	53	12	0.9	[0.43–1.89]	7	0.42	[0.18–1.01]
p for trend				0.98			0.21
Gasoline							
Never	2161	243	–		323	–	
Ever	510	96	1.11	[0.83–1.50]	100	0.93	[0.70–1.23]
CEI							
Low	257	54	1.19	[0.82–1.72]	51	0.89	[0.62–1.27]
Medium	205	32	1.02	[0.65–1.61]	46	1.19	[0.80–1.77]
High	48	10	0.93	[0.42–2.06]	3	0.23	[0.07–0.79]
p for trend				0.87			0.03
Special petroleum products							
Never	2439	300	–		384	–	
Ever	234	38	1.20	[0.79–1.82]	39	0.93	[0.63–1.39]
CEI							
Low	118	18	1.22	[0.68–2.20]	17	0.86	[0.48–1.54]
Medium	93	17	1.21	[0.65–2.24]	20	1.07	[0.61–1.89]
High	23	3	1.10	[0.29–4.17]	2	0.64	[0.14–2.94]
p for trend				0.55			0.75
Diesel, fuels and kerosene							
Never	1753	175	–		239	–	
Ever	918	164	1.19	[0.90–1.56]	184	1.05	[0.82–1.35]
CEI							
Low	460	80	1.12	[0.80–1.56]	88	1.01	[0.74–1.37]
Medium	366	69	1.36	[0.96–1.93]	80	1.21	[0.88–1.67]
High	92	15	0.92	[0.48–1.75]	16	0.80	[0.43–1.48]
p for trend				0.61			0.41
White spirits							
Never	1436	125	–		186	–	
Ever	1240	216	1.14	[0.82–1.58]	237	0.93	[0.70–1.24]
CEI							
Low	620	93	1.15	[0.80–1.67]	112	0.99	[0.71–1.37]
Medium	494	86	0.99	[0.67–1.47]	94	0.84	[0.59–1.20]
High	126	37	1.46	[0.88–2.43]	31	0.97	[0.58–1.60]
p for trend				0.09			0.70

Abbreviations: *CEI* Cumulative Exposure Index
[a]OR adjusted for age at interview, residence area, alcohol consumption, smoking status, frequency and duration of smoking, exposure to asbestos

ORs were slightly elevated for each solvent, on the order of 1.2, with no significant trend with cumulative exposure. The highest OR was found for the highest level of cumulative exposure to white spirits (OR = 1. 46; 95% CI [0.88–2.43]), with some indication of a dose-response relationship (p for trend = 0.09). For laryngeal cancer, the ORs were around the null value of 1 for all solvents.

Regarding exposure to oxygenated solvents (Table 3), ever exposure to tetrahydrofuran was associated with non-significantly elevated risks of hypopharyngeal and laryngeal cancer. There was some evidence of a dose-response relationship for hypopharyngeal cancer, with a higher OR for the highest level of cumulative exposure (OR = 2.63; 95 CI% [0.55–12.65]; p for trend = 0.07). We also observed a significant increased OR for laryngeal cancer risk among men with the lowest level of exposure to ethylene glycol (OR = 1.75; 95% CI [1.04–2.94]) with a significant negative trend with the level of exposure (p for trend = 0.04). No association appeared between exposure to other oxygenated solvents and hypopharyngeal or laryngeal cancer risk.

Further adjustment for socioeconomic status generally slightly decreased the ORs without any relevant change (see Additional file 3 for petroleum-based solvents and Additional file 4 for oxygenated solvents). Analyses considering exposure to combinations of petroleum solvents are shown in Table 4. Exclusive exposure to white spirits was associated with a non-statistically significantly elevated risk of hypopharyngeal cancer (OR = 1.40; 95% CI [0.85–2.32]), as well as other combinations including white spirits. Men exposed to the five petroleum solvents had an elevated risk of hypopharyngeal cancer (OR = 2.12; 95% CI [0.98–4.61]). An elevated risk of laryngeal cancer was found for exclusive exposure to diesel (OR = 1.62; 95% CI [0.89–2.96]), but not for exposure to diesel combined with other petroleum solvents. Combined exposure to benzene, special petroleum products and white spirits was associated with a decreased risk of laryngeal cancer (OR = 0.41; 95% CI [0.17–1.00]).

The analysis of exposure to combinations of oxygenated solvents (Table 5) showed that men exposed to ketones, alcohols and tetrahydrofuran had a significantly higher risk of hypopharyngeal cancer (OR = 2.79; 95% CI [1.12–6.95]); an increased OR of borderline significance was also observed for laryngeal cancer (OR = 2.25; 95% CI [0.94–5.38]). No increased risks were found for other combinations including alcohols and ketones. No subject was exposed solely to tetrahydrofuran.

Discussion

In this study, we investigated the associations between occupational exposure to petroleum-based or oxygenated

Table 3 Association between hypopharyngeal and laryngeal cancers and occupational exposure to oxygenated solvents

	Controls	Hypopharynx			Larynx		
	n	n	OR[a]	[95% CI]	n	OR[a]	[95% CI]
Ketones and esters							
Never	2055	238	–		297	–	
Ever	618	100	1.01	[0.74–1.37]	126	1.10	[0.84–1.45]
CEI							
Low	309	46	1.05	[0.71–1.56]	62	1.24	[0.88–1.75]
Medium	245	38	0.89	[0.58–1.35]	53	1.08	[0.74–1.56]
High	64	16	1.34	[0.70–2.59]	11	0.87	[0.42–1.79]
p for trend			0.52			0.62	
Alcohols							
Never	1775	225	–		290	–	
Ever	898	113	0.95	[0.72–1.27]	133	0.90	[0.70–1.17]
CEI							
Low	447	45	0.85	[0.59–1.25]	64	0.99	[0.71–1.37]
Medium	359	50	1.07	[0.74–1.55]	53	0.86	[0.60–1.22]
High	91	17	1.25	[0.68–2.31]	16	0.93	[0.51–1.72]
p for trend			0.31			0.87	
Diethyl ether							
Never	2580	333	–		419	–	
Ever	90	5	0.59	[0.20–1.70]	4	0.37	[0.12–1.11]
CEI							
Low	45	1	0.28	[0.04–2.19]	1	0.2	[0.03–1.53]
Medium	36	4	1.41	[0.43–4.67]	3	0.73	[0.20–2.65]
High	9	0	–	–	0	–	–
p for trend			0.90			0.41	
Ethylene glycol							
Never	2487	312	–		387	–	
Ever	183	26	0.82	[0.49–1.36]	36	1.00	[0.64–1.56]
CEI							
Low	92	15	1.08	[0.57–2.04]	28	1.75	[1.04–2.94]
Medium	72	11	0.83	[0.39–1.74]	6	0.39	[0.16–0.96]
High	19	0	–	–	2	0.34	[0.07–1.64]
p for trend			0.10			0.04	
Tetrahydrofuran							
Never	2603	319	–		406	–	
Ever	67	19	1.67	[0.87–3.21]	17	1.39	[0.73–2.63]
CEI							
Low	35	7	1.33	[0.53–3.35]	9	1.50	[0.66–3.35]
Medium	26	8	1.57	[0.61–4.08]	8	1.62	[0.65–4.07]
High	6	4	2.63	[0.55–12.65]	0	–	–
p for trend			0.07			0.80	

Abbreviations: *CEI* Cumulative Exposure Index
[a]OR adjusted for age at interview, residence area, alcohol consumption, smoking status, frequency and duration of smoking, exposure to asbestos

Table 4 Association between hypopharyngeal and laryngeal cancers and exposure to combinations of petroleum-based solvents

Exposure to petroleum-based solvents	Controls n = 2536	Hypopharynx n = 313		Larynx n = 396	
	n	n	OR[a] [95% CI]	n	OR[a] [95% CI]
None	1231	95	1	143	1
White spirits	316	46	1.40 [0.85–2.32]	55	0.98 [0.63–1.51]
Diesel	90	9	0.92 [0.41–2.11]	23	1.62 [0.89–2.96]
Ben, WS	74	19	1.55 [0.79–3.03]	26	1.27 [0.70–2.29]
WS, Diesel	242	44	1.47 [0.88–2.45]	46	0.90 [0.57–1.43]
Ben, SPP, WS	86	10	1.07 [0.47–2.45]	7	0.41 [0.17–1.00[
Gasoline, WS, Diesel	95	20	1.48 [0.75–2.90]	20	0.93 [0.50–1.73]
Ben, Gasoline, WS, Diesel	233	41	1.27 [0.75–2.15]	44	0.86 [0.54–1.39]
All petroleum-based solvents	55	15	2.12 [0.98–4.61]	14	1.28 [0.60–2.71]

Abbreviations: *WS* white spirits, *diesel* diesel, fuels and kerosene, *ben* benzene, *SPP* special petroleum products
[a]OR adjusted for age at interview, residence area, alcohol consumption, smoking status, frequency and duration of smoking, exposure to asbestos

solvents and hypopharyngeal or laryngeal cancer. We did not find any significant excess risk when exposure to a single solvent was considered. Overall, our results do not suggest a substantial role of exposure to petroleum-based or oxygenated solvents in hypopharyngeal or laryngeal cancer risk.

Research on occupational exposure to solvents and the risk of hypopharyngeal and laryngeal cancers has been limited so far. In a case-control study conducted in Southern Europe, a significant increased risk of hypopharyngeal and laryngeal cancers was reported among men exposed to organic solvents [8]. In a multicenter case-control study in Central and Eastern Europe, exposure to organic solvents was associated with a non-significantly elevated risk of hypopharyngeal cancer, but no association was found with laryngeal cancer [9]. Other epidemiological studies which considered exposure to solvents in general did not report excess risks of laryngeal cancer [9, 18–21]. Most of these studies were case-control studies, that adjusted for smoking and alcohol [8, 9, 18–21], with the exception of a cohort study of construction workers, in which alcohol consumption was not available [21].

Exposure to solvents was assessed by industrial hygienists from detailed occupational histories in one study [9], with a JEM in three studies [8, 20, 21], and was self-reported in two studies [18, 19]. Very few studies have previously investigated exposures to specific petroleum-based and oxygenated solvents, so comparison of our results with the literature is limited.

As in our study, moderate and non-significant associations have been previously reported between laryngeal cancer and exposure to gasoline [9, 19] or to diesel, fuels and kerosene [9].

Our findings provide limited evidence of an increased risk of hypopharyngeal cancer in men exposed to white spirits, with elevated ORs for the highest level of cumulative exposure, and for men exposed to white spirits only or in combination with other solvents. Analogously, we previously reported non-significantly increased risks of hypopharyngeal and laryngeal cancer in women exposed to white spirits [13]. To our knowledge, only one study reported results on the relationship between exposure to mineral spirits and laryngeal cancer and found no association [9].

Table 5 Association between hypopharyngeal and laryngeal cancers and exposure to combinations of oxygenated solvents

Exposure to oxygenated solvents	Controls n = 2670	Hypopharynx n = 338		Larynx n = 423	
	n	n	OR[a] [95% CI]	n	OR[a] [95% CI]
None	1684	207	1	268	1
Ket	36	9	1.40 [0.57–3.48]	10	1.26 [0.55–2.92]
Alc, Ket	305	45	0.95 [0.63–1.43]	66	1.15 [0.81–1.63]
Alc, Etg	314	29	1.02 [0.63–1.65]	24	0.64 [0.40–1.05]
Alc, Ket, THF	25	10	2.79 [1.12–6.95]	10	2.25 [0.94–5.38]
Alc, Ket, Etg	158	23	0.84 [0.49–1.45]	27	0.86 [0.52–1.41]

Abbreviations: *OR* odds-ratio, *CI* confidence intervals, *Ket* ketones and esters, *Alc* alcohols, *Etg* ethylene glycol, *THF* tetrahydrofuran
[a]OR adjusted for age at interview, residence area, alcohol consumption, smoking status, frequency and duration of smoking, exposure to asbestos

Our findings also suggest that exposure to tetrahydrofuran may increase the risk of hypopharyngeal cancer, and to a lesser extent the risk of laryngeal cancer. For hypopharyngeal cancer, the risk increased with cumulative exposure, and a significantly elevated OR was observed among men exposed to tetrahydrofuran, ketones and alcohols. The evidence is weaker for laryngeal cancer, with lower ORs and no indication of a dose-response relationship. Tetrahydrofuran has been recently classified by the International Agency for Research on Cancer as possibly carcinogenic to humans, with sufficient evidence of carcinogenicity in animals and no data in humans [22].

Overall, the associations between hypopharyngeal cancer and exposure to tetrahydrofuran and white spirits must be interpreted with caution and need to be replicated in other studies. Little information on possible underlying mechanisms is available. Exposure to tetrahydrofuran causes liver and renal tumors in rodents [22–24]. The mechanisms are not firmly established, but are probably different from that operating in the upper airways.

The evidence of carcinogenicity of white spirits in experimental animals remains limited [25]. Studies on the genotoxicity of tetrahydrofuran and white spirits are inconclusive [23–25] and mostly negative. The upper airways are nevertheless in direct contact with inhaled toxic agents. Respiratory tract irritation following inhalation exposure has been documented in humans and laboratory animals for both tetrahydrofuran [23, 24] and white spirits [25].

Chronic irritation, inflammation and increased cell proliferation is a possible mechanism, although there are no experimental data to support this hypothesis. Such mechanisms may be relevant to other parts of the upper respiratory tract and to the lower airways. It is worth noting that exposure to mineral spirits was previously found to be associated with squamous cell carcinomas of the lung [26] and oesophagus [27]. The association between exposure to tetrahydrofuran and cancer of the respiratory tract warrants further investigation.

Another possible mechanism is that eexposure to solvents may facilitate the penetration of carcinogens through the mucosa. To further investigate this hypothesis, we evaluate the presence of multiplicative interaction between smoking, alcohol drinking, asbestos exposure and exposure to white spirits and tetrahydrofuran. No significant interaction was found, but the statistical power was limited.

Our study has some limitations. We used JEMs to assess occupational exposures retrospectively. As JEMs do not take into account the heterogeneity of tasks within the same job title, they usually generate misclassification of exposure. On the other hand, JEMs assign exposure in a reproducible and automatic way, independently of the case or control status; consequently, misclassification of exposure is likely to be non-differential.

Non-differential misclassification of exposure leads to an average bias towards the null for dichotomous exposures, and tends to disrupt dose-response trends for multilevel exposure variables. Our positive findings are therefore unlikely to be explained by exposure misclassification [28].

We did not collect information about non-occupational solvent exposure, but the relative contribution of this source of exposure is likely to be minimal. Despite an overall large number of subjects, the prevalence of exposure to some solvents was low, resulting in large confidence intervals and limited ability for in-depth analyses.

Recall bias is possible, but was limited by the use of standardized questionnaires and the average number of reported jobs was similar in cases (4.2) and controls (4.6). Selection bias is probably not a major limitation of this study: controls had a distribution by socioeconomic status and lifetime prevalence of exposure to solvents comparable to that of the general population [16]; the distribution by age, sex and cancer site of the included cases was similar to that observed in France in the same period [29]. Finally, we assessed a large number of associations, and some findings may be due to chance.

Our study has important strengths. We used data from a large population-based case-control study, with sufficient statistical power to detect moderate associations. Availability of detailed information on lifelong occupational history allowed us to assess indices of cumulative exposure and to study dose-response relationships. We adjusted for smoking, alcohol consumption, the main non-occupational risk factors, as well as occupational exposure to asbestos. In additional analyses, we also took into account socioeconomic status and other occupational exposures, therefore residual confounding is likely to be minimal.

Conclusions

This study provides weak evidence for an association between hypopharyngeal cancer and exposure to white spirits and tetrahydrofuran. Our findings do not suggest that the other petroleum-based or oxygenated solvents cause hypopharyngeal or laryngeal cancers.

Additional files

Additional file 1: Categories of exposure indices.

Additional file 2: Spearman correlation coefficients between cumulative exposures to petroleum-based and oxygenated solvents.

Additional file 3: Association between hypopharyngeal and laryngeal cancers and exposure to petroleum-based solvents, with adjustment for socioeconomic status.

Additional file 4: Association between hypopharyngeal and laryngeal cancers and exposure to oxygenated solvents, with adjustment for socioeconomic status.

Abbreviations
Alc: Alcohols; ben: Benzene; CEI: Cumulative Exposure Index; CI: Confidence interval; diesel: Diesel, fuels and kerosene; Etg: Ethylene glycol; Ket: Ketones and esters; OR: Odds-ratio; SPP: Special petroleum products; THF: Tetrahydrofuran; WS: White spirits

Acknowledgements
The authors thank all members of the MatGéné working group from Santé Publique France and, in particular, Ms. Brigitte Dananché for providing job-exposure matrices.
Members of ICARE Study Group: Anne-Valérie Guizard (Registre des cancers du Calvados, France); Arlette Danzon, Anne-Sophie Woronoff (Registre des cancers du Doubs, France); Michel Velten (Registre des cancers du Bas-Rhin, France); Antoine Buemi, Émilie Marrer (Registre des cancers du Haut-Rhin, France); Brigitte Trétarre (Registre des cancers de l'Hérault, France); Marc Colonna, Patricia Delafosse (Registre des cancers de l'Isère, France); Paolo Bercelli, Florence Molinié (Registre des cancers de Loire-Atlantique-Vendée, France); Simona Bara (Registre des cancers de la Manche, France); Bénédicte Lapotre-Ledoux, Nicole Raverdy (Registre des cancers de la Somme, France); Sylvie Cénée, Oumar Gaye, Florence Guida, Farida Lamkarkach, Loredana Radoï, Marie Sanchez, Isabelle Stücker (INSERM, Centre for research in Epidemiology and Population Health (CESP), U1018, Environmental Epidemiology of Cancer Team, Villejuif, France); Matthieu Carton, Diane Cyr, Annie Schmaus (Inserm Epidemiologic Cohorts Unit—UMS 011 INSERM-UVSQ, Villejuif, France); Joëlle Févotte (University Lyon 1, UMRESTTE, Lyon, France); Corinne Pilorget (French Public Health Agency, Department of Occupational Health, Saint Maurice, France); Gwenn Menvielle (Sorbonne Universités, UPMC Univ Paris 06, INSERM,IPLESP UMRS 1136, Paris, France); Danièle Luce (INSERM U 1085-IRSET, Pointe-à-Pitre, France).

Funding
The ICARE study was funded by the French National Research Agency (ANR); French National Cancer Institute (INCA); French Agency for Food, Environmental and Occupational Health and Safety (ANSES); French Institute for Public Health Surveillance (InVS); Fondation pour la Recherche Médicale (FRM); Fondation de France; Fondation ARC pour la Recherche sur le Cancer; Ministry of Labour (Direction Générale du Travail); Ministry of Health (Direction Générale de la Santé).

Authors' contributions
DL and CB designed the current study, conducted the analyses and drafted the manuscript; MC, GM and LR contributed to the statistical analysis and interpretation of the results. CP was involved in exposure assessment. SB contributed to data collection and quality control. DL and IS are the principal investigators of the ICARE study, conceived this study and coordinated the original collection of the data. All the authors critically reviewed and revised the manuscript, and gave their approval for its final version.

Competing interests
The authors declare that they have no competing interests.

Author details
[1]Univ Rennes, Inserm, EHESP, Irset (Institut de recherche en santé, environnement et travail)-UMR_S 1085, Pointe-à-Pitre F-97110, France. [2]Univ Paris Sud, Paris Saclay University, Orsay, France. [3]Département de Biométrie, Institut Curie, DRCI, PSL Research University, Paris, France. [4]CESP, Cancer and Environment Team, INSERM U1018, Université Paris-Sud, Université Paris-Saclay, Villejuif, France. [5]Faculty of Dental Surgery, University Paris Descartes, Paris, France. [6]Sorbonne Universités, UPMC Univ Paris 06, INSERM, Institut Pierre Louis d'épidémiologie et de Santé Publique (IPLESP UMRS 1136), Paris, France. [7]The French Public Health Agency, Saint Maurice, France. [8]Ifsttar, UMRESTTE, UMR T_9405, Univ Lyon, Claude Bernard Lyon1 University, Lyon, France. [9]Manche Cancer Registry, Cotentin Hospital, Cherbourg-Octeville, France.

References
1. Forman D, Bray F, Brewster DH, Gombe Mbalawa C, Kohler B, Piñeros M, Steliarova-Foucher E, Swaminathan R, Ferlay J, editors. Cancer incidence in five continents, vol. X. IARC scientific publication no. 164. Lyon: International Agency for Research on Cancer; 2014.
2. Secretan B, Straif K, Baan R, Grosse Y, El Ghissassi F, Bouvard V, et al. A review of human carcinogens–part E: tobacco, areca nut, alcohol, coal smoke, and salted fish. Lancet Oncol. 2009;10:1033–4.
3. Hashibe M, Brennan P, Chuang SC, Boccia S, Castellsague X, Chen C, et al. Interaction between tobacco and alcohol use and the risk of head and neck Cancer: pooled analysis in the international head and neck Cancer epidemiology consortium. Cancer Epidemiol Biomark Prev. 2009;18:541–50.
4. Baan R, Grosse Y, Straif K, Secretan B, El Ghissassi F, Bouvard V, et al. A review of human carcinogens–part F: chemical agents and related occupations. Lancet Oncol. 2009;10:1143–4.
5. Straif K, Benbrahim-Tallaa L, Baan R, Grosse Y, Secretan B, El Ghissassi F, et al. A review of human carcinogens–part C: metals, arsenic, dusts, and fibres. Lancet Oncol. 2009;10:453–4.
6. Paget-Bailly S, Cyr D, Luce D. Occupational exposures to asbestos, polycyclic aromatic hydrocarbons and solvents, and cancers of the oral cavity and pharynx: a quantitative literature review. Int Arch Occup Environ Health. 2012;85:341–51.
7. Paget-Bailly S, Cyr D, Luce D. Occupational exposures and cancer of the larynx—systematic review and meta-analysis. J Occup Environ Med. 2012;54: 71–84.
8. Berrino F, Richiardi L, Boffetta P, Estéve J, Belletti I, Raymond L, et al. Occupation and larynx and hypopharynx cancer: a job-exposure matrix approach in an international case–control study in France, Italy, Spain and Switzerland. Cancer Causes Control. 2003;14:213–23.
9. Shangina O. Occupational exposure and laryngeal and Hypopharyngeal Cancer risk in central and Eastern Europe. Am J Epidemiol. 2006;164:367–75.
10. Barul C, Fayossé A, Carton M, Pilorget C, Woronoff A-S, Stücker I, et al. Occupational exposure to chlorinated solvents and risk of head and neck cancer in men: a population-based case-control study in France. Environ Health. 2017;16:77.
11. Paget-Bailly S, Guida F, Carton M, Menvielle G, Radoï L, Cyr D, et al. Occupation and head and neck cancer risk in men: results from the ICARE study, a French population-based case–control study. J Occup Environ Med. 2013;55:1065–73.
12. ICARE study group, Luce D, Stücker I. Investigation of occupational and environmental causes of respiratory cancers (ICARE): a multicenter, population-based case-control study in France. BMC Public Health. 2011;11:928.
13. Carton M, Barul C, Menvielle G, Cyr D, Sanchez M, Pilorget C, et al. Occupational exposure to solvents and risk of head and neck cancer in women: a population-based case-control study in France. BMJ Open. 2017;7:e012833.
14. International Labour Office. International standard classification of occupations (ISCO). Geneva: ILO; 1968.
15. Institut National de la Statistique et Des Etudes Economiques. Définitions et méthodes - Nomenclature d'activités française. Paris: INSEE; 2000.
16. Fevotte J, Dananche B, Delabre L, Ducamp S, Garras L, Houot M, et al. Matgene: a program to develop job-exposure matrices in the general population in France. Ann Occup Hyg. 2011;55:865–78.
17. Lacourt A, Leffondre K, Gramond C, Ducamp S, Rolland P, Gilg Soit Ilg A, et al. Temporal patterns of occupational asbestos exposure and risk of pleural mesothelioma. Eur Respir J. 2012;39:1304–12.
18. Ahrens W, Jöckel KH, Patzak W, Elsner G. Alcohol, smoking, and occupational factors in cancer of the larynx: a case-control study. Am J Ind Med. 1991;20: 477–93.
19. De Stefani E, Boffetta P, Oreggia F, Ronco A, Kogevinas M, Mendilaharsu M. Occupation and the risk of laryngeal cancer in Uruguay. Am J Ind Med. 1998;33:537–42.
20. Elci OC, Akpinar-Elci M, Blair A, Dosemeci M. Risk of laryngeal Cancer by occupational chemical exposure in Turkey. J Occup Environ Med. 2003;45: 1100–6.
21. Purdue MP, Järvholm B, Bergdahl IA, Hayes RB, Baris D. Occupational exposures and head and neck cancers among Swedish construction workers. Scand J Work Environ Health. 2006;32:270–5.

22. Grosse Y, Loomis D, Guyton KZ, El Ghissassi F, Bouvard V, Benbrahim-Tallaa L, et al. Some chemicals that cause tumours of the urinary tract in rodents. Lancet Oncol. 2017;18:1003–4.

23. Fowles J, Boatman R, Bootman J, Lewis C, Morgott D, Rushton E, et al. A review of the toxicological and environmental hazards and risks of tetrahydrofuran. Crit Rev Toxicol. 2013;43:811–28.

24. U.S Environmental Protection Agency. Toxicological Review of Tetrahydrofuran (CAS No. 109–99-9), Document Reference EPA/635/R-11/006F, Washington, 2012; Available from: www.epa.gov/iris. Accessed 4 Aug 2017.

25. Mckee RH, Adenuga MD, Carrillo J-C. Characterization of the toxicological hazards of hydrocarbon solvents. Crit Rev Toxicol. 2015;45:273–365.

26. Siemiatycki J, Dewar R, Nadon L, Gérin M, Richardson L, Wacholder S. Associations between several sites of cancer and twelve petroleum-derived liquids. Results from a case-referent study in Montreal. Scand J Work Environ Health. 1987;13:493–504.

27. Parent ME, Siemiatycki J, Fritschi L. Workplace exposures and oesophageal cancer. Occup Environ Med. 2000;57:325–34.

28. Blair A, Stewart P, Lubin JH, Forastiere F. Methodological issues regarding confounding and exposure misclassification in epidemiological studies of occupational exposures. Am J Ind Med. 2007;50:199–207.

29. Ligier K, Belot A, Launoy G, Velten M, Bossard N, Iwaz J, et al. Descriptive epidemiology of upper aerodigestive tract cancers in France: incidence over 1980–2005 and projection to 2010. Oral Oncol. 2011;47:302–7.

24

Frequency of HPV in oral cavity squamous cell carcinoma

Priscila Marinho de Abreu[1], Anna Clara Gregório Có[2], Pedro Leite Azevedo[2], Isabella Bittencourt do Valle[1], Karine Gadioli de Oliveira[3], Sônia Alves Gouvea[3], Melissa Freitas Cordeiro-Silva[4], Iúri Drummond Louro[1], José Roberto Vasconcelos de Podestá[5], Jeferson Lenzi[5], Agenor Sena[5], Elismauro Francisco Mendonça[6] and Sandra Lúcia Ventorin von Zeidler[1,2*]

Abstract

Background: The prevalence of high-risk human papillomavirus (HPV) DNA in cases of oral cavity squamous cell carcinoma (SCC) varies widely. The aim of this study is to investigate the frequency of high-risk HPV DNA in a large Brazilian cohort of patients with oral cavity SCC.

Methods: Biopsy and resected frozen and formalin-fixed paraffin-embedded specimens of oral cavity SCC were available from 101 patients who were recruited at two Brazilian centres. Stringent measures with respect to case selection and prevention of sample contamination were adopted to ensure reliability of the data. Nested PCR using MY09/MY11 and GP5$^+$/GP6$^+$ as well as PGMY09/11 L1 consensus primers were performed to investigate the presence of HPV DNA in the tumours. HPV-positive cases were subjected to direct sequencing. Shapiro–Wilk and Student t test were used to evaluate data normality and to compare the means, respectively. Qualitative variables were analysed by logistic regression.

Results: Our results demonstrate that the frequency of high-risk HPV types in oral cavity SCC is very low and is less than 4%. All HPV-positive cases were HPV16. In addition, our results do not show a significant association between the tumour clinical features and the risk factors (tobacco, alcohol and HPV) for oral cavity SCC.

Conclusion: In the current study, we observed an overlapping pattern of risk factors that are related to tumour development. This, along with a low frequency of high-risk HPV DNA, supports the findings that HPV is not involved in the genesis of oral cavity SCC in Brazilian population.

Keywords: Oral cancer, HPV, Frequency, Incidence, Oral cavity, Squamous cell carcinoma, Human papillomavirus

Background

Head and neck squamous cell carcinoma (HNSCC) is a significant cause of cancer morbidity worldwide as 650,000 new cases and 350,000 deaths occur every year [1]. HNSCC encompasses tumours of the oral cavity, oropharynx, hypopharynx and larynx, which are each associated with different risk factors and prognoses. Latin America has a relatively high incidence of these tumours [1]. It was estimated that 15,290 new cases of oral cavity squamous cell carcinoma (SCC) occurred in Brazil in 2015 [2]. The oral cavity is the most frequent site of cancer within the head and neck region and is in the "top ten" list of tumours with the highest incidences [1].

HNSCC is one of several cancers that is strongly associated with tobacco and alcohol use [3]. However, over the last 15 years, high-risk (HR) human papillomavirus (HPV) infection has also been aetiologically linked to a subset of HNSCCs. HPV involvement in oral and oropharyngeal carcinogenesis was first proposed by Syrjanen et al. in 1983 [4]. In 2007, the International Agency for Research on Cancer recognized human papillomavirus type 16 (HPV16) as the only carcinogenic type of HPV in sites other than the cervix uteri, including the anus, penis, vagina, vulva, oral cavity

* Correspondence: sandra.zeidler@ufes.br
[1]Programa de Pós-Graduação em Biotecnologia, Centro de Ciências da Saúde, Universidade Federal do Espirito Santo, Vitoria, Espirito Santo, Brazil
[2]Departamento de Patologia, Programa de Pós-graduação em Biotecnologia, Centro de Ciências da Saúde, Universidade Federal do Espirito Santo, Av. Marechal Campos, 1468 Maruípe, Vitória, ES 29.040-090, Brazil
Full list of author information is available at the end of the article

and oropharynx [5]. HPV16-associated carcinogenesis is mediated by expression of the viral E6 and E7 oncoproteins, which inactivate the tumour suppressor proteins p53 and retinoblastoma; this then disrupts cell cycle regulatory pathways [6]. Therefore, the lack of p53 mutations [7] and p16 protein accumulation [8–10], which occur as a result of the loss of transcriptional repression during early tumorigenesis, are considered to be hallmarks of HPV-related HNSCC [11].

Although the frequency of high-risk HPV that is detected may be higher in samples of HNSCC, substantial heterogeneity exists among studies in terms of the detection rates. A portion of this variation may be related to differences in the incidence among geographic locations and the head and neck subsites enrolled in the included studies [12]. Additionally, it is important to consider variations in the sample sources and the collection methods as well as in the HPV detection methods. Methods for the detection of HPV DNA include in situ hybridization and polymerase chain reaction (PCR), while methods for the detection of HPV E6/E7 RNA include quantitative reverse transcriptase PCR (qRT-PCR) and RNA in situ hybridization.

To support the involvement of HPV in head and neck tumours, few studies have been conducted to determine the frequency of HPV DNA exclusively in SCC of the oral cavity, specifically in Brazil [13, 14]. Most of the published studies have included multiple subsites of HNSCC, which have precluded the specific analysis of HPV involvement in oral carcinogenesis [15]. Furthermore, the frequency of HPV infection in oral cavity SCC exhibits much variation among studies worldwide as well in different regions within Brazil [13, 14, 16].

The aim of this study is to investigate the frequency of high-risk HPV in a large Brazilian cohort of patients with oral cavity SCC. The relevance of this study lies in our accuracy of the selection of tumour sites and in the collection of samples. We also used different HPV DNA detection methods and adopted stringent measures to prevent sample contamination, which ensures the reliability of the data.

Methods
Study subjects
This is a multicentre cross-sectional study conducted at the following two Brazilian centres: Santa Rita de Cassia Hospital and University Hospital Antonio Cassiano de Moraes, which are both located in Espírito Santo. This study was approved by the clinical centre ethics committees and by the National Commission on Ethics in Research (Protocols 318/2011 and 681/2011). Written consent was given by each patient prior to his or her participation in the study.

A total of 171 cases of oral cavity SCC that were diagnosed by histopathology between 2012 and 2015 were reviewed. The inclusion criteria included tumours from oral cavity that were diagnosed according to the International Classification of Diseases, version 10 [17] and patients who had not undergone any previous antineoplastic treatment. The anatomical subsites selected were: tongue (C02.0, C02.3, C02.8, C02.9); gum and alveolar ridge (C03.0, C03.1, C03.9); floor of the mouth (C04.0, C04.1, C04.8, C04.9); palate (C05.0, C05.8, C05.9); buccal mucosa (C06.0, C06.1); retromolar trigone (C06.2) and overlapping sites of other parts of mouth (C06.8, C06.9). Seventy cases were excluded for not presenting formalin-fixed paraffin-embedded or frozen tissues available.

Following patient consent, 82 fresh tumour specimens were collected at the time of biopsy or surgical resection into RNAlater® reagent (Qiagen, Valencia, CA, USA) and stored at − 80 °C until further processing. In addition, 19 formalin-fixed paraffin-embedded tumours were retrieved from the pathology archive at Santa Rita de Cassia Hospital.

Clinical and pathological data (i.e., age, gender, tumour site, TNM stage, alcohol consume and tobacco exposure) were obtained by interview and from the medical records. The clinical stage of the tumours was categorized as early (clinical stages I–II) or advanced clinical stages (clinical stages III–IV), and all tumours were classified according to the TNM classification system [18].

DNA extraction and integrity
Genomic DNA was obtained from frozen tissues and from four 10 μm-thick sections cut from the paraffin blocks. Formalin-fixed paraffin-embedded sections were placed in 2 ml microcentrifuge tubes and dewaxed with multiple washes of xylene and graded solutions of 100%, 95% and 70% ethanol. After overnight digestion with sodium dodecyl sulphate (SDS) and 5% of 20 mg/ml of K proteinase (Sigma, Saint Louis, USA) at 37 °C, DNA was extracted from both types of samples by standard phenol-chloroform-isoamylic alcohol and sodium acetate-ethanol precipitation. Rigorous efforts were made to avoid cross-contamination at every stage. A new microtome blade was used each time a new case was sectioned, and the components of the microtome were cleaned with xylene and ethanol after each sample was sectioned. In addition, aerosol tips were used for all pipetting steps, and separate rooms were used for pre- and post-PCR experimental steps.

DNA concentrations were estimated using a DyNA Quant 200 Fluorometer (Hoeffer Scientific, Holliston, MA, USA). To exclude false negative results derived from the degradation of DNA in samples that were overfixed, the integrity of the DNA was assessed by amplification of a fragment of the human β-globin gene using

PCO3 (5'-ACACAACTGTGTTCACTAGC-3') and PCO7 (5'-GAAAACATCAAGGGTCCCAT-3') primers, which result in a 509-bp DNA fragment [19]. All β-globin-negative samples were excluded from further analysis.

HPV DNA detection

Nested PCR using MY09/MY11 and GP5⁺/GP6⁺ primers

The detection of high-risk HPV was performed by nested PCR to amplify a part of the HPV L1 gene, which encodes the major capsid protein of several subtypes of HPV, as previously described by Jacob in 1995 [20]. Briefly, 50 ng of DNA from each sample was amplified with the consensus primers MY09/MY11 followed by amplification with general primers GP5⁺/GP6⁺ by two-step nested PCR. Standard PCR with the MY09/MY11 primers was performed as previously described [20, 21]. Each sample was amplified with 50 pmol each of the primers MY09 (5'-CGTCCMARRGGAWACTGATC-3') and MY11 (5'-GCMCAGGGWCATAAYAATGG-3') in the presence of 6 mM $MgCl_2$ buffer, 200 mmol (each) dATP, dCTP, and dGTP, 600 mmol dUTP, and 7.5 U of Hot Start Taq DNA polymerase (Invitrogen, Waltham, MA, USA). Then, PCR was performed using the product of the first reaction as a template in 50 mM KCl, 10 mM TrisHCl (pH 8.3), 200 mM of each deoxynucleoside triphosphate, 3.5 mM $MgCl_2$, 7.5 U of Hot Start Taq DNA polymerase (Invitrogen, Waltham, MA, USA), and 50 pmol each of the GP5⁺ (5'-TTTGTTACTGTGGT AGATACTAC-3') and GP6⁺ (3'-CTTATACTAAATGT CAAATAAAAAG-5') primers. Amplifications were performed in a Mastercycler Nexus (Eppendorf, Hamburg, DE) with an activation at 94 °C for 7 min and 25 cycles (first step) or 15 cycles (second step) at 94 °C for 45 s, 56 °C (first step) or 46 °C (second step) for 45 s and 72 °C for 1 min. This was followed by a final extension at 72 °C for 7 min, and storage at 4 °C.

PGMY09/11 L1 consensus PCR

Additionally, to ensure the reliability of the data, we subjected the samples to a second round of PCR using a consensus PGMY09/11 primer set. An equimolar mixture of each primer was added to the PCR master mix for a final concentration of 10 pmol of each oligonucleotide in the primer sets; the final $MgCl_2$ concentration was 4 mM. Then, the PCR buffers, reagents, and amplification profiles were identical to those described by Gravitt in 2000 [21]. Cycling conditions were as follows: 95 °C for 5 min, followed by 30 cycles at 95 °C for 1 min, 57 °C for 1 min, 72 °C for 1 min and a 7-min final extension period at 72 °C (Mastercycler Nexus, Eppendorf, Hamburg, DE).

Positive and negative controls were used for each amplification and consisted of a previously known HPV-positive cervical carcinoma and ultrapure water,

respectively. The products were then subjected to electrophoresis on an 8% polyacrylamide gel followed by a silver stain. Specimens were considered positive for HPV DNA using the MY09/MY11 and GP5⁺/GP6⁺ primer sets when they presented a 150-bp DNA fragment. This represents some of the low-risk genotypes (6, 11, 40, 42, 43, 44) or the high-risk genotypes (16, 18, 31, 33, 35, 39, 45, 51, 52, 56, 58, 59, 66, 68), as described by Jacobs (1995) [20]. Samples that were amplified using PGMY09/11 were considered HPV-positive if the PCR product was a 450-bp fragment. PGMY09/11 consensus primers allowed the detection of more than 30 HPV genotypes as follows: 6, 11,16, 18, 26, 31, 33, 35, 39, 40, 42, 45, 51, 52, 53, 54, 55, 56, 58, 59, 61, 62, 64, 66, 67, 68, 69, 70, 71, 72, 73, IS39, CP8304, CP6108, MM4, MM7, and MM8 [21].

DNA sequencing

PCR products were purified using the ExoSAP-IT PCR Clean-up Kit (GE Healthcare Life Sciences, Uppsala, SE) and were sequenced using the BigDye® Terminator v3. 1 Cycle Sequencing Kit (Applied Biosystems, Foster City, CA, USA). Capillary electrophoresis was performed in an ABI Prism 310 Genetic Analyzer (Applied Biosystems, Foster City, CA, USA). The sequences were analysed using the Basic Local Alignment Search Tool (BLAST) available online at National Center for Biotechnology Information (https://blast.ncbi.nlm.nih.gov/Blast. cgi).

Statistical analysis

Shapiro–Wilk test was used to evaluate data normality. Variables distribution were presented by mean, standard deviation. Student t test was used to compare the mean of ages between HPV-positive and HPV-negative individuals. Multiple logistic regression was applied in order to compare HPV status, tumour size, and nodal involvement with risk factors. The level of significance adopted in all analysis was 5% with a 95% confidence interval. For the data analysis the Statistical Package for the Social Sciences, version 17 for Windows (SPSS, Chicago, USA) was used.

Results

DNA from all 19 formalin-fixed paraffin-embedded specimens produced a β-globin PCR 509-bp fragment, as did the majority of the frozen specimens (71 of 82; 85.6%). DNA from 11 frozen biopsies which presented β-globin negative were excluded from the subsequent analysis. The reasons for the exclusion were the presence of degraded and low quality DNA from tiny fragments that could not be resubmitted to DNA extraction and the existence of PCR inhibitors. Thus, the HPV status was assessed in a total of 68 males and 22 females with a mean age at diagnosis of 57.9 years (range 30–93 years; standard deviation 12.2 years) and was reported as either positive or negative. The details concerning the clinical findings and the HPV status of the cases in our series are summarized in Table 1. Cases that exhibited HPV-positive status (3/90) were detected by nested PCR using the MY09/MY11 and GP5$^+$/GP6$^+$ primer sets, and the frequency of HPV infection was found to be 3.3%. Furthermore, 87 HPV-negative samples where enough DNA was present were also assessed by PGMY09/11; these samples presented a 100% concordance rate, which ensures the reliability of the previous results. The sequencing showed the presence of HPV16 in all HPV-positive cases originated from both formalin-fixed paraffin-embedded (1/19) and frozen tissues (2/71). No difference was observed considering the sample storage methods. Among the HPV-positive cases, two were heavy smokers and alcoholics males while the other was a female with no exposure to any of the known risk factors.

All HPV-positive cases were in advanced stage of the disease (III-IV) presenting tumour size (T3/T4) and lymph node metastasis (N$^+$) at the time of diagnosis. Besides that, there was no significant association among HPV status and TNM stage as well as gender, alcohol consumption, tobacco use or tumour site (Table 1). The mean age of HPV-positive patients was 61.0 years,

whereas the mean age of the HPV-negative patients was 57.5 years; this difference was not significant (Table 2). In addition, the most used prognostic factors tumour size and nodal involvement were not associated with alcohol consumption, tobacco use, or HPV infection. Therefore, these variables could not be considered risk or protection factors in our cohort (Tables 2 and 3).

Discussion

This study presented a cohort with a significant number of patients with oral cavity SCC. Our results demonstrate that the frequency of high-risk HPV types in oral cavity SCC is very low and is less than 4%. We believe that this result is significant, as we have assessed a precise anatomical site in our cohort. We have thus avoided bias related to the differences in the incidence of oral SCC in other sites, especially in the oropharynx where the prevalence of high-risk HPV has been reported to be high [22, 23]. Tumour sites were validated by verification of the database and the medical records; in the three HPV-positive cases, the tumours were located in the tongue and in the alveolar ridge (Table 1). In addition, rigorous efforts were taken to prevent sample contamination as previously described, which ensures the consistency of our results.

The reported prevalence of high-risk HPV DNA in oral cavity SCC varies widely. A large multicentre study

Table 1 Association of clinical findings and HPV status in oral cavity SCC (*n* = 90)

	HPV				OR (Adjusted)	95% CI	p-value**
	Positive		Negative				
	n	(%)	n	(%)			
Gender							
Male	2	(66.6)	66	(75.9)	1	–	–
Female	1	(33.4)	21	(24.1)	3.023	(0.135–67.544)	0.485
Tumour site							
Tongue	2	(66.7)	47	(54.0)	1,07E + 08	0	0.988
Floor of the mouth	0	(0.0)	22	(25.3)	1	–	–
Others^a	1	(33.3)	18	(20.7)	2,07E + 08	0	0.998
Alcohol Consumption							
No	1	(33.3)	37	(43.0)	1	–	–
Yes	2	(66.7)	49	(57.0)	2.446	0	0.637
Tobacco Consumption							
No	1	(33.3)	39	(45.3)	1	–	–
Yes	2	(66.7)	47	(54.7)	1.993	(0.045–88.793)	0.722
TNM Stage							
I/II	0	(0.0)	28	(32.9)	1	–	–
III/IV	3	(100.0)	57	(67.1)	1,30E + 08	0	0.998

Reference category of the dependent variable - HPV negative
OR Odds Ratio, *CI* Confidence interval; **. Multiple logistic regression (Adjusted to all variables)
^{a}Palate, retromolar trigone, gum, buccal mucosa, alveolar ridge
Data unknown: alcohol consumption - 1; tobacco consumption - 1; TNM stage - 2

Table 2 Comparison of the ages of the patients with HPV-positive and HPV-negative oral cavity SCC

HPV	n	Mean	STD[b]	CI (95%)	p
Negative	87	57.5	12.0	54.91–60.09	0.63[a]
Positive	3	61.0	16.0	46.00–79.00	

[a]*Student t test*
[b]*STD Standard deviation*

reported HPV DNA in 4% of 766 oral cancers using the consensus PCR primers GP5$^+$/GP6$^+$ [24]. Studies performed in United Kingdom and in the United States analysed large cohorts and found an HPV frequency of less than 2% and 5.6%, respectively [25, 26]. Moreover, in India, a study revealed an HPV infection rate of 46% in oral cavity SCC [27] while a meta-analysis published by Termine et al. (2008), in which 62 studies were analysed, revealed a 38.1% prevalence of HPV DNA in 4852 oral squamous cell carcinoma biopsy samples [28].

In Brazil, few studies have been conducted on the frequency of HPV in oral cavity SCC, and the data presented thus far are also discordant; data show a range of 0–19.2% frequency, which is mostly related to HPV16 infection [13, 16, 29]. Table 4 illustrates some of the consistent publications in recent years that have considered the frequency of HPV infection in oral cavity SCC.

Thus, to evaluate the involvement of HPV in the genesis of oral cavity SCC, the geographic distribution of the populations should be considered. Besides, the wide variation in HPV detection rates can be influenced by other factors, such as sensitivity of the HPV testing method, the coverage of HPV genotypes in the test panel, sample collection methods as well as sample storage conditions.

The most widely applied HPV detection methods are based on the PCR amplification of viral DNA. In the current study, we have used three different standard primer sets (MY09/MY11, GP5$^+$/GP6$^+$ and PGMY09/11) and nested PCR to detect HPV DNA in head and neck tumours, which increases the sensitivity compared to a single PCR reaction [30]. Some advantages of the PCR methods used are the high sensitivity to detect more than 30 HPV genotypes, wide availability, and cost-effectiveness [31]. A weakness of the standard PCR-based assay is that it can not distinguish oncogenic virus from biologically irrelevant virus because is not possible to identify integrated or episomal DNA [25, 28, 32]. In addition, PCR techniques have lower specificity compared with in situ hybridization and are technically troublesome to perform.

Although it is expected that HPV detection rate by PCR is usually higher in frozen tissues, in our study we did not find difference when we compared it to formalin-fixed paraffin-embedded tumours. Thus, we suggest that the use of nested PCR, which was adopted to avoid interference of small fragments from DNA degradation during fixation procedures could contribute to this result. In addition, other studies have used both clinical specimens and have not observed differences in HPV DNA detection rates using PCR-based methods [13, 25]. Furthermore, Lopes et al., (2011) [25] report that non-quantitative PCR methods, when subject to stringent quality control measures, such as the methodology adopted in our study, are effective methods to detect HPV DNA in those samples.

Studies have reported that patients with oral cavity SCC who do not present with a history of alcohol and tobacco consumption tend to be younger than patients who smoke and drink alcohol [16, 33]. Thus, the low frequency of HPV DNA in the present study might be related to the high mean age of our cohort, as no difference was observed between the mean age

Table 3 Association of prognostic features and the risk factors (n = 90)

	Tumour Size				OR (Adjusted)	95% CI	p-value**	Nodal Involvement[a]				OR (Adjusted)	95% CI	p-value**
	T1/T2		T3/T4					N0		N+				
	n	(%)	n	(%)				n	(%)	n	(%)			
HPV status														
Negative	36	(100.0)	48	(94.1)	1	–	–	48	(100.0)	36	(92.3)	1	–	–
Positive	0	(0.0)	3	(5.9)	1.18E + 09	0	0.999	0	(0.0)	3	(7.7)	2.04E + 09	0	0.999
Alcohol Drinkers														
No	16	(44.4)	21	(42.0)	1	–	–	21	(44.7)	16	(41.0)	1	–	–
Yes	20	(55.6)	29	(58.0)	0.708	(0.243–2.060)	0.526	26	(55.3)	23	(59.0)	0.626	(0.209–1.180)	0.404
Tobacco Users														
No	19	(52.8)	19	(38.0)	1	–	–	25	(53.2)	13	(33.3)	1	–	–
Yes	17	(47.2)	31	(62.0)	2173	(0.751–6.290)	0.152	22	(46.8)	26	(66.7)	2947	(0.977–8.887)	0.055

Reference category of the dependent variable Tumor size - T1/T2; Reference category of the dependent variable Nodal Involvement- N0; *OR* Odds Ratio
CI Confidence Interval; **. Multiple logistic regression (Adjusted to all variables);
[a]N0 - absence of lymph node metastasis; N+ – lymph node metastasis;
Data unknown: alcohol drinkers - 1; tobacco users - 1; tumour size - 3; nodal involvement - 3

Table 4 Prevalence of HPV in oral cavity SCC

Author / Year	Country	No. of cases	HPV (%)	Samples	Methods
Kaminagakura et al. [16] 2012	Brazil	114	19.2	FFPE	GP5+/GP6+
Attner et al. [40] 2011	Sweden	87	78.0	FFPE	GP5+/GP6+
Lopes et al. [25] 2011	United Kingdom	118	< 2.0	FT[b]/FFPE	GP5+/GP6+
Termine et al. [41] 2012	Italy	83	12.1	FFPE	Nested PCR[a] PGMY09/11
Smith et al. [42] 2012	USA	170	9.4	FFPE	GP5+/GP6+ PGMY09/11
Lee et al. [34] 2012	Taiwan	173	38.0	FFPE	MY11/GP6+
Duray et al. [43] 2012	Belgium	147	44.2	FFPE	GP5+/GP6+
Lingen et al. [26] 2013	USA	409	5.9	FFPE	SPF10
González-Ramírez et al. [44] 2013	Mexico	80	5.0	FT[b]	Nested PCR[a]
Lopez et al. [13] 2014	Brazil	121	6.6	FT/FFPE	PGMY09/11
Chakrobarty et al. [27] 2014	India	83	46.0	FT[b]	MY09/MY11

[a]Nested PCR, MY09/11 and GP5+/GP6+
[b]FT frozen tissue

of the individuals in the HPV-positive and HPV-negative groups. Moreover, most of our cases presented with an advanced stage of the disease and a history of long and intense exposure to known risk factors. Furthermore, no differences were observed among the anatomical subsites, tumour size, presence of lymph node metastasis and TNM stage among the HPV-positive and HPV-negative cases.

Furthermore, the frequency of HPV in our study is too close to the HPV DNA rates found in healthy individuals. The natural history of HPV infection has been extensively investigated in epidemiologic studies by PCR-based methods, HPV serology and DNA/RNA in situ hybridization [25, 34]. A review about epidemiological investigation on oral HPV prevalence in healthy individuals, published by Shigeishi & Sugiyama (2016), reported that HPV frequency in saliva of healthy individuals have shown low and variable rates in a period of time, which is related to each patient's immune response and can, therefore, be inconstant. In addition, rates of oncogenic HPV infection in the oral cavity of healthy people are also known to be low (around 2%) and the natural history of HPV in this anatomical site shows HPV acquisition is a rare event compared to genital or anal infections [35, 36].

Data from a database in the USA shows a reduction in tobacco use over the last several decades [37]. Although HNSCC is closely linked to tobacco and alcohol use, its increasing incidence indicates that HPV16-related HNSCC arises in the oropharynx [24, 33, 38]. In contrast, the incidence of oral cavity SCC has declined significantly between 1973 and 2004 at a yearly rate of 1.85% [39], which suggests that HPV is not related to oral carcinogenesis. These results are reinforced by the variation in the frequency of HPV DNA, as demonstrated in this work and in other studies [40–44].

Conclusion

In conclusion, in the current study, we observed an overlapping pattern of the risk factors tobacco and alcohol; this along with the low frequency of HPV DNA, supports the evidence that HPV is not involved in the development of oral cavity SCC in Brazilian population.

Abbreviations
HNSCC: Head and Neck Squamous Cell Carcinoma; HPV: Human Papillomavirus; HPV16: Human Papillomavirus type 16; HR: High Risk; PCR: Polymerase Chain Reaction; qRT-PCR: Quantitative Reverse Transcriptase-PCR; SCC: Squamous Cell Carcinoma; SDS: Sodium dodecyl sulphate

Acknowledgements
We thank the Laboratório Multiusuário de Análises Biomoleculares (LABIOM - UFES) and Professor Liliana Cruz Spano for all support on HR-HPV PCR.

Funding
This work was supported by Fundação de Amparo à Pesquisa do Estado do Espírito Santo (FAPES award number 60929073/2013) and Coordenação de Aperfeiçoamento de Pessoal de Nível Superior (Bolsista CAPES – Proc. n° 11780/13–4).

Authors' contributions
SZ and PMA conceived and conduced study design as well draft the manuscript. AC, IV and PLA carried out all laboratory experiments and cooperate to draft the manuscript. AS, JL, EM and JP conduced patient recruitment, supplied all samples, and had a revising critically the manuscript. SG and KO assisted on data quality control, statistical analysis and critical revision of the manuscript. MS and IL participated in data acquisition and critical revision of the manuscript. All authors read and approved the final manuscript and agreed to be accountable for all aspects of the work.

Competing interests
The authors declare that they have no competing interests.

Author details

[1]Programa de Pós-Graduação em Biotecnologia, Centro de Ciências da Saúde, Universidade Federal do Espirito Santo, Vitoria, Espirito Santo, Brazil.
[2]Departamento de Patologia, Programa de Pós-graduação em Biotecnologia, Centro de Ciências da Saúde, Universidade Federal do Espirito Santo, Av. Marechal Campos, 1468 Maruípe, Vitória, ES 29.040-090, Brazil.
[3]Departamento de Ciências Fisiológicas, Centro de Ciências da Saúde, Universidade Federal do Espirito Santo, Vitoria, Espírito Santo, Brazil.
[4]Faculdade Católica Salesiana do Espírito Santo, Vitória, Espírito Santo, Brazil.
[5]Programa de Prevenção e Detecção Precoce do Câncer Bucal, Setor de Cirurgia de Cabeça e Pescoço, Hospital Santa Rita de Cássia, Vitória, Espírito Santo, Brazil. [6]Faculdade de Odontologia, Universidade Federal de Goiás, Goiânia, Goiás, Brazil.

References

1. Ferlay J, Soerjomataram I, Dikshit R, Eser S, Mathers C, Rebelo M, Parkin DM, Forman D, Bray F. Cancer incidence and mortality worldwide: sources, methods and major patterns in GLOBOCAN 2012. Int J Cancer. 2015;136: E359–86.
2. Ministério da Saúde, INCA. Estimativa 2014: Incidência de Câncer no Brasil. Rio de Janeiro: INCA. p. 2014.
3. Leemans CR, Braakhuis BJM, Brakenhoff RH. The molecular biology of head and neck cancer. Nat Rev Cancer. 2011;11:9–22.
4. Syrjanen KJ, Pyrhonen S, Syrjanen SM, Lamberg MA. Immunohistochemical demonstration of human papilloma virus (HPV) antigens in oral squamous cell lesions. Br J Oral Surg. 1983;21:147–53.
5. IARC. IARC monographs on the evaluation of carcinogenic risks to humans. V 90. França: IARC; 2007.
6. Chaudhary AK, Singh M, Sundaram S, Mehrotra R. Role of human papillomavirus and its detection in potentially malignant and malignant head and neck lesions: updated review. Head Neck Oncol. 2009;1(1):22.
7. Westra WH, Taube JM, Poeta ML, Begum S, Sidransky D, Koch WM. Inverse relationship between human papillomavirus-16 infection and disruptive p53 gene mutations in squamous cell carcinoma of the head and neck. Clin Cancer Res. 2008;14:366–9.
8. Kumar B, Cordell KG, Lee JS, Worden FP, Prince ME, Tran HH, Wolf GT, Urba SG, Chepeha DB, Teknos TN, Tsien CI, Taylor JMG, Silva NJD, Yang K, Kurnit MD, Bauer JA, Bradford CR, Carey TE. EGFR, p16, HPV titer, Bcl-xL and p53, sex, and smoking as indicators of response to therapy and survival in oropharyngeal cancer. Clin Oncol. 2008;26:3128–37.
9. O'Regan EM, Toner ME, Finn SP, Fan CY, Ring M, Hagmar B, Timon C, Smyth P, Cahill S, Flavin R, Sheils OM, O'Leary JJ. p16INK4A genetic and epigenetic profiles differ in relation to age and site in head and neck squamous cell carcinomas. Hum Pathol. 2008;39:452–8.
10. Weinberger PM, Yu Z, Haffty BG, Kowalski D, Harigopal M, Brandsma J, Sasaki C, Joe J, Camp RL, Rimm DL, Psyrri A. Molecular classification identifies a subset of human papillomavirus – associated oropharyngeal cancers with favorable prognosis. J Clin Oncol. 2006;24:736–47.
11. Mroz EA, Baird AH, Michaud WA, Rocco JW. COOH-terminal binding protein regulates expression of the p16INK4A tumor suppressor and senescence in primary human cells. Cancer Res. 2008;68:6049–53.
12. Kreimer AR, Clifford GM, Boyle P, Franceschi S. Human papillomavirus types in head and neck squamous cell carcinomas worldwide: a systematic review. Cancer Epidemiol Biomark Prev. 2005;14:467–75.
13. López RVM, Levi JE, Eluf-Neto J, Koifman RJ, Koifman S, Curado MP, Michaluart-Junior P, Figueiredo DLA, Saggioro FP, de Carvalho MB, Kowalski LP, Abrahão M, de Góis-Filho F, Tajara EH, Waterboer T, Boffetta P, Brennan P, Wünsch-Filho V. Human papillomavirus (HPV) 16 and the prognosis of head and neck cancer in a geographical region with a low prevalence of HPV infection. Cancer Causes Control. 2014;25:461–71.
14. Soares RC, Oliveira MC, Souza LB, Costa AL, Medeiros SRB, Pinto LP. Human papillomavirus in oral squamous cells carcinoma in a population of 75 Brazilian patients. Am J Otolaryngol. 2007;28:397–400.
15. Paolini F, Rizzo C, Sperduti I, Pichi B, Mafera B, Rahimi SS, Vigili MG, Venuti A. Both mucosal and cutaneous papillomaviruses are in the oral cavity but only alpha genus seems to be associated with cancer. J Clin Virol. 2013;56:72–6.
16. Kaminagakura E, Villa LL, Andreoli MA, Sobrinho JS, Vartanian JG, Soares FA, Nishimoto IN, Rocha R, Kowalski LP. High-risk human papillomavirus in oral squamous cell carcinoma of young patients. Int J Cancer. 2012;130:1726–32.

17. World Health Organization. International Statistical Classification of Diseases and Related Health Problems. Tenth Revision. 2nd ed. v 2. Geneva: WHO; 2004.
18. Sobin LH, Gospodarowicz MK, Wittekind C. TNM: Classification of mMalignant Tumours. 7th ed. Oxford: Wiley-Blackwell; 2009.
19. Husman ADR, Snijders PJF, Stell HV, Brulel AJC Van De, Meijer C. Processing of long-stored archival cervical smears for human papillomavirus detection by the polymerase chain reaction. Br J Cancer. 1995; 72:412–417.
20. Jacobs MV, De Roda Husman AM, Van den Brule AJC, Snijders PJF, Meijer CJLM, Walboomers JMM. Group-specific differentiation between high- and low-risk human papillomavirus genotypes by general primer-mediated PCR and two cocktails of oligonucleotide probes. J Clin Microbiol. 1995;33:901–5.
21. Gravitt PE, Peyton CL, Alessi TQ, Wheeler CM, Coutlée F, Hildesheim A, Schiffman MH, Scott DR, Apple RJ. Improved amplification of genital human papillomaviruses. J Clin Microbiol. 2000;38:357–61.
22. Machado J, Reis PP, Zhang T, Simpson C, Xu W, Perez-Ordonez B, Goldstein DP, Brown DH, Gilbert RW, Gullane PJ, Irish JC, Kamel-Reid S. Low prevalence of human papillomavirus in oral cavity carcinomas. Head Neck Oncol. 2010;2(1):6.
23. St Guily JL, Jacquard AC, Prétet JL, Haesebaert J, Beby-Defaux A, Clavel C, Agius G, Birembaut P, Okaïs C, Léocmach Y, Soubeyrand B, Pradat P, Riethmuller D, Mougin C, Denis F. Human papillomavirus genotype distribution in oropharynx and oral cavity cancer in France-the EDiTH VI study. J Clin Virol. 2011;51:100–4.
24. Herrero R, Castellsagué X, Pawlita M, Lissowska J, Kee F, Balaram P, Rajkumar T, Sridhar H, Rose B, Pintos J, Fernández L, Idris A, Sánchez MJ, Neto A, Talamini R, Tavani A, Bosch FX, Reidel U, Snijders PJF, Meijer CJLM, Viscidi R, Muñoz N, Franceschi S. Human papillomavirus and oral Cancer: the International Agency for Research on Cancer multicenter study. J Natl Cancer Inst. 2003;95:1772–83.
25. Lopes V, Murray P, Williams H, Woodman C, Watkinson J, Robinson M. Squamous cell carcinoma of the oral cavity rarely harbours oncogenic human papillomavirus. Oral Oncol. 2011;47:698–701.
26. Lingen MW, Xiao W, Schmitt A, Jiang B, Pickard R, Kreinbrink P, Perez-Ordonez B, Jordan RC, Gillison ML. Low etiologic fraction for high-risk human papillomavirus in oral cavity squamous cell carcinomas. Oral Oncol. 2013;49:1–8.
27. Chakrobarty B, Roy JG, Majumdar S, Uppala D. Relationship among tobacco habits, human papilloma virus (HPV) infection, p53 polymorphism/mutation and the risk of oral squamous cell carcinoma. J Oral Maxillofac Pathol. 2014; 18:211–6.
28. Termine N, Panzarella V, Falaschini S, Russo A, Matranga D, Lo Muzio L, Campisi G. HPV in oral squamous cell carcinoma vs head and neck squamous cell carcinoma biopsies: a meta-analysis (1988-2007). Ann Oncol. 2008;19:1681–90.
29. Spíndula-Filho JV, Cruz AD, Oton-Leite AF, Batista AC, Leles CR, Alencar R de CG, Saddi VA, Mendonça EF. Oral squamous cell carcinoma versus oral verrucous carcinoma: an approach to cellular proliferation and negative relation to human papillomavirus (HPV). Tumor Biol. 2011;32:409–16.
30. Fuessel Haws AL, He Q, Rady PL, Zhang L, Grady J, Hughes TK, Stisser K, Konig R, Tyring SK. Nested PCR with the PGMY09/11 and GP5 +/6 + primer sets improves detection of HPV DNA in cervical samples. J Virol Methods. 2004;122:87–93.
31. Cantley RL, Gabrielli E, Montebelli F, Cimbaluk D, Gattuso P, Petruzzelli G. Ancillary studies in determining human papillomavirus status of squamous cell carcinoma of the oropharynx: a review. Patholog Res Int. 2011;2011:1–7.
32. Dayyani F, Etzel CJ, Liu M, Ho C-H, Lippman SM, Tsao AS. Meta-analysis of the impact of human papillomavirus (HPV) on cancer risk and overall survival in head and neck squamous cell carcinomas (HNSCC). Head Neck Oncol. 2010;2:1–11.
33. Marur S, Souza GD, Westra WH, Forastiere AA. HPV-associated head and neck cancer : a virus-related cancer epidemic. Lancet Oncol. 2010;11:781–9.
34. Lee LA, Huang CG, Liao CT, Lee LY, Hsueh C, Chen TC, Lin CY, Fan KH, Wang HM, Huang SF, Chen IH, Kang CJ, Ng SH, Yang SL, Tsao KC, Chang YL, Yen TC. Human papillomavirus-16 infection in advanced oral cavity cancer patients is related to an increased risk of distant metastases and poor survival. PLoS One. 2012;7:7–9.
35. Kreimer AR, Pierce Campbell CM, Lin H-Y, Fulp W, Papenfuss MR, Abrahamsen M, Hildesheim A, Villa LL, Salmerón JJ, Lazcano-Ponce E, Giuliano AR. Incidence and clearance of oral human papillomavirus infection in men: the HIM cohort study. Lancet. 2013;382:877–87.

36. Shigeishi H, Sugiyama M. Risk factors for oral human papillomavirus infection in healthy individuals: a systematic review and meta-analysis. J Clin Med Res. 2016;8:721–9.

37. Chaturvedi AK, Engels EA, Pfeiffer RM, Hernandez BY, Xiao W, Kim E, Jiang B, Goodman MT, Sibug-Saber M, Cozen W, Liu L, Lynch CF, Wentzensen N, Jordan RC, Altekruse S, Anderson WF, Rosenberg PS, Gillison ML. Human papillomavirus and rising oropharyngeal cancer incidence in the United States. J Clin Oncol. 2011;29:4294–301.

38. Smith EM, Ritchie JM, Summersgill KF, Klussmann JP, Lee JH, Wang D, Haugen TH, Turek LP. Age, sexual behavior and human papillomavirus infection in oral cavity and oropharyngeal cancers. Int J Cancer. 2004;108:766–72.

39. Chaturvedi AK, Engels EA, Anderson WF, Gillison ML. Incidence trends for human papillomavirus-related and -unrelated oral squamous cell carcinomas in the United States. J Clin Oncol. 2008;26:612–9.

40. Attner P, Du J, Näsman A, Hammarstedt L, Ramqvist T, Lindholm J, Marklund L, Dalianis T, Munck-Wikland E. Human papillomavirus and survival in patients with base of tongue cancer. Int J Cancer. 2011;128:2892–7.

41. Termine N, Giovannelli L, Rodolico V, Matranga D, Pannone G, Campisi G. Biopsy vs. brushing: comparison of two sampling methods for the detection of HPV DNA in squamous cell carcinoma of the oral cavity. Oral Oncol. 2012;48:870–5.

42. Smith EM, Rubenstein LM, Haugen TH, Pawlita M, Turek LP. Complex etiology underlies risk and survival in head and neck cancer human papillomavirus, tobacco, and alcohol: a case for multifactor disease. J Oncol. 2012;2012:1–9.

43. Duray A, Descamps G, Decaestecker C, Remmelink M, Sirtaine N, Lechien J, Ernoux-Neufcoeur P, Bletard N, Somja J, Depuydt CE, Delvenne P, Saussez S. Human papillomavirus DNA strongly correlates with a poorer prognosis in oral cavity carcinoma. Laryngoscope. 2012;122:1558–65.

44. González-Ramírez I, Irigoyen-Camacho ME, Ramírez-Amador V, Lizano-Soberón M, Carrillo-García A, García-Carrancá A, Sánchez-Pérez Y, Méndez-Martínez R, Granados-García M, Ruíz-Godoy LM, García-Cuellar CM. Association between age and high-risk human papilloma virus in Mexican oral cancer patients. Oral Dis. 2013;19:796–804.

25

Salivary extracellular vesicle-associated miRNAs as potential biomarkers in oral squamous cell carcinoma

Chiara Gai[1], Francesco Camussi[2], Roberto Broccoletti[2], Alessio Gambino[2], Marco Cabras[2], Luca Molinaro[1], Stefano Carossa[2], Giovanni Camussi[1] and Paolo G. Arduino[2*]

Abstract

Background: Several studies in the past have investigated the expression of micro RNAs (miRNAs) in saliva as potential biomarkers. Since miRNAs associated with extracellular vesicles (EVs) are known to be protected from enzymatic degradation, we evaluated whether salivary EVs from patients with oral squamous cell carcinoma (OSCC) were enriched with specific subsets of miRNAs.

Methods: OSCC patients and controls were matched with regards to age, gender and risk factors. Total RNA was extracted from salivary EVs and the differential expression of miRNAs was evaluated by qRT-PCR array and qRT-PCR. The discrimination power of up-regulated miRNAs as biomarkers in OSCC patients versus controls was evaluated by the Receiver Operating Characteristic (ROC) curves.

Results: A preliminary qRT-PCR array was performed on samples from 5 OSCC patients and 5 healthy controls whereby a subset of miRNAs were identified that were differentially expressed. On the basis of these results, a cohort of additional 16 patients and 6 controls were analyzed to further confirm the miRNAs that were up-regulated or selectively expressed in the previous pilot study. The following miRNAs: miR-302b-3p and miR-517b-3p were expressed only in EVs from OSCC patients and miR-512-3p and miR-412-3p were up-regulated in salivary EVs from OSCC patients compared to controls with the ROC curve showing a good discrimination power for OSCC diagnosis. The Kyoto Encyclopedia of Gene and Genomes (KEGG) pathway analysis suggested the possible involvement of the miRNAs identified in pathways activated in OSCC.

Conclusions: In this work, we suggest that salivary EVs isolated by a simple charge-based precipitation technique can be exploited as a non-invasive source of miRNAs for OSCC diagnosis. Moreover, we have identified a subset of miRNAs selectively enriched in EVs of OSCC patients that could be potential biomarkers.

Keywords: Oral squamous cell carcinoma (OSCC), Extracellular vesicles (EVs), microRNA (miRNA), miRNA-512-3p (miR-512), miRNA-412-3p (miR-412), miR-302b-3p (miR-302b), miR-517b-3p (miR-517b), miR-27a-3p (miR-27a), miR-494

Background

Oral squamous cell carcinoma (OSCC) is the most frequent cancer of the head and neck [1, 2]. Despite outstanding diagnostic and therapeutic improvements in oncology, OSCC still holds a poor prognosis with an estimated 5-year overall survival rate of 56% both in the United States and Western Europe [1, 2]. Specifically, in northern Italy, the 3-year and 5-year overall survival rate has been estimated to be 57% and 49% [3] with the latter decreasing dramatically when considering advanced or metastatic cases. Although, in recent years different biological and molecular factors have been described for the prognosis of OSCC, none of them have had a real impact on routine clinical care. Histopathological staging still remains the gold standard for post-operative management and prognosis of the disease [4]. Hence, more reliable and time saving diagnostic tools are needed.

---

* Correspondence: paologiacomo.arduino@unito.it
[2]Department of Surgical Sciences, University of Turin, Via Nizza 230, 10126 Turin, Italy
Full list of author information is available at the end of the article

In OSCC, metastasis spreads predominantly via a lymphatic route with cervical lymph nodes (LN) as the first location, whereas metastasis to distant sites is relatively uncommon [5]. Efficient detection and removal of LN metastasis is therefore crucial in the treatment and survival of patients with this form of carcinoma. Therefore, great expectations lie on the identification of specific predictive factors that could be used clinically for the diagnosis, prognosis and monitoring of the therapeutic response.

In the last decade, extracellular vesicles (EVs) have gained significant attention as a conceivable source of biomarkers. These small membrane-bound vesicles are categorized into 3 different types: exosomes, microvesicles or ectosomes, and apoptotic bodies [6]. EVs are secreted under different physiological and pathophysiological conditions into the extracellular milieu by a variety of cell types, including tumor cells. Tumor-derived EVs have been identified to influence the tumor environment by promoting cancer progression, survival, invasion, and angiogenesis [7]. However, as EVs carry biologically active proteins and nucleic acids from the parent cells, tumor-derived EVs could therefore act as molecular signatures of cancer cells from which they are derived [7, 8].

MicroRNAs (miRNAs) are small non-coding RNA molecules approximately 22 nucleotides in length, which act as regulatory gatekeepers of coding genes. MiRNAs are expressed in a tissue-specific manner, and changes in their expression within a tissue can be correlated with a disease status [9]. Furthermore, they can also modulate gene expression by regulating mRNA translation and/or degradation depending on complementarity between the miRNA and the mRNA [10]. MiRNAs can be secreted either through EVs and/or by forming protein-miRNA complexes with molecules such as high-density lipoproteins and AGO2, which are part of the RISC complex. However, miRNAs carried in EVs are more stable once released as the encapsulation provides protection from enzyme degradation. This therefore makes them more promising as next-generation biomarkers for cancer diagnosis and prognosis [8]. To date, cancer biomarkers carried by EVs have been studied in several types of tumors [9, 11–13], including head and neck cancer [14]. However, no work has been published on the expression of miRNAs in EVs from saliva of patients with OSCC.

The aim of the present study was therefore to evaluate whether salivary EVs of OSCC patients and healthy controls express a different pattern of miRNAs and whether the differentially expressed miRNAs could be applied as potential biomarkers for OSCC.

Methods

Selection of patients

The enrolled subjects were attending the Oral Medicine Section of the Department of Surgical Sciences, University of Turin, CIR-Dental School, between January and June 2015. Patients with biopsy-proven OSCC were involved in the study with the exclusion of patients with the following criteria: 1) < 18 years of age, 2) pregnant or breast feeding, 3) psychiatrically or mentally unstable. Local ethical committee approval (n° 310/2015, "A.O.U. Città della Salute e della Scienza di Torino", Turin, Italy) was obtained and all patients provided written informed consent. Demographic information, age at the time of diagnosis and gender, smoking, tumor site, and TNM classification [15] were recorded at baseline (Table 1 and Additional file 1: Table S1). Healthy subjects presenting no clinically detectable oral lesions matched for age, gender, and risk factors were recruited as controls (Table 1).

Saliva collection

As previously reported [16], all subjects were asked to refrain from: eating, drinking, or oral hygiene for at least one hour prior to collection (usually between 9 and 11 a.m.); they then rinsed their mouths with water and then waited for at least 5 min before spitting into a 50 ml Falcon tube. Participants were instructed not to cough or forcefully expectorate in order to collect unstimulated saliva samples.

HPV-16 in situ hybridization

In situ hybridization (ISH) for HPV was performed on hematoxylin and eosin sections using the Bond TM Ready-to-Use ISH HPV Probe (Leica Biosystems, Newcastle, UK) which targets the following subtypes: 16, 18, 31, 33, and 51. ISH was carried out following the manufacturer's instructions on the automated Leica BOND system (BOND-MAX, Leica Biosystems).

EV isolation

The sample of saliva from patients with OSCC and healthy controls was diluted 1:1 with PBS (phosphate buffered saline) and centrifuged at 3000 g for 15 min at room temperature to remove cells, debris and bacteria. The supernatant was filtered with 0.2 μm filters and

Table 1 Characteristics of OSCC patients and controls enrolled in the study

Characteristics	OSCC patients	Controls	P value
Number	21	11	
Age	65.75 [61; 73]	61.64 [61.5; 67.5]	0.381
Range	38–78	39–75	
Gender (male/female)	12 (57%)/9 (43%)	6 (55%)/5 (45%)	
Smokers	6 (28%)	3 (27%)	

For each group, the table indicates the total number of subjects, the mean age of each group and quartiles [Q1; Q3], the minimum and maximum age of enrolled subjects, number and percentage of male and female and of smokers. The differences in ages between the two groups were not statistically significant (Student's t test) transferred to a sterile tube after which, a precipitation solution (65 µL per 250 µL of saliva) was added and the mixture incubated at 4 °C overnight. The following day, samples were centrifuged at 3000 g for 30 min to precipitate EVs. The resulting supernatant was removed and samples re-centrifuged at 1500 g for 5 min to remove any remaining supernatant [17]. The pellet was resuspended in either: 100 µL of PBS for NanoSight analysis, or 100 µl of RIPA lysis buffer (Sigma Aldrich, Milan, IT) for protein extraction, or 600 µL of Lysis/Binding Buffer (mirVana Isolation Kit, Thermo Fisher Scientific, Waltham, MA, USA) and stored at − 80 °C for subsequent RNA extraction.

EV characterization

The EV samples isolated from saliva were diluted 1:200 in physiologic solution and analyzed by NanoSight LM-10 (Malvern Instruments Ltd., Malvern, UK). The average number and size of EVs were measured by Nanoparticle Tracking Analysis (NTA) software (Malvern Instruments Ltd). Transmission electron microscopy (TEM) of negatively stained EVs (NanoVan, Nanoprobes, Yaphank, NK, USA) was also performed as described previously [17] and the images were obtained using the Joel JEM 1010 electron microscope (Jeol, Tokyo, Japan).

Western blot analysis

Protein concentration in EV samples was measured by Bradford assay. Protein samples were loaded on polyacrylamide gel at the concentration of 30 µg/well and separated by SDS/PAGE, using 4–15% precast gel (Mini-PROTEAN® Precast Gels, Bio-Rad, Hercules, CA, USA). Proteins were transferred on nitrocellulose membranes by liquid electrophoresis. Membranes were immunoblotted by polyclonal antibodies anti-CD9, CD63, TSG101, and Alix (Santa Cruz Biotechnologies, Dalls, TX, USA). Protein-bands were detected by chemiluminescent Clarity™ ECL Western Blotting Substrate (Bio-Rad) and analyzed by ChemiDoc™ XRS + System (Bio-Rad).

RNA extraction and quantification

miRNAs were extracted from purified EVs by mirVana Isolation Kit (Thermo Fisher Scientific), according to the manufacturer's instruction. RNA concentration was measured by Nanodrop ND-1000 (Thermo Fisher Scientific), and the ratio 260/280 and 260/230 showed no contaminations. RNA integrity was assessed by a Bioanalyzer (Agilent, Santa Clara, CA) using the RNA 6000 Pico Kit (Agilent).

miRNA expression analysis by qRT-PCR array

To select differentially expressed miRNAs, qRT-PCR array analysis was performed on EVs isolated from five patients with OSCC and five healthy controls. The concentration of selected RNA samples was up to 20 ng/µl and 50 ng of total RNA were retro-transcribed to cDNA with TaqMan® MicroRNA Reverse Transcription Kit (Thermo Fisher Scientific). cDNA was pre-amplified with Megaplex™ RT Primers, Human Pool Set v3.0 and TaqMan® PreAmp Master Mix (Thermo Fisher Scientific) using a Veriti Thermal Cycler (Thermo Fisher Scientific). The expression profile of a panel of 754 human microRNAs was evaluated by a TaqMan® Array Human MicroRNA Card Set v3.0 (Thermo Fisher Scientific) using the real-time thermal cycler 7900HT (Thermo Fisher Scientific).

qRT-PCR

On the basis of results obtained from the array, we studied miRNAs up-regulated or selectively expressed by patients in a cohort of additional 16 OSCC patients and 6 controls. 500 ng of total RNA was retro-transcribed to cDNA with miScript II RT Kit (Qiagen, Hilden, D) and evaluated for the expression of five miRNAs up-regulated in patients compared to healthy controls (miR-412-3p, miR-489-3p, miR-512-3p, miR-597-5p, and miR-603). Furthermore, eight miRNAs exclusively expressed only in OSCC patients (miR-27a-3p, miR-302b-3p, miR-337-5p, miR-373-3p, miR-494-3p, miR-517b, and miR-520d-3p, miR-645) were also evaluated. Each sample was run in triplicate and each miRNA-specific primer was run in a separate reaction. SnoRNA RNU6B and miR-191 were used as endogenous control as previously described [18–20] due to their stable expression in saliva samples which was also confirmed in the current study by qRT-PCR in tested salivary EV samples.

The qRT-PCR reaction mix was composed of 2 ng of cDNA, 100 nM miScript Universal Primer (Qiagen), 100 nM miRNA-specific primer (Eurofins Genomics, Ebersberg, D), 5 µl QuantiTect SYBR Green PCR Master Mix (Qiagen), and nuclease free water (Qiagen) to reach a final reaction volume of 10 µl. The Real-Time Thermal Cycler Quant Studio 12 k (Thermo Fisher Scientific) was used for analysis.

Enrichment analysis

Enrichment analysis for biological pathways was performed for miRNAs that were found to be up-regulated ($p < 0.09$) or only expressed by OSCC patients. Kyoto Encyclopedia of Gene and Genomes (KEGG) pathway analysis was performed through the DIANA-mirPath v. 3.0 [21] online software and miRNA targets were searched on microT-CDS [22]. Results were merged by a "pathway-union" criterion. The p value was calculated by DIANA software online with: False Discovery Rate (FDR) correction, p value threshold at 0.05 and MicroT threshold at 0.8. Fisher's exact test was used as the statistical method for the enrichment analysis.

Discrimination power analysis

The discrimination power of the up-regulated miRNAs as biomarkers for OSCC diagnosis was evaluated by the Receiver Operating Characteristic (ROC) curves [23]. The ROC curves were constructed using the relative quantification (RQ) of the expression levels of controls and OSCC patients by the demo version of GraphPad Prism 6.01 software. Sensitivity, specificity, area under curve (AUC) and p value were calculated by the software. The optimal threshold value was decided using Youden's index (sensitivity + specificity-1) [24].

Statistical analysis

For array data analysis, SDS Software v.2.3 (Thermo Fisher Scientific) was used to calculate Raw Ct values, with an automatic baseline and threshold. Expression-Suite Software 1.1 (Thermo Fisher Scientific) was used to calculate RQ ($2^{-\Delta\Delta Ct}$) values. Data were normalized using global normalization, an algorithm that finds the assays common to every sample and then uses the median Ct of those assays as the normalization factor, on a per sample basis [25]. Ct values > 35 or with Amp score < 0.7 were excluded from the analysis. To identify candidate miRNAs differentially expressed between patients and controls, we selected miRNAs with low p values ($p \leq 0.05$). P values were calculated by the ExpressionSuite software using Student's t-test for sample group comparisons, without multiple test correction. Further to this, we screened the group for miRNAs expressed in every sample and with low variability among the same group.

For qRT-PCR data analysis, Excel software (Microsoft Office 365 ProPlus) was used to calculate ΔCt, $-\Delta\Delta Ct$, and RQ for patients and controls. Statistical analysis was performed on RQ values through the demo version of GraphPad Prism 6.01 software using an unpaired non-parametric two-sided Mann-Whitney test. Confidence level was set at 95% (p value ≤0.05).

Results

Patient characterization

A total of 21 patients with OSCC (12 men and 9 women) were analyzed (Table 1). The TNM staging system identified the following lesion categories: T1 ($n = 7$), T2 ($n = 8$), T3 ($n = 3$), T4 ($n = 3$); according to the histology, of biopsy specimens, three patients were identified as well differentiated, twelve as moderately differentiated and six as poorly differentiated. The lateral border of the tongue was the most commonly affected site (24%), followed by the floor of the mouth and gingiva (19% respectively), the palate (14%), the pelvis (9.5%) and lastly other sites (19%) (Additional file 1: Table S1). Five, out

of 21 patients, were positive for HPV (23.8%). A total of 11 controls (seven men and four women) were also analyzed. The subjects did not show oral lesions, infections, or tumor history. Controls and OSCC patients were matched based on gender, age and risk factor, as shown in Table 1.

EV characterization

According to NanoSight results, EVs isolated from saliva samples through charge-based precipitation appeared as a heterogeneous population with a size ranging from 100 to 300 nm (Fig. 1a). TEM analysis confirmed the characteristic shape, aspects, and dimensions of EVs (Fig. 1b). Furthermore, we observed that the size and concentration of salivary EVs from OSCC patients were slightly increased compared to healthy controls, however, the differences were not statistically significant. Western Blot analysis demonstrated the expression of the typical exosome markers: CD63, CD9, TSG 101, and Alix (Fig. 1c). Additionally, Western blot analysis performed in duplicate on samples from 10 OSCC patients and 8 controls was also positive for the exosome markers: CD63 and TSG 101 marker, confirming the reproducibility of the isolation method (Additional file 2: Figure S1). The expression of the exosome markers was similar for both OSCC patients and controls. According to Bioanalyzer results, RNA cargo is mainly constituted of RNAs ranging from 20 to 200 nucleotides, whereas the ribosomal RNAs 18 s and 28 s were absent (Figure 1d). No differences were observed between RNA profiles of OSCC patients and controls (Additional file 3: Figure S2).

miRNA expression analysis by qRT-PCR array

On analyzing the expression of miRNAs in salivary EVs, we identified five miRNAs to be up-regulated (miR-412-3p, miR-489-3p, miR-512-3p, miR-597-5p, and miR-603), and six miRNAs down-regulated (miR-193b-3p, miR-30e-3p, miR-376c-3p, miR-484, miR-720, and miR-93-3p) in tumor EVs compared to controls (Table 2). Moreover, eight miRNAs were exclusively detected in EVs from OSCC patients, while 14 miRNAs were specific only to EVs from controls (Table 3). The complete qRT-PCR array results are shown in Additional file 4: Table S2, reporting all miRNAs expressed in EVs of both groups of patients.

qRT-PCR expression analysis

After an initial screening by qRT-PCR array, we selected 11 miRNAs for subsequent analysis. We chose the five miRNAs up-regulated in OSCC patients (miR-412-3p, miR-489-3p, miR-512-3p, miR-597-5p, and miR-603) and eight miRNAs expressed only by OSCC patients (miR-27a-3p, miR-302b-3p, miR-337-5p, miR-373-3p, miR-494-3p, miR-517b, and miR-520d-3p, miR-645). The analysis of the up-regulated miRNAs showed a

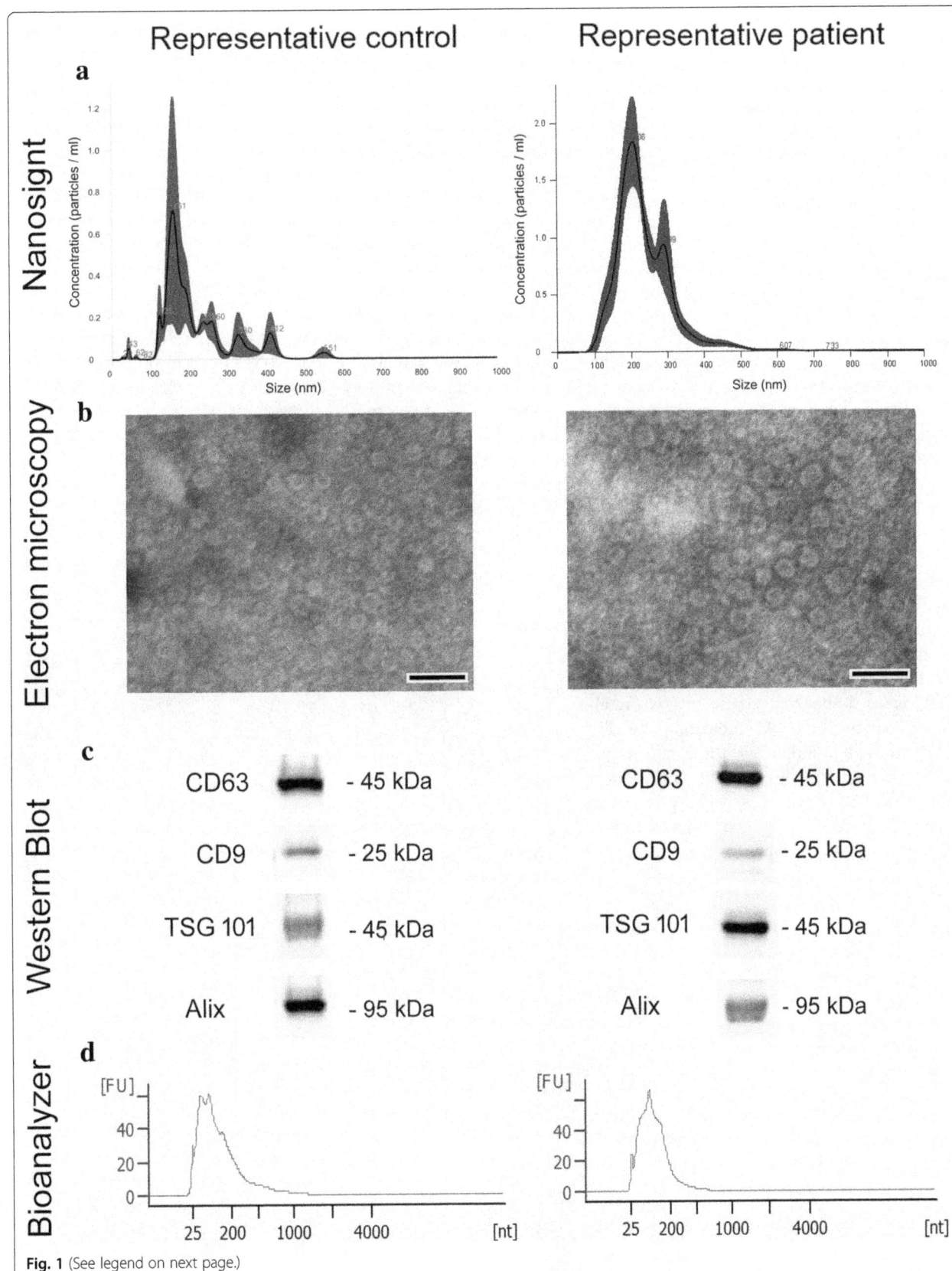

Fig. 1 (See legend on next page.)

Fig. 1 Characterization of salivary EVs. (**a**) Representative NanoSight image of isolated EVs showing particle size (nm)/concentration (10^8 particles/ml) of a representative control (left) and a representative OSCC patient (right). (**b**) Representative transmission electron microscopy image of purified EVs negatively stained with NanoVan (JEOL Jem-1010 electron microscope, black line = 200 nm) of a control (left) and a patient (right). (**c**) Representative western blots confirming the expression of the exosome markers: CD63, CD9, Tsg101, and Alix, on salivary EVs from a control (left) and a OSCC patient (right). (**d**) Representative profiles of RNA isolated from EVs of a healthy control (left) and a patient (right). The graphs show fluorescence intensity [FU]/nucleotide length [nt] and were obtained through bioanalyzer analysis. Four experiments were performed with similar results

significant up-regulation of miR-412-3p and miR-512-3p in OSCC patients with respect to controls (Fig. 2a). The qRT-PCR analysis of miRNAs detected only in OSCC patients through qRT-PCR array showed that miR-27a-3p, miR-337-5p, miR-373-3p, miR-494-3p, and miR-520d-3p were overexpressed in patients however still present in controls (Fig. 2b). MiR-27a-3p, miR-373-3p and miR-494-3p showed a p value lower than 0.1, indicating a conserved but not statistically significant trend of up-regulation in OSCC patients (Fig. 2b). MiR-302b-3p and miR-517b-3p were confirmed to be expressed only in patients (data not shown), while miR-645 expression level was comparable to controls (data not shown).

Discrimination power of miRNAs as OSCC biomarkers
ROC curves were constructed to evaluate the discrimination power of the two up-regulated miRNAs as potential biomarkers for OSCC diagnosis. For each miRNA, the ROC curves express the sensitivity (true positive rate) versus 1-specificity (false positive rate) at various cut-off values, the AUC, indicating the discrimination power of the biomarker, and the p value (Fig. 2c, d). The optimal threshold value was set as the maximum Youden's index (sensitivity + specificity-1) represented as a black circle. MiR-512-3p (Fig. 2c) and miR-412-3p (Fig. 2d) showed high sensitivity and specificity, with high

AUC values of 0.847 and 0.871 respectively, and p values lower than 0.02.

KEGG pathway enrichment analysis
The four miRNAs (miR-512-3p, miR-412-3p, miR-27a-3p, and miR-494-3p) confirmed to be up-regulated and the two miRNAs (miR-302b-3p and miR-517b-3p) confirmed to be expressed only in OSCC patients by qRT-PCR were selected for KEGG pathway enrichment analysis. Eight pathways were found to be significantly enriched for at least two of the tested miRNAs (Fig. 3a). Furthermore, Fig. 3b shows the number of predicted target genes involved in each pathway and Fig. 3c shows,

Table 2 miRNAs differentially expressed in salivary EVs of patients with OSCC compared to healthy controls

	miRNA	RQ	RQ Min	RQ Max	P value
UP	miR-412-3p	9.404	5.855	15.104	0.007
	miR-489-3p	35.07	17.47	70.41	0.020
	miR-512-3p	5.13	2.05	12.85	0.031
	miR-597-5p	3.62	1.83	7.14	0.026
	miR-603	2.36	1.30	4.28	0.042
DOWN	miR-193b-3p	0.26	0.05	1.27	0.042
	miR-30e-3p	0.21	0.07	0.65	0.010
	miR-376c-3p	0.17	0.08	0.32	0.035
	miR-484	0.44	0.23	0.85	0.048
	miR-720	0.29	0.09	0.96	0.017
	miR-93-3p	0.39	0.15	1.05	0.044

MiRNAs were considered up-regulated (UP) or down-regulated (DOWN) for p value < 0.05 and similar expression levels in each sample. Relative quantification (RQ) = $2^{-\Delta\Delta Ct}$

Table 3 miRNAs exclusively expressed in salivary EVs of the OSCC patients or the controls

	miRNA	Ct mean	St dev
Only patients	miR-27a-3p	29.5	1.33
	miR-302b-3p	33.9	0.34
	miR-337-5p	30.0	1.32
	miR-373-3p	30.9	0.40
	miR-494-3p	33.5	1.24
	miR-517b	32.2	1.57
	miR-520d-3p	31.2	1.42
	miR-645	34.2	0.40
Only controls	miR-126-5p	32.6	1.86
	miR-127-3p	32.1	1.39
	miR-1276	31.4	0.95
	miR-1289	33.8	1.34
	miR-144-5p	32.4	2.55
	miR-182-5p	32.2	1.11
	miR-30d-3p	31.3	1.22
	miR-520c-3p	32.1	1.70
	miR-550a-5p	32.1	0.29
	miR-628-3p	30.5	0.70
	miR-944	32.9	0.93
	miR-99a-3p	31.1	1.21
	miR-942	31.1	0.85
	RNU48	32.1	1.03

MiRNAs were considered as expressed only by patients or controls when at least 3 samples out of 5 have Ct > 35 or show no expression

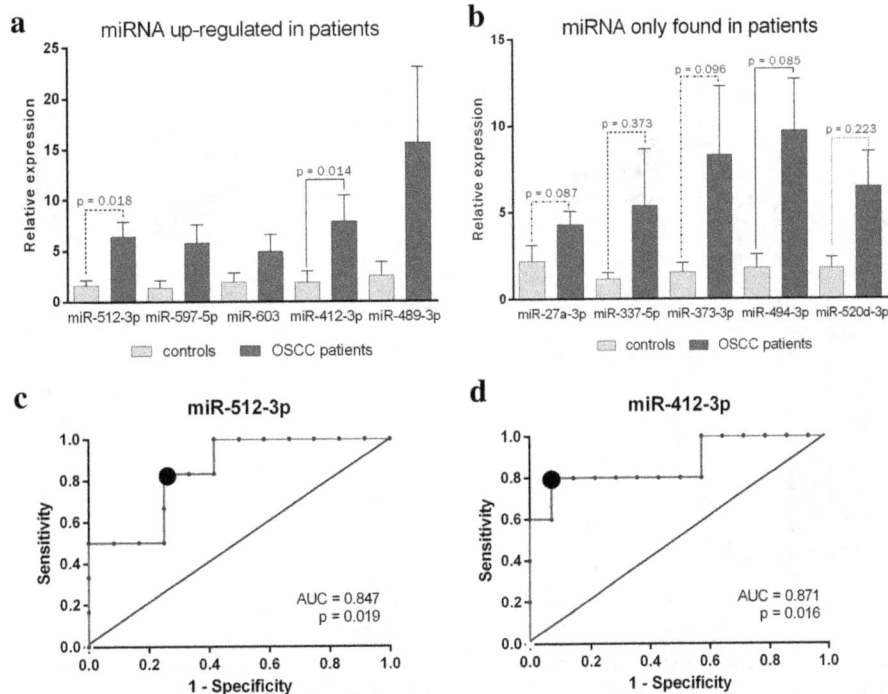

Fig. 2 miRNA relative expression detected by qRT-PCR in salivary EV samples from OSCC patients compared to normal subjects. (**a**) Expression levels of miRNAs that were significantly up-regulated in patients. (**b**) Expression levels of miRNAs that were exclusively expressed by OSCC patients. The bars represent mean relative expression ($2^\wedge-\Delta\Delta Ct$) of control and patient groups ± SEM, p value (two-sided Mann-Whitney test) are reported. ROC curve describing predictive potency of the up-regulated miRNAs as a diagnostic test. The curves represent specificity versus sensitivity of miR-512-3p (**c**), miR-412-3p (**d**). Data are derived from miRNAs' expression levels (RQ) of OSCC patients and controls. The big gray dots indicate the optimal threshold value of sensitivity and specificity determined by the maximum Youden's index (sensitivity+specificity-1)

for each miRNA, the number of predicted target genes in each pathway and the respective p value.

Discussion

The use of saliva as a diagnostic biofluid has been widely recognized, and it has many advantages over other specimens like blood, exfoliated cells and urine [26, 27]. Salivary biomarkers have the potential to serve as non-invasive, widely accessible screening tools. In fact, the collection is inexpensive and can be easily performed. Identifying the proper salivary biomarker profile could contribute to the current screening method of oral cancer, which is limited to physical exam and biopsy of suspicious lesions [26].

Several works describe the possibility to detect RNA biomarkers of numerous diseases in saliva [26–28] and, more specifically, miRNAs associated with oral cancer [26–31]. Evidence demonstrates that it is possible to isolate EV-associated RNA from saliva and oral samples [28, 32, 33]. However, to date, miRNA expression analysis in EVs from OSCC have never been reported.

In this work, according to previous evidence [17, 32–35], we successfully isolated EVs from saliva. A previous study [17] showed that most of the salivary RNA was associated with EVs. Through Bioanalyzer RNA profiles, we observed

that EVs were enriched with RNAs ranging from 20 to 200 nucleotides whereas ribosomal RNAs were nearly absent. Our results are in accordance with other published data of EV RNA cargo [33, 36, 37]. Molecular analysis of miRNAs revealed an up-regulation of miR-412-3p, miR-512-3p, miR-27a-3p, miR-373-3p, miR-494-3p in salivary EVs from OSCC patients. Furthermore, we found that miR-302b-3p and miR-517b-3p were expressed specifically only in samples from the OSCC group. KEGG pathway enrichment analysis based on predicted miRNA targets provides speculative information of miRNA functions. Eight pathways showed a statistically significant enrichment with each pathway predicted to involve two or more miRNAs. For instance, miR-512-3p and miR-27a-3p could target respectively 7 and 20 genes involved in the ErbB signaling pathway. The pathway is known to promote cell proliferation and survival in several solid tumors [38] and has been shown to be activated in OSCC as well [39–41]. MiR-512-3p, miR-27a-3p, and miR-302b-3p could target respectively 14, 30, and 14 genes regulating proteoglycan in cancer pathways. Evidence has shown that CD44, which can be targeted by both miR-512-3p and miR-302b-3p, and the downstream pathway promote cell invasion and migration upon c-Fos stimulation in OSCC [42]. Increased CD44 expression has been associated with ERK1/2 phosphorylation,

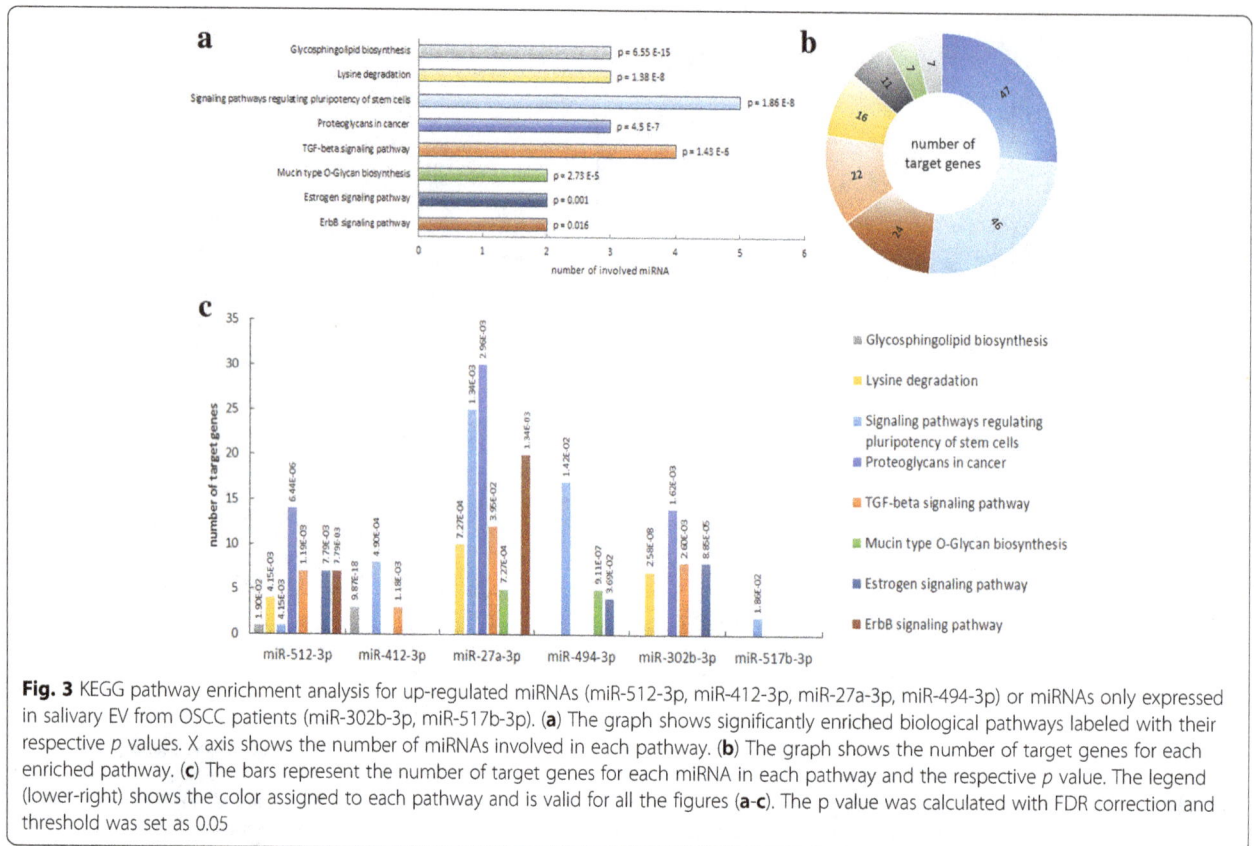

Fig. 3 KEGG pathway enrichment analysis for up-regulated miRNAs (miR-512-3p, miR-412-3p, miR-27a-3p, miR-494-3p) or miRNAs only expressed in salivary EV from OSCC patients (miR-302b-3p, miR-517b-3p). (**a**) The graph shows significantly enriched biological pathways labeled with their respective *p* values. X axis shows the number of miRNAs involved in each pathway. (**b**) The graph shows the number of target genes for each enriched pathway. (**c**) The bars represent the number of target genes for each miRNA in each pathway and the respective *p* value. The legend (lower-right) shows the color assigned to each pathway and is valid for all the figures (**a-c**). The p value was calculated with FDR correction and threshold was set as 0.05

and increased tumor aggressiveness [43]. Moreover, high CD44 levels have been described as a characteristic feature of cancer stem-like cells in OSCC [44]. In addition, miR-512-3p, miR-412-3p, miR-27a-3p, and miR-302b-3p could target several genes of the TGFβ signaling pathway, including TGFβR2 gene. Interestingly, it has been previously reported that TGFβR2 is commonly reduced in oral epithelium and stroma in OSCC patients [45]. In line with cancer stem like cells, 46 genes involved in signaling pathways regulating pluripotency of stem cells can also be targeted by miR-512-3p, miR-27a-3p, miR-494-3p, miR-517b-3p, and miR-412-3p. The overexpression of Bmi1, which can be targeted by miR-494 and miR-27a-3p, has been shown to promote formation, growth, migration, and metastasis in a subpopulation of tumor cells of the HNSCC [46]. Basing on these observations, we speculate that the increase of miRNA that target genes involved in tumor progression in salivary EVs might represent a defenses mechanism of tumor cells to eliminate anti-tumor miRNAs. However, due to the speculative nature of this analysis, the relation between miRNAs and target genes and pathways should be further proven experimentally.

To better evaluate the discrimination power of the up-regulated miRNAs as OSCC biomarkers, we constructed ROC curves. MiR-512-3p and miR-412-3p resulted to be

either sensitive and specific, as shown by high AUC values (0.847 and 0.871 respectively, with *p* values < 0.02) and maximum Youden's Index. This indicates that the two miRNAs are good predictors and can be suggested as new candidate biomarkers for OSCC, which can be evaluated through further studies on a larger population. On the other hand, the up-regulation of miR-27a-3p and miR-494-3p can be used as indicators, but are not sufficient as diagnostic biomarkers. Nevertheless, the involvement of miR-494-3p and miR-27a-3p in OSCC is supported by the literature. MiR-494 has been previously isolated from blood of OSCC patients and proposed as a biomarker [47]. MiR-27a-3p is involved in the progression of OSCC by targeting YAP1 and therefore inhibiting epithelial to mesenchymal transition processes [48]. Furthermore, miR-27a-3p can also target MCPH1, which acts as an onco-suppressor gene [49]. It has also been proposed that high levels of miR-27a increase heat sensitivity in OSCC cells, enhancing hyperthermia-induced-cell death [50]. Moreover, miR-27a-3p seems to play a role in progression and metastasis of nasopharyngeal carcinoma [51], gastric cancer [52], esophageal cancer [53], and has been proposed as an EV-associated biomarker for colorectal cancer [54]. No evidence has been reported confirming the involvement of miR-412-3p, miR-512-3p, miR-302b-3p, and miR-517b-3p in OSCC, thus our work provides new insights about the dysregulation of miRNAs in the tumor environment. It is worth mentioning that miR-512-3p has been reported to be up-regulated in metastatic prostate cancer [55], and conversely shown anti-tumor activity in non-small cell lung cancer [56] and hepatocellular carcinoma [57].

On the other hand, our molecular analysis revealed the expression, although not statistically significant, of several miRNAs that have been reported in the literature as up-regulated in whole saliva or plasma of OSCC patients and have been proposed as biomarkers. For example, we observed the expression of both miR-31-5p and miR-31-3p in OSCC patients, however the levels were comparable with controls (Additional file 4: Table S2). Several studies have reported that miR-31 is overexpressed and/or involved in OSCC [58–63]. MiR-184, expressed in OSCC patients and controls, has been reported to have a good diagnostic value [30]. MiR-708 is up-regulated in progressing oral pre-malignant lesions [29] and was increased but without any statistically significant up-regulation in our group of patients (Additional file 4: Table S2). The discrepancies among the miRNAs up-regulated in our study and in other studies in the literature may be due to the relatively small number of recruited patients and controls and to the different geographical origin of the group of cases enrolled in each study. Moreover, most of the studies detected miRNAs in whole saliva [18, 20, 29, 30] or plasma [58], instead of salivary EVs. This may lead to different results since miRNAs can be differentially represented in whole saliva and salivary EVs, as it has been previously described for total plasma or plasma-derived EVs [64, 65].

Conclusions

In this work, we demonstrated the possibility to use salivary EVs as a non-invasive source of miRNAs for OSCC diagnosis and we identified two miRNAs (miR-412-3p and miR-512-3p) overexpressed in OSCC patients and two miRNAs (miR-302b-3p and miR-517b-3p) selectively enriched in EVs from OSCC patients. These four miRNAs have the potential to be used as biomarkers.

Additional files

Additional file 1: Table S1. Characteristics and tumor staging of OSCC patients enrolled in the study.

Additional file 2: Figure S1. Protein expression analysis of exosome markers CD63 and TSG101. For each protein, the picture shows two western blot experiments performed on salivary EVs from 10 OSCC patients (left) and 8 controls (right).

Additional file 3: Figure S2. Bioanalyzer RNA profiles. Profiles of RNA isolated from salivary EVs of four controls (left) and four patients (right) in duplicate (a, b). The graphs show fluorescence intensity [FU]/nucleotide length [nt] and were obtained by bioanalyzer analysis.

Additional file 4: Table S2. miRNAs expressed in both controls and OSCC patients.

Abbreviations

AGO2: protein argonaute-2; EVs: Extracellular vesicles; HNSCC: Head and neck squamous-cell carcinoma; KEGG: Kyoto Encyclopedia of Gene and Genomes; LN: lymph node; miRNA: microRNA; OSCC: Oral squamous cell carcinoma; RISC: RNA-induced silencing complex; ROC: Receiver Operating Characteristic; RQ: Relative quantification; TEM: Transmission electron microscopy

Acknowledgements

The authors thank Unicyte for providing the precipitation solution to purify EVs. The authors thanks Dr. Sharad Kholia for the revision of English.

Funding

This work was supported by the Associazione Italiana Ricerca Cancro (grant number AIRC IG 2015.16973) to GC and by "Fondi Universitari ex-60% 2014" to PGA. Funding agencies had not any influence in the design of the study, collection, analysis, and interpretation of data and in writing the manuscript.

Authors' contributions

CG, GC, SC, and PGA performed the study design. AG and MC recruited the patients and performed HPV tests on saliva. Data acquisition was operated by CG, FC, PGA, LM, quality control of data and algorithms was performed by CG and PGA. CG and GC performed data analysis and interpretation, CG and RB performed statistical analysis. The manuscript was prepared by CG, FC, RB, AG, MC, LM, SC, GC and PGA. All authors read and approved the final manuscript.

Competing interests

GC is named as inventors in a related patent application. All other authors declare no conflict of interest.

Author details

[1]Department of Medical Sciences, University of Turin, C.so Dogliotti, 14 – 10126 Turin, Italy. [2]Department of Surgical Sciences, University of Turin, Via Nizza 230, 10126 Turin, Italy.

References

1. Moore S, Johnson N, Pierce A. The epidemiology of mouth cancer: a review of global incidence. Oral Dis. 2000;6(2):65–74.
2. Bagan J, Sarrion G, Jimenez Y. Oral cancer: clinical features. Oral Oncol. 2010;46(6):414–7.
3. Arduino PG, Carrozzo M, Chiecchio A, Broccoletti R, Tirone F, Borra E, et al. Clinical and histopathologic independent prognostic factors in oral squamous cell carcinoma: a retrospective study of 334 cases. J Oral Maxillofac Surg. 2008;66(8):1570–9.

4. Woolgar JA. Histopathological prognosticators in oral and oropharyngeal squamous cell carcinoma. Oral Oncol. 2006;42(3):229–39.

5. Zanaruddin SN, Saleh A, Yang YH, Hamid S, Mustafa WM, Khairul Bariah AA, et al. Four proteins signature accurately predicts lymph node metastasis and survival in oral squamous cell carcinoma. Hum Pathol. 2013;44(3):417–26.

6. Raposo G, Stoorvogel W. Extracellular vesicles: exosomes, microvesicles, and friends. J Cell Biol. 2013;200(4):373–83.

7. Javeed N, Mukhopadhyay D. Exosomes and Their role in the micro–/macro-environment: a comprehensive review. J Biomed Res 2016 Mar 15;30. https://doi.org/10.7555/JBR.30.20150162. [Epub ahead of print] Review. PubMed PMID: 2829018210.

8. Kinoshita T, Yip KW, Spence T, Liu FF. MicroRNAs in extracellular vesicles: potential cancer biomarkers. J Hum Genet 2017 Jan;62(1):67–74. https://doi.org/10.1038/jhg.2016.87. Epub 2016 Jul 7. Review. PubMed PMID: 27383658.

9. Hutvagner G, Zamore PD. A microRNA in a multiple-turnover RNAi enzyme complex. Science. 2002;297(5589):2056–60.

10. He Y, Lin J, Kong D, Huang M, Xu C, Kim TK, Etheridge A, Luo Y, Ding Y, Wang K. Current state of circulating MicroRNAs as Cancer biomarkers. Clin Chem 2015 Sep;61(9):1138–1155. https://doi.org/10.1373/clinchem.2015. 241190. Epub 2015 Aug 3. Review.

11. Nawaz M, Camussi G, Valadi H, Nazarenko I, Ekström K, Wang X, et al. The emerging role of extracellular vesicles as biomarkers for urogenital cancers. Nat Rev Urol. 2014;11(12):688–701.

12. Sadovska L, Eglītis J, Linē A. Extracellular vesicles as biomarkers and therapeutic targets in breast Cancer. Anticancer Res. 2015;35(12):6379–90.

13. Melo SA, Luecke LB, Kahlert C, Fernandez AF, Gammon ST, Kaye J, et al. Glypican-1 identifies cancer exosomes and detects early pancreatic cancer. Nature. 2015;523(7559):177–82.

14. Bergmann C, Strauss L, Wieckowski E, Czystowska M, Albers A, Wang Y, et al. Tumor-derived microvesicles in sera of patients with head and neck cancer and their role in tumor progression. Head Neck. 2009;31(3):371–80.

15. Hermanek P, Sobin L. Classification of malignant tumors. Forth. Berlin: Springer-Verlag; 1988.

16. Arduino PG, Menegatti E, Cappello N, Martina E, Gardino N, Tanteri C, et al. Possible role for interleukins as biomarkers for mortality and recurrence in oral cancer. Int J Biol Markers. 2015;30(2):262–6.

17. Deregibus MC, Figliolini F, D'Antico S, Manzini PM, Pasquino C, Lena De, et al. Charge-based precipitation of extracellular vesicles. Int J Mol Med. 2016; 38(5):1359–66.

18. Park NJ, Zhou H, Elashoff D, Henson BS, Kastratovic DA, Abemayor E, et al. Salivary microRNA: discovery, characterization, and clinical utility for oral cancer detection. Clin Cancer Res. 2009;15(17):5473–7.

19. Sauer E, Madea B, Courts C. An evidence based strategy for normalization of quantitative PCR data from miRNA expression analysis in forensically relevant body fluids. Forensic Sci Int Genet. 2014;11:174–81.

20. Momen-Heravi F, Trachtenberg AJ, Kuo WP, Cheng YS. Genomewide study of salivary MicroRNAs for detection of oral Cancer. J Dent Res. 2014;93(7 Suppl):86S–93S.

21. Vlachos IS, Zagganas K, Paraskevopoulou MD, Georgakilas G, Karagkouni D, Vergoulis T, et al. DIANA-miRPath v3.0: deciphering microRNA function with experimental support. Nucleic Acids Res. 2015;43(1):460–6.

22. Paraskevopoulou MD, Georgakilas G, Kostoulas N, Vlachos IS, Vergoulis T, Reczko M, Filippidis C, Dalamagas T, Hatzigeorgiou AG. DIANA-microT web server v5.0: service integration into miRNA functional analysis workflows. Nucleic Acids Res. 2013 Jul;41(Web Server issue):W169–73. https://doi.org/10.1093/nar/gkt393.

23. Hajian-Tilaki K. Receiver operating characteristic (ROC) curve analysis for medical diagnostic test evaluation. Caspian J Intern Med. 2013;4(2):627–35.

24. Ruopp MD, Perkins NJ, Whitcomb BW, Schisterman EF. Youden index and optimal cut-point estimated from observations affected by a lower limit of detection. Biom J. 2008;50(3):419–30.

25. Mestdagh P, Van Vlierberghe P, De Weer A, Muth D, Westermann F, Speleman F, Vandesompele J. A novel and universal method for microRNA RT-qPCR data normalization. Genome Biol. 2009;10(6):R64. https://doi.org/10.1186/gb-2009-10-6-r64.

26. Kaczor-Urbanowicz KE, Martin Carreras-Presas C, Aro K, Tu M, Garcia-Godoy F, Wong DT. Saliva diagnostics - current views and directions. Exp Biol Med (Maywood). 2017;242(5):459–72.

27. Li Y, St John MA, Zhou X, Kim Y, Sinha U, Jordan RC, et al. Salivary transcriptome diagnostics for oral cancer detection. Clin Cancer Res. 2004;10:8442–50.

28. Michael A, Bajracharya SD, Yuen PS, Zhou H, Star RA, Illei GG, et al. Exosomes from human saliva as a source of microRNA biomarkers. Oral Dis. 2010;16(1):34–8.

29. Yang Y, Li YX, Yang X, Jiang L, Zhou ZJ, Zhu YQ. Progress risk assessment of oral premalignant lesions with saliva miRNA analysis. BMC Cancer. 2013;13:129.

30. Zahran F, Ghalwash D, Shaker O, Al-Johani K, Scully C. Salivary microRNAs in oral cancer. Oral Dis. 2015;21(6):739–47.

31. Zhou Y, Kolokythas A, Schwartz JL, Epstein JB, Adami GR. microRNA from brush biopsy to characterize oral squamous cell carcinoma epithelium. Cancer Med. 2017;6(1):67–78.

32. Yap T, Vella LJ, Seers C, Nastri A, Reynolds E, Cirillo N, et al. Oral swirl samples - a robust source of microRNA protected by extracellular vesicles. Oral Dis. 2017;23(3):312–7.

33. Lässer C, Alikhani VS, Ekström K, Eldh M, Paredes PT, Bossios A, Sjöstrand M, Gabrielsson S, Lötvall J, Valadi H. Human saliva, plasma and breast milk exosomes contain RNA: uptake by macrophages. J Transl Med. 2011;9:9. https://doi.org/10.1186/1479-5876-9-9.

34. Marzesco AM, Janich P, Wilsch-Bräuninger M, Dubreuil V, Langenfeld K, Corbeil D, et al. Release of extracellular membrane particles carrying the stem cell marker prominin-1 (CD133) from neural progenitors and other epithelial cells. J Cell Sci. 2005;118(13):2849–58.

35. Ogawa Y, Kanai-Azuma M, Akimoto Y, Kawakami H, Yanoshita R. Exosome-like vesicles with dipeptidyl peptidase IV in human saliva. Biol Pharm Bull. 2008;31(6):1059–62.

36. Willms E, Johansson HJ, Mäger I, Lee Y, Blomberg KE, Sadik M, Alaarg A, Smith CI, Lehtiö J, El Andaloussi S, Wood MJ, Vader P. Cells release subpopulations of exosomes with distinct molecular and biological properties. Sci Rep. 2016;6:22519. https://doi.org/10.1038/srep22519.

37. Santonocito M, Vento M, Guglielmino MR, Battaglia R, Wahlgren J, Ragusa M, Barbagallo D, Borzì P, Rizzari S, Maugeri M, Scollo P, Tatone C, Valadi H, Purrello M, Di Pietro C. Molecular characterization of exosomes and their microRNA cargo in human follicular fluid: bioinformatic analysis reveals that exosomal microRNAs control pathways involved in follicular maturation. Fertil Steril. 2014;102(6):1751–61.e1. https://doi.org/10.1016/j.fertnstert.2014. 08.005.

38. Appert-Collin A, Hubert P, Crémel G, Bennasroune A. Role of ErbB receptors in Cancer cell migration and invasion. Front Pharmacol. 2015;6:283.

39. Li X, Sun R, Geng X, Wang S, Zen D, Pei J, et al. A comprehensive analysis of candidate gene signatures in oral squamous cell carcinoma. Neoplasma. 2017;64(2):167–74.

40. Ohnishi Y, Yasui H, Kakudo K, Nozaki M. Lapatinib-resistant cancer cells possessing epithelial cancer stem cell properties develop sensitivity during sphere formation by activation of the ErbB/AKT/cyclin D2 pathway. Oncol Rep. 2016;36(5):3058–64.

41. Li SX, Yang YQ, Jin LJ, Cai ZG, Sun Z. Detection of survivin, carcinoembryonic antigen and ErbB2 level in oral squamous cell carcinoma patients. Cancer Biomark. 2016;17(4):377–82.

42. Dong C, Ye DX, Zhang WB, Pan HY, Zhang ZY, Zhang L. Overexpression of c-fos promotes cell invasion and migration via CD44 pathway in oral squamous cell carcinoma. J Oral Pathol Med. 2015;44(5):353–60.

43. Judd NP, Winkler AE, Murillo-Sauca O, Brotman JJ, Law JH, Lewis JS Jr, et al. ERK1/2 regulation of CD44 modulates oral cancer aggressiveness. Cancer Res 2012;72(1):365–374.

44. Ghuwalewala S, Ghatak D, Das P, Dey S, Sarkar S, Alam N, et al. CD44(high)CD24(low) molecular signature determines the Cancer stem cell and EMT phenotype in oral squamous cell carcinoma. Stem Cell Res. 2016;16(2):405–17.

45. Meng W, Xia Q, Wu L, Chen S, He X, Zhang L, et al. Downregulation of TGF-beta receptor types II and III in oral squamous cell carcinoma and oral carcinoma-associated fibroblasts. BMC Cancer. 2011;11:88.

46. Liu W, Feng JQ, Shen XM, et al. Two stem cell markers, ATP-binding cassette, G2 subfamily (ABCG2) and BMI-1, predict the transformation of oral leukoplakia to cancer: a long-term follow-up study. Cancer. 2012;118:1693–700.

47. Ries J, Vairaktaris E, Agaimy A, Kintopp R, Baran C, Neukam FW, et al. miR-186, miR-3651 and miR-494: potential biomarkers for oral squamous cell carcinoma extracted from whole blood. Oncol Rep. 2014;31(3):1429–36.

48. Zeng G, Xun W, Wei K, Yang Y, Shen H. MicroRNA-27a-3p regulates epithelial to mesenchymal transition via targeting YAP1 in oral squamous cell carcinoma cells. Oncol Rep. 36(3):1475–82.

49. Venkatesh T, Nagashri MN, Swamy SS, Mohiyuddin SM, Gopinath KS, Kumar A. Primary microcephaly gene MCPH1 shows signatures of tumor suppressors and is regulated by miR-27a in oral squamous cell carcinoma. PLoS One. 2013;8(3):e54643. https://doi.org/10.1371/journal.pone.0054643.

50. Kariya A, Furusawa Y, Yunoki T, Kondo T, Tabuchi Y. A microRNA-27a mimic sensitizes human oral squamous cell carcinoma HSC-4 cells to hyperthermia through downregulation of Hsp110 and Hsp90. Int J Mol Med. 2014;34(1):334–40.

51. Li L, Luo Z. Dysregulated miR-27a-3p promotes nasopharyngeal carcinoma cell proliferation and migration by targeting Mapk10. Oncol Rep. 2017; https://doi.org/10.3892/or.2017.5544.

52. Zhou L, Liang X, Zhang L, Yang L, Nagao N, Wu H, et al. MiR-27a-3p functions as an oncogene in gastric cancer by targeting BTG2. Oncotarget. 2016;7(32):51943–54.

53. Wu XZ, Wang KP, Song HJ, Xia JH, Jiang Y, Wang YL. MiR-27a-3p promotes esophageal cancer cell proliferation via F-box and WD repeat domain-containing 7 (FBXW7) suppression. Int J Clin Exp Med. 2015;8(9):15556–62.

54. Ostenfeld MS, Jensen SG, Jeppesen DK, Christensen LL, Thorsen SB, Stenvang J, et al. miRNA profiling of circulating EpCAM(+) extracellular vesicles: promising biomarkers of colorectal cancer. J Extracell Vesicles. 2016;5:31488.

55. Sadeghi M, Ranjbar B, Ganjalikhany MR, M Khan F, Schmitz U, Wolkenhauer O, Gupta SK. MicroRNA and transcription factor gene regulatory network analysis reveals key regulatory elements associated with prostate Cancer progression. PLoS One. 2016 Dec 22;11(12):e0168760. https://doi.org/10.1371/journal.pone.0168760.

56. Chen F, Zhu HH, Zhou LF, Wu SS, Wang J, Chen Z. Inhibition of c-FLIP expression by miR-512-3p contributes to taxol-induced apoptosis in hepatocellular carcinoma cells. Oncol Rep. 2010;23(5):1457–62.

57. Zhu X, Gao G, Chu K, Yang X, Ren S, Li Y, et al. Inhibition of RAC1-GEF DOCK3 by miR-512-3p contributes to suppression of metastasis in non-small cell lung cancer. Int J Biochem Cell Biol. 2015;61:103–14.

58. Liu CJ, Kao SY, Tu HF, Tsai MM, Chang KW, Lin SC. Increase of microRNA miR-31 level in plasma could be a potential marker of oral cancer. Oral Dis. 2010;16(4):360–4.

59. Lu WC, Kao SY, Yang CC, Tu HF, Wu CH, Chang KW, et al. EGF up-regulates miR-31 through the C/EBPβ signal cascade in oral carcinoma. PLoS One. 2014;9(9):e108049.

60. Siow MY, Ng LP, Vincent-Chong VK, Jamaludin M, Abraham MT. Abdul Rahman Zaet al. Dysregulation of miR-31 and miR-375 expression is associated with clinical outcomes in oral carcinoma. Oral Dis. 2014;20(4):345.

61. Hung PS, Tu HF, Kao SY, Yang CC, Liu CJ, Huang TY, et al. miR-31 is up-regulated in oral premalignant epithelium and contributes to the immortalization of normal oral keratinocytes. Carcinogenesis. 2014;35(5):1162–71.

62. Yan ZY, Luo ZQ, Zhang LJ, Li J, Liu JQ. Integrated analysis and MicroRNA expression profiling identified seven miRNAs associated with progression of oral squamous cell carcinoma. J Cell Physiol. 2016; https://doi.org/10.1002/jcp.25728.

63. Hung KF, Liu CJ, Chiu PC, Lin JS, Chang KW, Shih WY, et al. MicroRNA-31 up-regulation predicts increased risk of progression of oral potentially malignant disorder. Oral Oncol. 2016;53:42–7.

64. Cheng L, Sharples RA, Scicluna BJ, Hill AF. Exosomes provide a protective and enriched source of miRNA for biomarker profiling compared to intracellular and cell-free blood. J Extracell Vesicles. 2014;3 https://doi.org/10.3402/jev.v3.23743.

65. Endzeliņš E, Berger A, Melne V, Bajo-Santos C, Soboļevska K, Ābols A, et al. Detection of circulating miRNAs: comparative analysis of extracellular vesicle-incorporated miRNAs and cell-free miRNAs in whole plasma of prostate cancer patients. BMC Cancer. 2017;17(1):730. https://doi.org/10.1186/s12885-017-3737-z.

26

AKT1 restricts the invasive capacity of head and neck carcinoma cells harboring a constitutively active PI3 kinase activity

Sanja Brolih[1†], Scott K. Parks[1†], Valérie Vial[1], Jérôme Durivault[1], Livio Mostosi[1], Jacques Pouysségur[1], Gilles Pagès[1,2] and Vincent Picco[1*] (iD)

Abstract

Background: In mammals, the AKT/PKB protein kinase family comprises three members (AKT1–3). PI3-Kinase (PI3K), a key oncogene involved in a wide variety of cancers, drives AKT activity. Constitutive activation of the PI3K/AKT pathway has been associated with tumorigenic properties including uncontrolled cell proliferation and survival, angiogenesis, promotion of cellular motility, invasiveness and metastasis. However, AKT1 activity has also been recently shown to repress the invasive properties of breast cancer cells in specific contexts.

Methods: This study used both pharmacological and shRNA approaches to inhibit AKT function, microscopy to characterize the cellular morphology, 3D spheroid models to assess migratory and invasive cellular capacities and a phenotypic screening approach based on electrical properties of the cells.

Results: Here we demonstrate that the alternative action of AKT1 on invasive properties of breast cancers can be extended to head and neck carcinomas, which exhibit constitutive activation of the PI3K/AKT pathway. Indeed, inhibition of AKT1 function by shRNA or a specific pharmacological inhibitor resulted in cellular spreading and an invasive phenotype. A phenotypic screening approach based on cellular electrical properties corroborated microscopic observations and provides a foundation for future high-throughput screening studies. This technique further showed that the inhibition of AKT1 signaling is phenocopied by blocking the mTORC1 pathway with rapamycin.

Conclusion: Our study suggests that the repressive action of PI3K/AKT1 on cellular invasive properties may be a mechanism common to several cancers. Current and future studies involving AKT inhibitors must therefore consider this property to prevent metastases and consequently to improve survival.

Keywords: Cancer, Metastasis, AKT/PKB, Head and neck squamous cell carcinoma, Phenotypic screening, Epithelial-mesenchymal transition, Adhesion, Migration, Invasion

Background

The serine/threonine kinase AKT promotes the epithelial-mesenchymal transition (EMT), cellular motility and invasion in a wide variety of physiological and pathological conditions. In developing vertebrate embryos, the EMT events leading to the formation of mesoderm during gastrulation rely on AKT activity and its upstream activator phosphatidylinositol 3-kinase (PI3K) [1–3]. AKT activity is also associated with EMT, migration and invasion in a diverse range of tumor cell models [4–6]. Furthermore, AKT is a major mediator of cell survival through direct inhibition of pro-apoptotic proteins. Based on these observations, AKT was proposed to be a suitable target for anticancer therapies and clinical trials using inhibitors of PI3K or AKT have been performed previously and are ongoing [7].

Among the most recent clinically suitable AKT inhibitors, MK-2206, an allosteric inhibitor targeting AKT isoforms 1–3 with an affinity in the nanomolar range, has undergone phase II clinical trials in several cancer types [8–11]. Despite acceptable tolerance and promising

* Correspondence: vpicco@centrescientifique.mc
†Equal contributors
[1]Centre Scientifique de Monaco, Department of Medical Biology, 8 Quai Antoine Ier, Monaco, Principality of Monaco
Full list of author information is available at the end of the article

preclinical results, none of the clinical trials have shown favorable effects for MK-2206 treatment [8–24]. Interestingly, the different AKT isoforms can display drastically different functions, especially with regards to cell migration. For example, preclinical data suggested that AKT2 promotes metastasis in ovarian and breast cancer cell models [25, 26] while AKT1 was proposed to inhibit the migration and metastasis of breast cancers [27–30]. Collectively, these results raise concerns over the clinical outcomes of pan-AKT inhibitors and indicate the potential benefits of pursuing isoform-specific inhibitors.

In the present study, we extend recent results showing that AKT1 restricts the invasive potential of breast tumor cells [27–30] to head and neck squamous cell carcinoma (HNSCC) cells. In these HNSCC model cell lines, AKT1 inhibition induced a drastic change in the cellular morphology of the CAL33 oral cancer cell line that is associated with increased migratory and invasive capacities. By means of phenotypic screening based on electrical cellular properties, we identified other HNSCC cell lines that either demonstrated the same phenotype (Detroit562) or an absence of drug sensitivity (CAL27). We next screened for other anti-cancer compounds and showed that the mTORC1 inhibitor rapamycin induces a comparable modification of the cellular electrical properties and modification of CAL33 and Detroit562 cell morphology. Our results therefore extend the concept that AKT1 exerts an anti-metastatic effect. Finally, our results suggest that some anti-cancer drugs may induce a pro-metastatic effect and proposes an efficient in vitro screen to evaluate this effect. This unexpected detrimental effect of anti-cancer drugs should be considered with caution and emphasizes the need for personalized therapies.

Methods

Cell lines, shRNAs and pharmacological inhibitors

All cell lines used in this study were cultured in Dulbecco's Modified Eagle's Medium (DMEM, Invitrogen) supplemented with 7.5% heat-inactivated fetal calf serum (FCS) at 37 °C in an atmosphere of 5% CO_2. The three human head and neck cancer cell lines used in this study, CAL33, CAL27 and Detroit562 were provided through a Material Transfer Agreement with the Oncopharmacology Laboratory, Centre Antoine Lacassagne (Nice, France) where they had initially been isolated [31]. For knockdown experiments, the cells were infected using a lentiviral vector containing non-target control or two independent sequences of shRNA targeting the product of the AKT1 gene (shAKT1.1 5′- GGACAAGGACGGGCACAT TAA -3′ and shAKT1.2 5′- CTATGGCGCTGAGATTG TGTC -3′) cloned in pLKO.1 puro, (gift from Bob Weinberg, Addgene plasmid #8453) according to the protocol available at www.addgene.com. A total population of cells was generated by selection with 10 µg/mL puromycin for

10–15 days. MK-2206 (S1078, Selleck Chemicals) AKT inhibitor was used at a final concentration of 5 µM. Rapamycin (S1039, Sellek Chemicals) mTORC1 inhibitor was used at a final concentration of 5 µM. Erlotinib (S7786, Selleck Chemicals) EGFR inhibitor was used at a final concentration of 5 µM.

Phalloidin staining and e-cadherin immunostaining

Cells were grown at low density on glass coverslips or 24-well plates and fixed with PBS-4% paraformaldehyde (PFA) for 10 min followed by saturation for 30 min in PBS-3% skim milk-0.1% Triton X-100. Cells were then stained with phalloidin actin-stain 555 (Euromedex) according to the manufacturer's protocols. In certain preparations, immunostaining was then performed afterwards by incubating the cells overnight at 4 °C in the dark in a 1/100 dilution of an e-cadherin antibody (14,472, Cell Signaling Technology). Cells were then washed 3 times in PBS, incubated for 2 h at room temperature in the dark in a 1/500 dilution of an anti-mouse Alexa Fluor 488 conjugated antibody (4408, Cell Signaling Technology) and washed 3 times in PBS. The nuclear DNA was counterstained with Hoechst 33,342 (4082, Cell Signaling Technology) according to the manufacturer's protocols. Cells grown on coverslips were mounted onto slides with Prolong Gold Antifade moutant (Thermo Fischer Scientitifc) and images were captured using a Leica DMI-4000 microscope (Leica Microsystems) equipped with a Zyla 5.5 sCMOS camera (Andor). Measurement of the surface area of the cell colonies, the cell-cell contact e-cadherin staining and counting of the nuclei were performed with ImageJ 1.51j8 software (National Institute of Health). Graphic representations and statistical analyses were generated using Prism 5 (Graphpad Software).

Immunoblotting

The following antibodies were used for immunoblotting: anti-phospho AKT pS473 (Cell Signalling Technology, Cat. No. 4051S), anti-pan-AKT (Cell Signalling Technology, Cat. No. 9272S), anti-AKT1 and AKT2 (sc-5270 and sc-1618 respectively, Santa Cruz Biotechnology) and anti-GAPDH (Thermo Fischer Scientific, Cat. No. MA5–15738).

Cell migration and invasion

Four thousand cells were seeded in 20 µL hanging drops of DMEM supplemented with 7.5% FCS to obtain spheroids. After 7 days, they were transferred in DMEM-3% FCS supplemented with 1 µg/mL Matrigel (Corning Inc) and cultured for 8 days. Pictures were taken with an AMG Evos microscope 40× objective (Thermo Fisher Scientific Inc) and spheroid surface areas were measured using ImageJ 1.51j8 software (National Institute of Health).

Electrical cell impedance measurements

Electrode-containing arrays 8W10E+ (Ibidi, Cat. No.72040) were equilibrated with 400 μL of DMEM-7.5% FCS for 1 h on the ECIS Z Theta apparatus (Ibidi). 200 μL of medium was then removed and replaced by 200 μL of cell suspension containing 250.000 cells +/- 10 μM MK-2206 (Selleck Chemicals, Cat. No.S1078), 10 μM Rapamycin (Selleck Chemicals, Cat. No.S1039) or 10 μM Erlotinib (Selleck Chemicals, Cat. No.S7786). Electrical properties of the cells were then measured for 15 h. Raw data were exported from the ECIS software and used to generate graphical representations with the Prism software (Additional files 1, 2, 3, 4, 5, 6, 7, 8 and 9). Phenotypic differences were determined via analyses over a 4 h period of the most robust increase in electrode resistance (measured at 4000 Hz) during the cell attachment phase (Additional file 9).

Cell viability and proliferation assays

The viability of CAL33 cells was measured after 48 h of cell culture +/- 10 μM MK-2206 or 5 μM Rapamycin with an Adam apparatus (NanoEntek) according to the manufacturer's instructions. For proliferation assays, 25,000 cells were seeded in duplicate in 60 mm diameter dishes in DMEM-7.5% FCS. Twenty-four hours later, medium was replaced with DMEM-7.5% FCS in the presence or absence of MK-2206 (5 μM) or Rapamycin (5 μM). Cells were counted with a Z Series Coulter (Beckman Coulter Life Sciences) on day 3 and 4.

Statistical methods

Statistical analyses presented in the figures were performed on at least 3 independent replicates. One-way ANOVA with Bonferroni's post-test was performed using GraphPad Prism v5.03 (GraphPad Software) to determine significance of the observed effects.

Results

Inhibition of AKT1 induces morphological changes in CAL33 cells

Inhibition of AKT activity in the PI3K/AKT constitutively active CAL33 cell line was performed with either MK-2206, a pharmacological inhibitor that targets AKT isoforms 1–3 or with two independent AKT1-specific shRNA sequences. Both methods of AKT inhibition resulted in strong alterations of cellular morphology as revealed by staining of the actin cytoskeleton with Alexa555-coupled phalloidin (Fig. 1a). CAL33 cells increased spreading, formed looser cell-cell contacts and exhibited a significantly increased surface area when AKT was inhibited (Fig. 1b). Decreased gene expression levels of AKT1 by two independent shRNA sequences specific to AKT1 strongly reduced both total AKT protein expression and AKT activity as revealed by reduced phosphorylation at the S473 site (Fig. 1c). Similarly, cells treated with the

AKT inhibitor experienced an even stronger reduction of AKT phosphorylation (Fig. 1c). Moreover, western blots performed with antibodies specific to either AKT1 or AKT2 revealed that AKT1 is the major isoform expressed in the CAL33 cells (Additional file 10: Figure S1). The observed morphological changes induced by the inhibition of AKT in CAL33 cells are typical of a loss of epithelial phenotype. We observed disruption of the epithelial marker e-cadherin expression and membrane localization in these conditions, suggesting the occurrence of an EMT-like process (Fig. 1d and e and Additional file 11: Figure S2). Combined, these results indicate that AKT1 activity is necessary to maintain CAL33 cells epithelial morphology.

Inhibition of AKT1 increases invasion capacity of CAL33 cells

The increased spreading of the CAL33 cells induced by AKT1 inhibition suggested that their invasive capacities may be increased as well under these conditions. We tested this hypothesis in a 3D spheroid invasion assay in purified extracellular matrix (Matrigel, Corning). Inhibition of AKT1 via both shRNA and pharmacology strongly increased cell spreading from the spheroids into the extracellular matrix after eight days (Fig. 2a and b) thus suggesting an increased cellular ability to invade and migrate through a matrix.

Electrical property-based cell phenotype screening

To further characterize the phenotype induced by AKT1 inhibition, we measured the electrical properties of cells (impedance, resistance and capacitance) that were seeded at high density on an electrode [32]. Time-course experiments of CAL33 monolayers revealed that treatment with MK-2206 at the time of spreading or knockdown of AKT1 significantly decreased the rate of resistance increase during the cell-adhesion phase (~ 4-8 h following cell plating, Fig. 3a). These changes are not likely to be due to cell death or proliferative defects as MK-2206 only slightly reduced cell viability at 48 h and proliferation rates were not affected by any of the treatments at this time point (Additional file 12: Figure S3A and B). We then performed a phenotypic-based screening for compounds that may induce the same phenotype as the AKT inhibitor. mTOR is one of the downstream effectors of AKT [33] and the EGF receptor is an upstream activator of the PI3K/AKT pathway mutated in approximately 90% of HNSCC cases [34, 35]. We therefore used the classical mTOR targeting drug rapamycin and the EGFR inhibitor erlotinib in this screening. Rapamycin phenocopied the effect of AKT inhibition while erlotinib did not alter the electrical properties of the cells (Fig. 3b). Although erlotinib is a potent cytotoxic drug for HNSCC cell lines [35, 36], the absence of an

AKT1 restricts the invasive capacity of head and neck carcinoma cells harboring a constitutively active...

219

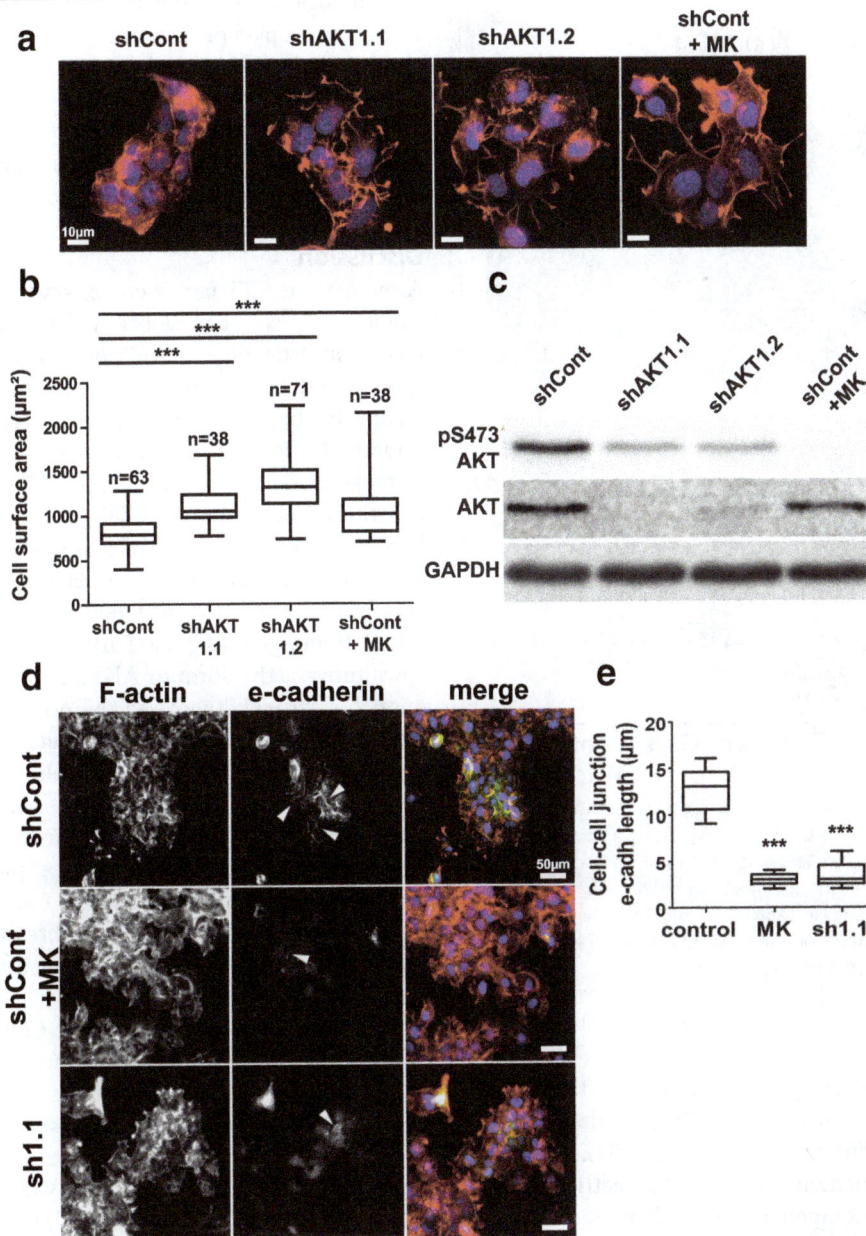

Fig. 1 AKT1 inhibition induces CAL33 cell spreading. **a** Alexa555-phalloidin (red) staining of the actin cytoskeleton in CAL33 cells expressing a control shRNA (shCont), two independent shRNA sequences targeting AKT1 (shAKT1.1 and shAKT1.2) or control cells treated with the pan-AKT inhibitor MK-2206 (shCont+MK). Nuclear DNA was counterstained with Hoechst 33,342 (blue). **b** Average cell surface areas were measured by dividing the surface of cell colonies by the number of nuclei in the colonies. **c** AKT activity and expression levels were evaluated by immunoblot with an anti-phospho-AKT antibody (pS473-AKT) and an anti-pan-AKT antibody. GAPDH was used as a loading control. **d** Immunostaining of e-cadherin (green) and Alexa555-phalloidin (red) staining of the actin cytoskeleton (F-actin) in CAL33 cells expressing a control shRNA (shCont), an shRNA sequences targeting AKT1 (sh1.1) or control cells treated with the pan-AKT inhibitor MK-2206 (shCont+MK). Nuclear DNA was counterstained with Hoechst 33,342 (blue). White arrows indicate examples of cell-cell junction e-cadherin staining. **e** Measurements of the mean length of cell-cell junctional e-cadherin per cell. Box-and-whisker plots presented in the figure extend from the 25th to 75th percentiles with whiskers displaying the whole range of the dataset and horizontal bars representing the median. The number of measurements from at least three independent experiments is displayed above each plot; one-way ANOVA with Bonferroni's post-test: *** $p < 0.001$ as compared to shCont

observed phenotype indicates that this electrical screening technique can delineate specific differences between compounds with respect to morphological or cytotoxic alterations. We next used the same assay to screen additional HNSCC cell lines based on their response to AKT inhibition (Fig. 3c). Treatment of CAL27 cells with MK-2206 did not induce significant changes in their electrical properties whereas Detroit562 cells displayed a

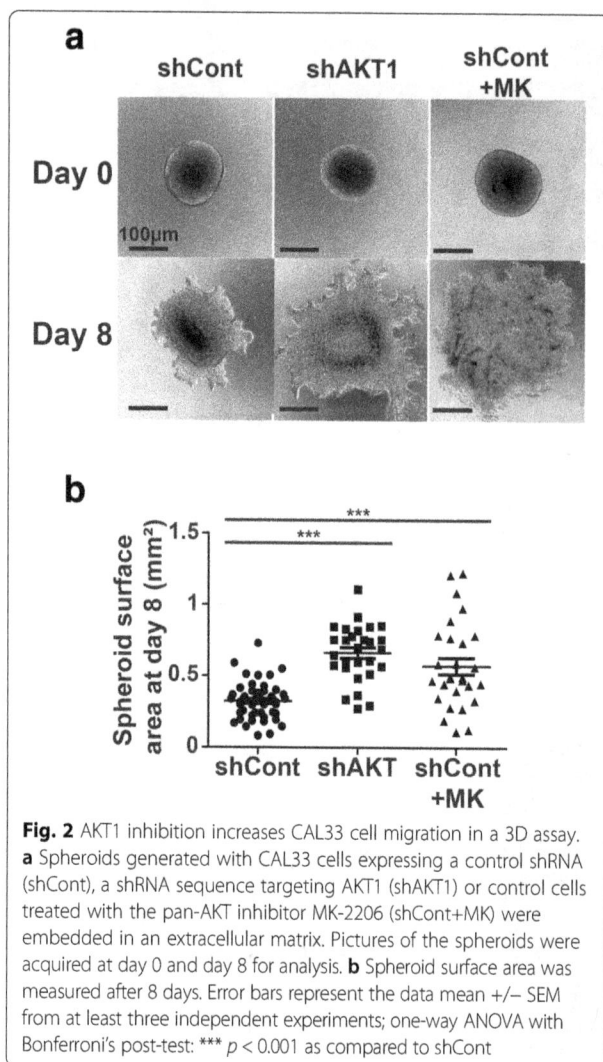

Fig. 2 AKT1 inhibition increases CAL33 cell migration in a 3D assay. **a** Spheroids generated with CAL33 cells expressing a control shRNA (shCont), a shRNA sequence targeting AKT1 (shAKT1) or control cells treated with the pan-AKT inhibitor MK-2206 (shCont+MK) were embedded in an extracellular matrix. Pictures of the spheroids were acquired at day 0 and day 8 for analysis. **b** Spheroid surface area was measured after 8 days. Error bars represent the data mean +/− SEM from at least three independent experiments; one-way ANOVA with Bonferroni's post-test: *** $p < 0.001$ as compared to shCont

phenotypic change comparable to that of the CAL33 cells upon inhibition of AKT (Fig. 3c, Additional file 11: Figure S2 and Additional file 13: Figure S4). Taken together, our results demonstrate that the electrical phenotype screening of compounds and cell lines allows the discovery of potential treatment-induced EMT-like processes in HNSCC cell lines.

Validation of results obtained via electrical phenotypic screening

In order to confirm the results described above, we assessed the ability of rapamycin to induce a phenotypic change in Detroit562 cells. Electrical resistance increase was strongly impaired with both the AKT inhibitor MK-2206 and the mTOR inhibitor rapamycin (Fig. 4a). This result is consistent both with the ability of MK-2206 to induce a phenotypic change in Detroit562 cells and the ability of rapamycin to induce comparable changes in CAL33 cells (Fig. 2b and c). Finally, in order to confirm the correlation between the electrical property modifications and the

morphological alterations, cells were stained with Alexa555-coupled phalloidin to observe the actin cytoskeleton of both CAL33 and Detroit562 cells treated with either MK-2206 or rapamycin (Fig. 4b). Quantitative validation of our phenotypic screening approach showed that cell spreading of both cell lines was significantly increased upon treatment with the two compounds (Fig. 4c).

Discussion

Although the AKT family comprises three isoforms, most studies only consider global AKT1–3 activity. However, recent investigations have now elegantly revealed the specific effects mediated by AKT1 and AKT2 isoforms in both the ErbB2-driven and the polyoma middle T (PyMT)-driven mammary adenocarcinoma transgenic mouse models [26, 27, 37]. In these models, constitutive activation of AKT1 in the mammary epithelium accelerated the onset of tumorigenesis but drastically decreased the number of metastatic lesions [27]. Conversely, removal of the *akt1* gene strongly delayed the onset of tumorigenesis [37]. Furthermore, expression of a constitutive active form of AKT2 had no effect on tumor onset but strongly increased the occurrence of lung metastases [26]. Combined, these results suggest that AKT1 and AKT2 may play opposite roles in the metastatic process and that differential AKT isoform activities require further consideration in cancer studies. The relevance of these findings in mouse models have been recently reported for human breast tumors [29, 30]. Gene expression datasets obtained from breast cancer cell lines and clinical samples revealed a strong association between high *akt1* expression, low expression of mesenchymal markers and better patient survival. Collectively, these results strongly suggest that AKT1 activity promotes early stages of tumorigenesis but restricts the tumor cell metastatic potential. However, these results have never been extended to non-breast cancer models. Our study suggests that AKT1 specific activity is also involved in the maintenance of the epithelial phenotype of HNSCC cells. An important implication is that AKT1 may also be predictive of the invasive capacities and aggressiveness of HNSCCs. Enhanced AKT/mTOR activity is common in oral carcinomas [38] and alterations of the PI3K/Akt/mTOR pathway are found in a large majority of HNSCCs [39]. As the consensus from the literature is that these pathways promote cell survival and metastasis, a great effort has been placed on pharmacological targeting of the PI3K pathway in HNSCC [34, 40]. The majority of previous in vitro studies on HNSCCs have focused on classical readouts such as association of AKT activity with cell survival and lower sensitivity to radiotherapy and chemotherapy [41–44]. Other research has indicated that increased AKT activity may promote a mesenchymal phenotype [45]. However, none of the previous in vitro (or in vivo) studies on

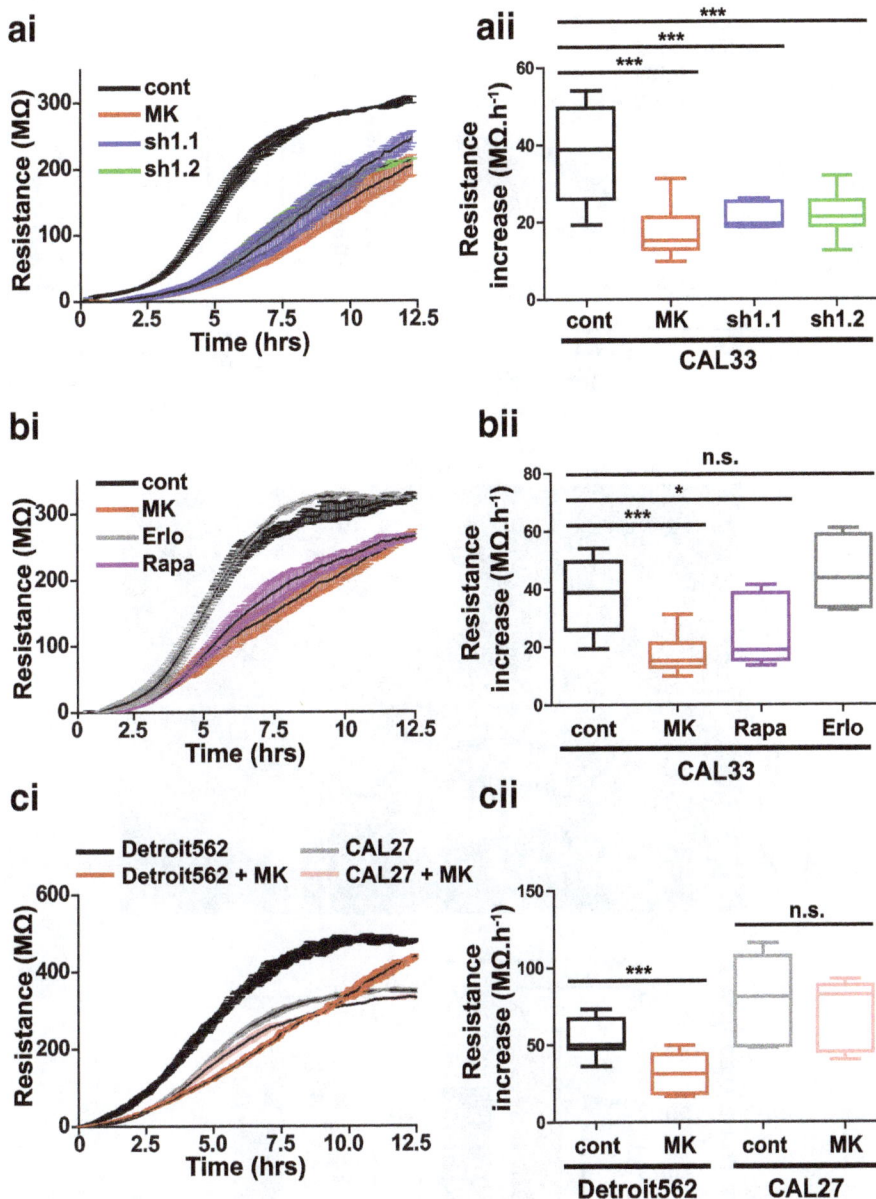

Fig. 3 AKT1 inhibition modifies cellular electrical properties. **ai, aii** Electrode resistance measured at 4000 Hz for CAL33 cells expressing a control shRNA (cont), two independent shRNA sequences targeting AKT1 (sh1.1 and sh1.2) or control cells treated with a pan-AKT inhibitor (MK) was observed for up to 12.5 h (ai). The cell spreading/attachment phase was determined via calculation of the increased electrical resistance during the period of 4-8 h following cell plating (aii). **bi, bii** Electrode resistance measured at 4000 Hz for CAL33 cells treated with the pan-AKT inhibitor MK-2206 (MK), the mTORC1 inhibitor Rapamycin (Rapa) or the EGF receptor inhibitor Erlotinib (Erlo) was observed for up to 12.5 h (bi). Changes in electrical resistance between 4 and 8 h after cell spreading were then quantified (bii). **ci, cii** Electrode resistance measured at 4000 Hz for Detroit562 or CAL27 cells +/− MK-2206 (MK) was observed for up to 12.5 h (ci). As above, changes in electrical resistance between 4 and 8 h after cell spreading were then quantified (cii). Each dataset was generated from at least three independent experiments. One-way ANOVA with Bonferroni's post-test: *** $p < 0.001$, *$p < 0.05$, n.s.: non-significant as compared to control

HNSCCs have considered the influence that specific AKT isoform expression could have on the outcome of AKT inhibition. Here we have observed that in certain subtypes of HNSCCs, which predominantly express AKT1 in comparison to AKT2, AKT1 inhibition leads to a more invasive phenotype. Therefore, it appears that, as has been recently revealed in an extensive body of work for breast cancer [26, 27, 29, 30], additional cancer types such as HNSCC may require AKT isoform analysis to predict the outcome of pan-AKT inhibitors. Despite encouraging results obtained with mTOR inhibitors [46–48], most of the clinical trials involving agents targeting the PI3K/Akt/mTOR pathway have failed to pass phase II. Consistently, a phase II clinical trial with the pan-AKT inhibitor

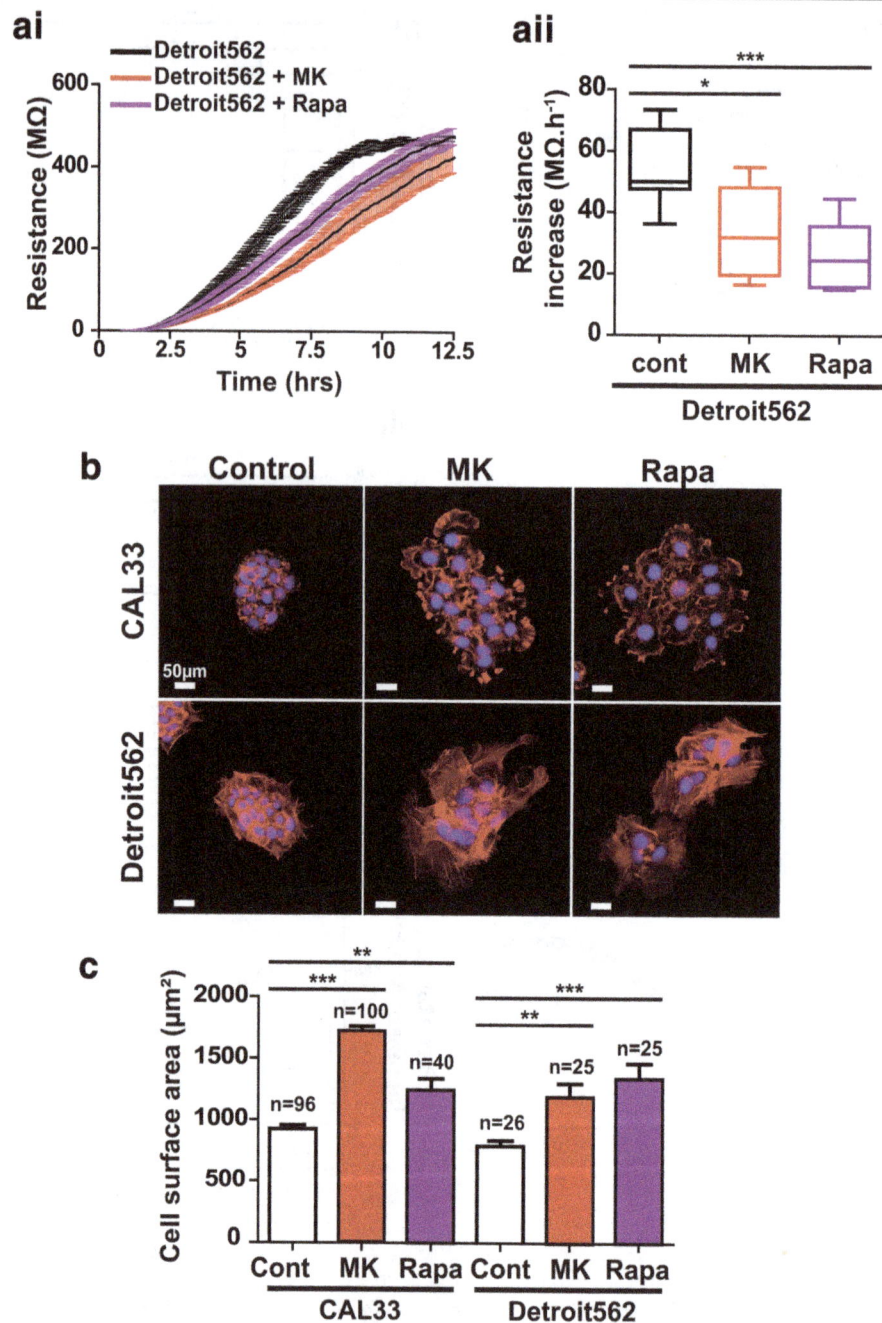

Fig. 4 Further experiments validating the use of electrical properties screening for uncovering of phenotypic differences. **ai**, **aii** Electrode resistance measured at 4000 Hz for Detroit562 cells treated with the pan-AKT inhibitor MK-2206 (MK) or the mTORC1 inhibitor Rapamycin (Rapa) was measured for up to 12.5 h (ai). Combined values for the resistance increase from 4 to 8 h after cell spreading (aii). **b** Staining of the actin cytoskeleton with Alexa555-phalloidin (red) for CAL33 and Detroit562 cells treated with either MK-2206 (MK) or Rapamycin (Rapa). Nuclear DNA was counterstained with Hoechst 33,342 (blue). **c** Average cell surface areas were measured by dividing the surface of cell colonies by the number of nuclei in the colonies. The number of measurements from at least three independent experiments is displayed above the histograms. Data represent mean +/− SEM, one-way ANOVA with Bonferroni's post-test: *** $p < 0.001$, ** $p < 0.01$, *$p < 0.05$ as compared to control

MK2206 on recurrent and metastatic HNSCC resulted in a partial response and was not moved to phase III so far (ClinicalTrials.gov identifier NCT01349933). A significant consideration is that treatments targeting the PI3K or all AKT isoforms may promote the invasive capacities of cancer cells in some cases. These counterintuitive results may explain why PI3K and AKT inhibitors are not included yet in clinical practices [49]. The possibility that some targeted therapies may increase the invasive and thus metastatic potential despite a reduction of the tumor burden should therefore be scrutinized.

We described a screening technique to determine potential pro-metastatic effects of a drug by electrical properties measurements. This method is mostly used for established models such as maintenance of endothelial cell-cell junctions or wound healing on confluent cell monolayers [50, 51]. Components of the electrical changes observed during the early phase of cell attachment can be more difficult to confidently interpret. Linking such electrical measurements to a given biological effect therefore requires complementary experiments. We observed that the increase of electrical resistance during the attachment phase is lower when AKT1 is inhibited in some but not all HNSCC cell lines. Conventional morphology and invasion assays indicated that these differences in electrical properties correlated with cell spreading, decreased cell-cell contact and acquisition of an invasive phenotype. We thus envision this technique becoming a valuable tool for high-throughput screening of drug-induced metastatic potential.

Alterations in the PI3K/AKT/mTOR pathway occur in 38% of all cancers as demonstrated on nearly 20,000 tumors of diverse origins [52]. More specifically in HNSCCs, pooled results from several databases showed that the PIK3CA gene, encoding the p110alpha catalytic subunit of the PI3K, is amplified in approximately 70% of HNSCC cell lines and 20% of HNSCCs clinical cases analyzed [53]. These results pinpoint the importance of the PI3K/AKT pathway dysregulation in cancers. The CAL33 and Detroit562 cell lines that adopted a mesenchymal phenotype upon AKT or mTORC1 inhibition bear a H1047R activating mutation in PIK3CA. Conversely, the CAL27 cell line does not bear this mutation and does not display comparable modifications in the same experimental conditions. Maintenance of the epithelial phenotype of CAL33 and Detroit562 cells could rely on the constitutive activity of the PI3K/AKT1 axis that is absent in CAL27 cells. In this case, the presence of both AKT1 amplification and constitutive PI3K activity would be a prognostic marker for pro-metastatic effects of pan-AKT inhibitors.

Conclusions

In summary, we extended the role of AKT1 specific activity in the maintenance of an epithelial phenotype to a new cancer type. This suggests that the differential role of AKT isoforms may be widespread in cancer. Furthermore, we have established an electrical screening protocol that correlates with metastatic cellular phenotypes. We believe that our method will be valuable for future efforts involving high-throughput screening of new pharmacological compounds and for the detection of potential

deleterious effects of drugs that are currently approved for clinical use. Finally, future efforts are required to delineate specific functions of AKT isoforms to avoid unwanted outcomes from the use of pan-AKT inhibitors or to develop specific AKT2/3 inhibitors.

Additional files

Additional file 1: CAL33-shControl cells treated with Erlotinib, Rapamycin and MK-2206 electrical resistance measurements. Raw output file of the ECIS measurement of resistance in MΩ at a frequency of 4000 Hz.

Additional file 2: CAL33-shControl cells untreated or treated with Rapamycin and MK-2206 electrical resistance measurements. Raw output file of the ECIS measurement of resistance in MΩ at a frequency of 4000 Hz.

Additional file 3: CAL33-shControl cells untreated or treated with MK-2206 and CAL33-shAKT1.1 and 1.2 cells electrical resistance measurements. Raw output file of the ECIS measurement of resistance in MΩ at a frequency of 4000 Hz.

Additional file 4: CAL33-shControl cells untreated or treated with MK-2206 and CAL33-shAKT1.1 and 1.2 cells electrical resistance measurements. Raw output file of the ECIS measurement of resistance in MΩ at a frequency of 4000 Hz.

Additional file 5: CAL33-shControl cells untreated or treated with MK-2206 and CAL33-shAKT1.1 and 1.2 cells electrical resistance measurements. Raw output file of the ECIS measurement of resistance in MΩ at a frequency of 4000 Hz.

Additional file 6: Detroit562 and CAL27 cells untreated or treated with MK-2206 electrical resistance measurements. Raw output file of the ECIS measurement of resistance in MΩ at a frequency of 4000 Hz.

Additional file 7: Detroit562 cells untreated or treated with MK-2206 or Rapamycin electrical resistance measurements. Raw output file of the ECIS measurement of resistance in MΩ at a frequency of 4000 Hz.

Additional file 8: Detroit562 cells untreated or treated with MK-2206 or Rapamycin electrical resistance measurements. Raw output file of the ECIS measurement of resistance in MΩ at a frequency of 4000 Hz.

Additional file 9: Electrical data used to generate the figures. The ECIS measurements of resistance in MΩ at a frequency of 4000 Hz were normalized to the first measurement and plotted in the Graphpad Prism software to generate the traces shown in Figs. 3a-c and 4a. The quantification data were obtained by measuring the mean resistance increase during the cell attachment phase (from 4 to 8 h after cell spreading).

Additional file 10: Figure S1. AKT1 and AKT2 isoform expression in CAL33, Detroit562 and CAL27 cells. AKT1 and AKT2 expression levels were evaluated by immunoblot with specific anti-AKT antibody in CAL33 cells expressing a control shRNA (shCont), two independent shRNA sequences targeting AKT1 (sh1.1 and sh1.2) and in Detroit562 and CAL27 cells. GAPDH was used as a loading control.

Additional file 11: Figure S2 Analysis of e-cadherin expression and localization by immunofluorescence in CAL33 cells. Immunostaining of e-cadherin (green) and Alexa555-phalloidin (red) staining of the actin cytoskeleton (F-actin) in CAL33 cells expressing a control shRNA (shCont), an shRNA sequences targeting AKT1 (sh1.2) or control cells treated with the pan-AKT inhibitor MK-2206 (MK), Rapamycin (Rapa) or Erlotinib (Erlo). Nuclear DNA was counterstained with Hoechst 33,342 (blue).

Additional file 12: Figure S3 Cell viability and proliferation assays. (A) The viability of CAL33 cells expressing a control shRNA (CAL33), two independent shRNA sequences targeting AKT1 (shAKT1.1 and shAKT1.2) or treated with the pan-AKT inhibitor MK-2206 (MK) or the mTORC1 inhibitor Rapamycin (Rapa) was measured after 48 h. Statistical analysis was performed using one-way ANOVA with Bonferroni's post-test: *** $p < 0.001$, n.s.: non-significant. (B) CAL33 cell proliferation assays of the same experimental manipulations as described in part (A). Cell proliferation is represented as a fold-increase over the starting number of cells and was measured after 3 and 4 days of treatment.

Additional file 13: Figure S4 Analysis of e-cadherin expression and localization by immunofluorescence in CAL27 and Detroit562 cells. Immunostaining of e-cadherin (green) and Alexa555-phalloidin (red) staining of the actin cytoskeleton (F-actin) in CAL27 and Detroit562 cells treated with the pan-AKT inhibitor MK-2206 (MK), Rapamycin (Rapa) or Erlotinib (Erlo). Nuclear DNA was counterstained with Hoechst 33,342 (blue).

Abbreviations

DMEM: Dulbecco's modified Eagle's medium; ECIS: Electrical impedance cell sensing; EGFR: Epithelial growth factor receptor; EMT: Epithelium-to-mesenchyme transition; FCS: Fetal calf serum; GAPDH: Glyceraldehyde 3-phosphate dehydrogenase; HNSCC: Head and neck squamous cell carcinoma; mTOR: mammalian target of rapamycin; PFA: paraformaldehyde; PI3K: Phosphoinositide 3-kinase; PyMT: Polyoma middle T; shRNA: short hairpin ribonucleic acid

Acknowledgements

The authors are grateful to the Oncopharmacology Lab, Antoine Lacassagne Anticancer Center, Nice, France who isolated and kindly provided the cell lines used in this study. The authors are grateful to the middle school trainees who helped to analyze some of the imaging data.

Funding

This work was funded by the Centre Scientifique de Monaco and the Government of the Principality of Monaco. The funding bodies did not participate in any aspect of the design of the study and collection, analysis, and interpretation of data and in writing the manuscript.

Authors' contributions

SB, SKP, LM and VP performed and analyzed the cell staining and cellular electrical properties experiments; VV performed the immunoblot experiments; JD generated the shRNA cell lines; VP and SKP made the figures and wrote the manuscript; JP and GP edited the manuscript and were the recipients of the funding. All authors read and approved the final manuscript.

Competing interests

The authors declare that they have no competing interests.

Author details

¹Centre Scientifique de Monaco, Department of Medical Biology, 8 Quai Antoine Ier, Monaco, Principality of Monaco. ²UCA, Université Côte d'Azur, Nice-Sophia-Antipolis, Institute for Research on Cancer and Aging of Nice, CNRS-UMR 7284-Inserm U1081, Nice, France.

References

1. Montero JA, Kilian B, Chan J, Bayliss PE, Heisenberg CP. Phosphoinositide 3-kinase is required for process outgrowth and cell polarization of gastrulating mesendodermal cells. Current biology : CB. 2003;13(15):1279–89.

2. Yang X, Chrisman H, Weijer CJ. PDGF signalling controls the migration of mesoderm cells during chick gastrulation by regulating N-cadherin expression. Development. 2008;135(21):3521–30.

3. Yeh CM, Liu YC, Chang CJ, Lai SL, Hsiao CD, Lee SJ. Ptenb mediates gastrulation cell movements via Cdc42/AKT1 in zebrafish. PLoS One. 2011;6(4):e18702.

4. Grille SJ, Bellacosa A, Upson J, Klein-Szanto AJ, van Roy F, Lee-Kwon W, Donowitz M, Tsichlis PN, Larue L. The protein kinase Akt induces epithelial mesenchymal transition and promotes enhanced motility and invasiveness of squamous cell carcinoma lines. Cancer Res. 2003;63(9):2172–8.

5. Govindarajan B, Sligh JE, Vincent BJ, Li M, Canter JA, Nickoloff BJ, Rodenburg RJ, Smeitink JA, Oberley L, Zhang Y, et al. Overexpression of Akt converts radial growth melanoma to vertical growth melanoma. J Clin Invest. 2007; 117(3):719–29.

6. Tang H, Massi D, Hemmings BA, Mandala M, Hu Z, Wicki A, Xue G. AKT-ions with a TWIST between EMT and MET. Oncotarget. 2016;7(38):62767–77.

7. Liu P, Cheng H, Roberts TM, Zhao JJ. Targeting the phosphoinositide 3-kinase pathway in cancer. Nat Rev Drug Discov. 2009;8(8):627–44.

8. Ramanathan RK, McDonough SL, Kennecke HF, Iqbal S, Baranda JC, Seery TE, Lim HJ, Hezel AF, Vaccaro GM, Blanke CD. Phase 2 study of MK-2206, an allosteric inhibitor of AKT, as second-line therapy for advanced gastric and gastroesophageal junction cancer: a SWOG cooperative group trial (S1005). Cancer. 2015;121(13):2193–7.

9. Ma BB, Goh BC, Lim WT, Hui EP, Tan EH, Lopes Gde L, Lo KW, Li L, Loong H, Foster NR, et al. Multicenter phase II study of the AKT inhibitor MK-2206 in recurrent or metastatic nasopharyngeal carcinoma from patients in the mayo phase II consortium and the cancer therapeutics research group (MC1079). Investig New Drugs. 2015;33(4):985–91.

10. Ahn DH, Li J, Wei L, Doyle A, Marshall JL, Schaaf LJ, Phelps MA, Villalona-Calero MA, Bekaii-Saab T. Results of an abbreviated phase-II study with the Akt inhibitor MK-2206 in patients with advanced biliary cancer. Sci Rep. 2015;5:12122.

11. Oki Y, Fanale M, Romaguera J, Fayad L, Fowler N, Copeland A, Samaniego F, Kwak LW, Neelapu S, Wang M, et al. Phase II study of an AKT inhibitor MK2206 in patients with relapsed or refractory lymphoma. Br J Haematol. 2015;171(4):463–70.

12. Yap TA, Yan L, Patnaik A, Fearen I, Olmos D, Papadopoulos K, Baird RD, Delgado L, Taylor A, Lupinacci L, et al. First-in-man clinical trial of the oral pan-AKT inhibitor MK-2206 in patients with advanced solid tumors. J Clin Oncol. 2011;29(35):4688–95.

13. Hudis C, Swanton C, Janjigian YY, Lee R, Sutherland S, Lehman R, Chandarlapaty S, Hamilton N, Gajria D, Knowles J, et al. A phase 1 study evaluating the combination of an allosteric AKT inhibitor (MK-2206) and trastuzumab in patients with HER2-positive solid tumors. Breast cancer research : BCR. 2013;15(6):R110.

14. Brana I, Berger R, Golan T, Haluska P, Edenfield J, Fiorica J, Stephenson J, Martin LP, Westin S, Hanjani P, et al. A parallel-arm phase I trial of the humanised anti-IGF-1R antibody dalotuzumab in combination with the AKT inhibitor MK-2206, the mTOR inhibitor ridaforolimus, or the NOTCH inhibitor MK-0752, in patients with advanced solid tumours. Br J Cancer. 2014; 111(10):1932–44.

15. Fouladi M, Perentesis JP, Phillips CL, Leary S, Reid JM, McGovern RM, Ingle AM, Ahern CH, Ames MM, Houghton P, et al. A phase I trial of MK-2206 in children with refractory malignancies: a Children's oncology group study. Pediatr Blood Cancer. 2014;61(7):1246–51.

16. Janku F, Hong DS, Fu S, Piha-Paul SA, Naing A, Falchook GS, Tsimberidou AM, Stepanek VM, Moulder SL, Lee JJ, et al. Assessing PIK3CA and PTEN in early-phase trials with PI3K/AKT/mTOR inhibitors. Cell Rep. 2014;6(2):377–87.

17. Konopleva MY, Walter RB, Faderl SH, Jabbour EJ, Zeng Z, Borthakur G, Huang X, Kadia TM, Ruvolo PP, Feliu JB, et al. Preclinical and early clinical evaluation of the oral AKT inhibitor, MK-2206, for the treatment of acute myelogenous leukemia. Clin Cancer Res. 2014;20(8):2226–35.

18. Molife LR, Yan L, Vitfell-Rasmussen J, Zernhelt AM, Sullivan DM, Cassier PA, Chen E, Biondo A, Tetteh E, Siu LL, et al. Phase 1 trial of the oral AKT inhibitor MK-2206 plus carboplatin/paclitaxel, docetaxel, or erlotinib in patients with advanced solid tumors. J Hematol Oncol. 2014;7:1.

19. Davies BR, Guan N, Logie A, Crafter C, Hanson L, James V, Dudley P, Jacques K, Ladd B, et al. Tumors with AKT1E17K mutations are rational targets for single agent or combination therapy with AKT inhibitors. Mol Cancer Ther. 2015;14(11):2441–51.

20. Do K, Speranza G, Bishop R, Khin S, Rubinstein L, Kinders RJ, Datiles M, Eugeni M, Lam MH, Doyle LA, et al. Biomarker-driven phase 2 study of MK-

AKT1 restricts the invasive capacity of head and neck carcinoma cells harboring a constitutively active...

225

2206 and selumetinib (AZD6244, ARRY-142886) in patients with colorectal cancer. Investig New Drugs. 2015;33(3):720–8.

21. Doi T, Tamura K, Tanabe Y, Yonemori K, Yoshino T, Fuse N, Kodaira M, Bando H, Noguchi K, Shimamoto T, et al. Phase 1 pharmacokinetic study of the oral pan-AKT inhibitor MK-2206 in Japanese patients with advanced solid tumors. Cancer Chemother Pharmacol. 2015;76(2):409–16.

22. Gonzalez-Angulo AM, Krop I, Akcakanat A, Chen H, Liu S, Li Y, Culotta KS, Tarco E, Piha-Paul S, Moulder-Thompson S, et al. SU2C phase Ib study of paclitaxel and MK-2206 in advanced solid tumors and metastatic breast cancer. J Natl Cancer Inst. 2015;107(3)

23. Gupta S, Argiles G, Munster PN, Hollebecque A, Dajani O, Cheng JD, Wang R, Swift A, Tosolini A, Piha-Paul SA. A phase i trial of combined ridaforolimus and mk-2206 in patients with advanced malignancies. Clin Cancer Res. 2015;21(23):5235–44.

24. Chung V, McDonough S, Philip PA, Cardin D, Wang-Gillam A, Hui L, Tejani MA, Seery TE, Dy IA, Al Baghdadi T, et al. Effect of Selumetinib and MK-2206 vs Oxaliplatin and fluorouracil in patients with metastatic pancreatic cancer after prior therapy: SWOG S1115 study randomized clinical trial. JAMA oncology. 2017;3(4):516–22.

25. Arboleda MJ, Lyons JF, Kabbinavar FF, Bray MR, Snow BE, Ayala R, Danino M, Karlan BY, Slamon DJ. Overexpression of AKT2/protein kinase Bbeta leads to up-regulation of beta1 integrins, increased invasion, and metastasis of human breast and ovarian cancer cells. Cancer Res. 2003;63(1):196–206.

26. Dillon RL, Marcotte R, Hennessy BT, Woodgett JR, Mills GB, Muller WJ. Akt1 and akt2 play distinct roles in the initiation and metastatic phases of mammary tumor progression. Cancer Res. 2009;69(12):5057–64.

27. Hutchinson JN, Jin J, Cardiff RD, Woodgett JR, Muller WJ. Activation of Akt-1 (PKB-alpha) can accelerate ErbB-2-mediated mammary tumorigenesis but suppresses tumor invasion. Cancer Res. 2004;64(9):3171–8.

28. Irie HY, Pearline RV, Grueneberg D, Hsia M, Ravichandran P, Kothari N, Natesan S, Brugge JS. Distinct roles of Akt1 and Akt2 in regulating cell migration and epithelial-mesenchymal transition. J Cell Biol. 2005;171(6):1023–34.

29. Li CW, Xia W, Lim SO, Hsu JL, Huo L, Wu Y, Li LY, Lai CC, Chang SS, Hsu YH, et al. AKT1 inhibits epithelial-to-mesenchymal transition in breast cancer through phosphorylation-dependent Twist1 degradation. Cancer Res. 2016; 76(6):1451–62.

30. Riggio M, Perrone MC, Polo ML, Rodriguez MJ, May M, Abba M, Lanari C, Novaro V. AKT1 and AKT2 isoforms play distinct roles during breast cancer progression through the regulation of specific downstream proteins. Sci Rep. 2017;7:44244.

31. Gioanni J, Fischel JL, Lambert JC, Demard F, Mazeau C, Zanghellini E, Ettore F, Formento P, Chauvel P, Lalanne CM, et al. Two new human tumor cell lines derived from squamous cell carcinomas of the tongue: establishment, characterization and response to cytotoxic treatment. Eur J Cancer Clin Oncol. 1988;24(9):1445–55.

32. Giaever I, Keese CR. A morphological biosensor for mammalian cells. Nature. 1993;366(6455):591–2.

33. Porta C, Paglino C, Mosca A. Targeting PI3K/Akt/mTOR signaling in cancer. Front Oncol. 2014;4:64.

34. Wong KK, Engelman JA, Cantley LC. Targeting the PI3K signaling pathway in cancer. Curr Opin Genet Dev. 2010;20(1):87–90.

35. Barzegar M, Ma S, Zhang C, Chen X, Gu Y, Shang C, Jiang X, Yang J, Nathan CA, Yang S, et al. SKLB188 inhibits the growth of head and neck squamous cell carcinoma by suppressing EGFR signalling. Br J Cancer. 2017;117(8):1154–63.

36. Benhamou Y, Picco V, Raybaud H, Sudaka A, Chamorey E, Brolih S, Monteverde M, Merlano M, Lo Nigro C, Ambrosetti D, et al. Telomeric repeat-binding factor 2: a marker for survival and anti-EGFR efficacy in oral carcinoma. Oncotarget. 2016;7(28):44236–51.

37. Maroulakou IG, Oemler W, Naber SP, Tsichlis PN. Akt1 ablation inhibits, whereas Akt2 ablation accelerates, the development of mammary adenocarcinomas in mouse mammary tumor virus (MMTV)-ErbB2/neu and MMTV-polyoma middle T transgenic mice. Cancer Res. 2007;67(1):167–77.

38. Martins F, de Sousa SC, Dos Santos E, Woo SB, Gallottini M. PI3K-AKT-mTOR pathway proteins are differently expressed in oral carcinogenesis. J Oral Pathol Med. 2016;45(10):746–52.

39. Grandis JR HD, El-Naggar AK, and The Cancer Genome Atlas Group Comprehensive genomic characterization of squamous cell carcinoma of the head and neck. TCGA 2nd annual scientific symposium 2012.

40. Simpson DR, Mell LK, Cohen EE. Targeting the PI3K/AKT/mTOR pathway in squamous cell carcinoma of the head and neck. Oral Oncol. 2015;51(4):291–8.

41. Hehlgans S, Eke I, Cordes N. Targeting FAK radiosensitizes 3-dimensional grown human HNSCC cells through reduced Akt1 and MEK1/2 signaling. Int J Radiat Oncol Biol Phys. 2012;83(5):e669–76.

42. Stegeman H, Span PN, Peeters WJ, Verheijen MM, Grenman R, Meijer TW, Kaanders JH, Bussink J. Interaction between hypoxia, AKT and HIF-1 signaling in HNSCC and NSCLC: implications for future treatment strategies. Future science OA. 2016;2(1):FSO84.

43. Silva-Oliveira RJ, Melendez M, Martinho O, Zanon MF, de Souza Viana L, Carvalho AL, Reis RM. AKT can modulate the in vitro response of HNSCC cells to irreversible EGFR inhibitors. Oncotarget. 2017;8(32):53288–301.

44. Cheng Y, Wang Y, Li J, Chang I, Wang CY. A novel read-through transcript JMJD7-PLA2G4B regulates head and neck squamous cell carcinoma cell proliferation and survival. Oncotarget. 2017;8(2):1972–82.

45. Chang JW, Jung SN, Kim JH, Shim GA, Park HS, Liu L, Kim JM, Park J, Koo BS. Carboxyl-terminal modulator protein positively acts as an oncogenic driver in head and neck squamous cell carcinoma via regulating Akt phosphorylation. Sci Rep. 2016;6:28503.

46. Fury MG, Sherman E, Haque S, Korte S, Lisa D, Shen R, Wu N, Pfister D. A phase I study of daily everolimus plus low-dose weekly cisplatin for patients with advanced solid tumors. Cancer Chemother Pharmacol. 2012;69(3):591–8.

47. Fury MG, Lee NY, Sherman E, Ho AL, Rao S, Heguy A, Shen R, Korte S, Lisa D, Ganly I, et al. A phase 1 study of everolimus + weekly cisplatin + intensity modulated radiation therapy in head-and-neck cancer. Int J Radiat Oncol Biol Phys. 2013;87(3):479–86.

48. Fury MG, Sherman E, Ho AL, Xiao H, Tsai F, Nwankwo O, Sima C, Heguy A, Katabi N, Haque S, et al. A phase 1 study of everolimus plus docetaxel plus cisplatin as induction chemotherapy for patients with locally and/or regionally advanced head and neck cancer. Cancer. 2013;119(10):1823–31.

49. Nitulescu GM, Margina D, Juzenas P, Peng Q, Olaru OT, Saloustros E, Fenga C, Spandidos D, Libra M, Tsatsakis AM. Akt inhibitors in cancer treatment: the long journey from drug discovery to clinical use (review). Int J Oncol. 2016;48(3):869–85.

50. Gong H, Liu M, Klomp J, Merrill BJ, Rehman J, Malik AB. Method for dual viral vector mediated CRISPR-Cas9 gene disruption in primary human endothelial cells. Sci Rep. 2017;7:42127.

51. Ochoa-Callejero L, Pozo-Rodrigalvarez A, Martinez-Murillo R, Martinez A. Lack of adrenomedullin in mouse endothelial cells results in defective angiogenesis, enhanced vascular permeability, less metastasis, and more brain damage. Sci Rep. 2016;6:33495.

52. Millis SZ, Ikeda S, Reddy S, Gatalica Z, Kurzrock R. Landscape of Phosphatidylinositol-3-kinase pathway alterations across 19784 diverse solid tumors. JAMA oncology. 2016;2(12):1565–73.

53. Li H, Wawrose JS, Gooding WE, Garraway LA, Lui VW, Peyser ND, Grandis JR. Genomic analysis of head and neck squamous cell carcinoma cell lines and human tumors: a rational approach to preclinical model selection. Molecular cancer research : MCR. 2014;12(4):571–82.

27

In vitro and in silico validation of *CA3* and *FHL1* downregulation in oral cancer

Cláudia Maria Pereira[1,2], Ana Carolina de Carvalho[3,6], Felipe Rodrigues da Silva[4], Matias Eliseo Melendez[3], Roberta Cardim Lessa[1,2], Valéria Cristina C. Andrade[5], Luiz Paulo Kowalski[1], André L. Vettore[2,6] and André Lopes Carvalho[1,3,7*]

Abstract

Background: Aberrant methylation is a frequent event in oral cancer.

Methods: In order to better characterize these alterations, a search for genes downregulated by aberrant methylation in oral squamous cell carcinoma (OSCC) was conducted through the mining of ORESTES dataset. Findings were further validated in OSCC cell lines and patients' samples and confirmed using TCGA data. Differentially expressed genes were identified in ORESTES libraries and validated in vitro using RT-PCR in HNSCC cell-lines and OSCC tumor samples. Further confirmation of these results was performed using mRNA expression and methylation data from The Cancer Genome Atlas (TCGA) data.

Results: From the set of genes selected for validation, *CA3* and *FHL1* were downregulated in 60% (12/20) and 75% (15/20) of OSCC samples, respectively, and in HNSCC cell lines. The treatment of cell lines JHU-13 and FaDu with the demethylating agent 5'-aza-dC was efficient in restoring *CA3* and *FHL1* expression. TCGA expression and methylation data on OSCC confirms the downregulation of these genes in OSCC samples and also suggests that expression of *CA3* and *FHL1* is probably regulated by methylation. The downregulation of *CA3* and *FHL1* observed in silico was validated in HNSCC cell lines and OSCC samples, showing the feasibility of integrating different datasets to select differentially expressed genes in silico.

Conclusions: These results showed that the downregulation of *CA3* and *FHL1* data observed in the ORESTES libraries was validated in HNSCC cell lines and OSCC samples and in a large cohort of samples from the TCGA database. Moreover, it suggests that expression of *CA3* and *FHL1* could probably be regulated by methylation having an important role the oral carcinogenesis.

Keywords: OSCC, Gene expression, Methylation, *CA3*, *FHL1*

Background

Squamous cell carcinoma (SCC) is the most frequent histological subtype of oral cavity cancers. This disease originates from the epithelial tissue that covers the entire aero digestive tract and accounts for more than 90% of all malignancies in that anatomical region [1]. This cancer site is among the most common worldwide and a major cause of morbidity and mortality [2]. Despite extensive research and improvements in diagnostic methods and treatment approaches, the five-year overall survival rate for oral squamous cell carcinoma (OSCC) patients have only improved marginally. Investigation of molecular targets and signaling pathways to design appropriate therapeutic, follow-up and monitoring strategies may have the potential to improve survival [3].

Several studies in oral carcinogenesis point to an important relationship between aberrant DNA methylation at the promoter of tumor suppressor genes and their inactivation [4–9]. DNA methylation is a frequent epigenetic event that occurs by the addition of a methyl group (-CH$_3$) to a cytosine (C) situated at a 5′ position of a guanine (G) in CpG dinucleotides of superior eukaryotic cells [10, 11]. Genetic and epigenetic events

* Correspondence: carvalhoal@gmail.com
[1]Department of Head and Neck Surgery, A. C. Camargo Cancer Hospital, São Paulo, Brazil
[3]Molecular Oncology Research Center, Barretos Cancer Hospital, Barretos, Brazil
Full list of author information is available at the end of the article

can confer competitive advantages to a cell leading to a cancer phenotype [12, 13], therefore a wide transcriptome analysis revealing the molecular mechanisms underlying cancer environment is important [14, 15].

The integration of different data sets such as serial analysis of gene expression (SAGE), expressed sequence tags (ESTs) and open reading expressed sequence tags (ORESTES), provide powerful platforms to evaluate gene expression data in cancer tissues [16]. The ORESTES data set was developed by a Brazilian research group during the Human Cancer Genome Project, yielding more than 1 million sequences representing parts of mRNAs expressed in different tumors [17]. This technology allowed the acquisition of sequences from the central codifying region of transcripts by using random primers [18] and was used to identify differentially expressed genes and several transcriptomes [15, 17, 19–21]. All sequences produced in these projects are available in public databases.

The Cancer Genome Atlas (TCGA) Research Network is a multi-institutional consortium focused on the comprehensive clinical and molecular profiling of 32 different tumor types [22]. Head and neck squamous cell carcinoma (HNSCC) sample collection from TCGA data portal contains 528 cases, including samples from oral cavity, larynx, tonsils, base of tongue, pharynx and lips [22].

The use of gene expression based molecular markers as tools to improve the understanding of the biological mechanisms involved in oral cancer carcinogenesis opens the potential for the discovery of new therapy targets, better prediction of patient outcome, therapy choice and surveillance strategies, improving patient quality of life and survival rates. Thus, in this study, we used bioinformatics analysis from head and neck ORESTES libraries to identify differentially expressed genes in oral cancer and to investigate whether gene downregulation was a consequence of aberrant methylation. To validate the findings, we performed the pharmacological unmasking of OSCC cell lines through their treatment with a demethylating agent, and analyzed the gene-expression level of selected genes in patients' samples. We further confirmed the results by analyzing methylation and RNA expression data from the TCGA database.

Methods

In silico analysis of ORESTES data
Downregulated transcripts were selected from ORESTES data available at the National Center for Biotechnology Information (NCBI) database. A bioinformatic analysis generated a list of differentially expressed genes in different head and neck squamous cell carcinoma subsites in comparison to their correspondent normal tissue. The program BlastN was used to compare the 946,260 ORESTES sequences deposited at NCBI with the 29,529

reference sequences of human genes presented at the RefSeq database [23]. The best hit of an ORESTES sequence with a human gene was selected to define from which gene this sequence was generated, with no visual inspection. Only hits with e-values better than 1×10^{-10} were considered, thus, 570,214 ORESTES were included in this analysis. Results were then loaded into a relational database.

Only normal and tumor head and neck ORESTES libraries were analyzed (see Additional file 1: Table S1) which were compared by three ways: (1) normal larynx libraries plus normal hypopharynx libraries were compared with oral cavity tumor library; (2) normal larynx libraries were compared with larynx tumor libraries; and (3) normal hypopharynx libraries were compared with hypopharynx tumor libraries. The Fisher Exact Test was applied to identify genes differentially expressed and a p-value < 0.05 was used to consider statistical significance.

Downregulated candidate genes selection
By using available web tools (see Additional file 2: Table S2), several criteria were applied to define the best downregulated candidate genes such as: (1) the presence of CpG island in the promoter region; (2) ESTs expression evaluation in head and neck tissue; and (3) data from a literature review. In this last criterion, genes with biologic functions related to carcinogenesis and those described as downregulated in other tumors were included, while genes previously described as oncogenes or overexpressed were excluded.

OSCC specimen and control samples
Twenty primary OSCC specimens from patients surgically treated at the Department of Head and Neck Surgery, A. C. Camargo Hospital and available at the Tumor Bank of this institution were included. All tissues were subjected to intraoperative frozen section evaluation to select necrosis and calcification-free areas and immediately stored at − 80°C until nucleic acid extraction. Ten histologically normal oral mucosa samples were collected from healthy donors undergoing dental and pre-prosthetic surgeries and were used as control tissue. Written informed consent was obtained from all OSCC patients and healthy donors at the time of enrollment and all aspects of this investigation were approved by the Ethics Committees of A. C. Camargo Hospital (process number 737/05).

Tumor cell lines
HNSCC cell lines JHU-12, JHU-13, JHU-19, JHU-28 were kindly provided by Dr. Joseph Califano (Department of Otolaryngology and Head and Neck Surgery - Jonhs Hopkins University). FaDu cell line was acquired from ATCC (American Type Cell Collection – Rockville, MD).

JHU-12, JHU-13, JHU-19, JHU-28 cell lines were maintained in RPMI medium and FaDu in MEM medium, supplemented with 10% fetal bovine serum in the presence of antibiotics at 37 °C with 5% CO_2.

5′-aza-2′-deoxycytidine treatment

To investigate a possible role of epigenetic in the downregulation of selected genes, 10^5 JHU-13 and FaDu cells were seeded on day 0 and treated with 1 μM of the demethylating agent 5-aza-dC (Sigma-Aldrich, St. Louis, MO) for 3, 5 and 7 days. DNA and RNA were extracted at days 0, 3, 5 and 7 and stored at – 80°C. The level of gene expression of the genes selected was tested before and after treatment with the demethylating agent, following the procedures described next.

RNA extraction and cDNA synthesis

Total RNA from normal and tumor samples was extracted using the TRIzol Reagent (Invitrogen, Carlsbad, CA, USA) according to the manufacturer's protocol. Total RNA from HNSCC cell lines was extracted by cesium chloride gradient ultracentrifugation method. Briefly, cells were homogenized in 9 mL of lyses solution (4 M guanidinium isothiocyanate, 2 mM sodium citrate pH 7.0; 0.1 M β-mercaptoethanol). The cell lysate was then transferred to an ultracentrifuge tube with 4 mL of cesium chloride solution (5.7 M CsCl; 1 M sodium acetate) and submitted to 29,000 rpm for 20 h at 20°C. Following centrifugation, the RNA pellet was dissolved in 100 μL of RNAse-free water. All extracted RNA samples were quantified in the spectrophotometer

NanoDrop-ND 1000 (Thermo Scientific, Wilmington, DE) and analyzed by electrophoresis in 1% agarose gel stained by 0.5 μg/mL ethidium bromide.

Two micrograms of template RNA were used for first-strand cDNA synthesis using oligo (dT) primers and the reverse transcriptase Superscript III (Invitrogen, Carlsbad, CA) following manufacturer's instructions. The cDNA product was diluted 10 times prior to use. Quality cDNA control was performed by the amplification of an *ACTB* (NM 001101) fragment using forward (5′-CACTGTGTT G GCGTACAGGT-3′ and reverse primers (5′-TCATC ACCATTGGCAATGAG-3′). Reactions were carried out under the following conditions: 94 °C for 2 min, followed by 35 cycles at 94 °C for 30 s, 58 °C for 45 s, 72 °C for 45 s and 72 °C for 7 min. PCR products were evaluated by electrophoresis in 1% agarose gel stained with 0.5 μg/mL ethidium bromide.

Validation of mRNA expression changes in HNSCC cell lines by RT-PCR

The expression level of ten genes (*CA3, FHL1, HMGN4, FSTL1, NFE2L1, SAR1B, C9orf64, ANXA6, WDR26, CC N1*) was evaluated by Reverse Transcription PCR (RT-PCR) in five HNSCC cell lines. Primer sequences, amplicon sizes, $MgCl_2$ concentration and annealing temperatures are available in Table 1.

Real-time quantitative RT-PCR (qRT-PCR) analysis

To validate the expression profile data from HNSCC cell lines in clinical samples, mRNA levels of the selected candidate genes *CA3 and FHL1* were tested by qRT-

Table 1 Primer sequences, product size, $MgCl_2$ concentration and annealing temperatures used in RT-PCR analyses

Gene	Primer sequence (5′-3′)	Product size (bp)	$MgCl_2$ (mM)	Annealing temperature (°C)
CA3	F: TGAAGCAGCGCGATGGGAT R: GTCAGAGCTCACGGTCATGGGC	260	2	66
FHL1	F: CCGCTTCTGGCATGACACCT R: ACGGTCCCCTTGTACTCCACG	189	2	66
ANXA6	F: -CCGGCACAGATGAAAAGGCTC R: TTCTCCTCCCTCCTCACGATGC	191	2	66
WDR26	F: TGCCAATTGCGGAGCTGACA R: CGTCTGCTCCAAATTCACCATCAA	196	2	66
HMGN4	F: CCTTCCCTCGCCTTCCTGTTCC R: TGTCCTCCTCACGCGTGTTCCTGG	182	1	66
C9orf64	F: AGGCTCTTTTCTCAACTGCGTCCGT R: AGCAGCCATCTCCTTTTCCTTCCA	191	2	66
FSTL1	F: CCCAGACCCAGACAGAGGAGGAG R: ACTGGTGATTTGGCGACTGTAGCA	203	2	66
CCN1	F: GCAATTCAGAGGATCCATG R: GGTGTGCTTGAGGGGACGGTAG	220	3	55
SAR1B	F: ACCACGAAAGGCTGTTAGAGTCAAAA R: AACCAAACATCTCTCGCAACCTCTC	146	2	66
NFE2L1	F: ACGGAACCTGCTAGTGGATGGAGA R: CTGTTATGCTGGAAATGTCTGCTGGA	167	1	70

PCR on 20 OSCC cases and 10 normal oral samples. All qRT-PCR analyses were performed on an ABI 7000 Sequence Detection System (Applied Biosystems, Foster City, CA) using SYBR Green (Applied Biosystems, Faster City, CA) for detection. Tests for optimal annealing conditions, as well as melting curve analysis to confirm amplification specificity were conducted for each set of gene-specific primers.

The amplification reactions were carried out using 2 µL of cDNA template in a final volume of 20 µL containing: 1 U of Platinum Taq DNA Polymerase (Invitrogen, Grand Island, NY), 1X polymerase buffer, 2 mM $MgCl_2$, 200 µM of each dNTP, 20 pmol of each primer, 5% DMSO and 0.2 µL of SYBR Green I (working dilution 1:100; Applied Biosystems, Faster City, CA). The standard amplification protocol consisted of an initial denaturation step for 2 min at 95 °C, followed by 40 amplification cycles at 95 °C for 15 s, annealing at 68 °C (CA3) or 72 °C (FHL1) for 30 s and extension at 72°C for 30 s.

Experiments were performed in triplicates and mean values were used for gene expression calculations. The relative gene expression level was estimated using the $2^{-\Delta\Delta Ct}$ method [24]. Each sample data was normalized on the basis of the expression of three reference genes RPLO, PPIA and TBP [21]. The results were expressed as n-fold differences in the relative expression of the reference genes in tumor and the normal samples. A gene was considered downregulated when the expression level was below the arbitrary cut-off adopted (2-fold change downregulation).

In silico TCGA data analysis

We decided to further validate the results from the selected genes by analyzing the TCGA data on gene expression and methylation available for HNSCC (UNC_IlluminaHiSeq_RNASeqV2 for RNA sequencing data; JHU-USC_HumanMethylation450, for DNA methylation data; and Biotab for clinical data). The data from 14 normal and 312 OSCC samples were all obtained from the TCGA data portal (http://www.cbioportal.org/study?-id=hnsc_tcga#summary). Samples included are described in Additional file 3: Table S3. Methylation data for both genes analyzed were targeted by multiple probes, but only mean β-values for each gene were used in statistical analysis. Expression and methylation differences between tumor and normal OSCC samples were tested with independent t-test at 5% significance level. Pearson's correlation test was performed for CA3 and FHL1 mRNA expression and methylation, at 5% significance level. For the heatmap graphical representations, CA3 and FHL1 mRNA expression levels were dichotomized at 250 and 2300 (normalized counts), respectively. These values were chosen arbitrarily in order to best maximize the capacity of distinction between OSCC and healthy subjects, based in the box-plot graphs presented in Fig. 4. Statistical analyses were performed in SPSS v19. Graphical heatmap representations were constructed with heatmap3 package of R statistical software [25, 26].

Results
Selection of downregulated genes in HNSCC

The program Blastn was run for 946,260 ORESTES against the RefSeq database of human genes, resulting in 570,214 ORESTES selected in this analysis. Comparisons of normal and tumor head and neck ORESTES libraries using Fisher's Exact Test generated a list with 75 differentially expressed genes (64 downregulated and 11 upregulated genes). The 64 downregulated genes are listed in Additional file 4: Table S4 and the accession numbers for the libraries used are listed in Additional file 5: Table S5. Thirty of these candidates presented CpG islands at their promoter sites and their expression in head and neck was validated by using the Virtual Northern tool from SAGE Anatomic Viewer - Cancer Genome Anatomy Project (SAV-CGAP). This analysis confirmed 24 candidates as downregulated in HNSCC. After a review of the literature data, genes with biologic functions related to carcinogenesis or described as downregulated in other tumors were selected. By the end, we were able to select 10 genes for the assessment of gene expression in HNSCC cell lines (CA3, FHL1, ANXA6, WDR26, HMGN4, C9orf64, FSTL1, CCN1, NFE2L1 and SAR1B).

Evaluation of selected genes expression in head and neck cell lines

Due to the scarcity of RNA obtained from many samples evaluated in the following steps and the high number of genes selected, it would be virtually impossible to evaluate all possible candidate-genes in all samples. Therefore, we performed a first assessment of the expression of these 10 selected genes in cell lines and picked up only the most promising candidates to be evaluated in further experiments with patients' samples. The results showed that CA3 was expressed in four of the cell lines evaluated, whereas no mRNA was detected in the JHU-13 cell line, suggesting that this gene is downregulated in this cell line. FHL1 showed reduced mRNA expression only in FaDu cell line, being expressed in the other cell lines evaluated. The eight remaining genes (ANXA6, WDR26, HMGN4, C9orf64, FSTL1, CCN1, SAR1B and NFE2L1) were expressed in all five HNSCC cell lines evaluated (Fig. 1).

Validation of mRNA expression in OSCC samples by qRT-PCR

After observing the CA3 and FHL1 downregulation in HNSCC cell lines, we sought to test the expression level of these genes in 20 OSCC samples. Clinical and

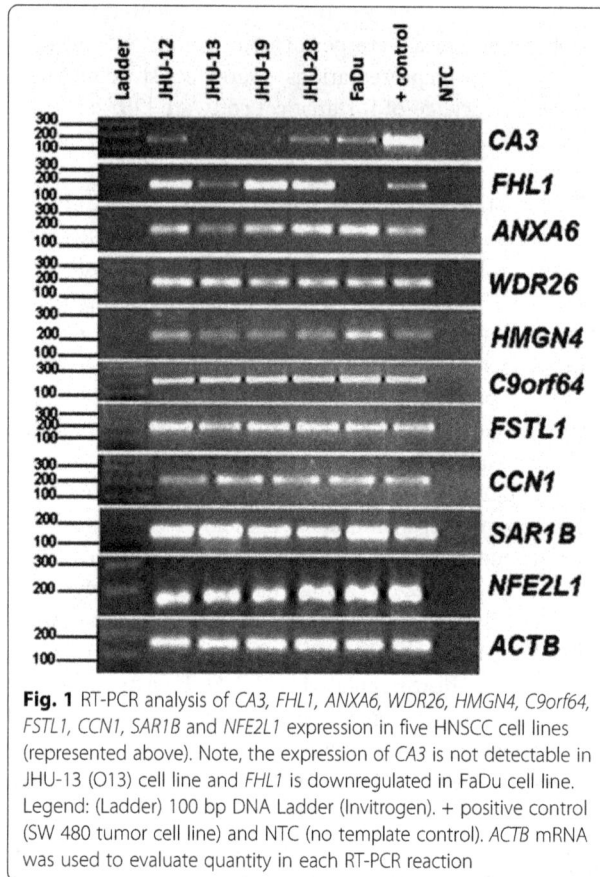

Fig. 1 RT-PCR analysis of *CA3, FHL1, ANXA6, WDR26, HMGN4, C9orf64, FSTL1, CCN1, SAR1B* and *NFE2L1* expression in five HNSCC cell lines (represented above). Note, the expression of *CA3* is not detectable in JHU-13 (O13) cell line and *FHL1* is downregulated in FaDu cell line. Legend: (Ladder) 100 bp DNA Ladder (Invitrogen). + positive control (SW 480 tumor cell line) and NTC (no template control). *ACTB* mRNA was used to evaluate quantity in each RT-PCR reaction

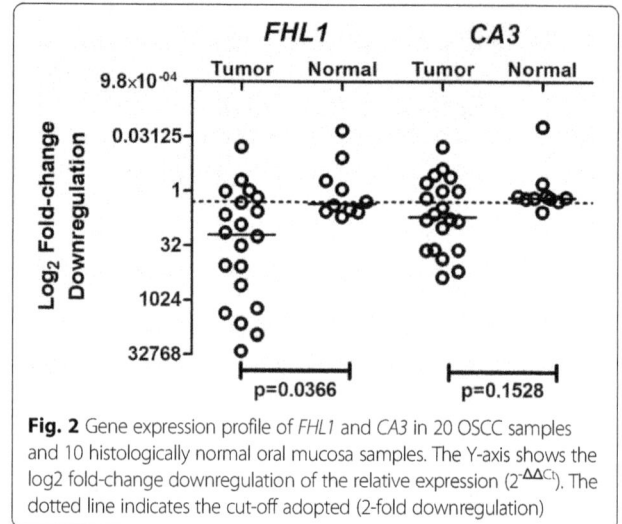

Fig. 2 Gene expression profile of *FHL1* and *CA3* in 20 OSCC samples and 10 histologically normal oral mucosa samples. The Y-axis shows the log2 fold-change downregulation of the relative expression ($2^{-\Delta\Delta Ct}$). The dotted line indicates the cut-off adopted (2-fold downregulation)

pathological data of the 20 OSCC patients enrolled in this study are as follows: the mean age was 59.4 years, 80% of the patients were male, 70% were tobacco users, 60% had advanced stage tumors (II-IV) and 75% of the tumors were in the oral tongue followed by 20% in the floor of the mouth and 5% in the alveolar ridge. Seventy-five percent (15/20) of the samples showed downregulation of *FHL1* while *CA3* was downregulated in 60% (12/20) of the samples (Fig. 2). The Mann-Whitney test was performed to assess the difference between the expression levels of these two genes between OSCC and normal samples. Results showed a statistically significant difference between these two groups for FHL1 ($p = 0.0366$), but not for CA3 ($p = 0.1528$).

In silico TCGA validation

To validate the results obtained with the 20 OSCC patient samples and cell lines in a larger cohort, we analyzed publicly available TCGA data of DNA methylation and mRNA expression (Figs. 3 and 4). Supervisionized heatmap (by sample type) of *CA3* methylation β-values showed a clear separation in samples, where normal samples were frequently hypomethylated for most of the probes (Fig. 3). *FHL1* methylation heatmap did not show

a clear separation (Fig. 3). Statistical analysis of mean methylation β-values supports these observations, for *CA3* and *FHL1* ($p < 0.0001$ and $p = 0.055$, respectively; Fig. 4a and c). In addition, mRNA expression values also showed a clear discrimination of normal and tumoral samples, where most of the tumor samples presented downregulation of both *CA3* and *FHL1* genes ($p < 0.0001$ – Fig. 4b and d). Pearson's correlation analysis showed a significant correlation between mRNA expression and mean methylation for the *CA3* gene ($r = -0.176$; $p = 0.001$ – Fig. 4b) and a trend on this correlation for *FHL1* ($r = -0.100$; $p = 0.071$ – Fig. 4d). Although statistical analysis of *FHL1* methylation was not significant, all results toghether suggest that expression of *CA3* and *FHL1* is probably regulated by methylation.

Expression evaluation after 5'-aza-dC treatment

In order to evaluate if methylation may contribute to the silencing of gene *CA3* and *FHL1*, the cell lines JHU-13 and FaDu were submitted to 5'-aza-dC treatment. RT-PCR showed that *CA3* downregulation in JHU-13 cell line at day 0 (without 5'-aza-dC treatment) was reverted by 3-day treatment with 1 μM of 5'-aza-dC and the gene expression was gradually recovered until day 7 of treatment (Fig. 5a). *FHL1* gene was not expressed in FaDu cell line, but the 3-day treatment with 1 μM of 5'-aza-dC restored the gene expression (Fig. 5b). Once again, these results suggest that expression of *CA3* and *FHL1* could be regulated by methylation of the promoter region.

Discussion

A detailed analysis from ORESTES libraries data may be useful on the identification of differentially expressed genes [12, 15, 21, 27]. Based on this concept, this

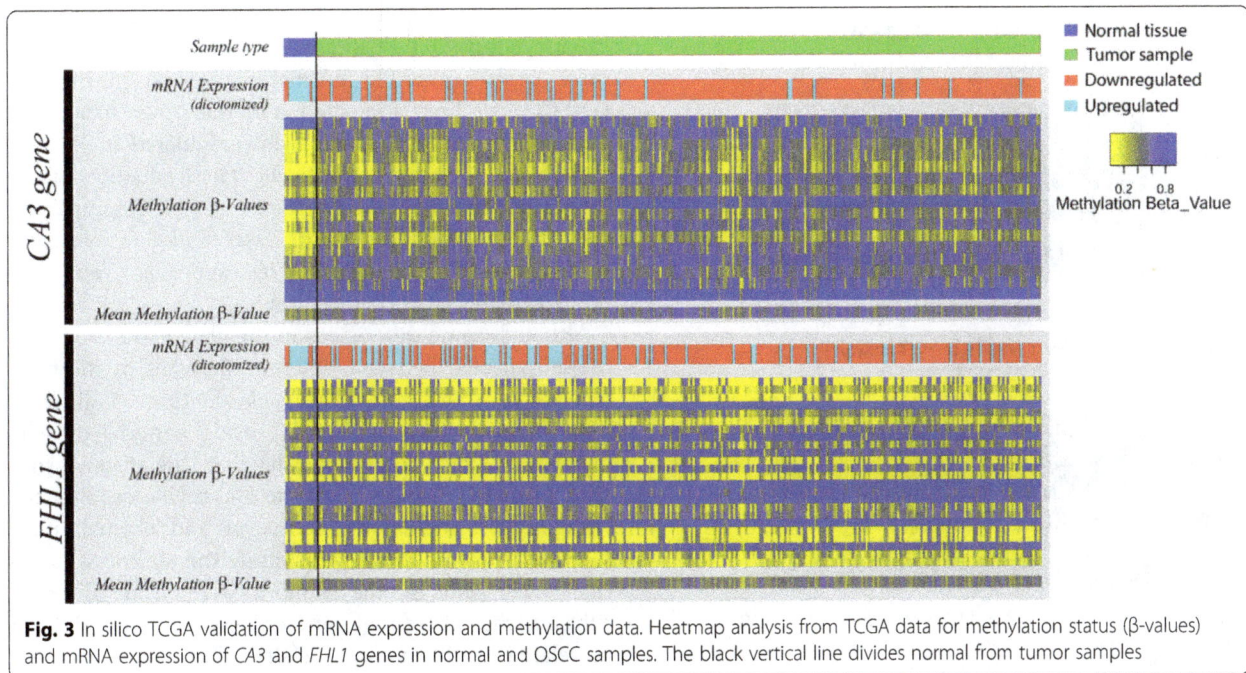

Fig. 3 In silico TCGA validation of mRNA expression and methylation data. Heatmap analysis from TCGA data for methylation status (β-values) and mRNA expression of *CA3* and *FHL1* genes in normal and OSCC samples. The black vertical line divides normal from tumor samples

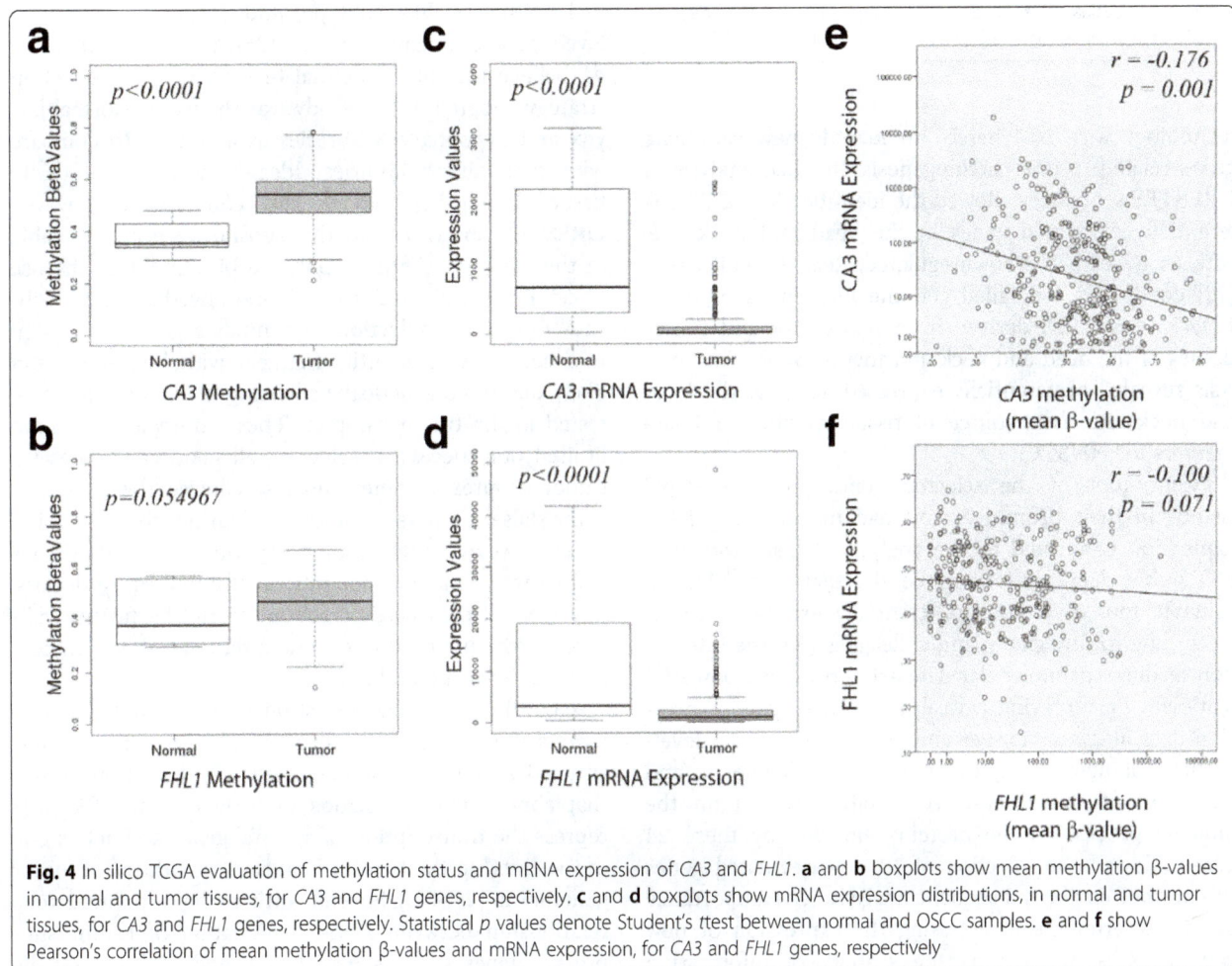

Fig. 4 In silico TCGA evaluation of methylation status and mRNA expression of *CA3* and *FHL1*. **a** and **b** boxplots show mean methylation β-values in normal and tumor tissues, for *CA3* and *FHL1* genes, respectively. **c** and **d** boxplots show mRNA expression distributions, in normal and tumor tissues, for *CA3* and *FHL1* genes, respectively. Statistical *p* values denote Student's *t*test between normal and OSCC samples. **e** and **f** show Pearson's correlation of mean methylation β-values and mRNA expression, for *CA3* and *FHL1* genes, respectively

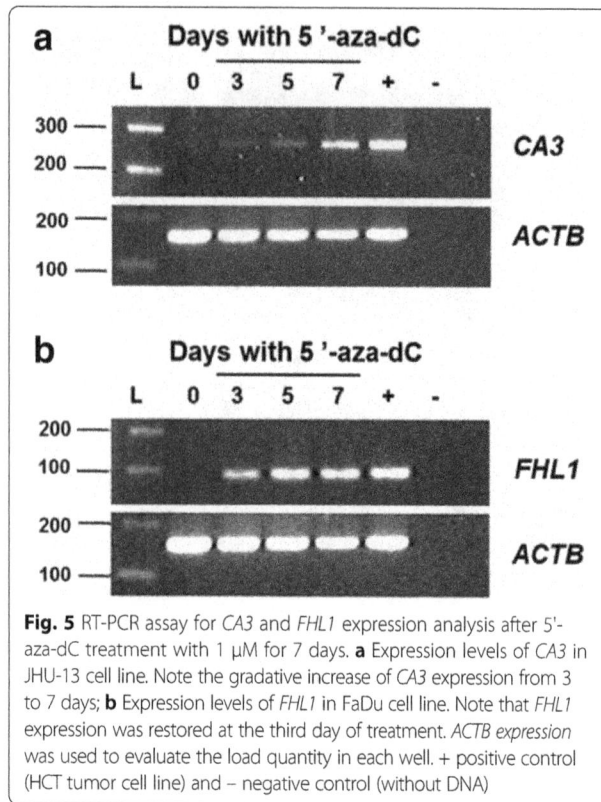

Fig. 5 RT-PCR assay for *CA3* and *FHL1* expression analysis after 5'-aza-dC treatment with 1 μM for 7 days. **a** Expression levels of *CA3* in JHU-13 cell line. Note the gradative increase of *CA3* expression from 3 to 7 days; **b** Expression levels of *FHL1* in FaDu cell line. Note that *FHL1* expression was restored at the third day of treatment. *ACTB expression* was used to evaluate the load quantity in each well. + positive control (HCT tumor cell line) and – negative control (without DNA)

about genes involved on the molecular events of oral carcinogenesis. RT-PCR analysis showed that eight of these genes presented normal expression in the five HNSCC cell lines evaluated. On the other hand, two genes, *CA3* and *FHL1*, were downregulated in JHU-13 and FaDu cell lines, respectively. The evaluation of the expression level of these two genes in OSCC samples by qRT-PCR and in a series of cases and controls from TCGA, demonstrated that *FHL1* and *CA3* were also downregulated in patients' samples.

Although some differences in the gene expression profile is expected between different subtypes of the head and neck, Chung and colleagues identified 4 different molecular subtypes of HNSCC using patterns of gene expression which were not related to the distinct subsites evaluated (tumors from the oral cavity, oropharynx, hypopharynx and larynx, moreover and normal tissue samples from tonsils). In this study the authors showed that, even though the tumors were from different subsites, the differential gene expression profile did not correlated with tumor subsites but with different molecular and histological features such as EGFR-pathway signature, mesenchymal-enriched subtype, normal epithelium-like subtype, and a subtype with high levels of antioxidant enzymes [28]. In spite of that, we do believe that one potential bias of the gene selection strategy adopted in this study was the use of normal larynx and hypopharynx libraries as a control to compare with oral cancer libraries. Ideally, normal oral cavity tissue should be used in this comparison, however, ORESTES libraries from this subsite were not available in the database. Another putative bias could be the use of cell lines originated from different head and neck subsites during the selection of candidate genes. This step was necessary to identify markers with low expression likely due to epigenetically silencing in tumor cells to be tested in the tumor samples. These strategies may have limited our success in selecting all good candidates for tumor suppressor genes and also allowed the choose of some false positive candidates. During the validation process, we avoid this issue comparing oral cavity tissues from tumor and normal mucosa from healthy donors, however, all data here presented should be further validated with larger dataset containing normal and tumors samples from the oral cavity.

According to previous studies, the most frequent targets for methylation events are the CpG islands situated at gene promoter regions [7]. It is well known that abnormal CpG islands methylation can efficiently repress the transcription of specific genes and act as one of the "hits" in the two-hit Knudson hypothesis of tumor generation [29–31]. Several authors have pointed to a relationship between DNA methylation of tumor suppressor genes such as *p16*, *DAPK* and *MGMT* and the

technology was used hereby to identify new candidate genes related to oral carcinogenesis. In silico analysis of ORESTES sequences allowed the identification of 75 differentially expressed genes in the head and neck site, with 64 genes being downregulated. Reis and colleagues [12] conducted a detailed genome mapping analysis of 134,495 ORESTES derived from non-tumor and tumor tissues of the head and neck and thyroid sites. This analysis revealed preferentially expressed genes at the head and neck site as a source of tissue-specific candidate markers for HNSCC.

Twenty-four of the selected genes presented CpG islands in their promoters and had the downregulated expression confirmed by the analysis of head and neck EST public data, reinforcing the idea that ORESTES is a valuable tool to identify differentially expressed genes. According to Strausberg and colleagues [16] the integration of different molecular data sets provides a powerful platform for surveying a wealth of cancer gene expression data in cancer tissues and contributes to the development of new strategies of detection, diagnostic and treatment of this disease. A literature search on the biologic process of the proteins encoded by these 24 genes allowed the selection of 10 downregulated genes to continue in the subsequent analysis. The importance of the experiments in assessing the expression of new candidates is justified by the scarcity of information development and progression of head and neck cancers, including oral cancer [32–39]. We therefore reasoned whether aberrant methylation in promoter sites could be the cause of the downregulation observed in the genes selected from the HNSCC ORESTES libraries and started checking for this relationship using in vitro and in silico models. To answer that, we performed the pharmacological unmasking of these cell lines through their treatment with a demethylating agent and observed an upregulation of these genes in the treated cell lines. In silico analysis of TCGA data for normal and OSCC samples showed similar results, with clear-mirrored methylation/expression profiles for both CA3 and FHL1 genes. These results reinforced the data, initially obtained from the ORESTES analysis.

The CA3 gene (carbonic anhydrase III) is a member of a multigene family that encodes carbonic anhydrase isozymes that catalyze the reversible hydration of carbon dioxide to form carbonic acid [40, 41]. Downregulation of this gene was observed in human hepatocelular carcinoma [42] and, according to these authors, the relationship between CA3 and the response to oxidative stress suggests a role of this gene as a possible mediator of apoptosis or programmed cellular death.

The protein encoded by FHL1 (Four-and-a-Half LIM-domains 1) seems to act as a transcriptional factor, and to be associated to focal adherence and intercellular junctions [43]. FHL1 expression was found downregulated in melanoma and leukemia cell lines [44]. Immunohistochemistry analysis revealed the absence of FHL1 expression in astrocitoma, breast carcinoma, renal carcinoma, hepatocarcinoma, pulmonary adenocarcinoma, prosthatic carcinoma and melanoma tumor samples compared to their corresponding normal tissues [45]. According to these authors, due to its ability in inhibiting specific aspects of tumor cellular growth, FHL1 could have a tumor suppressor activity [45].

The identification of hypermethylated genes in cancer is extremely important, since silencing confers benefits to the survival of these cells, contributing to a neoplastic phenotype and tumor progression, through the accumulation of genetic and epigenetic hits [11]. In the present study, the treatment of JHU-13 and FaDu cell lines with the demethylating agent 5-aza-2′-deoxycytidine was able to restore CA3 and FHL1 expression, possibly showing a link between CA3 and FHL1 downregulation and aberrant methylation in their promoter sites and a role of methylation in the regulation of these two genes.

Moreover, a recently published study found a significant association of FHL1 downregulation and its promoter methylation in OSCC cell lines and tumor samples, also suggesting that inactivation of the FHL1 in OSCCs is through DNA methylation of the promoter region [46].

Conclusion

In conclusion, our results showed that the downregulation of CA3 and FHL1 data observed in silico were validated in HNSCC cell lines and OSCC samples and also suggests that expression of CA3 and FHL1 could possibly be regulated by methylation having an important role in the oral carcinogenesis. Moreover, these results warrant further studies for the evaluation of the gene expression and methylation profile of CA3 and FHL1 in larger number of samples with clinical and demographic data available to allow the investigation of relevant associations with patient outcome.

Additional files

Additional file 1: Table S1. List of ORESTES Libraries included in this study.

Additional file 2: Table S2. Websites used in the selection of downregulated genes.

Additional file 3: Table S3. TCGA sample description.

Additional file 4: Table S4. Downregulated genes in head and neck tumors according to the analysis of the ORESTES dataset.

Additional file 5: Table S5. List of accession numbers for the ORESTES data used in the study.

Abbreviations

5-aza-dC: 5-aza-2′-deoxycytidine; BlastN: Basic Local Alignment Search Tool Nucleotide; CA3: Carbonic anhydrase III; cDNA: Complementary DNA; CpG: 5′-C-phosphate-G-3′; CsCl: Cesium Chloride; Ct: Cycle threshold; DMSO: Dimethyl sulfoxide; dNTP: Deoxynucleotides triphosphates; ESTs: Expressed sequence tags; FHL1: Four-and-a-Half LIM-domains 1; HNSCC: Head and Neck Squamous Cell Carcinoma; MEM: Minimum Essential Media; MgCl₂: Magnesium chloride; mRNA: Messenger RNA; NCBI: National Center for Biotechnology Information; ORESTES: Open Reading Expressed Sequence Tags; OSCC: Oral Squamous Cell Carcinoma; qRT-PCR: Quantitative Reverse transcription polymerase chain reaction; RefSeq: Reference Sequences; RPMI: Roswell Park Memorial Institute; RT-PCR: Reverse transcription polymerase chain reaction; SAGE: Serial analysis of gene expression; SAV-CGAP: SAGE Anatomic Viewer - Cancer Genome Anatomy Project; SCC: squamous cell carcinoma; TCGA: The Cancer Genome Atlas

Acknowledgments

C. M. P. was a recipient of fellowship from Fundação António Prudente (FAP). A.L.V. and A.L.C. had a CNPq scholarship.

Funding

This work was financially supported by Conselho Nacional de Pesquisa (CNPq) grant 476586/2006-2 (to A.L.C.) and by Fundação de Amparo à Pesquisa do Estado de São Paulo (FAPESP) grant 05/02580-8 (to A.L.V.). The funding body had no role in the design of the study and collection, analysis, and interpretation of data and in writing the manuscript.

Authors' contributions

CMP carried out the molecular biology studies and data analyzes. ACC helped in the data analyzes and in the draft of the manuscript. FRS performed the bioinformatics analyzes. MEM performed the bioinformatics analyzes and helped in the draft of the manuscript. RCL and VCCA helped in the molecular biology studies LPK participated in study design, recruited patients and collected tissue samples. ALV and ALC participated in study design and coordination and helped to draft the manuscript. All authors read and approved the final manuscript.

Competing interests

The authors declare that they have no competing interests.

Author details

[1]Department of Head and Neck Surgery, A. C. Camargo Cancer Hospital, São Paulo, Brazil. [2]Laboratory of Cancer Genetics, Ludwig Institute for Cancer Research, Sao Paulo, Branch, Brazil. [3]Molecular Oncology Research Center, Barretos Cancer Hospital, Barretos, Brazil. [4]Embrapa Informatica Agropecuaria, Campinas, Brazil. [5]Discipline of Hematology and Hemotherapy, Universidade Federal de São Paulo, UNIFESP, São Paulo, Brazil. [6]Department of Science Biology, Universidade Federal de São Paulo, UNIFESP, Diadema, Brazil. [7]Department of Head and Neck Surgery, Barretos Cancer Hospital, Barretos, São Paulo, Brazil.

References

1. Barasch A, Safford M, Eisenberg E. Oral cancer and oral effects of anticancer therapy. The Mount Sinai J Med, New York. 1998;65(5–6):370–7.
2. Das BR, Nagpal JK. Understanding the biology of oral cancer. Medical science monitor : international medical journal of experimental and clinical research. 2002;8(11):RA258–67.
3. Chakraborty S, Mohiyuddin SM, Gopinath KS, Kumar A. Involvement of TSC genes and differential expression of other members of the mTOR signaling pathway in oral squamous cell carcinoma. BMC Cancer. 2008;8:163.
4. Arantes LM, de Carvalho AC, Melendez ME, Carvalho AL, Goloni-Bertollo EM. Methylation as a biomarker for head and neck cancer. Oral Oncol. 2014; 50(6):587–92.
5. Sailasree R, Abhilash A, Sathyan KM, Nalinakumari KR, Thomas S, Kannan S. Differential roles of p16INK4A and p14ARF genes in prognosis of oral carcinoma. Cancer epidemiol, biomarkers & prev: a publ Am Asso Cancer Res, cosponsored by the Am Soc of Prev Oncol. 2008;17(2):414–20.
6. Ha PK, Califano JA. Promoter methylation and inactivation of tumour-suppressor genes in oral squamous-cell carcinoma. The lancet oncol. 2006; 7(1):77–82.
7. Viswanathan M, Tsuchida N, Shanmugam G. Promoter hypermethylation profile of tumor-associated genes p16, p15, hMLH1, MGMT and E-cadherin in oral squamous cell carcinoma. Int J Cancer. 2003;105(1):41–6.
8. Lee JK, Kim MJ, Hong SP, Hong SD. Inactivation patterns of p16/INK4A in oral squamous cell carcinomas. Exp Mol Med. 2004;36(2):165–71.
9. Arantes LM, de Carvalho AC, Melendez ME, Centrone CC, Gois-Filho JF, Toporcov TN, Caly DN, Tajara EH, Goloni-Bertollo EM, Carvalho AL. Validation of methylation markers for diagnosis of oral cavity cancer. Eur J Cancer. 2015;51(5):632–41.
10. Jones PA, Baylin SB. The fundamental role of epigenetic events in cancer. Nat Rev Genet. 2002;3(6):415–28.
11. Baylin SB, Ohm JE. Epigenetic gene silencing in cancer - a mechanism for early oncogenic pathway addiction? Nat Rev Cancer. 2006;6(2):107–16.
12. Reis EM, Ojopi EP, Alberto FL, Rahal P, Tsukumo F, Mancini UM, Guimaraes GS, Thompson GM, Camacho C, Miracca E, et al. Large-scale transcriptome analyses reveal new genetic marker candidates of head, neck, and thyroid cancer. Cancer Res. 2005;65(5):1693–9.
13. Lallemant B, Evrard A, Chambon G, Sabra O, Kacha S, Lallemant JG, Lumbroso S, Brouillet JP. Gene expression profiling in head and neck squamous cell carcinoma: clinical perspectives. Head Neck. 2010;32(12): 1712–9.
14. Brentani H, Caballero OL, Camargo AA, da Silva AM, da Silva WA, Jr., Dias Neto E, Grivet M, Gruber A, Guimaraes PE, Hide W et al: The generation and utilization of a cancer-oriented representation of the human transcriptome by using expressed sequence tags. Proc Natl Acad Sci U S A 2003, 100(23): 13418–13423.
15. Mello BP, Abrantes EF, Torres CH, Machado-Lima A, Fonseca Rda S, Carraro DM, Brentani RR, Reis LF, Brentani H. No-match ORESTES explored as tumor markers. Nucleic Acids Res. 2009;37(8):2607–17.
16. Strausberg RL, Camargo AA, Riggins GJ, Schaefer CF, de Souza SJ, Grouse LH, Lal A, Buetow KH, Boon K, Greenhut SF, et al. An international database and integrated analysis tools for the study of cancer gene expression. Pharmacogenomics J. 2002;2(3):156–64.
17. Camargo AA, Samaia HP, Dias-Neto E, Simao DF, Migotto IA, Briones MR, Costa FF, Nagai MA, Verjovski-Almeida S, Zago MA, et al. The contribution of 700,000 ORF sequence tags to the definition of the human transcriptome. Proc Natl Acad Sci U S A. 2001;98(21):12103–8.
18. Dias Neto E, Correa RG, Verjovski-Almeida S, Briones MR, Nagai MA, da Silva W Jr, Zago MA, Bordin S, Costa FF, Goldman GH, et al. Shotgun sequencing of the human transcriptome with ORF expressed sequence tags. Proc Natl Acad Sci U S A. 2000;97(7):3491–6.
19. Lockyer AE, Spinks JN, Walker AJ, Kane RA, Noble LR, Rollinson D, Dias-Neto E, Jones CS. Biomphalaria Glabrata transcriptome: identification of cell-signalling, transcriptional control and immune-related genes from open reading frame expressed sequence tags (ORESTES). Dev Comp Immunol. 2007;31(8):763–82.
20. Maia RM, Valente V, Cunha MA, Sousa JF, Araujo DD, Silva WA Jr, Zago MA, Dias-Neto E, Souza SJ, Simpson AJ, et al. Identification of unannotated exons of low abundance transcripts in Drosophila Melanogaster and cloning of a new serine protease gene upregulated upon injury. BMC Genomics. 2007;8:249.
21. Lessa RC, Campos AH, Freitas CE, Silva FR, Kowalski LP, Carvalho AL, Vettore AL. Identification of upregulated genes in oral squamous cell carcinomas. Head Neck. 2013;35(10):1475–81.
22. TCGA: The Cancer Genome Atlas. http://cancergenome.nih.gov/.
23. Pruitt KD, Tatusova T, Maglott DR. NCBI reference sequence (RefSeq): a curated non-redundant sequence database of genomes, transcripts and proteins. Nucleic Acids Res. 2005;33(Database issue):D501–4.
24. Livak KJ, Schmittgen TD. Analysis of relative gene expression data using real-time quantitative PCR and the 2(−Delta Delta C(T)) method. Methods. 2001;25(4):402–8.
25. Dessau RB, Pipper CB. "R"–project for statistical computing. Ugeskr Laeger. 2008;170(5):328–30.
26. Zhao S, Guo Y, Sheng Q, Shyr Y. Heatmap3: an improved heatmap package with more powerful and convenient features. BMC Bioinf. 2014;15(Suppl 10):P16.
27. Leerkes MR, Caballero OL, Mackay A, Torloni H, O'Hare MJ, Simpson AJ, de Souza SJ. In silico comparison of the transcriptome derived from purified normal breast cells and breast tumor cell lines reveals candidate upregulated genes in breast tumor cells. Genomics. 2002;79(2):257–65.
28. Chung CH, Parker JS, Karaca G, Wu J, Funkhouser WK, Moore D, Butterfoss D, Xiang D, Zanation A, Yin X, et al. Molecular classification of head and neck squamous cell carcinomas using patterns of gene expression. Cancer Cell. 2004;5(5):489–500.
29. Jones PA, Laird PW. Cancer epigenetics comes of age. Nat Genet. 1999; 21(2):163–7.
30. Baylin SB, Herman JG. DNA hypermethylation in tumorigenesis: epigenetics joins genetics. Trends Genet. 2000;16(4):168–74.
31. Robertson KD. DNA methylation, methyltransferases, and cancer. Oncogene. 2001;20(24):3139–55.
32. Nakahara Y, Shintani S, Mihara M, Ueyama Y, Matsumura T. High frequency of homozygous deletion and methylation of p16(INK4A) gene in oral squamous cell carcinomas. Cancer Lett. 2001;163(2):221–8.
33. Nakayama S, Sasaki A, Mese H, Alcalde RE, Tsuji T, Matsumura T. The E-cadherin gene is silenced by CpG methylation in human oral squamous cell carcinomas. Int J Cancer. 2001;93(5):667–73.
34. Shintani S, Nakahara Y, Mihara M, Ueyama Y, Matsumura T. Inactivation of the p14(ARF), p15(INK4B) and p16(INK4A) genes is a frequent event in human oral squamous cell carcinomas. Oral Oncol. 2001;37(6):498–504.
35. Ogi K, Toyota M, Ohe-Toyota M, Tanaka N, Noguchi M, Sonoda T, Kohama G, Tokino T. Aberrant methylation of multiple genes and clinicopathological features in oral squamous cell carcinoma. Clin Cancer Res. 2002;8(10):3164–71.
36. McGregor F, Muntoni A, Fleming J, Brown J, Felix DH, MacDonald DG, Parkinson EK, Harrison PR. Molecular changes associated with oral dysplasia progression and acquisition of immortality: potential for its reversal by 5-azacytidine. Cancer Res. 2002;62(16):4757–66.
37. Cao J, Zhou J, Gao Y, Gu L, Meng H, Liu H, Deng D. Methylation of p16 CpG island associated with malignant progression of oral epithelial dysplasia: a prospective cohort study. Clin Cancer Res. 2009;15(16):5178–83.
38. Wiklund ED, Gao S, Hulf T, Sibbritt T, Nair S, Costea DE, Villadsen SB,

Bakholdt V, Bramsen JB, Sorensen JA, et al. MicroRNA alterations and associated aberrant DNA methylation patterns across multiple sample types in oral squamous cell carcinoma. PLoS One. 2011;6(11):e27840.

39. Bhatia V, Goel MM, Makker A, Tewari S, Yadu A, Shilpi P, Kumar S, Agarwal SP, Goel SK. Promoter region Hypermethylation and mRNA expression of MGMT and p16 genes in tissue and blood samples of human premalignant oral lesions and oral squamous cell carcinoma. Biomed Res Int. 2014;2014: 248419.

40. Fraser P, Cummings P, Curtis P. The mouse carbonic anhydrase I gene contains two tissue-specific promoters. Mol Cell Biol. 1989;9(8):3308–13.

41. Cabiscol E, Levine RL. The phosphatase activity of carbonic anhydrase III is reversibly regulated by glutathiolation. Proc Natl Acad Sci U S A. 1996;93(9): 4170–4.

42. Kuo WH, Chiang WL, Yang SF, Yeh KT, Yeh CM, Hsieh YS, Chu SC. The differential expression of cytosolic carbonic anhydrase in human hepatocellular carcinoma. Life Sci. 2003;73(17):2211–23.

43. Brown S, McGrath MJ, Ooms LM, Gurung R, Maimone MM, Mitchell CA. Characterization of two isoforms of the skeletal muscle LIM protein 1, SLIM1. Localization of SLIM1 at focal adhesions and the isoform slimmer in the nucleus of myoblasts and cytoplasm of myotubes suggests distinct roles in the cytoskeleton and in nuclear-cytoplasmic communication. J Biol Chem. 1999;274(38):27083–91.

44. Morgan MJ, Whawell SA. The structure of the human LIM protein ACT gene and its expression in tumor cell lines. Biochem Biophys Res Commun. 2000; 273(2):776–83.

45. Shen Y, Jia Z, Nagele RG, Ichikawa H, Goldberg GS. SRC uses Cas to suppress Fhl1 in order to promote nonanchored growth and migration of tumor cells. Cancer Res. 2006;66(3):1543–52.

46. Koike K, Kasamatsu A, Iyoda M, Saito Y, Kouzu Y, Koike H, Sakamoto Y, Ogawara K, Tanzawa H, Uzawa K. High prevalence of epigenetic inactivation of the human four and a half LIM domains 1 gene in human oral cancer. Int J Oncol. 2013;42(1):141–50.

28

Investigation of the *SLC22A23* gene in laryngeal squamous cell carcinoma

Seda Ekizoglu[1], Didem Seven[1], Turgut Ulutin[1], Jalal Guliyev[2] and Nur Buyru[1]*

Abstract

Background: Laryngeal squamous cell carcinoma (LSCC) is the second most common cancer of the head and neck. In order to identify differentially expressed genes which may have a role in LSCC carcinogenesis, we performed GeneFishing Assay. One of the differentially expressed genes was the *SLC22A23* (solute carrier family 22, member 23) gene.

SLC22A23 belongs to a family of organic ion transporters that are responsible for the absorption or excretion of many drugs, xenobiotics and endogenous compounds in a variety of tissues. SLC22A23 is expressed in a various tissues but no substrates or functions have been identified for it. Although the exact function is unknown, single nucleotide polymorphisms (SNPs) which are located in *SLC22A23* gene were associated with inflammatory bowel disease (IBD), endometriosis-related infertility and the clearance of antipsychotic drugs. On the other hand *SLC22A23* is identified as a prognostic gene to predict the recurrence of triple-negative breast cancer.

Methods: To understand the role of the *SLC22A23* gene in laryngeal carcinogenesis, we investigated its mRNA expression level in laryngeal tumor tissue and adjacent non-cancerous tissue samples obtained from 83 patients by quantitative real-time PCR. To understand the association between SNPs in *SLC22A23* and LSCC, selected genetic variations (rs4959235, rs6923667, rs9503518) were genotyped.

Results: We found that *SLC22A23* expression was increased in 46 of 83 tumor tissues (55.4%) and was decreased in 30 of 83 (36.1%) tumor tissues compared to normal tissues. 77.2% of patients were homozygote for genotype rs9503518-AA and they most frequently had histological grade 2 and 3 tumors. We also found that rs9503518-AA genotype is associated with increased *SLC22A23* expression.

Conclusions: Our results indicate that *SLC22A23* may play a role in the development of laryngeal cancer.

Keywords: Laryngeal cancer, GeneFishing, SLC22A23, Expression, Genotyping

Background

Laryngeal squamous cell carcinoma (LSCC) is the second most common cancer of the head and neck [1]. It has been proposed that LSCC is a complex disease caused by the interaction of genetic and environmental factors. Smoking, high alcohol consumption and human papillomavirus infections have been considered as the major environmental factors [2, 3]. Although, early detection and diagnosis of LSCC can greatly increase the success of treatment by surgery, chemotherapy and radiothearapy, the 5-year survival rates vary between 40 and 80% depending on the anatomical location [4].

Therefore, a better understanding of the mechanisms underlying LSCC is of great importance and several studies have addressed the identification of target genes involved in LSCC pathogenesis.

Solute carrier (SLC) transporters comprise one of the two membrane transporters with more than 300 members which have been divided into 52 families [5, 6]. The main functions of these proteins is to transfer a wide range of substrates such as amino acids, lipids, inorganic ions, peptides, saccharides, metal ions, proteins, xenobiotics and drugs [7, 8]. Therefore, the effect of each transporter on the cell behaviour depends on the type of the molecule it transports. While some of the members such as organic anion transporters are involved in chemoresistance, some may play a role in cell survival and cell

---

* Correspondence: nbuyru@yahoo.com
[1]Cerrahpasa Medical Faculty, Department of Medical Biology, Istanbul University, Kocamustafapasa, 34098 Istanbul, Turkey
Full list of author information is available at the end of the article

cycle progression because of their function in nutrient transportation [9]. One of the known functions of the SLC proteins is to facilitate the uptake of nutrients and removal of metabolites. It is well known that cancer cells need extra metabolic requirements during rapid cell cycles. Accumulating evidence supports that many SLC transporters are up-regulated in various cancers to supply the increasing demand of the tumor cells [9, 10]. SLC22A23 (solute carrier family 22, member 23) belongs to the SLC family of organic ion transporters that are responsible for the uptake or excretion of many compounds including drugs, toxins and endogenous metabolites in a variety of tissues [11]. SLC22A23 is expressed in various tissues but no substrates or functions have yet been identified for it [12].

Single nucleotide polymorphisms (SNPs) are variations in individual nucleotides which occur within a gene or in a regulatory region near a gene. They may affect the gene's function or may have predict an individual's response to certain drugs, susceptibility to environmental factors and risk of developing particular diseases. SNPs also affect the gene expression rates by changing the nucleotide sequence in the transcription factor bindig domain or the sequence of non-coding RNA binding sites. Several SNPs have been identified in the *SLC22A23* locus previously [13–16]. Therefore, in this study we aimed to investigate the expression levels and probable role of the *SLC22A23* gene SNPs in LSCC.

Methods
Samples
A total of 83 patients diagnosed with LSCC were included in this study. Fresh tumors and matching non-cancerous tissue samples were obtained from patients undergoing surgery in the Department of Otorhinolaryngology, Cerrahpasa Medical Faculty. 2 ml of venous blood was collected into EDTA-containing tubes from all patients. There were 80 men (96.4%) and 3 women (3.6%). The mean age at diagnosis was 59 ± 9 years. The clinical characteristics, including stage, histological type, histological grade, smoking status, age and gender are shown in Table 1.

The study was approved by the Cerrahpasa Medical Faculty Ethics Committee (Approval number: 83045809/604.01/02-235,918), and has been performed in accordance with the ethical standarts laid down in the 2013 Declaration of Helsinki. Signed informed consent was obtained from all patients.

Identification of differentially expressed genes (DEGs) by GeneFishing
RNA isolation and GeneFishing reverse transcription
Total RNA was isolated from both tumors and adjacent non-cancerous tissues of 4 patients using the miRCURY

Table 1 Clinicopathological characteristics of patients

Parameters	Variable	n (%)
Clinical stage	Early stage (I+ II)	8 (9.6)
	Advanced stage (III+ IV)	74 (89.2)
	Unknown	1 (1.2)
Histology	Squamous cell carcinoma (SCC)	79 (95.2)
	Non-SCC	3 (3.6)
	Unknown	1 (1.2)
Histological grade	Grade 1	2 (2.4)
	Grade 2	35 (42.2)
	Grade 3	32 (38.6)
	Grade 4	7 (8.4)
	Unknown	7 (8.4)
Smoking	Smoker	69 (83.1)
	Non-smoker	12 (14.5)
	Unknown	2 (2.4)
Gender	Female	3 (3.6)
	Male	80 (96.4)
Age	≤50	13 (15.7)
	> 50	69 (83.1)
	Unknown	1 (1.2)

RNA Isolation Kit (Exiqon, Vedbaek, Denmark) according to the manufacturer's instructions. First strand cDNA was prepared from 3 µg of total RNA and reverse transcription was carried out for 90 min at 42 °C and 2 min at 94 °C in a final volume of 20 µl containing 1 µM dT-ACP1 (provided in the GeneFishing DEG Premix Kit, Seegene, Seoul, Korea), 1xRT buffer (Invitrogen, Carlsbad, CA, USA), 0.5 mM dNTP, 20 U RNase inhibitor (BIOMATIK, Wilmington, DE, USA) and 200 U M-MLV reverse transcriptase (Invitrogen, Carsbad, CA, USA). First strand cDNA was diluted by adding 80 µl of DNase-free water.

ACP-based GeneFishing polymerase chain reaction
GeneFishing PCRs were performed using a primer set consisting of 20 different arbitrary ACPs (Annealing Control Primers) provided in the GeneFishing DEG Premix Kit (Seegene, Seoul, Korea). The reaction conditions were: diluted first-strand cDNA (50 ng), 0.5 µM arbitrary ACP (one of the arbitrary ACPs), 0.5 µM dT-ACP2 and 1xSeeAmp ACP master mix in a 20 µl final volume. PCR was performed at 94 °C for 5 min, 50 °C for 3 min, 72 °C for 1 min, followed by 40 cycles of 94 °C for 40 s, 65 °C for 40 s and 72 °C for 40 s and a final step for 5 min at 72 °C. The amplified PCR products were separated on 2% agarose gels and the differentially expressed bands were purified from the gels using the Zymoclean Gel DNA Recovery Kit (Zymo Research, Irvine, CA, USA).

Cloning and sequencing

Purified PCR products were directly cloned into the pCR™4-TOPO vector using the TOPO TA Cloning Kit for Sequencing (Invitrogen, Carlsbad, CA, USA). Following the cloning reaction, the pCR™4-TOPO construct was transformed into competent *E. coli* (One Shot TOP 10) cells according to the One Shot chemical transformation protocol provided in the kit. *E. coli* cells were cultured overnight at 37 °C in LB (Luria-Bertani) agar plates containing 50 µg/ml kanamycin. 2-6 colonies were taken and cultured overnight at 37 °C in LB medium containing 50 µg/ml kanamycin. For identification of the inserted PCR product, the plasmid DNA was isolated using the PureLink Quick Plasmid Miniprep Kit (Invitrogen, Carlsbad, CA, USA) and sequenced on an ABI Prism 3100-Avant™ Genetic Analyzer (Applied Biosystems, Foster City, CA, USA) using the ABI Prism BigDye Terminator v3.1 Cycle Sequencing Kit (Applied Biosystems, Foster City, CA, USA). Sequences were analyzed by searching for similarities using the Basic Local Alignment Search Tool (BLAST) program.

Quantitative real time polymerase chain reaction (qRT-PCR) analysis of *SLC22A23*

Total RNA was isolated from 83 tumors and adjacent non-cancerous tissues using the PureLink RNA Mini Kit (Ambion, Carlsbad, CA, USA). cDNA was synthesized from 400 ng of total RNA using the RevertAid First-Strand cDNA Synthesis Kit (Thermo Scientific, Waltham, MA, USA).

Expression levels of the *SLC22A23* gene were analyzed by qRT-PCR using the LightCycler 480-II system (Roche Diagnostics, Mannheim, Germany). PCR was performed in a final volume of 15 µl containing 1× master PCR mix (SolGent, Daejeon, South Korea) with EvaGreen (Biotium, Fremont, CA, USA), 600 nM gene-specific primers, nuclease free water and cDNA. The sequences of the primers are shown in Table 2. The PCR amplification protocol was an initial denaturation of 15 min at 95 °C, 40 cycles of amplification at 95 °C for 15 s, 59 °C for 30 s, and 72 °C for 30 s followed by a cooling step of 10 s at 50 °C. The reference gene used for normalization was *Beta-2-microglobulin (B2M)* and relative mRNA levels were calculated by the comparative $2^{-\Delta\Delta Ct}$ method [17].

Genotyping

Genomic DNA was isolated from blood using the High Pure PCR Template Preparation Kit (Roche Diagnostics, Mannheim, Germany) and was kept at – 80 °C until use. The SNPs rs9503518, rs4959235 and rs6923667 within the human *SLC22A23* gene were genotyped using TaqMan SNP Genotyping Assays (Assay ID C__25960793_20, C__27912010_10, C__29004073_10) (Applied Biosystems, Foster City, CA, USA) and the Applied Biosystems 7500 Fast Real-Time PCR System. PCRs were performed in a final reaction volume of 20 µl per well containing 1× TaqMan Genotyping Master Mix (Applied Biosystems, Foster City, CA, USA), 1× SNP TaqMan SNP Genotyping Assay (Applied Biosystems, Foster City, CA, USA) and 20 ng DNA. The reaction conditions included an initial step of 1 min at 60 °C, an enzyme activation step of 10 min at 95 °C and 40 cycles at 95 °C for 15 s and 60 °C for 1 min. Allelic discrimination was determined using the 7500 Fast Real-Time PCR software version 2.3 and FAM and VIC fluorescence probes. The dye used as the passive reference was ROX.

Statistical analysis

Statistical analyses were performed using IBM SPSS Statistics 20 software (IBM Corp., Armonk, NY, USA). Wilcoxon test and Pearson's chi-square test are used to calculate p values. $p < 0.05$ was considered statistically significant.

Results

Identification of differentially expressed genes

To identify Differentially Expressed Genes (DEGs) in LSCC, we compared the mRNA expression profiles of the tumor tissues with those of normal tissues using ACP-based GeneFishing PCR with a combination of 20 arbitrary primers and two anchored oligo (dT) primers (dT-ACP1 and dT-ACP2). The analysis was performed with 4 pairs of tumor and normal tissues.

Twenty-seven DEGs were identified, including 15 down-regulated and 12 up-regulated DEGs in tumor tissue compared with normal tissue. Among these 27 DEGs, 12 DEGs were isolated, cloned, sequenced and searched in the GenBank.

We identified the *SLC22A23* gene by sequence analysis of one of the up-regulated DEGs by homology searching using the Basic Local Alignment Search Tool (BLAST) program. GeneFishig PCR results observed on an agarose gel for *SLC22A23* are shown in Fig. 1.

Confirmation of the expression pattern of *SLC22A23* by real-time PCR

We examined the altered expression level of the *SLC22A23* gene using Real-Time PCR in 83 tumor samples and adjacent non-cancerous tissue samples. We

Table 2 Primer sequences used for qRT-PCR

Gene	Primer	Sequence
SLC22A23	Forward	5′-ACCCCGACGGTGATAAGGTGT-3′
	Reverse	5′-TCTGGTTGTGCAGCTCGATGAT-3′
B2M	Forward	5′-CTCGCGCTACTCTCTCTTTCTGG-3′
	Reverse	5′-GCTTACATGTCTCGATCCCACTTAA-3′

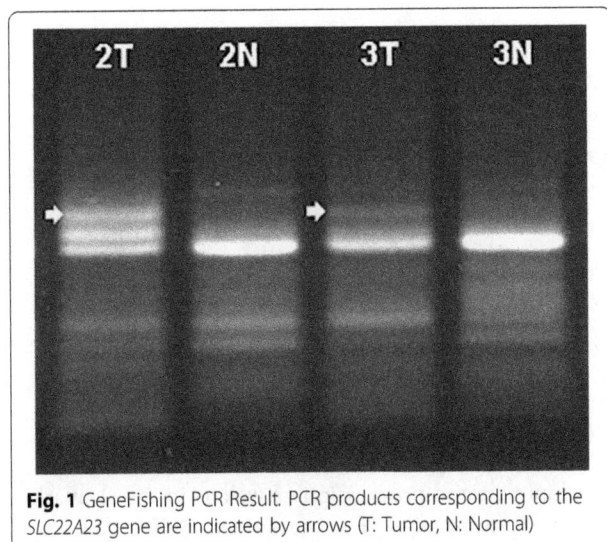

Fig. 1 GeneFishing PCR Result. PCR products corresponding to the SLC22A23 gene are indicated by arrows (T: Tumor, N: Normal)

observed increased *SLC22A23* mRNA expression in 46 of 83 tumor tissues (55.4%) and decreased expression in 30 tissues (36.1%) when compared to their normal counterparts. No change was detected in 7 samples. The $2^{-\Delta\Delta Ct}$ levels were 1.55 and 1 for the tumor and the normal tissue samples, respectively (Table 3). Statistically, significant upregulation of the *SLC22A23* mRNA was observed in laryngeal tumor tissues ($p = 0.001$). No significant correlation was found between *SLC22A23* expression and clinicopathological parameters such as the clinical stage ($p = 0.329$), histology ($p = 0.067$), sex ($p = 0.286$), age ($p = 0.482$), histological grade ($p = 0.649$) and smoking status ($p = 0,977$).

Genotyping of the *SLC22A23* polymorphisms

Genotyping of the *SLC22A23* rs9503518, rs4959235 and rs6923667 polymorphisms was carried out by real-time PCR allelic discrimination analysis. Genotype and allele frequencies for each SNP are shown in Table 4.

We observed that 77.2% of patients carried the homozygote AA-genotype for rs9503518, and 43.8% of patients carried the heterozygote CT-genotype for rs6923667. 84.1% of patients were homozygous for rs4959235-CC and 15.9% were heterozygous for rs4959235-CT but we didn't observe rs4959235-TT homozygotes in our study group. We didn't find any association between the rs4959235-CC/CT, rs6923667-CC/CT/TT genotypes and clinicopathological

Table 3 Expression values of the *SLC22A23* gene in tumors and normal tissues

	SLC22A23 Ct (Median)	B2M Ct (Median)	ΔCt (Median)	ΔΔCt	$2^{-\Delta\Delta Ct}$	p^a
Tumor	26.7	21.7	5	−0.6	1.55	0.014
Normal	27.6	22.3	5.3	0	1	

[a]Statistical analyses were performed using the Wilcoxon test

parameters such as the clinical stage, histology, sex, age, histological grade and smoking status. But we observed that patients who were homozygous for rs9503518-AA most frequently had histological grade 2 and 3 tumors and the association was statistiacally significant (Table 5).

Moreover, we investigated if SNPs of the *SLC22A23* gene play a role in the expression level of the gene and found that 52.2% of homozygote patients for genotype rs9503518-AA had increased *SLC22A23* gene expression (Table 6). The association between rs9503518-AA and *SLC22A23* expression level was statistically significant ($p = 0.046$). No significant association was found between the *SLC22A23* gene expression and rs4959235-CC/CT and rs6923667-CC/CT/TT genotypes.

Discussion

SLC transporters is one the largest membrane transporter families with more than 300 members and 52 subfamilies [5, 6]. They play a major role in the transport of many different charged and uncharged organic molecules in addition to inorganic ions [7, 8]. The SLC22 subfamily is responsible for the transport of organic ions and has been clustered in three different subgroups based on function and sequence homology such as organic cation transporters (OCTs), organic anion transporters (OATs) and organic zwitterion transporters (OCTNs) [18, 19].

Most of the OATs generally facilitate the movement of organic anions into the epithelial cells and are known as influx transporters [20]. Depending on their location OATs function in the uptake, reabsorption and excretion of drugs, nutrients and metabolites [18]. The best investigated OAT is *OAT1 (SLC22A6)* which has been cloned in 1996 as a kidney transporter [21]. Although OATs are also present in all barrier epithelia of the body, in liver, plasenta and brain; most of the SLC22A investigations have focused on the kidney. Accumulating evidence suggests that OATs are up-regulated in malignant tumors probably to supply the increased nutritional demand of the tumor cells. On the other hand, many members of the solute carriers have been associated with the uptake, distribution and excretion of several drugs [22–26]. It has been reported that renal drug excretion in proximal tubules is mediated by SLC22 family transporters [27, 28]. Shinatsar et al. investigated mRNA expression levels of some members of the SLCA22A family in renal cell carcinoma cell lines and reported that expression of *SLC22A3* increases the chemosensitivity to some drugs in kidney carcinoma cell lines [29]. Some other members of the SLC22A have been associated with pathological characteristics of the tumor cells. For example, a high level of *SLC22A18* has been associated with the smaller tumor size while lower levels of *SLC22A1* and *SLC22A11* have been associated with angioinvasion in

Table 4 Genotypes and allele frequencies

Variation number	Genotype	n	Genotype Frequency	Allele	Allele Frequency
rs9503518	AA	61	0.772	A	0.842
	GG	7	0.089	G	0.158
	AG	11	0.139		
rs4959235	CC	58	0.841	C	0.920
	TT	0	0	T	0.080
	CT	11	0.159		
rs6923667	CC	28	0.384	C	0.603
	TT	13	0.178	T	0.397
	CT	32	0.438		

pancreatic ductal adenocarcinoma (PDAC) [30]. Database analysis has also shown that *SLC22A7* expression is associated with multicentric tumor occurence in hepatocellular carcinoma [31]. Depending upon Triple Negative Breast (TNB) cancer prediction and pathway analysis Chen et al. identified 6 genes, one of these being *SLC22A23* [32]. However, detailed information is not available on the *SLC22A23* gene or its substrate. The first analysis of SLC22A23 has been performed by Bennet et al. who isolated the *SLC22A23* gene as a human homolog of the rat organic cation transporter by rapid amplification of cDNA ends (RACE) [12]. Additionally they also analyzed expression of the *SLC22A23* gene in cell lines. Performing functional expression analysis they proposed that SLC22A23 requires additional molecules or co-factors to show functional activity in the membrane transport. So far there is no study in the literature investigating the expression rate of the *SLC22A23* gene in cancer. Therefore, in view of our DEGs results we investigated expression levels of the *SLC22A23* gene in larynx tumor samples and observed up-regulation of the *SLC22A23* mRNA levels in a significant proportion of the tumors.

In recent years, it has been shown that SNPs in the membrane transporter genes may be involved in tumor development and progression as well as in the regulation of drug resistance. For example, SNPs *SLC22A1*, *SLC22A2*, *SLC22A6* and *SLC22A8* have been reported to be implicated in altered drug response [22, 33, 34]. Therefore, we also investigated three SNPs of the *SLC22A23* gene. One of these polymorphisms (rs9503518) has been associated with increased risk of cardiac arythmias. Some other polymorphisms of the *SLC22A23* gene have also been associated with complex diseases that have an inflammatory component such as IBD, endometriosis-related infertility which is an indicator of the transporter activity of the *SLC22A23* gene [13–15]. On the other hand, Aberq et al. attributed the QTc prolongation to the presence of rs4959235 polymorphism in the *SLC22A23* gene [16]. They proposed that rs4959235 mediates the effects of quetiapine via clearence of the drug from the heat or shuttling of the molecules which are involved in cardiac function. In our study group we observed an association between the rs9503518 polymorphism and the histological grade of the tumor. This indicates that *SLC22A23* may function in supplying of the nutritional needs of the cell. However, there is no data in the literature yet about the substrate of this transporter molecule.

Table 5 Association of rs9503518 with histological grade

		rs9503518			
		AA n (%)	GG n (%)	AG n (%)	p^a
Histological Grade	Grade 1	0 (0)	2 (2.5)	0 (0)	0.002
	Grade 2	24 (30.4)	3 (3.8)	6 (7.6)	
	Grade 3	26 (32.9)	2 (2.5)	3 (3.8)	
	Grade 4	6 (7.6)	0 (0)	1 (1.3)	
	Unknown	5 (6.3)	0 (0)	1 (1.3)	

[a]Statistical analyses were performed using the Pearson's chi-square test

Table 6 Association between the *SLC22A23* polymorphisms and gene expression

Variation number	Genotype	*SLC22A23* Gene Expression			
		No change n (%)	Decreased n (%)	Increased n (%)	p^a
rs9503518	A/A	6 (7.6)	23 (29.1)	32 (40.5)	0.046
	G/G	0 (0)	0 (0)	7 (8.9)	
	A/G	0 (0)	7 (8.9)	4 (5.1)	
rs4959235	C/C	5 (7.2)	19 (27.5)	34 (49.3)	0.360
	C/T	1 (1.4)	6 (8.7)	4 (5.8)	
rs6923667	C/C	1 (1.4)	12 (16.4)	15 (20.5)	0.556
	T/T	1 (1.4)	4 (5.5)	8 (11)	
	C/T	5 (6.8)	11 (15.1)	16 (21.9)	

[a]Statistical analyses were performed using the Pearson's chi-square test

Conclusions

In conclusion, as a preliminary report our results indicate that *SLC22A23* acts as one of the membrane transporters in larynx cancer which warrants further investigation in larynx cancer.

Abbreviations

ACP: Annealing Control Primer; B2M: Beta-2-microglobulin; BLAST: Basic Local Alignment Search Tool; DEG: Differently expressed gene; EDTA: Ethylenediaminetetraacetic acid; IBD: Inflammatory bowel disease; LB: Luria-Bertani; LSCC: Laryngeal squamous cell carcinoma; OAT: Organic anion transporter; OCT: Organic cation transporter; OCTN: Organic zwitterion transporter; PDAC: Pancreatic ductal adenocarcinoma; qRT-PCR: Quantitative real time polymerase chain reaction; RACE: Rapid Amplification of cDNA Ends; SLC: Solute carrier; SLC22A23: Solute carrier family 22, member 23; SNP: Single nucleotide polymorphism; TNB: Triple negative breast

Funding

The present study was supported by the Scientific Research Projects Coordination Unit of Istanbul University (Project numbers: 49005 and 24305).

Authors' contributions

SE performed GeneFishing assay, expression analysis experiments and participated in analysis and interpretation of data, also contributed to writing of the manuscript. DS performed genotyping assays. TU participated in the coordination of the study. JG provided tissue samples and clinical data. NB conceived the study, participated in its design and coordination, interpreted the data, and contributed to writing of the manuscript. All authors read and approved the final manuscript.

Competing interests

The authors declare that they have no competing interest.

Author details

[1]Cerrahpasa Medical Faculty, Department of Medical Biology, Istanbul University, Kocamustafapasa, 34098 Istanbul, Turkey. [2]Cerrahpasa Medical Faculty, Department of Otorhinolaryngology, Istanbul University, Istanbul, Turkey.

References

1. Siegel RL, Miller KD, Jemal A. Cancer statistics, 2016. CA Cancer J Clin. 2016; 66:7–30.
2. Bray I, Brennan P, Boffetta P. Projections of alcohol- and tobacco-related cancer mortality in Central Europe. Int J Cancer. 2000;87:122–8.
3. Li X, Gao L, Li H, Gao J, Yang Y, Zhou F, et al. Human papillomavirus infection and laryngeal cancer risk: a systematic review and meta-analysis. J Infect Dis. 2013;207:479–88.
4. Ferlay J, Steliarova-Foucher E, Lortet-Tieulent J, Rosso S, Coebergh JW, Comber H, et al. Cancer incidence and mortality patterns in Europe: estimates for 40 countries in 2012. Eur J Cancer. 2013;49:1374–403.
5. Fredriksson R, Nordström KJ, Stephansson O, Hägglund MG, Schiöth HB. The solute carrier (SLC) complement of the human genome: phylogenetic classification reveals four major families. FEBS Lett. 2008;582:3811–6.
6. Hägglund MG, Sreedharan S, Nilsson VC, Shaik JH, Almkvist IM, Bäcklin S, et al. Identification of SLC38A7 (SNAT7) protein as a glutamine transporter expressed in neurons. J Biol Chem. 2011;286:20500–11.
7. Rask-Andersen M, Masuram S, Fredriksson R, Schiöth HB. Solute carriers as drug targets: current use, clinical trials and prospective. Mol Asp Med. 2013; 34:702 10.
8. He L, Vasiliou K, Nebert DW. Analysis and update of the human solute carrier (SLC) gene superfamily. Hum Genomics. 2009;3:195–206.
9. Nakanishi T, Tamai I. Putative roles of organic anion transporting polypeptides (OATPs) in cell survival and progression of human cancers. Biopharm Drug Dispos. 2014;35:463–84.
10. Jong NN, McKeage MJ. Emerging roles of metal solute carriers in cancer mechanisms and treatment. Biopharm Drug Dispos. 2014;35:450–62.
11. Hediger MA, Romero MF, Peng JB, Rolfs A, Takanaga H, Bruford EA. The ABCs of solute carriers: physiological, pathological and therapeutic implications of human membrane transport proteinsIntroduction. Pflugers Arch. 2004;447:465–8.
12. Bennett KM, Liu J, Hoelting C, Stoll J. Expression and analysis of two novel rat organic cation transporter homologs, SLC22A17 and SLC22A23. Mol Cell Biochem. 2011;352:143–54.
13. Barrett JC, Hansoul S, Nicolae DL, Cho JH, Duerr RH, Rioux JD, et al. Genome-wide association defines more than 30 distinct susceptibility loci for Crohn's disease. Nat Genet. 2008;40:955–62.
14. Franke A, McGovern DP, Barrett JC, Wang K, Radford-Smith GL, Ahmad T, et al. Genome-wide meta-analysis increases to 71 the number of confirmed Crohn's disease susceptibility loci. Nat Genet. 2010;42:1118–25.
15. Zhao ZZ, Croft L, Nyholt DR, Chapman B, Treloar SA, Hull ML, et al. Evaluation of polymorphisms in predicted target sites for micro RNAs differentially expressed in endometriosis. Mol Hum Reprod. 2011;17: 92–103.
16. Aberg K, Adkins DE, Liu Y, McClay JL, Bukszár J, Jia P, et al. Genome-wide association study of antipsychotic-induced QTc interval prolongation. Pharmacogenomics J. 2012;12:165–72.
17. Schmittgen TD, Livak KJ. Analyzing real-time PCR data by the comparative C(T) method. Nat Protoc. 2008;3:1101–8.
18. Roth M, Obaidat A, Hagenbuch B. OATPs, OATs and OCTs: the organic anion and cation transporters of the SLCO and SLC22A gene superfamilies. Br J Pharmacol. 2012;165:1260–87.
19. Gründemann D, Gorboulev V, Gambaryan S, Veyhl M, Koepsell H. Drug excretion mediated by a new prototype of polyspecific transporter. Nature. 1994;372:549–52.
20. Kullak-Ublick GA, Hagenbuch B, Stieger B, Schteingart CD, Hofmann AF, Wolkoff AW, et al. Molecular and functional characterization of an organic anion transporting polypeptide cloned from human liver. Gastroenterology. 1995;109:1274–82.
21. Lopez-Nieto CE, You G, Barros EJ, Beier DR, Nigam SK, et al. J Am Soc Nephrol. 1996;7:1301.
22. Nigam SK, Bush KT, Martovetsky G, Ahn SY, Liu HC, Richard E, et al. The organic anion transporter (OAT) family: a systems biology perspective. Physiol Rev. 2015;95:83–123.
23. Nigam SK. What do drug transporters really do? Nat Rev Drug Discov. 2015; 14:29–44.
24. Koepsell H. The SLC22 family with transporters of organic cations, anions and zwitterions. Mol Asp Med. 2013;34:413–35.
25. Srimaroeng C, Perry JL, Pritchard JB. Physiology, structure, and regulation of the cloned organic anion transporters. Xenobiotica. 2008;38:889–935.
26. Emami Riedmaier A, Nies AT, Schaeffeler E, Schwab M. Organic anion transporters and their implications in pharmacotherapy. Pharmacol Rev. 2012;64:421–49.
27. Burckhardt BC, Burckhardt G. Transport of organic anions across the basolateral membrane of proximal tubule cells. Rev Physiol Biochem Pharmacol. 2003;146:95–158.
28. Wright SH, Dantzler WH. Molecular and cellular physiology of renal organic cation and anion transport. Physiol Rev. 2004;84:987–1049.
29. Shnitsar V, Eckardt R, Gupta S, Grottker J, Müller GA, Koepsell H, et al. Expression of human organic cation transporter 3 in kidney carcinoma cell lines increases chemosensitivity to melphalan, irinotecan, and vincristine. Cancer Res. 2009;69:1494–501.
30. Mohelnikova-Duchonova B, Brynychova V, Hlavac V, Kocik M, Oliverius M, Hlavsa J, et al. The association between the expression of solute carrier transporters and the prognosis of pancreatic cancer. Cancer Chemother Pharmacol. 2013;72:669–82.
31. Kudo A, Mogushi K, Takayama T, Matsumura S, Ban D, Irie T, et al. Mitochondrial metabolism in the noncancerous liver determine the occurrence of hepatocellular carcinoma: a prospective study. J Gastroenterol. 2014;49:502–10.
32. Chen LH, Kuo WH, Tsai MH, Chen PC, Hsiao CK, Chuang EY, et al. Identification of prognostic genes for recurrent risk prediction in triple negative breast cancer patients in Taiwan. PLoS One. 2011;6:e28222.

29

CD31 and VEGF are prognostic biomarkers in early-stage, but not in late-stage, laryngeal squamous cell carcinoma

Anke Schlüter[1], Patrick Weller[1], Oliver Kanaan[1], Ivonne Nel[2,4], Lukas Heusgen[1,5], Benedikt Höing[1], Pia Haßkamp[1], Sebastian Zander[1], Magis Mandapathil[1,6], Nina Dominas[1], Judith Arnolds[1], Boris A. Stuck[1,7], Stephan Lang[1], Agnes Bankfalvi[3] and Sven Brandau[1,8*] [iD]

Abstract

Background: Patients suffering from squamous cell carcinoma of the larynx (LSCC) with lymphatic metastasis have a relatively poor prognosis and often require radical therapeutic management. The mechanisms which drive metastasis to the lymph nodes are largely unknown but may be promoted by a pro-angiogenic tumor microenvironment. In this study, we examined whether the number of microvessels and the expression level of vascular endothelial growth factor (VEGF) in the primary tumor are correlated with the degree of lymph node metastasis (N-stage), tumor staging (T) and survival time in LSCC patients.

Methods: Tissue-Microarrays of 97 LSCC patients were analyzed using immunohistochemistry. The expression of VEGF was scored as intensity of staining (low vs high) and the number of CD31-positive vessels (median $</\geq 7$ vessels per visual field) was counted manually. Scores were correlated with N-stage, T-stage and 5-year overall survival rate.

Results: A high expression of angiogenic biomarkers was not associated with poor overall survival in the overall cohort of patients. Instead high CD31 count was associated with early stage cancer ($p = 0.004$) and in this subgroup high VEGF expression correlated with poor survival ($p = 0.032$). Additionally, in early stage cancer a high vessel count was associated with an increased recurrence rate ($p = 0.004$).

Conclusion: Only in the early stage subgroup a high expression of angiogenic biomarkers was associated with reduced survival and an increased rate of recurrence. Thus, biomarkers of angiogenesis may be useful to identify high risk patients specifically in early stage LSCC.

Keywords: Angiogenesis, Laryngeal squamous cell carcinoma, Biomarkers, VEGF, CD31

Background

Head and neck carcinomas with lymphatic metastasis usually require radical therapeutic management and are associated with poor prognosis. This is particularly true for squamous cell carcinoma of the larynx (LSCC). In addition, patients with lymph node (LN) involvement have a worse prognosis compared to patients without LN metastasis [1]. The identification of early stage LSCC patients at high risk therefore could help improving prognosis and treatment selection and preventing recurrence [2, 3]. Although clinically of high importance, the mechanisms which drive metastasis to the lymph nodes in LSCC are still largely unknown. It has been suggested that a pro-angiogenic tumor microenvironment may promote lymphatic metastasis [4–6]. The presence of neovascularization around neoplastic tissue is a typical finding in many solid tumors. Angiogenesis seems to be an important biological parameter implicated in tumor growth, metastasis and progression [4, 5]. However, in LSCC controversial data with respect to the impact of

* Correspondence: sven.brandau@uk-essen.de
[1]Department of Otorhinolaryngology, Head and Neck Surgery, University Hospital Essen, Essen, Germany
[8]Experimental and Translational Research, Department of Otorhinolaryngology, University Hospital Essen, Hufelandstrasse 55, 45147 Essen, Germany
Full list of author information is available at the end of the article

CD31 and VEGF are prognostic biomarkers in early-stage, but not in late-stage, laryngeal squamous cell...

243

angiogenesis on metastasis have been reported. Some studies suggested angiogenesis as a precursor for regional lymph node metastasis [6] and implicated microvessel density in local tumor progression [7]. In contrast, other studies did not show any prognostic relation between angiogenesis and prognosis, especially in patients with LSCC [8–11].

Well defined markers of angiogenesis are CD31 and vascular endothelial growth factor (VEGF). CD31 is highly expressed on the surface of endothelial cells and well established for the monitoring of vessel density in malignant tissue. It is a member of the Immunoglobulin-superfamily PECAM-1 [12] and it was reported that CD31 is involved in angiogenesis for example in early breast cancer [13]. CD31 was even used as a prognostic marker for nasopharyngeal cancer [14]. Sion-Vaardy et al. found a significantly increased number of vessels in head and neck tumors with deeper invasion [15]. Kyzas et al., however, have questioned the role of CD31 for the prognosis of LSCC in their study on 69 patients with LSCC and oral cancer. They rather suggested that the expression of VEGF might have prognostic significance in these patients [16].

VEGF is an important growth factor and signaling molecule involved in vasculogenesis and angiogenesis [17]. VEGF was reported to influence the pathogenesis of LSCC as a parameter of angiogenesis [16, 18–21]. In addition, a gene polymorphism of VEGF was suspected to be a risk factor for LSCC [22]. Chen et al. found as well that VEGF influenced the pathogenesis of head and neck cancer and supposed an important role of VEGF as a serological biomarker [23]. In contrast, Burian et al. were not able to demonstrate a relevant impact of elevated VEGF in the prognostic relevance of LSCC [8].

The controversial results regarding the role of these angiogenic factors may be due to the heterogeneity of the patient cohorts with regard to early or late stage disease. The aim of this study therefore was to investigate a possible relation between markers of angiogenesis, N-stage, T-stage, overall survival and recurrence rates in a cohort of 97 patients with LSCC with a special emphasis on tumor stage.

Methods

Study population and ethics approval

Patients with LSCC treated in the Department of Otorhinolaryngology, Head and Neck Surgery at the University Hospital Essen between 1995 and 2004 were included in this study. Samples of tumor tissue were collected during diagnostic biopsies or tumor resection and were stored for later analysis. Preparation of tissue and immunohistochemistry were performed between March 2014 and December 2014. Patient characteristics and data on survival were retrospectively assessed by extracting the corresponding data from the patient medical charts. Analysis of experimental data was performed in a completely anonymous fashion. The study was approved by the local ethics committee of the Medical Faculty of the University Duisburg-Essen (12–5192-BO) and was performed according to Declaration of Helsinki. Based on the retrospective and anonymous character of the study the approval contained a waiver for written informed consent. Tumor staging was performed according to the criteria of the Tumor-Node-Metastasis staging system, first reported by Pierre Denoix in the 1940's and adapted and compiled by the International Union against Cancer (UICC) [24]. Treatment regimens were planned according to tumor stage, surgical possibilities and patients´ decision. Patients with low T stage (T1 and T2) underwent mostly surgical therapy (70%). For patients with high T-stage (T3 + T4) surgery followed by RTX was chosen in the majority of cases (66%); more details on the treatment regimens are listed in Table 1.

Recurrence was defined as local relapse or cervical lymph node metastasis within 5 years after diagnosis. Overall recurrence rate was 27% (16 out of 59 patients from whom recurrence data were available, Table 1).

Preparation of tissue microarrays and immunohistochemistry

For preparation of tissue microarrays whole slides were inspected by a trained pathologist and regions of interest containing malignant tissue areas were marked. The tissue cores of 3 mm thickness were extracted from formalin-fixed/paraffin-embedded tumor tissue blocks using a skin biopsy punch (PFM, Cologne, Germany) and cut into 5 μm sections. Subsequently, the cores were de-parafinised and the antigens were retrieved by HIAR (heat-induced antigen retrieval) in citrate buffer pH 6.0 (Sigma–Aldrich, Taufkirchen, Germany). Samples were incubated with the primary antibodies (monoclonal mouse anti-human CD31, eBioscience, San Diego, USA and polyclonal rabbit anti-human VEGF, Millipore, Schwalbach, Germany) at 4 °C overnight. Then samples were incubated with peroxidase-coupled secondary antibodies for 30 min at room temperature and developed with AEC solution (Invitrogen, Karlsruhe, Germany) for 10 min. Nuclei were stained with haematoxylin (Carl Roth, Karlsruhe, Germany) for 1 min. Samples were covered with Kaisers glycerin gelatin (Merck, Darmstadt, Germany) and analyzed with a Zeiss Axioscope 2 microscope (Zeiss, Jena, Germany) at 200-fold magnification. Three trained scientists independently performed blinded scoring. VEGF expression was scored as intensity of the staining reaction in the samples and the immune reactive score (IRS) was calculated as mean IRS score of the three independent observers. VEGF was scored as *negative, weak, medium* and *strong* and subsequently categorized into low and high expression grade

Table 1 Patient Demographics

Demographic	Patients (n = 97)	
	No.	%
Tumor Staging		
T1	21	21
T2	29	30
T3	24	25
T4	23	24
Lymph nodes (N-stage)		
N0	67	70
N1	9	9
N2	20	20
N3	1	1
Gender		
male	86	89
female	11	11
Therapeutical Treatment		
Surgery	44	45
Surgery+RCTX	8	8
Surgery+RTX	40	41
RCTX	2	2
RTX	3	3
	Patients (n = 59)	
Recurrence No. of Patients	yes	no
T1	3	14
T2	9	9
T3	3	7
T4	1	13
Distribution Data (Total no.)	VEGF	CD31
No. of patients (97)	87	89
Recurrence total (59)	50	52
T-stage low (50)	42	46
Recurrence T-stage low (34)	27	30
N0 (67)	58	59
Recurrence N0 (44)	39	41

Patients with LSCC who were treated between 1995 and 2004 in our department were consecutively included in this study (n = 97). Distribution of T-stage, N-stage, gender and treatment of the patients is shown. For patients with available recurrence data a correlation between expression of VEGF/CD31 and the rate of recurrence during 5 year follow up was performed. The lower panel of the table indicates the number of patients eligible for analysis of recurrence in the respective groups. Recurrence was defined as local relapse or cervical lymph node metastasis within 5 years after diagnosis. Number of recurrences and break-up according to T stage are also shown

(Fig. 1a). Absolute numbers of CD31-positive vessels were quantified in four visual microscopic fields per sample and were expressed as mean per sample (Fig. 1b and c). Scores were correlated with N-stage, T-stage, recurrence and 5-year overall survival rate.

Statistical analysis

Statistical analyses were performed using SPSS© (Statistical Package for the Social Sciences, IBM©) statistical software version 20.0. The level of significance was set to $p < 0.05$. All P-values were based on two sided tests. The 5-years-survival curves were plotted according to the Kaplan–Meier method. Significance was tested using the log-rank test. Kruskal-Wallis-test and Mann-Whitney-U test were used to correlate clinical-pathological parameters such as T- and N-stage, respectively, with the number of CD31-positive vessels and VEGF expression. Chi square test was performed to analyze recurrence rates and CD31/VEGF expression in patients with early stage LSCC.

Results
Patient cohort

Ninety-seven patients were included in the study and for all patients complete clinical and immunohistochemical data was available. Patients were predominantly male (89%) and tumor stage equally distributed from T1 to T4. VEGF staining was evaluable in 87/97 patients and CD31 data in 89/97 patients. Follow up data were available for 59 (out of 97 patients) in the overall cohort, 34 (out of 50) patients with low T-stage and 44 (out of 67) patients with negative N-stage. Patient demographics are described in Table 1.

Immunohistochemical scores for VEGF and CD31

VEGF was scored as described above and the number of CD31 positive intratumoral vessels per visual field was quantified and ranged between 0 and 30 (example shown in Fig. 1a+b). Patients were divided into two groups according to the median of CD31-positive vessels, which was calculated as 7.3 (fig. 1c). In subsequent analyses patients with low (< 7) vs high (≥7) vessel count were compared.

A high number of CD31-positive vessels correlates with low T-stage and negative N-stage

As expected, a positive N-stage significantly correlated with high T-stage in our cohort ($p = 0.001$; Fig. 2a). Interestingly, a high number of CD31-positive vessels was significantly associated with lower T-stage (T1 + T2) ($p = 0.004$; Fig. 2b). In addition, the number of CD31-positive vessels also correlated with N-stage. Interestingly, a high vessel count was rather associated with the absence of lymph node metastasis (N0 status) and not with N+ status (Fig. 2c, $p = 0.028$). These data show that low stage LSCC is characterized by high vessel density. VEGF staining intensity was not significantly associated with T- or N-stage (data not shown).

Prognostic relevance of angiogenic biomarkers

The potential prognostic value of the two biomarkers in the total cohort of LSCC patients was tested. However,

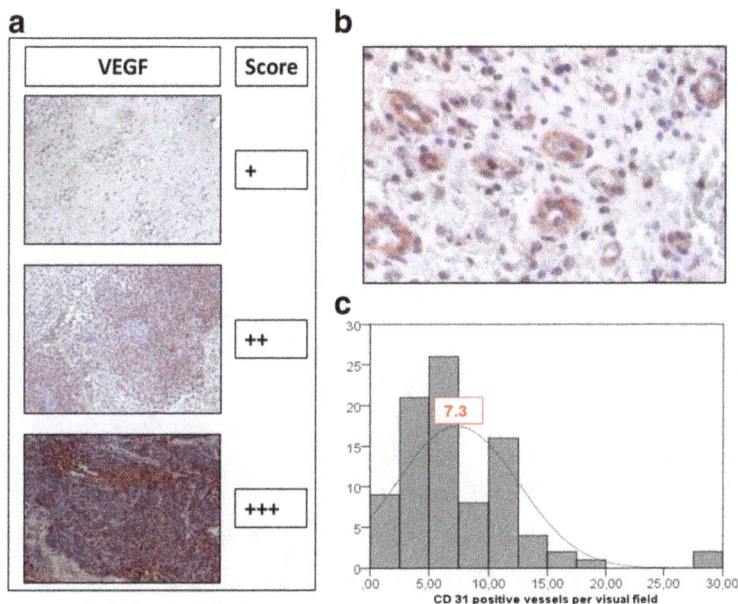

Fig. 1 Immunohistochemical staining and analysis. Immunohistochemical staining of VEGF (**a**) and CD31 (**b**) was evaluated. The immune reactive score (IRS) of VEGF was calculated as intensity of the staining reaction, evaluated by three independent observers. VEGF was scored as absent (−), *weak (+)*, *medium (++)*, and *strong (+++)* (Magnification = 200×) and categorized in low and high. Low includes −/+ and high includes ++/+++. CD31 was scored by absolute vessel counting per visual field (**b**). The median of the counted CD31-positive vessels was 7.3 per visual field (**c**) and was used as a cut-off to categorize patients into low (< 7) vs high (≥7)

neither vessel density nor VEGF expression were associated with overall survival in the total cohort (data not shown). Based on these results a potential correlation of VEGF and CD31 with overall survival was assessed separately in patients with early (T1 and T2, N0) and late (T3 and T4, N+) stage LSCC using Kaplan-Meier analysis. Strong VEGF expression was associated with poor survival in N0 patients, although not reaching statistical significance ($p = 0.116$; Fig. 3a). No association was found in patients with positive N-stage ($p = 0.927$, not shown). Strong VEGF expression also correlated with poor survival in patients with low T-stage (T1 and T2; $p = 0.032$; Fig. 3a). Again no correlation was found in patients with high T-stage (T3 and T4; $p = 0.846$; not shown). Thus, strong VEGF expression was associated with poor survival in early stage but not in late stage LSCC. In contrast, CD31 vessel count was not associated with overall survival in this LSCC cohort, neither in

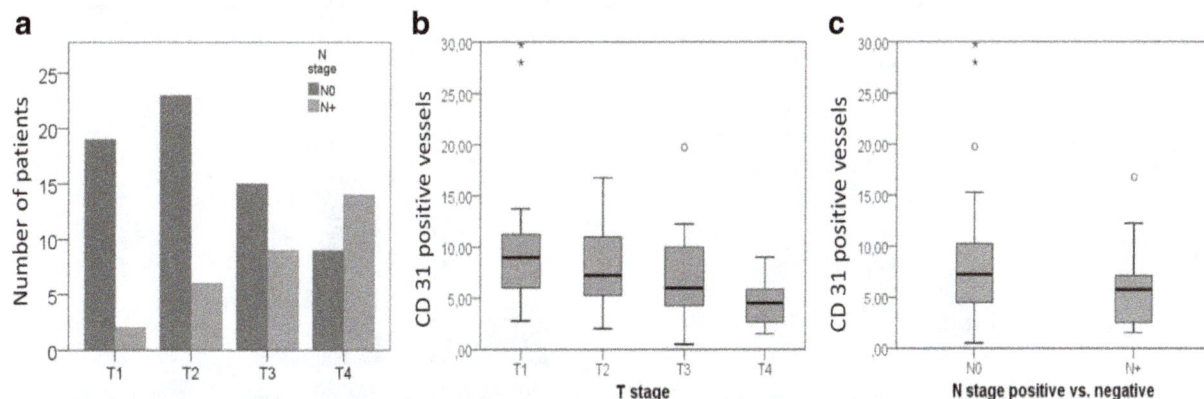

Fig. 2 Vessel density is increased in early stage LSCC. T-stage was determined in LSCC patients ($n = 97$). The number of patients without (N0) or with lymph node metastasis (N+) was determined for each T-stage. High T-stage correlated with positive node status (Kruskal-Wallis test; $p = 0.001$) (**a**). The absolute number of vessels per microscopic visual field was determined by immunohistochemistry and correlated with tumor T-stage (**b**) and N-stage (**c**). A high vessel count correlated with low T-stage (Kruskal-Wallis test; $p = 0.004$) and the absence of lymph node metastasis (Mann-Whitney-U test; $p = 0.028$). Data are depicted as box-plots indicating mean and absolute numbers of CD31 positive vessels and error bars

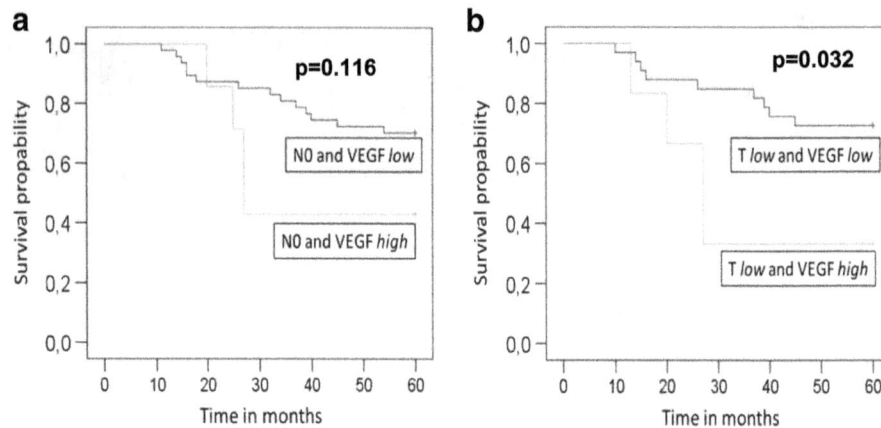

Fig. 3 Reduced expression of VEGF correlates with improved survival in early stage LSCC. Patients with negative N-stage ($n = 67$) (**a**) and low T-stage (T1 + T2, $n = 50$) (**b**) were grouped into either VEGF high or VEGF low and further examined in terms of their survival. Kaplan Meier analysis of survival and log rank test were performed

patients with early nor late stage disease (data not shown). Finally, we analyzed a potential link between CD31/VEGF and recurrence-free survival. No correlation was found between the VEGF score and the number of recurrences in early stage LSCC within the 5-year follow-up period. In contrast, our analyses revealed a potential link between vessel count and recurrence rate. As shown in fig. 4a patients with low T-stage and a low number of CD31-positive vessels had a tendency for better recurrence free survival compared to patients with low T-stage and high CD31-positive vessel number, although not reaching statistical significance (Fig. 4a, $p= 0.098$). Low CD31 vessel count significantly correlated with reduced recurrence rate in patients with negative N-stage ($p = 0.004$) (Fig. 4b).

Collectively, these data show that low expression of angiogenic biomarkers seems to be associated with improved clinical outcome in early stage, but not in advanced LSCC.

Discussion

A potential role for angiogenesis in the prognosis of cancer has been demonstrated in previous studies for different cancer types [5, 25–32]. It was the aim of this study to provide new information about the relation between angiogenesis, tumor stage and prognosis of LSCC.

Angiogenic biomarkers are particularly associated with early tumor stages

In non-laryngeal HNSCC, studies by Gleich et al. reported an association of angiogenesis with increasing T and N stage in oropharyngeal cancer (OPC) (higher T-stages here defined as T2-T4) [30], but there was no statistical correlation between tumor aggressiveness and

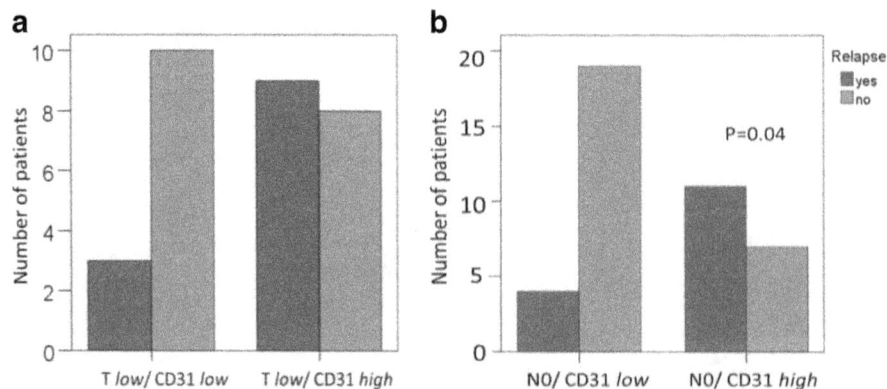

Fig. 4 High vessel count is associated with an increased recurrence rate in early stage LSCC. Chi-square-Test was applied to comparerelapse rates and vessel count in patients with (**a**) low T-stage or (**b**) negative N-stage. Patients with a high number of CD31-positive vessels early stage LSCC had a significantly higher relapse rate compared to patients with early LSCC and low number of CD 31-positive vessels. **a** Patients were grouped according to T-stage and vessel count. Number of patients with relapse within 5 years is indicated. Chi-square test; $p = 0.098$. **b** Patients were grouped according to N-stage and vessel count. Number of patients with relapse within 5 years is indicated. Chi-square test; $p = 0.004$

tumor angiogenesis in low T stages (here defined as T1) [33]. For LSCC, the literature provides controversial information whether angiogenesis is an early event in LSCC development or whether it is associated with increased tumor stages [24, 29, 34]. Some studies did not show any relation between angiogenesis and prognosis, especially in patients with LSCC [8–11]. In our study we demonstrated a significant correlation of CD31-positive vessels with early T-stages and the absence of LN metastasis (N0 status). There is a controversy in the literature regarding a direct relation between tumor stage and VEGF, another potential marker of angiogenesis. Some studies did not show any association [35] while others revealed significant correlations especially between N-stage and VEGF [27, 36–38]. Interestingly, Wang et al. even reported a strong association of VEGF expression with lymph node metastasis in primary laryngeal carcinomas [27]. In contrast, other studies did not reveal any association of angiogenesis with the presence of LN metastasis [25, 28]. In our analysis there was no direct correlation between T- or N-stage and VEGF.

Angiogenic biomarkers and their influence on prognosis

As mentioned above the VEGF expression of patients with LSCC is not directly related to T- or N-stage when analyzing the entire cohort. We noted, however, that patients with initial negative N-stage and low T-stage who have a strong VEGF expression showed reduced overall survival. This is in line with findings by Krecicki et al. who reported that a pro-angiogenic tumor microenvironment may promote lymphatic metastasis [6] and consecutively shorter survival. They identified vessel endothelial cells with antibodies against factor VIII and analyzed the vessel density (VD) per image in 55 patients with laryngeal cancer. In their study VD correlated with the existence of nodal metastases ($P = 0.02$) in contrast to histological grading of the tumor or the T-stage. The authors hypothesized that angiogenesis in laryngeal cancer may be of some value in predicting N-stage. In another study, Kupisz et al. found a direct correlation between increased tumor angiogenesis and increased T-stage, histologic grade and a shorter survival rate [25]. Teknos et al. reported that highly-vascularized tumors were associated with worse survival [26]. Williams et al. detected a higher regional recurrence rate in tumors with high angiogenesis and used it as an independent prognostic indicator [39]. Pignataro et al. as well showed that patients with poorly vascularized tumors had a tendency for better prognosis. Similar to our study, no relation between microvessel density and clinical pathological features or prognosis in the later tumor stages was found. The authors suggested that angiogenesis might be an early event in laryngeal tumorigenesis [29]. In our study positive N-stage was not associated with

high expression of angiogenic biomarkers in the primary tumor lesion suggesting that that these events are not directly spatiotemporally linked. Instead we found a potential link between angiogenesis and shorter survival exclusively in patients with early stage LSCC. A possible explanation for our findings would be that early stage tumors, which are highly angiogenic prepare the tumor for metastasis. However, these metastasis become clinically detectable at far later time points, when the microenvironment of the primary tumor is no longer characterized by highly expressed angiogenic biomarkers.

In patients with early tumor stage, we also investigated the recurrence rate and found that early recurrence was associated with a higher number of CD31-positive vessels, indicative of a pro-angiogenic microenvironment. Similarly, Bolzoni Villaret et al. analyzed angiogenesis and lymphangiogenesis using immunohistochemistry with antibodies against CD31 and podoplanin. Twenty seven patients with poor outcome were identified and compared with a selected sample of 28 patients. Based on analysis of these groups they concluded that patients with early T-stages of laryngeal cancer showing a pro-angiogenic microenvironment had a significantly higher rate of relapse [2]. Using semiquantitative scoring analysis Murray et al. [40] reported that angiogenesis (CD31 IHC) might be a significant predictor for relapse in patients with negative N-stage. In our study we can substantiate these findings using a large cohort of LSSC patients and exact absolute counting of vessels.

Relevance of presence of angiogenic biomarkers in early tumor stages in prognosis

In summary in this study we identified VEGF and CD31 as prognostic factors for the clinical outcome of patients with early stage laryngeal cancer. In particular, we demonstrated a significant correlation of CD31-positive vessels with early T-stages and the absence of LN metastasis (N0 status), respectively, but higher relapse rate and we identified strong VEGF expression as a marker of poor survival in patients with a low T-stage and a negative N-stage. Based on these data one could hypothesize that angiogenesis is of special clinical relevance at non-metastatic early tumor stages and determines later tumor progression already at this stage. Based on the data presented in this study we postulate that the quantification of high VEGF and CD31 in early tumor stages could be a useful tool to identify patients with poor prognosis at early tumor and lymph node stages. This could help to improve the clinical management of these patients. As several anti-angiogenic drugs have been developed in the past years [41] these drugs can be considered as additional therapeutic options in high risk LSCC patients with highly angiogenic cancers. Along this line, Beatrice et al. suggested to perform a special anti-angiogenic RCTX in patients with high capillary count even in case of surgical R0 resection. Our results further underscore the hypothesis that a proangiogenic microenvironment in early, non-metastatic stages might prepare the tumor for recurrence. Furthermore it indicates that high vessel densities, as well as strong VEGF expression, are characteristic for smaller tumors and might precede the development of metastasis at later stages. These findings would argue in favor of a more radical treatment of a small subgroup of patients with a highly angiogenic tumor microenvironment. However, further studies, ideally in a prospective design, should be performed to substantiate these findings.

Conclusion

Patients with low T-stage and negative N-stage are generally known to have a good five-year survival rate. However, our study identified a subgroup of patients with strong VEGF expression and high CD31-positive vessel number, which was linked to poor prognosis and increased risk for relapse. Thus, our study provides further evidence that quantification of angiogenesis in a subgroup of patients with laryngeal cancer could help to predict patient outcome and to better guide therapeutic decisions in this cancer entity.

Abbreviations

IRS: Immune Reactive Score; LN: Lymph Node; LSCC: laryngeal squamous cell carcinoma; VEGF: vascular endothelial growth factor

Acknowledgements

The authors wish to thank Petra Altenhoff (Department of Otorhinolaryngology, University Hospital Essen) for excellent technical support and Ulrike Krahn (University Hospital Essen, IMIBE = Institute of medical informatics, biometry and epidemiology) for support with the statistical analyses.

Funding

This research did not receive any specific grant from funding agencies in the public, commercial, or not-for-profit sectors. The funding body had no role in the design of the study and collection, analysis, and interpretation of data and in writing the manuscript.

Authors' contributions

Conception and design: SB. Provision of study materials or patients: AB, SZ, ND, JA, MM, SL. Collection and assembly of data: AS, PW, OK, LH, PH, BH. Data analysis and interpretation: AS, IN, PW, SB. Manuscript writing: AS, PW, IN, BAS, SB. Final approval of manuscript: all authors. All authors read and approved the final manuscript.

Competing interests

The authors declare that they have no competing interests.

Author details

[1]Department of Otorhinolaryngology, Head and Neck Surgery, University Hospital Essen, Essen, Germany. [2]Molecular Oncology Risk-Profile Evaluation, Department of Medical Oncology, West German Cancer Center, University Duisburg-Essen, 45122 Essen, Germany. [3]Institute for Pathology, University Hospital Essen, Essen, Germany. [4]Present address: ABA GmbH & Co.KG, BMZ2, 44227 Dortmund, Germany. [5]Present address: Martha-Maria Hospital Munich Solln, Munich, Germany. [6]Present address: Department of Otorhinolaryngology, Head and Neck Surgery, Asklepios Kliniken Hamburg, Hamburg, Germany. [7]Present address: Department of Otorhinolaryngology, Head and Neck Surgery, University Hospital Marburg, Marburg, Germany. [8]Experimental and Translational Research, Department of Otorhinolaryngology, University Hospital Essen, Hufelandstrasse 55, 45147 Essen, Germany.

References

1. Boffeta P, Merletti F, Faggiano F, Migliaretti G, Ferro G, Zanetti R, Terracini B. Prognostic factors and survival of laryngeal cancer patients from Turin, Italy. A population-based study. Am J Epidemiol. 1997;145:1100–5.
2. Bolzoni Villaret A, Barbieri D, Peretti G, et al. Angiogenesis and lymphangiogenesis in early-stage laryngeal carcinoma: prognostic implications. Head Neck. 2013;35:1132–7.
3. Lionello M, Staffieri A, Marioni G. Potential prognostic and therapeutic role for angiogenesis markers in laryngeal carcinoma. Acta Otolaryngol. 2012; 132:574–82.
4. Beatrice F, Cammarota R, Giordano C, et al. Angiogenesis: prognostic significance in laryngeal cancer. Anticancer Res. 1998;18:4737–40.
5. Liotta LA, Steeg PS, Stetler-Stevenson WG. Cancer metastasis and angiogenesis: an imbalance of positive and negative regulation. Cell. 1991;64:327–36.
6. Krecicki T, Dus D, Kozlak J, et al. Quantitative evaluation of angiogenesis in laryngeal cancer by digital image measurement of the vessel density. Auris Nasus Larynx. 2002;29:271–6.
7. Lentsch EJ, Goudy S, Sosnowski J, Major S, Bumpous JM. Microvessel density in head and neck squamous cell carcinoma primary tumors and its correlation with clinical staging parameters. Laryngoscope. 2006;116:397–400.
8. Burian M, Quint C, Neuchrist C. Angiogenic factors in laryngeal carcinomas: do they have prognostic relevance? Acta Otolaryngol. 1999;119:289–92.
9. Teppo H, Soini Y, Melkko J, Koivunen P, Alho O. Prognostic factors in laryngeal carcinoma: the role of apoptosis, p53, proliferation (Ki-67) and angiogenesis. APMIS. 2003;111:451–7.
10. Rodrigo JP, Cabanillas R, Chiara MD, Garcia Pedrero J, Astudillo A, Suarez Nieto C. Prognostic significance of angiogenesis in surgically treated supraglottic squamous cell carcinomas of the larynx. Acta Otorrinolaringol Esp. 2009;60:272–7.
11. Hagedorn HG, Nerlich AG. Microvessel density and endothelial basement membrane composition in laryngeal squamous cell carcinomas. Acta Otolaryngol. 2000;120:891–8.
12. Gumina RJ, Kirschbaum NE, Rao PN, vanTuinen P, Newman PJ. The human PECAM1 gene maps to 17q23. Genomics. 1996;34:229–32.
13. Jong JS. De, van Diest PJ, Baak JP. Heterogeneity and reproducibility of microvessel counts in breast cancer. Lab Investig. 1995;73:922–6.
14. Rubio L, Burgos JS, Morera C, Vera-Sempere FJ. Morphometric study of tumor angiogenesis as a new prognostic factor in nasopharyngeal carcinoma patients. Pathol Oncol Res. 2000;6:210–6.
15. Sion-Vardy N, Fliss DM, Prinsloo I, Shoham-Vardi I, Benharroch D. Neoangiogenesis in squamous cell carcinoma of the larynx - biological and prognostic associations. Pathol Res Pract. 2001;197:1–5.
16. Kyzas PA, Stefanou D, Batistatou A, Agnantis NJ. Prognostic significance of VEGF immunohistochemical expression and tumor angiogenesis in head and neck squamous cell carcinoma. J Cancer Res Clin Oncol. 2005;131:624–30.
17. Yla-Herttuala S, Rissanen TT, Vajanto I, Hartikainen J. Vascular endothelial growth factors: biology and current status of clinical applications in cardiovascular medicine. J Am Coll Cardiol. 2007;49:1015–26.
18. Sawatsubashi M, Yamada T, Fukushima N, Mizokami H, Tokunaga O, Shin T. Association of vascular endothelial growth factor and mast cells with angiogenesis in laryngeal squamous cell carcinoma. Virchows Arch. 2000;436:243–8.

19. Chen G, Liu Y, Wang J, et al. Expression of vascular endothelial growth factor and cyclooxygenase-2 in laryngeal squamous cell carcinoma and its significance. J Huazhong Univ Sci Technolog Med Sci. 2006;26:105–7.

20. Denhart BC, Guidi AJ, Tognazzi K, Dvorak HF, Brown LF. Vascular permeability factor/vascular endothelial growth factor and its receptors in oral and laryngeal squamous cell carcinoma and dysplasia. Lab Investig. 1997;77:659–64.

21. Neuchrist C, Quint C, Pammer A, Burian M. Vascular endothelial growth factor (VEGF) and microvessel density in squamous cell carcinomas of the larynx: an immunohistochemical study. Acta Otolaryngol. 1999;119:732–8.

22. Unal ZN, Unal M, Bagdatoglu OT, Polat G, Atik U. Genetic polymorphism of VEGF-1154 (a/G) in laryngeal squamous cell carcinoma. Arch Med Res. 2008; 39:209–11.

23. Chen Z, Malhotra PS, Thomas GR, et al. Expression of proinflammatory and proangiogenic cytokines in patients with head and neck cancer. Clin Cancer Res. 1999;5:1369–79.

24. Bernier J. Head and neck Cancer: multimodality management. New York: Springer; 2011.

25. Kupisz K, Chibowski D, Klatka J, Klonowski S, Stepulak A. Tumor angiogenesis in patients with laryngeal cancer. Eur Arch Otorhinolaryngol. 1999;256:303–5.

26. Teknos TN, Cox C, Barrios MA, et al. Tumor angiogenesis as a predictive marker for organ preservation in patients with advanced laryngeal carcinoma. Laryngoscope. 2002;112:844–51.

27. Wang Z, Chen Y, Li X, et al. Expression of VEGF-C/VEGFR-3 in human laryngeal squamous cell carcinomas and its significance for lymphatic metastasis. Asian Pac J Cancer Prev. 2012;13:27–31.

28. Bonhin RG, Rocha VBC, De Carvalho GM, et al. Correlation between vascular endothelial growth factor expression and presence of lymph node metastasis in advanced squamous cell carcinoma of the larynx. Braz J Otorhinolaryngol. 2015;81:58–62.

29. Pignataro L, Carboni N, Midolo V, et al. Clinical relevance of microvessel density in laryngeal squamous cell carcinomas. Int J Cancer. 2001;92:666–70.

30. Gleich LL, Biddinger PW, Duperier FD, Gluckman JL. Tumor angiogenesis as a prognostic indicator in T2-T4 oral cavity squamous cell carcinoma: a clinical-pathologic correlation. Head Neck. 1997;19:276–80.

31. Chaudhury TK, Lerner MP, Nordquist RE. Angiogenesis by human melanoma and breast cancer cells. Cancer Lett. 1980;11:43–9.

32. Frank R, Saclarides TJ, Leurgans S, Speziale NJ, Drab EA, Rubin DB. Tumor angiogenesis as a predictor of recurrence and survival in patients with node-negative Colon Cancer. Ann Surg. 1995;222(6):695–9.

33. Gleich LL, Biddinger PW, Pavelic ZP, Gluckman JL. Tumor angiogenesis in T1 oral cavity squamous cell carcinoma: role in predicting tumor aggressiveness. Head Neck. 1996;18:343–6.

34. Laitakari J, Nayha V, Stenback F. Size, shape, structure, and direction of angiogenesis in laryngeal tumour development. J Clin Pathol. 2004;57:394–401.

35. Akdeniz O, Akduman D, Haksever M, Ozkarakas H, Muezzinoglu B. Relationships between clinical behavior of laryngeal squamous cell carcinomas and expression of VEGF, MMP-9 and E-cadherin. Asian Pac J Cancer Prev. 2013;14:5301–10.

36. Baek S, Jung K, Lee S, et al. Prognostic significance of vascular endothelial growth factor-C expression and lymphatic vessel density in supraglottic squamous cell carcinoma. Laryngoscope. 2009;119:1325–30.

37. Sullu Y, Gun S, Atmaca S, Karagoz F, Kandemir B. Poor prognostic clinicopathologic features correlate with VEGF expression but not with PTEN expression in squamous cell carcinoma of the larynx. Diagn Pathol. 2010;5:35.

38. Hinojar-Gutierrez A, Fernandez-Contreras M, Gonzalez-Gonzalez R, et al. Intratumoral lymphatic vessels and VEGF-C expression are predictive factors of lymph node relapse in T1-T4 N0 laryngopharyngeal squamous cell carcinoma. Ann Surg Oncol. 2007;14:248–57.

39. Williams JK, Carlson GW, Cohen C, DeRose PB, Hunter S, Jurkiewicz MJ. Tumor angiogenesis as a prognostic factor in oral cavity tumors. Am J Surg. 1994;168:373–80.

40. Murray JD, Carlson GW, McLaughlin K, et al. Tumor angiogenesis as a prognostic factor in laryngeal cancer. Am J Surg. 1997;174:523–6.

41. Rajeev S, Shevde LA. Recent advances in anti-Angiogenic therapy of Cancer. Oncotarget. 2011;2(3):122–34.

Permissions

All chapters in this book were first published in CANCER, by BioMed Central; hereby published with permission under the Creative Commons Attribution License or equivalent. Every chapter published in this book has been scrutinized by our experts. Their significance has been extensively debated. The topics covered herein carry significant findings which will fuel the growth of the discipline. They may even be implemented as practical applications or may be referred to as a beginning point for another development.

The contributors of this book come from diverse backgrounds, making this book a truly international effort. This book will bring forth new frontiers with its revolutionizing research information and detailed analysis of the nascent developments around the world.

We would like to thank all the contributing authors for lending their expertise to make the book truly unique. They have played a crucial role in the development of this book. Without their invaluable contributions this book wouldn't have been possible. They have made vital efforts to compile up to date information on the varied aspects of this subject to make this book a valuable addition to the collection of many professionals and students.

This book was conceptualized with the vision of imparting up-to-date information and advanced data in this field. To ensure the same, a matchless editorial board was set up. Every individual on the board went through rigorous rounds of assessment to prove their worth. After which they invested a large part of their time researching and compiling the most relevant data for our readers.

The editorial board has been involved in producing this book since its inception. They have spent rigorous hours researching and exploring the diverse topics which have resulted in the successful publishing of this book. They have passed on their knowledge of decades through this book. To expedite this challenging task, the publisher supported the team at every step. A small team of assistant editors was also appointed to further simplify the editing procedure and attain best results for the readers.

Apart from the editorial board, the designing team has also invested a significant amount of their time in understanding the subject and creating the most relevant covers. They scrutinized every image to scout for the most suitable representation of the subject and create an appropriate cover for the book.

The publishing team has been an ardent support to the editorial, designing and production team. Their endless efforts to recruit the best for this project, has resulted in the accomplishment of this book. They are a veteran in the field of academics and their pool of knowledge is as vast as their experience in printing. Their expertise and guidance has proved useful at every step. Their uncompromising quality standards have made this book an exceptional effort. Their encouragement from time to time has been an inspiration for everyone.

The publisher and the editorial board hope that this book will prove to be a valuable piece of knowledge for researchers, students, practitioners and scholars across the globe.

List of Contributors

Timothy M. Hoggard
University of South Florida Morsani College of Medicine, 12901 Bruce B Downs Blvd., Tampa, FL 33612, USA

Evita Henderson-Jackson and Marilyn M. Bui
Department of Anatomic Pathology, 12901 Bruce B Downs Blvd., Tampa, FL 33612, USA
Sarcoma Department, 12901 Bruce B Downs Blvd., Tampa, FL 33612, USA

Jamie Caracciolo
Department of Diagnostic Imaging, 12901 Bruce B Downs Blvd., Tampa, FL 33612, USA

Jamie K. Teer
Department of Biostatistics and Bioinformatics, 12901 Bruce B Downs Blvd., Tampa, FL 33612, USA

Sean Yoder
Molecular Genomics Core Facility, 12901 Bruce B Downs Blvd., Tampa, FL 33612, USA

Ricardo J. Gonzalez and Andrew S. Brohl
Sarcoma Department, 12901 Bruce B Downs Blvd., Tampa, FL 33612, USA

Odion Binitie
Sarcoma Department, 12901 Bruce B Downs Blvd., Tampa, FL 33612, USA
Adolescent and Young Adult Program; H. Lee Moffitt Cancer Center and Research Institute, 12901 Bruce B Downs Blvd., Tampa, FL 33612, USA

Damon R. Reed
Sarcoma Department, 12901 Bruce B Downs Blvd., Tampa, FL 33612, USA
Chemical Biology and Molecular Medicine Program, 12901 Bruce B Downs Blvd., Tampa, FL 33612, USA
Adolescent and Young Adult Program; H. Lee Moffitt Cancer Center and Research Institute, 12901 Bruce B Downs Blvd., Tampa, FL 33612, USA

Francisco Bárbara Abreu Barros, Agnes Assao, Natália Galvão Garcia and Denise Tostes Oliveira
Department of Stomatology, Area of Pathology, Bauru School of Dentistry, University of São Paulo, Alameda Octávio Pinheiro Brisolla, 9-75, Bauru, São Paulo 17012-901, Brazil

Suely Nonogaki
Adolfo Lutz Institute, Pathology Division, São Paulo, Brazil

André Lopes Carvalho
Fundação Pio XII Institution – Cancer Hospital of Barretos, Barretos, São Paulo, Brazil

Fernando Augusto Soares
Rede D'Or Hospitals Network - Pathology Division São Paulo, Brazil

Luiz Paulo Kowalski
Department of Head and Neck Surgery and Otorhinolaringology, A.C.Camargo Cancer Center Hospital, São Paulo, Brazil

Cédric Panje, Oliver Riesterer and Christoph Glanzmann
Department of Radiation Oncology, University Hospital Zurich, Rämistrasse 100, CH-8091 Zürich, Switzerland

Gabriela Studer
Department of Radiation Oncology, University Hospital Zurich, Rämistrasse 100, CH-8091 Zürich, Switzerland
Cantonal Hospital Lucerne, Spitalstrasse, CH-6000 Lucerne, Switzerland

Mushfiq H. Shaikh
School of Dentistry and Oral Health, Griffith University, Gold Coast, QLD 4222, Australia
School of Medical Science, Griffith University, Gold Coast, QLD 4222, Australia
Understanding Chronic Conditions Program, Menzies Health Institute Queensland, Gold Coast, QLD 4222, Australia

Daniel T. W. Clarke and Nigel A. J. McMillan
School of Medical Science, Griffith University, Gold Coast, QLD 4222, Australia
Understanding Chronic Conditions Program, Menzies Health Institute Queensland, Gold Coast, QLD 4222, Australia

Aminul I. Khan
Department of Pathology, National Medical College and Hospital, Dhaka 1100, Bangladesh

Anwar Sadat
Department of Oral and Maxillo-facial Surgery, Dhaka Dental College and Hospital, Dhaka 1216, Bangladesh

Ahmed H. Chowdhury
Department of Neuro-medicine, Dhaka Medical College and Hospital, Dhaka 1000, Bangladesh

Shahed A. Jinnah
Department of Pathology, Dhaka Medical College and Hospital, Dhaka 1000, Bangladesh

Vinod Gopalan and Alfred K. Lam
School of Medicine, Griffith University, Gold Coast, QLD 4222, Australia

Newell W. Johnson
School of Dentistry and Oral Health, Griffith University, Gold Coast, QLD 4222, Australia
Understanding Chronic Conditions Program, Menzies Health Institute Queensland, Gold Coast, QLD 4222, Australia
Dental Institute, King's College London, London, UK
Menzies Health Institute Queensland and School of Dentistry and Oral Health, Griffith University, Building G40, Room 9.16, Gold Coast Campus, Gold Coast, QLD 4222, Australia

Verena Ruhlmann, Thorsten D. Poeppel, Andreas Bockisch and Ken Herrmann
Department of Nuclear Medicine, University Duisburg-Essen, Medical Faculty, University Hospital Essen, Hufelandstrasse 55, 45147 Essen, Germany

Johannes Veit and Thomas K. Hoffmann
Department of Oto-Rhino-Laryngology, Head and Neck Surgery, University Hospital Ulm, Frauensteige 12, 89070 Ulm, Germany

James Nagarajah
Department of Nuclear Medicine, Radboud University Nijmegen Medical Centre, Geert Grooteplein 8, 6525, GA, Nijmegen, the Netherlands

Lale Umutlu
Department of Diagnostic and Interventional Radiology and Neuroradiology, University Duisburg Essen, University Hospital Essen, Hufelandstrasse 55, 45147 Essen, Germany

Wolfgang Sauerwein
Department of Radiation Oncology, University Duisburg-Essen, University Hospital Essen, Hufelandstrasse 55, 45147 Essen, Germany

Joost H. van Ginkel
Department of Oral and Maxillofacial Surgery, University Medical Center Utrecht, Utrecht, The Netherlands
Department of Pathology, University Medical Center Utrecht, Heidelberglaan 100, 3584 CX Utrecht, The Netherlands

Manon M. H. Huibers and Stefan M. Willems
Department of Pathology, University Medical Center Utrecht, Heidelberglaan 100, 3584 CX Utrecht, The Netherlands

Robert J. J. van Es
Department of Oral and Maxillofacial Surgery, University Medical Center Utrecht, Utrecht, The Netherlands
Department of Head and Neck Surgical Oncology, UMC Utrecht Cancer Center, University Medical Center Utrecht, Utrecht, The Netherlands

Remco de Bree
Department of Head and Neck Surgical Oncology, UMC Utrecht Cancer Center, University Medical Center Utrecht, Utrecht, The Netherlands

Manuel Weber, Jutta Ries, Patrick Moebius, Raimund Preidl, Friedrich W. Neukam and Falk Wehrhan
Department of Oral and Maxillofacial Surgery, Friedrich-Alexander University Erlangen-Nürnberg, Glueckstrasse 11, 91054 Erlangen, Germany

Maike Büttner-Herold
Institute of Pathology, Department of Nephro-pathology, Friedrich-Alexander University Erlangen-Nürnberg, Erlangen, Germany

Luitpold Distel
Department of Radiation Oncology, Friedrich-Alexander University Erlangen-Nürnberg, Erlangen, Germany

Carol I. Geppert
Institute of Pathology, Friedrich-Alexander University Erlangen-Nürnberg, Erlangen, Germany

Sang-Yeon Kim and Min-Sik Kim
Department of Otolaryngology-Head and Neck Surgery, College of Medicine, The Catholic University of Korea, Seoul, Republic of Korea

Young-Soo Rho and Min Woo Park
Department of Otorhinolaryngology-Head and Neck Surgery, Ilsong Memorial Institute of Head and Neck Cancer, Hallym University, College of Medicine, Seoul, Republic of Korea

Eun-Chang Choi and Da-Hee Kim
Department of Otorhinolaryngology, Yonsei University, College of Medicine, Seoul, Republic of Korea

Joo-Hyun Woo
Department of Otolaryngology Head and Neck Surgery, Gachon University Gil Hospital, Incheon, Korea

Dong Hoon Lee
Department of Otolaryngology-Head and Neck Surgery, Chonnam National University Medical School and Chonnam National University Hwasun Hospital, Hwasun, Korea

Eun Jae Chung
Department of Otorhinolaryngology–Head and Neck Surgery, Seoul National University College of Medicine, Seoul, Korea

Young-Hoon Joo
Department of Otolaryngology-Head and Neck Surgery, College of Medicine, The Catholic University of Korea, Seoul, Republic of Korea
Department of Otolaryngology, Head and Neck Surgery, Bucheon St. Mary's Hospital, College of Medicine, The Catholic University of Korea, 2 Sosa-dong, Wonmi-gu, Bucheon, Kyounggi-do 420-717, Republic of Korea

Shan-Shan Guo, Wen Hu, Qiu-Yan Chen, Jian-Mei Li, Shi-Heng Zhu, Yan He, Jia-Wen Li, Le Xia, Lu Ji, Cui-Ying Lin, Li-Ting Liu, Lin-Quan Tang, Ling Guo, Hao-Yuan Mo, Chong Zhao, Xiang Guo, Ka-Jia Cao, Chao-Nan Qian, Yu-Ying Fan and Hai-Qiang Mai
State Key Laboratory of Oncology in South China, Collaborative Innovation Center for Cancer Medicine, Sun Yat-Sen University Cancer Center, Guangzhou 510060, People's Republic of China
Department of Nasopharyngeal Carcinoma, Sun Yat-Sen University Cancer Center, 651 Dongfeng Road East, Guangzhou 510060, People's Republic of China

Mu-Sheng Zeng
State Key Laboratory of Oncology in South China, Collaborative Innovation Center for Cancer Medicine, Sun Yat-Sen University Cancer Center, Guangzhou 510060, People's Republic of China

Ming-Huang Hong
State Key Laboratory of Oncology in South China, Collaborative Innovation Center for Cancer Medicine, Sun Yat-Sen University Cancer Center, Guangzhou 510060, People's Republic of China
Good Clinical Practice center, Sun Yat-Sen University Cancer Center, 651 Dongfeng Road East, Guangzhou 510060, People's Republic of China

Jian-Yong Shao
State Key Laboratory of Oncology in South China, Collaborative Innovation Center for Cancer Medicine, Sun Yat-Sen University Cancer Center, Guangzhou 510060, People's Republic of China
Department of Molecular Diagnostics, Sun Yat-Sen University Cancer Center, 651 Dongfeng Road East, Guangzhou 510060, People's Republic of China

Ying Sun and Jun Ma
State Key Laboratory of Oncology in South China, Collaborative Innovation Center for Cancer Medicine, Sun Yat-Sen University Cancer Center, Guangzhou 510060, People's Republic of China

Department of Radiation Oncology, Sun Yat-Sen University Cancer Center, Guangzhou 510060, People's Republic of China

Gerhard Dyckhoff and Peter K. Plinkert
Department of Otorhinolaryngology, Head and Neck Surgery, University of Heidelberg, Im Neuenheimer Feld 400, 69120 Heidelberg, Germany

Heribert Ramroth
Institute of Public Health, University of Heidelberg, INF 324, 69120 Heidelberg, Germany

Arutha Kulasinghe and Chamindie Punyadeera
The School of Biomedical Sciences, Institute of Health and Biomedical Innovation, Queensland University of Technology, Kelvin Grove, QLD, Australia
Translational Research Institute, Brisbane, Australia

Chris Perry
Department of Otolaryngology, Princess Alexandra Hospital, QLD, Woolloongabba, Australia

Liz Kenny
School of Medicine, University of Queensland, Brisbane, QLD, Australia
Royal Brisbane and Women's Hospital, Brisbane, QLD, Australia
Central Integrated Regional Cancer Service, Queensland Health, Brisbane, QLD, Australia

Majid E. Warkiani
School of Mechanical and Manufacturing Engineering, Australian Centre for NanoMedicine, University of New South Wales, Sydney, Australia
Garvan Institute for Biomedical Research, Sydney, Australia
School of Medical Sciences, Edith Cowan University, Joondalup, Perth, WA 6027, Australia

Colleen Nelson
Australian Prostate Cancer Research Centre - Queensland, Institute of Health and Biomedical Innovation, Queensland University of Technology, Princess Alexandra Hospital, Translational Research Institute Brisbane, Brisbane, Australia

Ayumi Sakuramoto, Yoko Hasegawa, Kazuma Sugahara, Kana Hasegawa, Mai Kurashita, Junya Sakai and Hiromitsu Kishimoto
Department of Dentistry and Oral Surgery, Hyogo College of Medicine, 1-1 Mukogawa-cho, Nishinomiya, Hyogo 663-8501, Japan

Yoshiyuki Komoda
Department of Chemical Science and Engineering, Graduate School of Engineering, Kobe University, Kobe, Hyogo 657-8501, Japan

Shinichi Hikasa
Department of Pharmacy, Hyogo College of Medicine, 1-1 Mukogawa-cho, Nishinomiya, Hyogo 663-8501, Japan

Masahiro Arita
Division of Occlusion and Maxillofacial Reconstruction, Department of Oral Function, School of Dentistry, Kyushu Dental University, Kitakyushu, Fukuoka 803-8580, Japan

Kazuhiro Yasukawa
Medical Research Group, Development Department. Takiron Co., Ltd., Osaka, Japan

Lu-Lu Zhang, Guan-Qun Zhou, Zhen-Yu Qi, Ling-Long Tang, Yan-Ping Mao and Ying Sun
Department of Radiation Oncology, Sun Yat-sen University Cancer Center, State Key Laboratory of Oncology in South China, Collaborative Innovation Center for Cancer Medicine, 651 Dongfeng Road East, Guangzhou 510060, People's Republic of China

Xiao-Jun He
Department of Clinical Medicine, School of Public Health, Sun Yat-sen University, Guangzhou, People's Republic of China

Jia-Xiang Li
Department of Oncology, First People's Hospital of Zhaoqing City, Guangdong, People's Republic of China

Ai-Hua Lin
Department of Oncology, First People's Hospital of Zhaoqing City, Guangdong, People's Republic of China
Department of Medical Statistics and Epidemiology, School of Public Health, Sun Yat-sen University, Guangzhou, People's Republic of China

Jun Ma
Department of Radiation Oncology, Sun Yat-sen University Cancer Center, State Key Laboratory of Oncology in South China, Collaborative Innovation Center for Cancer Medicine, 651 Dongfeng Road East, Guangzhou 510060, People's Republic of China
Department of Medical Statistics and Epidemiology, School of Public Health, Sun Yat-sen University, Guangzhou, People's Republic of China

Lina Wang
The State Key Laboratory Breeding Base of Basic Science of Stomatology (Hubei-MOST) and Key Laboratory of Oral Biomedicine Ministry of Education, School and Hospital of Stomatology, Wuhan University, 237 Luoyu road, Wuhan 430079, China

Department of Endodontics, College of Stomatology, Dalian Medical University, Dalian 116044, China

Wei Yin
The State Key Laboratory Breeding Base of Basic Science of Stomatology (Hubei-MOST) and Key Laboratory of Oral Biomedicine Ministry of Education, School and Hospital of Stomatology, Wuhan University, 237 Luoyu road, Wuhan 430079, China

Chun Shi
Department of Endodontics, College of Stomatology, Dalian Medical University, Dalian 116044, China

Go Omura and Kenya Kobayashi
Department of Otolaryngology-Head and Neck Surgery, Faculty of Medicine, The University of Tokyo, 7-3-1 Hongo, Bunkyo-ku, Tokyo 113-8655, Japan
2Department of Head and Neck Surgery, National Cancer Center Hospital, Tokyo, Japan

Mizuo Ando, Yuki Saito, Fukuoka, Ken Akashi, Osamu Masafumi Yoshida and Tatsuya Yamasoba
Department of Otolaryngology-Head and Neck Surgery, Faculty of Medicine, The University of Tokyo, 7-3-1 Hongo, Bunkyo-ku, Tokyo 113-8655, Japan

Yasuhiro Ebihara
Department of Otolaryngology-Head and Neck Surgery, Faculty of Medicine, The University of Tokyo, 7-3-1 Hongo, Bunkyo-ku, Tokyo 113-8655, Japan
Department of Head and Neck Surgery, Saitama Medical University International Medical Center, Saitama, Japan

Takahiro Asakage
Department of Otolaryngology-Head and Neck Surgery, Faculty of Medicine, The University of Tokyo, 7-3-1 Hongo, Bunkyo-ku, Tokyo 113-8655, Japan
Department of Head and Neck Surgery, Faculty of Medicine, Tokyo Medical and Dental University, Tokyo, Japan

Yi Su, Qiu-hong Yu, Xiang-yun Wang, Zong-feng Wang, Ying-chun Cao and Jian-dong Li
Department of E.N.T., Dongying People's Hospital, Shandong 257091, China

Li-ping Yu
Department of E.N.T., Kenli People's Hospital, Shandong, China

Koji Harada, Tarannum Ferdous and Yoshiya Ueyama
Department of Oral and Maxillofacial Surgery, Yamaguchi University Graduate School of Medicine, 1-1-1 Minamikogushi, Ube 755-8505, Japan

Frank K. Leusink and Eleftherios Koudounarakis
Department of Head and Neck Oncology and Surgery, Netherlands Cancer Institute – Antoni van Leeuwenhoek, Plesmanlaan 121, 1066, CX, Amsterdam, The Netherlands

Michael H. Frank and Ronald Koole
Department of Oral and Maxillofacial Surgery, University Medical Centre Utrecht, Heidelberglaan 100, 3584, CX, Utrecht, The Netherlands

Paul J. van Diest and Stefan M. Willems
Department of Pathology, University Medical Centre Utrecht, Heidelberglaan 100, 3584, CX, Utrecht, The Netherlands

Ye Tao, Yang Zhang and Zhigang Huang
Department of Otolaryngology-Head and Neck Surgery, Key Laboratory of Otolaryngology Head and Neck Surgery, Beijing Tongren Hospital, Capital Medical University, Beijing 100730, China

Neil Gross and Guojun Li
Department of Head and Neck Surgery, The University of Texas MD Anderson Cancer Center, Houston, TX 77030, USA

Xiaojiao Fan, Maikun Teng and Xu Li
Hefei National Laboratory for Physical Sciences at Microscale, Innovation Centre for Cell Signaling Network, School of Life Science, University of Science and Technology of China, Hefei, Anhui 230026, People's Republic of China

Jianming Yang
Department of Otolaryngology-Head and Neck Surgery, the Second Affiliated Hospital of Anhui Medical University, Hefei 230601, China

Yalian Yu, Aihui Yan, Xinyao Li and Wei Li
Department of Otorhinolaryngology, the First Affiliated Hospital of China Medical University, Shenyang, Liaoning Province, People's Republic of China.

Hongbo Wang
Department of Radiology, Shengjing Hospital of China Medical University, Shenyang, Liaoning Province, People's Republic of China

Hailong Wang
Department of Clinical Epidemiology and Center of Evidence Based Medicine, the First Affiliated Hospital of China Medical University, Shenyang, Liaoning Province, People's Republic of China

Jiangtao Liu
Department of Cardiovascular Surgery and Electro-chemotherapy, China-Japan Friendship Hospital, Beijing, People's Republic of China

Corinne Vannimenus, Olivier Le Rouzic and Arnaud Scherpereel
Service de Tabacologie, Clinique de Pneumologie, Hôpital Calmette, CHRU de Lille CS70001, 59037 Lille cedex, France

Hélène Bricout
Centre de Référence Régionale en Cancérologie, Lille, France

François Mouawad and Dominique Chevalier
Service d'Oto-rhino-laryngologie, CHRU de Lille, Lille, France

Eric Dansin, Laurence Rotsaert and Gautier Lefebvre
Département de Cancérologie Cervico-Faciale, Centre de Lutte Contre le Cancer Oscar Lambret, Lille, France

Olivier Cottencin
Service d'Addictologie, CHRU de Lille, Lille, France

Henri Porte
Clinique de Chirurgie Thoracique, CHRU de Lille, Lille, France

Florence Richard
Santé Publique et Epidémiologie, Institut Pasteur, Université de Lille, INSERM UMR744, Lille, France

Benjamin Rolland
Univ Lyon; UCBL; INSERM U1028 ; CNRS UMR5292; Service Universitaire d'Addictologie de Lyon, CH le Vinatier, Lyon, France

Tadej Dovšak, Vojko Didanovič, Andrej Kansky, Miha Verdenik and Nataša Ihan Hren
Clinical Department of Maxillofacial and Oral Surgery, |University Medical Center, Ljubljana, Slovenia
Department of Maxillofacial and Oral Surgery, Faculty of Medicine, University of Ljubljana, Vrazov trg 2, 1104 Ljubljana, Slovenia

Alojz Ihan
Institute of Microbiology and Immunology, Faculty of Medicine, University of Ljubljana, Ljubljana, Slovenia

Danièle Luce
Univ Rennes, Inserm, EHESP, Irset (Institut de recherche en santé, environnement et travail)-UMR_S 1085, Pointe-à-Pitre F-97110, France

Christine Barul
Univ Rennes, Inserm, EHESP, Irset (Institut de recherche en santé, environnement et travail)-UMR_S 1085, Pointe-à-Pitre F-97110, France
Univ Paris Sud, Paris Saclay University, Orsay, France

Matthieu Carton
Département de Biométrie, Institut Curie, DRCI, PSL Research University, Paris, France

Isabelle Stücker
CESP, Cancer and Environment Team, INSERM U1018, Université Paris-Sud, Université Paris-Saclay, Villejuif, France

Loredana Radoï
CESP, Cancer and Environment Team, INSERM U1018, Université Paris-Sud, Université Paris-Saclay, Villejuif, France
Faculty of Dental Surgery, University Paris Descartes, Paris, France

Gwenn Menvielle
Sorbonne Universités, UPMC Univ Paris 06, INSERM, Institut Pierre Louis d'épidémiologie et de Santé Publique (IPLESP UMRS 1136), Paris, France

Corinne Pilorget
The French Public Health Agency, Saint Maurice, France
Ifsttar, UMRESTTE, UMR T_9405, Univ Lyon, Claude Bernard Lyon1 University, Lyon, France

Simona Bara
Manche Cancer Registry, Cotentin Hospital, Cherbourg-Octeville, France

Priscila Marinho de Abreu, Isabella Bittencourt do Valle and Iúri Drummond Louro
Programa de Pós-Graduação em Biotecnologia, Centro de Ciências da Saúde, Universidade Federal do Espirito Santo, Vitoria, Espirito Santo, Brazil

Anna Clara Gregório Có and Pedro Leite Azevedo
Departamento de Patologia, Programa de Pós-graduação em Biotecnologia, Centro de Ciências da Saúde, Universidade Federal do Espirito Santo, Av. Marechal Campos, 1468 Maruípe, Vitória, ES 29.040-090, Brazil

Sandra Lúcia Ventorin von Zeidler
Programa de Pós-Graduação em Biotecnologia, Centro de Ciências da Saúde, Universidade Federal do Espirito Santo, Vitoria, Espirito Santo, Brazil
Departamento de Patologia, Programa de Pós-graduação em Biotecnologia, Centro de Ciências da Saúde, Universidade Federal do Espirito Santo, Av. Marechal Campos, 1468 Maruípe, Vitória, ES 29.040-090, Brazil

Karine Gadioli de Oliveira and Sônia Alves Gouvea
Departamento de Ciências Fisiológicas, Centro de Ciências da Saúde, Universidade Federal do Espirito Santo, Vitoria, Espirito Santo, Brazil

Melissa Freitas Cordeiro-Silva
Faculdade Católica Salesiana do Espírito Santo, Vitória, Espírito Santo, Brazil

José Roberto Vasconcelos de Podestá, Jeferson Lenzi and Agenor Sena
Programa de Prevenção e Detecção Precoce do Câncer Bucal, Setor de Cirurgia de Cabeça e Pescoço, Hospital Santa Rita de Cássia, Vitória, Espírito Santo, Brazil

Elismauro Francisco Mendonça
Faculdade de Odontologia, Universidade Federal de Goiás, Goiânia, Goiás, Brazil

Chiara Gai, Luca Molinaro and Giovanni Camussi
Department of Medical Sciences, University of Turin, C.so Dogliotti, 14 – 10126 Turin, Italy

Francesco Camussi, Roberto Broccoletti, Alessio Gambino, Marco Cabras, Stefano Carossa, and Paolo G. Arduino
Department of Surgical Sciences, University of Turin, Via Nizza 230, 10126 Turin, Italy

Sanja Brolih, Scott K. Parks, Valérie Vial, Jérôme Durivault, Livio Mostosi, Jacques Pouysségur and Vincent Picco
Centre Scientifique de Monaco, Department of Medical Biology, 8 Quai Antoine Ier, Monaco, Principality of Monaco

Gilles Pagès
Centre Scientifique de Monaco, Department of Medical Biology, 8 Quai Antoine Ier, Monaco, Principality of Monaco
UCA, Université Côte d'Azur, Nice-Sophia-Antipolis, Institute for Research on Cancer and Aging of Nice, CNRS-UMR 7284-Inserm U1081, Nice, France

Luiz Paulo Kowalski
Department of Head and Neck Surgery, A. C. Camargo Cancer Hospital, São Paulo, Brazil

Cláudia Maria Pereira and Roberta Cardim Lessa
Department of Head and Neck Surgery, A. C. Camargo Cancer Hospital, São Paulo, Brazil
Laboratory of Cancer Genetics, Ludwig Institute for Cancer Research, Sao Paulo, Branch, Brazil

Matias Eliseo Melendez
Molecular Oncology Research Center, Barretos Cancer Hospital, Barretos, Brazil

Felipe Rodrigues da Silva
Embrapa Informatica Agropecuaria, Campinas, Brazil

Valéria Cristina C. Andrade
Discipline of Hematology and Hemotherapy, Universidade Federal de São Paulo, UNIFESP, São Paulo, Brazil

Ana Carolina de Carvalho
Molecular Oncology Research Center, Barretos Cancer Hospital, Barretos, Brazil
Department of Science Biology, Universidade Federal de São Paulo, UNIFESP, Diadema, Brazil

André L. Vettore
Laboratory of Cancer Genetics, Ludwig Institute for Cancer Research, Sao Paulo, Branch, Brazil
Department of Science Biology, Universidade Federal de São Paulo, UNIFESP, Diadema, Brazil

André Lopes Carvalho
Department of Head and Neck Surgery, A. C. Camargo Cancer Hospital, São Paulo, Brazil
Molecular Oncology Research Center, Barretos Cancer Hospital, Barretos, Brazil
Department of Head and Neck Surgery, Barretos Cancer Hospital, Barretos, São Paulo, Brazil

Seda Ekizoglu, Didem Seven, Turgut Ulutin and Nur Buyru
Cerrahpasa Medical Faculty, Department of Medical Biology, Istanbul University, Kocamustafapasa, 34098 Istanbul, Turkey

Jalal Guliyev
Cerrahpasa Medical Faculty, Department of Otorhinolaryngology, Istanbul University, Istanbul, Turkey

Anke Schlüter, Patrick Weller, Oliver Kanaan, Benedikt Höing, Pia Haßkamp, Sebastian Zander, Nina Dominas, Judith Arnolds and Stephan Lang
Department of Otorhinolaryngology, Head and Neck Surgery, University Hospital Essen, Essen, Germany

Ivonne Nel
Molecular Oncology Risk-Profile Evaluation, Department of Medical Oncology, West German Cancer Center, University Duisburg-Essen, 45122 Essen, Germany
ABA GmbH and Co.KG, BMZ2, 44227 Dortmund, Germany

Agnes Bankfalvi
Institute for Pathology, University Hospital Essen, Essen, Germany

Lukas Heusgen
Department of Otorhinolaryngology, Head and Neck Surgery, University Hospital Essen, Essen, Germany
Martha-Maria Hospital Munich Solln, Munich, Germany

Magis Mandapathil
Department of Otorhinolaryngology, Head and Neck Surgery, University Hospital Essen, Essen, Germany
Department of Otorhinolaryngology, Head and Neck Surgery, Asklepios Kliniken Hamburg, Hamburg, Germany

Boris A. Stuck
Department of Otorhinolaryngology, Head and Neck Surgery, University Hospital Essen, Essen, Germany
Department of Otorhinolaryngology, Head and Neck Surgery, University Hospital Marburg, Marburg, Germany

Sven Brandau
Department of Otorhinolaryngology, Head and Neck Surgery, University Hospital Essen, Essen, Germany
Experimental and Translational Research, Department of Otorhinolaryngology, University Hospital Essen, Hufelandstrasse 55, 45147 Essen, Germany

Index